Neurotransmitter Actions
in the Vertebrate Nervous System

Neurotransmitter Actions

in the Vertebrate Nervous System

Edited by
Michael A. Rogawski
and
Jeffery L. Barker

National Institute of Neurological and Communicative
  Disorders and Stroke
National Institutes of Health
Bethesda, Maryland

PLENUM PRESS • NEW YORK AND LONDON

Library of Congress Cataloging in Publication Data

Main entry under title:

Neurotransmitter actions in the vertebrate nervous system.

Includes bibliographies and index.
1. Neurotransmitters. 2. Nervous system—Vertebrates. I. Rogawski, Michael A. II.
Barker, Jeffery L. [DNLM: 1. Neuroregulators—physiology. QV 126 N4938]
QP364.7.N465 1985   596'.0188   85-16784
ISBN-13: 978-1-4684-4963-1   e-ISBN-13: 978-1-4684-4961-7
DOI: 10.1007/978-1-4684-4961-7

Cover: Upper traces show continuous recording of elementary Cl⁻ ion-channel currents activated by the transmitter GABA in a patch of membrane excised from the cell body of a cultured mouse spinal cord neuron and held at -60 mV. Lower trace reflects a synaptically activated Cl⁻ current recorded at -60 mV in another cultured mouse spinal cord neuron that is most likely mediated by GABA. The time scales of the illustrated pharmacological and physiological activities are similar. The elementary ion-channel events are about one picoampere (pA) in amplitude, while the synaptic current peak is about 400 pA. Thus, the peak of the synaptic current is comprised of some 400 ion channels and the time course of decay reflects the histogram of ion channel durations with most channels staying open briefly and fewer and fewer remaining open for longer and longer periods. This broad spectrum of channel durations can easily be seen in the patch-clamp recording. (G. A. Redmann, H. Lecar, R. N. McBurney, and J. L. Barker, unpublished observations. See Chapter 3 for further details.)

©1985 Plenum Press, New York
Softcover reprint of the hardcover 1st edition 1985
A Division of Plenum Publishing Corporation
233 Spring Street, New York, N.Y. 10013

Contributors

B. E. ALGER • Department of Physiology, University of Maryland School of Medicine, Baltimore, Maryland 21201

JEFFERY L. BARKER • Laboratory of Neurophysiology, National Institute of Neurological and Communicative Disorders and Stroke, National Institutes of Health, Bethesda, Maryland 20892

BENJAMIN S. BUNNEY • Departments of Psychiatry and Pharmacology, Yale University School of Medicine, New Haven, Connecticut 06510

ROBERT A. DAVIDOFF • Department of Neurology, University of Miami School of Medicine, and Neurology Service, Veteran's Administration Medical Center, Miami, Florida 33101

JOHN R. DELFS • The William P. Arnold Pain Treatment and Research Center, New England Deaconess Hospital, and Departments of Neurology, Harvard Medical School, Beth Israel Hospital, and Children's Hospital, Boston, Massachusetts 02115

MARC A. DICHTER • Departments of Neurology, Harvard Medical School and Beth Israel Hospital, and Department of Neuroscience, Children's Hospital, Boston, Massachusetts 02115

RAYMOND DINGLEDINE • Department of Pharmacology, University of North Carolina, Chapel Hill, North Carolina 27514

J. J. DREIFUSS • Department of Physiology, University Medical Center, Geneva, Switzerland

NAE J. DUN • Department of Pharmacology, Loyola University, Stritch School of Medicine, Maywood, Illinois 60153

ANTHONY A. GRACE • Departments of Psychology and Psychiatry, The University of Pittsburgh, Pittsburgh, Pennsylvania 15260

HELMUT L. HAAS • Neurophysiology Laboratory, Neurochirurgische Universitätsklinik, CH-8091 Zurich, Switzerland

JOHN C. HACKMAN • Department of Neurology, University of Miami School of Medicine, and Neurology Service, Veteran's Administration Medical Center, Miami, Florida 33101

BARBARA K. HENON • Division of Neuroscience, Beckman Research Institute of the City of Hope, Duarte, California 91010

LILY YEH JAN • Department of Physiology, University of California, San Francisco, San Francisco, California 94143

YUH NUNG JAN • Department of Physiology, University of California, San Francisco, San Francisco, California 94143

JOHN S. KELLY • Department of Pharmacology, The University of Edinburgh, Edinburgh EH8 9JZ, England

SHIRO KONISHI • Department of Pharmacology, Faculty of Medicine, Tokyo Medical and Dental University, Bunkyo-ku, Tokyo 113, Japan

MARK L. MAYER • Laboratory of Developmental Neurobiology, National Institute of Child Health and Human Development, National Institutes of Health, Bethesda, Maryland 20892

DONALD A. McAFEE • Division of Neuroscience, Beckman Research Institute of the City of Hope, Duarte, California 91010

MICHEL MÜHLETHALER • Department of Physiology, University Medical Center, Geneva, Switzerland

ANDREA NISTRI • Department of Pharmacology, St. Bartholomew's Hospital Medical College, University of London, London EC.1M 6BQ, England

MARIO RAGGENBASS • Department of Physiology, University Medical Center, Geneva, Switzerland

MICHAEL A. ROGAWSKI • National Institute of Neurological and Communicative Disorders and Stroke, National Institutes of Health, Bethesda, Maryland 20892

C. P. VANDERMAELEN • Preclinical CNS Research, Pharmaceutical Research and Development, Bristol-Myers Company, Evansville, Indiana 47721

GARY L. WESTBROOK • Laboratory of Developmental Neurobiology, National Institute of Child Health and Human Development, National Institutes of Health, Bethesda, Maryland 20892

Preface

Intercellular communication via bioactive substances occurs in virtually all multicellular systems. Chemical neurotransmission in the vertebrate nervous system represents a form of signaling of this type. The biology of chemical neurotransmission is complex, involving transmitter synthesis, transport, and release by the presynaptic neuron; signal generation in the target tissue; and mechanisms for termination of the response. The focus of this book is on one aspect of this scheme: the diverse electrophysiological effects induced by different neurotransmitters on targets cells.

In recent years, astonishing progress has been made in elucidating the specific physiological signals mediated by neurotransmitters in the vertebrate nervous system, yet, in our view, this has not been adequately recognized, perhaps because the new concepts have yet to filter into neuroscience textbooks. Nevertheless, the principles of neurotransmitter action are critical to advances in many areas of neuroscience, including molecular neurobiology, neurochemistry, neuropharmacology, physiological psychology, and clinical neuroscience. It was the need for a sourcebook that prompted us to engage a group of neurophysiologists to prepare the chapters in this volume. However, there was an additional reason for this book: more and more it seemed that the field, if not yet having reached maturity, at least was approaching adolescence, with strengths in some areas and healthy conflicts in others. At this stage of development a textbook can help to define a field, clarify problems to be resolved, and identify areas for future investigation.

This book is organized into five parts, each containing one or more chapters on chemically related transmitter agents: amino acids, acetylcholine, biogenic amines, neuropeptides, and purines. In keeping with the broad audience to which the book is directed, most chapters contain introductory material on the anatomy, neurochemistry, and receptor pharmacology of the transmitter system whose physiology is discussed, and the main discussion is directed to the nonspecialist. Nevertheless, readers will require familiarity with standard concepts in neurophysiology, and as such this volume complements, but does not replace, presently available textbooks. For the most part, this book leaves discussion of transmitter actions at the skeletal neuromuscular junction and in autonomic effector tissues to these textbooks, and focuses on the less familiar context of the central nervous system and peripheral ganglia. The actions of well established transmitters—such as GABA, norepinephrine, and acetylcholine—are explored in this new territory as are a host of novel chemical agents, including neuropeptides and purines. However, many more putative transmitter substances have been discovered using histochemical, biochemical, and, more recently, molecular biological techniques than are covered in these chapters. We have of necessity only included chapters on those substances that have been studied most extensively using neurophysiological techniques.

We have also decided to limit our coverage to vertebrates, although in some chapters comparisons are made with invertebrate systems. Recent technical developments and the advent of new preparations of the vertebrate nervous system have made vertebrate neurons as accessible to microelectrode recording as invertebrate cells, and this has allowed the field of vertebrate neurotransmitter physiology to flourish on equal footing with work in invertebrates. For those who are interested, neurotransmitter actions in invertebrates have been covered in a number of excellent books and reviews.

We are grateful to those authors who have allowed figures from their original publications to be reproduced in this book and who have generously provided preprints of papers in press. We thank the following individuals for reading and providing useful comments on some of the chapters: B. E. Alger, R. J. Dingledine, J. M. Lakoski, M. R. Martin, and G. L. Westbrook. Finally, our editor at Plenum, Kirk Jensen, deserves special acknowledgment for his advice, support, and forebearance throughout the years that this book evolved from concept to reality.

Michael A. Rogawski
Jeffery L. Barker

Bethesda, Maryland

Contents

2. GABA and Glycine: Postsynaptic Actions

B. E. Alger

3. GABA and Glycine: Ion Channel Mechanisms

Jeffery L. Barker

PART II.   ACETYLCHOLINE

6. Acetylcholine

John S. Kelly and Michael A. Rogawski

PART III. BIOGENIC AMINES

7. Serotonin

C. P. VanderMaelen

8. Norepinephrine

Michael A. Rogawski

9. Dopamine

Anthony A. Grace and Benjamin S. Bunney

10. Histamine

Helmut L. Haas

PART IV. NEUROPEPTIDES

11. Opioid Peptides: Central Nervous System

Raymond Dingledine

12. Opioid Peptides: Peripheral Nervous System

Shiro Konishi

13. Substance P

Nae J. Dun

14. Somatostatin

John R. Delfs and Marc A. Dichter

PART V.   ADENOSINE AND ATP

17. **Adenosine and ATP**

   Donald A. McAfee and Barbara K. Henon

Introduction

1. THE FOUNDATIONS OF CHEMICAL NEUROTRANSMISSION

In the early part of this century, the theory that neurons were independent units gained acceptance over the concept that they formed a syncytium connected to each other by protoplasmic bridges. It thus became necessary to explain how excitation was transmitted across the gap between two neurons. Cajal, an early proponent of the independent neuron theory, established that nerve cells come in contact at morphologically specialized zones, which Sherrington referred to as *synapses*. In the succeeding decades, a precise understanding of some of the cellular mechanisms underlying transmission at synapses evolved from studies in several model systems. This introduction highlights some key points in the historical development of this field and gives an overview of the most important experimental preparations and methods. Further details regarding these topics can be found in the selected texts listed on page xxv.

The earliest speculations regarding the nature of synaptic transmission were those of DuBois-Reymond who, in the mid-19th century, proposed that nervous excitation of muscle was electrically mediated, although he also stated the alternative hypothesis that the secretion by nerve of an excitatory substance induced contraction in the muscle. Both electrical and chemical transmission are now known to occur, but the possibility that chemical neurotransmission might operate at the nerve–muscle junction and in the CNS was only seriously considered after the concept had been firmly established in the autonomic nervous system by pharmacological experiments in the whole animal and organ bath (see Chapters 6 and 8).

Further advances in the development of the concept of chemical neurotransmission relied upon the technique of intracellular recording with glass microelectrodes that was developed in the 1950s. It was shown that presynaptic nerve stimulation generated *synaptic potentials* in the postsynaptic cell (also known as *end plate potentials* in skeletal muscle). At the neuromuscular junction, evidence that acetylcholine mediated the end plate potential gained support from the pharmacological studies of Kuffler and Eccles.

An important technical advance for studying transmitter action at the neuromuscular junction was the development of iontophoresis by Nastuk. Acetylcholine, a positively charged ion in aqueous solution, could be ejected from a glass micropipette by the passage of positive electrical current. When applied in this manner close to the cell membrane, acetylcholine caused a depolarization of the muscle fiber that mimicked the effects of motor nerve stimulation. The observations made with intracellular recording and iontophoresis were difficult to reconcile with the theories of electrical transmission that had been proposed by Eccles and others, and the concept of chemical transmission at synapses was gradually accepted. Ironically, in 1959, Furshpan and Potter described a synapse in the crayfish that did operate by electrical transmission. Subsequently, many other examples of electrical transmission have been uncovered, in vertebrates as well as invertebrates. An introduction to this topic can be found in the text by Kuffler, Nicholls and Martin (1984) and it will not be considered further in this volume.

The nature of the end plate potential at the vertebrate neuromuscular junction was first investigated by Fatt and Katz. On the basis of microelectrode recordings in frog muscle, it was proposed that the potential change induced in the muscle cell by motor nerve stimulation results from a brief increase in permeability of the membrane at the junctional region to small ions, followed by a passive electrotonic spread and decay of the charge across the membrane. The ionic current at the end plate was subsequently measured directly using the voltage clamp technique. The essential question to be answered concerned which ions were involved in the generation of the end plate potential. It was concluded that acetylcholine acts by increasing the permeability of the postjunctional membrane to cations so that sodium ions flow inward and potassium ions flow outward. The molecular analysis of cholinergic excitation was begun in the 1970s by Katz and Miledi who, using the noise analysis technique (see Chapter 3), developed the hypothesis that acetylcholine activates two-state (closed–open) ion channels in the end plate membrane. This hypothesis has recently been confirmed by patch clamp measurements of the discrete transitions in ionic permeability occurring with activation of acetylcholine receptor-coupled channels. Thus, much of our present day understanding of chemical neurotransmission has been derived from the detailed investigation of synaptic mechanisms in skeletal muscle fibers. Similar experimental protocols were subsequently used in the more complex peripheral ganglia.

2. STUDIES ON NEURONS IN THE MAMMALIAN CENTRAL NERVOUS SYSTEM

The pioneering experiments on the physiology and pharmacology of central neurons were carried out concurrently with those in peripheral systems. While the basic methods of analysis were similar, the complexity of CNS tissue necessitated the development of different experimental strategies. Most early studies focused entirely on the pharmacological responsiveness of central neurons, with little attempt to investigate the revelance of these responses to the physiology of synaptic transmission. Initially, drugs were administered to the whole animal and the effects on field responses of populations of neurons and on the spontaneous firing of single neurons recorded with microelectrodes were examined. Subsequently, the method of iontophoresis was adapted for use in the CNS by Curtis and Eccles. Multibarrel micropipettes permitted extracellular (and even intracellular) recording of potentials from cells, while substances were ejected into their immediate microenvironment. A mass of data was accumulated, however interpretation was problematic due to the difficulty of deciding whether an observed response to an iontophoretically applied compound could be related to the synaptic effect of an endogenously released transmitter. With this in mind, researchers focused attention on target cells of "chemically identified" neuronal pathways, i.e., on systems whose presumed transmitter substance was defined by histochemical techniques.

An important advance was the ability to record from isolated CNS preparations *in vitro*. Although the methods were initially developed using tissue from cold-blooded amphibians, in the mid-1960s Yamamoto demonstrated that reliable synaptic field potentials could be evoked from mammalian brain slices and it was subsequently found that intracellular recordings were also possible in these preparations. Brain slices offer several unique advantages, in addition to the relative ease of obtaining stable intracellular recordings, including the ability to position recording and stimulating electrodes under direct visual inspection. In a laminated structure such as the hippocampus, it is possible to impale specific regions of individual neurons (dendrites and soma), map the transmitter sensitivity over the surface of the neuron by localized iontophoretic applications, or stimulate specific synaptic pathways. Moreover, using a modification of the slice technique it is now feasible to acutely isolate individual neurons for the recording of single transmitter-gated channels using the patch clamp method.

Tissue culture has also been used to study the action of transmitters on CNS neurons. Although the first intracellular studies of cultured neurons utilized explanted preparations, later workers have focused on primary dissociated monolayer cultures, which allow the highest degree of experimental accessibility to individual neurons. Cultures have been prepared from virtually all levels of the central and peripheral nervous systems. Cells grown in dissociated culture appear morphologically similar to neurons in the intact nervous system, form functional synapses, and have excitable membrane properties comparable to neurons *in situ*. However, with a few exceptions, it has proved difficult to identify specific cell types in cultures prepared from heterogeneous tissues. Moreover, growth in culture may be accompanied by modification of the cell biological characteristics of neurons, including their responsiveness to neurotransmitters. These problems have limited the applicability of dissociated cultures for the study of neurotransmitter actions, although they have been useful in certain circumstances, for example, the analysis of the electropharmacology of GABA (see Chapter 3).

3. PERSPECTIVE

The key principles for the investigation of transmitter action set forth in the classical studies of the neuromuscular junction have served as a model for physiologists seeking to identify the cellular mechanisms of transmitters in diverse systems. Although the fundamental methods of analysis have changed little over the past three decades, there have been revolutionary changes in our understanding of how transmitters interact with target cells. It is now well recognized that the example of a transmitter opening voltage-independent ion channels over a rapid time scale, as at the vertebrate neuromuscular junction, is just one of the multitude of mechanisms that exist. Thus, transmitters can close ion channels or the channels involved may have a strong voltage dependence. These channels may have important functions apart from mediating the effects of transmitters, such as maintenance of the resting potential, regulating the responsiveness of the cell to stimuli, or in the endogenous generation of repetitive activity (pacemaker or bursting patterns). By modifying the activity of ongoing ionic mechanisms, transmitters can alter the excitability of target cells in a wide variety of complex ways that complement the actions of conventional synaptic potentials. Another new mode of transmitter action occurs when a substance released from the same or adjacent nerve terminals indirectly modulates the signal mediated by a second transmitter. Such an interaction can occur by either pre- or postsynaptic mechanisms. Finally, it is now apparent that the time course of synaptic actions can vary over four orders of magnitude, from milliseconds to minutes and possibly longer. Recognizing this diversity of possible mechanisms, it is evident that unless experiments are carefully planned they may fail to detect the critical actions of a transmitter. For example, there are now several examples where transmitters modify conductances that are inactive at rest, and are brought into play only when the cell is polarized from the resting potential.

Each of the unique actions of a transmitter depends upon the specific transmitter receptor and the ionic channels to which it is coupled. The chemical class of the transmitter molecule itself—whether amino acid, biogenic amine, peptide or other substance—cannot be used to infer the nature of the synaptic signal, for a single transmitter molecule can have multiple actions depending upon the type of synaptic receptor activated.

This diversity of synaptic actions provides a rich vocabulary for the language of interneuronal communication. Nevertheless, despite the diversity, several general themes are easily recognizable in this volume. Among the many transmitter substances and neuronal systems that have been examined, the commonality arises because of the limited repertoire of responses that can be displayed by an excitable cell, or more properly, that our present day equipment can record. Excitation can be induced by an *increase* in membrane permeability to sodium or calcium or nonspecifically to all cations, so that the cell depolarizes toward the threshold for spike generation. Alternatively, neurons can be excited by a *decrease* in resting potassium conductance that tends to drive the membrane potential away from the equilibrium potential for potassium ions in the depolarized direction. On the other hand, synaptic inhibition can occur due to an increase in permeability to either potassium or chloride; in either case the membrane is shunted (held near the equilibrium potential for these ions) and depolarizing synaptic potentials are opposed. In invertebrate neurons, inhibitory potentials probably can occur by inhibition of resting cation conductance, but such an effect has been difficult to confirm in vertebrates. Finally, it has been proposed that transmitters can activate the electrogenic Na^+-K^+ pump, and thus induce a hyperpolarization since at each cycle three sodium ions are expelled for every two potassium ions pumped in.

In addition to these effects on passive membrane properties (and possibly on electrogenic ion pumps), it is now recognized that transmitters can influence the membrane channels that are intimately involved in the shaping of neuronal excitability properties, such as voltage-activated calcium channels, calcium-activated potassium channels, or novel voltage-dependent potassium channels (M channels, see Chapter 6; or A channels, see Chapter 8). The discussion of these more recently described forms of transmitter action constitutes an important part of this book. In the future, additional modes of transmitter action will surely be uncovered. Some of these will be variations on the themes that are already well understood. However, others will require new forms of experimental analysis and fresh approaches for their interpretation. For example, in the retina, dopamine, acting through the second messenger cyclic AMP, seems to uncouple electrical synapses (gap junctions, see Chapter 9). This unexpected action is a prelude to what will undoubtedly be a host of nonconventional synaptic actions to be described in years to come.

The discovery of new modes of transmitter action have raised fundamental questions regarding the link between activation of the receptor and induction of the physiological response. Whereas at the neuromuscular junction, the acetylcholine receptor and cation channel form a single macromolecular complex in the cell membrane, the situation seems to be different for other transmitter systems where several intermediate biochemical steps may be involved in the transduction process. As yet, in only selected systems have there been attempts to define these intermediate reactions and even in the most successful circumstances the details are incomplete.

4. CRITERIA FOR THE IDENTIFICATION OF CHEMICAL TRANSMITTERS

As the concept of chemical neurotransmission developed, certain logical criteria were proposed to identify a suspected chemical substance as being the endogenous transmitter agent. Despite the explosion of information regarding novel modes of transmitter action, these criteria are still applicable. However, they must been applied cautiously since it is well recognized that more than one transmitter can coexist in a single presynaptic neuron and a target cell can respond to the same transmitter in several ways depending upon the specific receptor that is activated. The criteria are listed below since they form the basis of many of the studies considered in this volume.

1. The substance must be present in the presynaptic neuron.
2. The neuron must be capable of synthesizing the substance and possess the necessary precursors and intermediates.
3. Upon stimulation, the substance must be released by the neuron.
4. There may be systems for the inactivation of the transmitter, such as enzymatic modification or uptake into pre- or postsynaptic structures.
5. When applied to the target cell, the substance should mimic the action of the synaptically released transmitter. If ion channel activity is modified by the transmitter, there should be a correspondence between the pharmacological effects of the transmitter on ion channels and the behavior of the synaptically gated channels.
6. Pharmacological agents which interact with the synaptically released transmitter should interact with the suspected transmitter in an identical manner.

From the physiologist's point of view, the last two criteria are of fundamental importance and are emphasized in the chapters of this book. Evidence in favor of the supporting criteria (1–4) are generally summarized in the introduction to each chapter.

Michael A. Rogawski
Jeffery L. Barker

Bethesda, Maryland

SELECTED TEXTS

Aidley, D. J., 1981, *The Physiology of Excitable Cells*, 2nd Edition, Cambridge University Press, Cambridge.

Dingledine, R. (ed.), 1984, *Brain Slices*, Plenum Press, New York.

Eccles, J. C., 1964, *The Physiology of Synapses*, Academic Press, New York.

Hille, B., 1984, *Ionic Channels of Excitable Membranes*, Sinauer Associates, Sunderland, Mass.

Jack, J. J. B., Noble, D. and Tsien, R. W., 1983, *Electric Current Flow in Excitable Cells*, Clarendon Press, Oxford.

Junge, D., 1981, *Nerve and Muscle Excitation*, 2nd Edition, Sinauer Associates, Sunderland, Mass.

Katz, B., 1966, *Nerve, Muscle and Synapse*, McGraw-Hill, New York.

Kuffler, S. W., Nicholls, J. G., and Martin, A. R., 1984, *From Neuron to Brain: A Cellular Approach to the Function of the Nervous System*, 2nd Edition, Sinauer Associates, Sunderland, Mass.

Phillis, J. W., 1970, *The Pharmacology of Synapses*, Pergamon Press, Oxford.

Sakmann, B. and Neher, E. (eds.), 1983, *Single-Channel Recording*, Plenum Press, New York.

Neurotransmitter Actions
in the Vertebrate Nervous System

PART I
AMINO ACIDS

1

GABA: Presynaptic Actions

ROBERT A. DAVIDOFF and JOHN C. HACKMAN

1. INTRODUCTION

Activation of afferent spinal inputs not only excites secondary neurons (interneurons) and motoneurons but also results in inhibition of the transmission of other sensory impulses.* Although the mechanism of this inhibition has been the focus of considerable controversy in the past two decades, there is agreement that much of the effect—designated "presynaptic inhibition"—is produced at the level of the presynaptic terminal of afferent fibers.

Presynaptic inhibition is still an imperfectly understood phenomenon. It is known, however, that GABA (γ-aminobutyric acid) is capable of affecting the membrane properties of afferent terminals, and it is believed that the amino acid is responsible for presynaptic inhibition because GABA satisfies certain of the minimal criteria required of a substance before it can be said to be a transmitter (see reviews by Levy, 1977; Nistri, 1983). This chapter discusses the evidence supporting the role of GABA in presynaptic inhibition. In addition, mention will be made of possible presynaptic roles of the amino acid in locations other than the spinal cord.

2. PRESYNAPTIC INHIBITION

Frank and Fuortes (1957) first reported that conditioning stimulation of certain afferent fibers entering the cord in dorsal roots resulted in a reduction

---

*This inhibition presumably occurs when the axon of an interneuron excited by an afferent sensory input forms an inhibitory axo-axonic synapse with the terminals of a primary afferent fiber.

of the amplitude of excitatory postsynaptic potentials (EPSPs) recorded in motoneurons—a reduction that was unaccompanied by detectable changes in the motoneuron membrane potential or excitability. These observations have been confirmed, and it is now known that depression of the EPSP is a long-lasting phenomenon that reaches a maximum decrease at 10–20 msec following the conditioning stimulus and decays over more than 100 msec. One explanation offered for this phenomenon was that it resulted from a decrease in the presynaptic release of excitatory transmitter from afferent terminals, i.e., the inhibition was "presynaptic."

3. PRIMARY AFFERENT DEPOLARIZATION

Volleys of afferent impulses also produce a slow depolarization of the terminals of primary afferent fibers—a process termed primary afferent depolarization (PAD). PAD is electrotonically conducted from the presynaptic terminal region out along afferent fibers. Its existence can therefore be measured by determining the potential of afferent fibers (see Schmidt, 1971, for review). The most frequently used method is to record dorsal root potentials (DRPs) from a dorsal root or rootlet (Fig. 1A). DRPs are usually recorded by means of two electrodes placed upon a dorsal root, one close to, but not

---

Figure 1. Primary afferent depolarization and presynaptic inhibition. (A) Dorsal root potential (DRP) recorded from a cat lumbar dorsal root in response to a cutaneous volley. Note dorsal root reflex. Calibration marked in 10 msec. (From Wall, 1958, with permission.) (B) DRPs recorded from dorsal root of isolated frog spinal cord in sucrose gap apparatus. Superimposed oscilloscope traces of DRPs evoked by supramaximal stimulation of adjacent dorsal root (larger trace) and ventral root of same spinal segment (smaller trace). (From Davidoff and Hackman, 1978, with permission.) (C) Depression of monosynaptic excitatory postsynaptic potentials (EPSPs) by "presynaptic inhibition." CON: control EPSP in a plantaris motoneuron. Subsequent EPSPs depressed by four conditioning volleys in the nerve to the hamstring muscles. The graph indicates the time course of the depression of the EPSP (as a percentage of the control amplitude) for the experiment partially illustrated in the upper traces. (Modified from Eccles et al., 1961, with permission.) (D) Primary afferent depolarization (PAD) recorded intracellularly from a large myelinated dorsal root fiber in the frog spinal cord and produced by stimulation of an adjacent dorsal root. Recording from same fiber shown at two different oscilloscope sweep speeds. (From Padjen and Hashiguchi, 1983, with permission.) (E) Intracellularly recorded PAD from fiber in frog spinal cord. The resting membrane potential of the fiber was -72 mV. Superimposed film records show increase of PAD in recordings made at three different levels of hyperpolarization produced by passing current through the recording microelectrode. (From Padjen and Hashiguchi, 1983, with permission.) (F) Sucrose gap recordings of DRPs from isolated frog spinal cord. Control records in normal Ringer's solution and low $[Cl^-]_o$ records obtained after superfusion with Ringer's solution in which 95% of the Cl^- was replaced with isethionate. Note reduction of early phase of dorsal root potential (DRP) produced by stimulation of a dorsal root (DR-DRP), appearance of a late component of the DR-DRP, and almost complete abolition of the DRP evoked by stimulation of a ventral root (VR-DRP) (unpublished observations of J. C. Hackman and R. A. Davidoff). (G) Changes in extracellular K^+ activity recorded with a K^+-sensitive microelectrode placed in the cat dorsal horn. The posterior tibialis nerve was stimulated at various frequencies. (Modified from Kříž et al., 1974.)

touching, the spinal cord (proximal electrode) and the other out near the cut distal end of the root (distal electrode). It is customary to express the sign of the potential with reference to the proximal electrode. A negativity of the proximal electrode indicates a depolarization of the intraspinal portion of the afferent fibers contained in the root and is conventionally recorded upwards. The duration of the DRP varies depending upon the type of recording

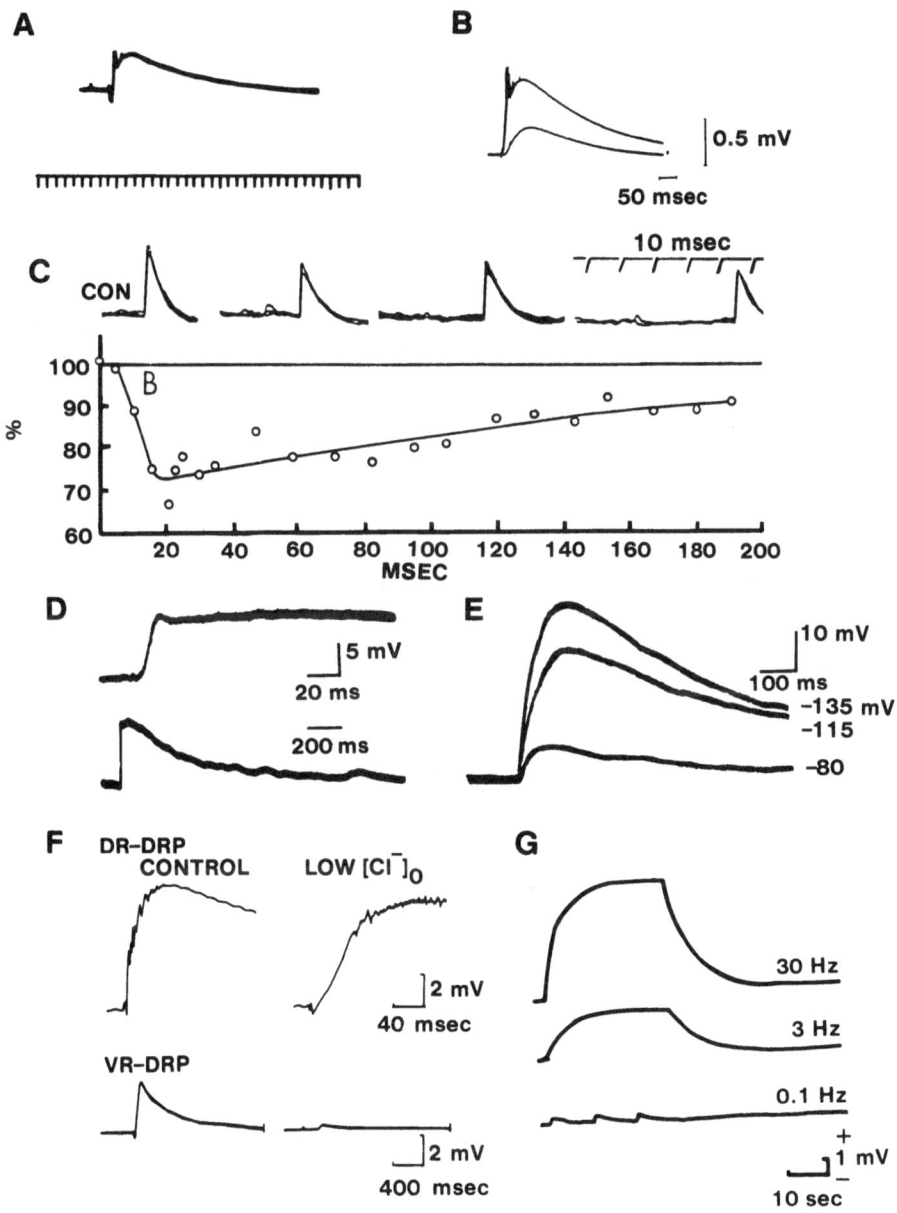

situation. In the cat spinal cord the DRP recorded with an amplifier time constant of 1 sec lasts about 200–300 msec, but the potential is considerably longer in the frog spinal cord when DC amplification is used and may reach a duration of 1000 msec.

In mammalian and in amphibian spinal cords, DRPs can be elicited by stimulation of afferent fibers in peripheral nerves or roots. In the frog, DRPs may also be elicited by antidromic firing of motoneuron axons contained in ventral roots (Fig. 1B). Furthermore, in all vertebrates depolarization of primary afferent terminals can also be evoked by stimulation of various supraspinal structures. PAD, as indicated by field potentials and excitability measurements (*vide infra*) is prominent in another site of termination of afferent fibers—the dorsal column nuclei.

4. THE ECCLES' HYPOTHESIS

An extensive series of investigations conducted in the early 1960s by Sir John Eccles and his colleagues led them to formulate a relationship between PAD and presynaptic inhibition (see Eccles, 1964, for review). This idea was based on the finding of a precise correlation between the time course of PAD and the presynaptic inhibition of EPSPs evoked by stimulation of the Ia fibers in motor nerves (Fig. 1C). Furthermore, it was postulated that presynaptic depolarization is the *causal* factor in the inhibition responsible for the EPSP reduction.

PAD was hypothesized to be produced by the action of an inhibitory chemical transmitter acting on the presynaptic terminal to produce a high ionic permeability. The inhibitory transmitter was assumed to be released from axo-axonic synapses located on, or close to, the synaptic terminals of afferent fibers. Later, Eccles and his co-workers postulated that GABA was the responsible transmitter (Eccles et al., 1963). Over the past two decades the ideas promulgated by Eccles have been subjected to extensive experimental testing. Some provisions have been fully accepted; some are still in dispute (cf. Burke and Rudomín, 1977; Nicoll and Alger, 1979; Davidoff and Hackman, 1984).

5. MECHANISMS OF PAD

At present there are two major hypotheses regarding the genesis of PAD: (1) PAD is caused by the action of a specific chemical transmitter, or (2) PAD is attributable to an increase in the K^+ concentration in the extracellular space surrounding the afferent terminals. The two hypotheses are not mutually exclusive—depolarization of primary afferent terminals could be caused by elevated K^+ and by release of a transmitter.

There is a great deal of evidence that at least part of PAD is a synaptic process caused by the action of a transmitter. Axo-axonic synapses are present on the terminals of afferent fibers. PAD has a central latency of several milliseconds—a latency compatible with a synaptic process involving at least two synapses (Jankowska et al., 1981). In addition, in the isolated frog cord PAD is substantially (>90%) reduced by exposure of the cord to Ringer's solution containing Mg^{2+} or Mn^{2+} ions in concentrations sufficient to block synaptic transmission. However, it should be noted that all of this evidence is indirect and while all of it is necessary, none of it is sufficient to confirm the hypothesis that PAD is a synaptic process.

If PAD is synaptically generated, it should have properties similar to those of a variety of other depolarizing chemical synaptic processes. There should be a change in the ionic conductance and the depolarization should have an equilibrium or reversal potential more positive than the resting membrane potential. However, precise analysis of PAD is made difficult by the complexity of the intact spinal cord. As a result, unequivocal data with regard to the ionic mechanisms of PAD is not available.

PAD can be recorded intracellularly by means of a microelectrode, but such recording is possible only in the dorsal region of the cord where the afferent fibers are relatively coarse (Fig. 1D). Such recordings have demonstrated that PAD is augmented by hyperpolarizing the fiber (Fig. 1E), and decreased by depolarizing it and that PAD is accompanied by a significant increase in the conductance of the afferent fiber membrane (Padjen and Hashiguchi, 1983). However, it has not been possible to reverse PAD by manipulations that depolarize afferent fiber terminals because of the rectifying properties of the membrane of afferent fibers (Padjen and Hashiguchi, 1983). It has been hypothesized that PAD could be caused by an increased permeability to Na^+ and/or Cl^- ions, and attempts have been made at defining the mechanism of PAD by means of ion substitution. The DRP in the frog cord has been reported to vary linearly with the logarithmic Na^+ concentration in the extracellular fluid (Carlson, 1964), but this phenomenon probably results from the effects that changes in Na^+ concentration have on impulse activity in the afferent fibers and on EPSPs in the interneurons producing the DRP, rather than from a direct action on the ionic process generating PAD. Superfusion of the isolated frog cord with Cl^--free Ringer's solution reduces an early component of the DRP evoked by stimulation of a dorsal root (Fig. 1F). This result is compatible with the idea that the early part of PAD is the result of a change in Cl^- permeability of the afferent terminal membrane. The DRP, however, is also markedly prolonged, and this prolongation is probably not the result of a direct action on PAD, but rather is caused by a block of Cl^--dependent spinal postsynaptic inhibition resulting in increased interneuronal activity of the cord. On the other hand, the DRP induced by ventral root stimulation in the frog cord is abolished by exposure to low Cl^--containing solutions (Fig. 1F) (Barker and Nicoll, 1973).

5.1. K$^+$ and PAD

Not only does afferent stimulation result in an increase in the concentration of K$^+$ ions in the extracellular space of the spinal gray matter (for review see Somjen, 1983), but the increase is highest in the dorsal horn and intermediate nucleus—those loci of the cord where PAD is generated. In addition, intraspinal afferent terminals are sensitive to changes in extracellular K$^+$ levels. As a result of these findings, the idea that PAD is produced by an alteration in extracellular K$^+$ concentration has received much recent attention.

There are a number of arguments against the idea that increases in K$^+$ concentration are responsible for generating *all* of the potential change in PAD. In particular, although substantial quantities of the cation are released by tetanic afferent stimulation (4–9.0 mM above resting levels) (Fig. 1G), only small amounts (<0.5 mM) are accumulated following single afferent volleys. Moreover, some pharmacological agents cause opposite effects on PAD and on K$^+$ accumulation. For example, barbiturates prolong, and sometimes increase, the amplitude of the DRP, but reduce the release of K$^+$ by afferent stimuli. On the other hand, a small DRP and a small increment in the extracellular K$^+$ concentration can be elicited in the frog spinal cord when all synaptic transmission has been blocked by bathing the cord in high concentrations of Mg^{2+} ions. On the basis of such data it has been calculated that the increment in extracellular K$^+$ evoked by a single dorsal root volley could account for 10–30% of the potential change underlying the DRP.

5.2. Two Components to PAD

As the data summarized above suggest, it now appears that more than one mechanism is involved in the generation of PAD. An early component of PAD—lasting approximately 100 msec—is most likely a synaptic process produced by the action of a chemical transmitter—presumably GABA—which increases the Cl$^-$ conductance of the membrane of primary afferent terminals. A later, slow phase may be caused by an accumulation of interstitial K$^+$ ions. It is also possible that the later part of PAD is produced by the action of another transmitter.

6. DISTRIBUTION OF GABA IN THE SPINAL CORD

The mammalian spinal cord contains a considerable amount of GABA with the highest levels found in the dorsal and lateral portions of the dorsal horn in laminae III and IV (Fig. 2). This distribution is consistent with a role for GABA in the production of PAD since this is an area of the cord where electron micrographs have demonstrated axo-axonic synapses formed by the

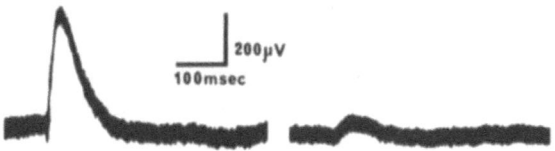

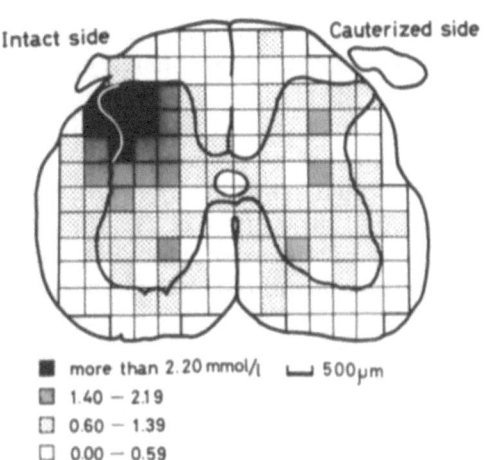

Figure 2. GABA content and dorsal root potentials in cat spinal cord. DRPs recorded from L_7 rootlet 7 days after unilateral cauterization of blood vessels supplying the dorsal horn. The spinal cord was removed after the recordings had been obtained, microdissected into 500 μm blocks and the GABA content in each block determined by an enzymic assay. (Modified from Miyata and Otsuka, 1975.)

terminals of interneurons making contact with the presynaptic terminals of primary afferent fibers (Conradi, 1969) and where the last interneurons intercalated in the pathway for PAD of cutaneous fibers are believed to be located (Jankowska et al., 1981). The contention that GABA is mainly concentrated in interneurons in the dorsal horn is based on the finding that infarction of the dorsal horn by cauterization of the blood vessels supplying that region reduces or abolishes the DRP recorded from an appropriate dorsal root, and decreases both the number of neurons in the dorsal horn and the concentration of GABA there (Fig. 2).

7. GABA AND AFFERENT TERMINALS

Many workers have demonstrated that GABA depolarizes primary afferent fibers by a direct action of the amino acid on specific receptors located on the terminals. Extensive efforts have been made to determine the mechanism of this depolarization using several different physiological preparations. These include the cat spinal cord *in vivo*, the isolated, superfused frog and rat spinal cords, and the dorsal root ganglion, intact and in culture.

7.1. Afferent Terminals in the Cat Spinal Cord

The effect of GABA on the terminals of single afferent fibers in the cat spinal cord has been determined by testing the effect of the amino acid on fiber excitability. In such experiments, single fiber terminals are excited to fire by the passage of small pulses of negative current through a microelectrode placed intraspinally in the vicinity of the terminals. The current is adjusted so that it is at threshold to produce an antidromic spike in a single afferent fiber (Fig. 3A). GABA (and other compounds) can then be ejected iontophoretically from a multibarrel micropipette located in the same spinal location. The effect of GABA is assessed by determining the amount of threshold current required to evoke an impulse in the terminal before and after the application of the amino acid.

When applied in this manner, GABA increases the excitability of afferent terminals (Fig. 3B) (Curtis et al., 1977). It is assumed that an increased excitability indicates a depolarization since, in general, an increased excitability reflects a membrane depolarization. In most fibers, the amino acid-evoked changes are reversible and dose dependent. Furthermore, although iontophoretically applied GABA does have some effects on afferent fibers proximal to the terminal region, larger amounts of GABA are needed to excite the proximal parts of fibers when compared to terminals—a finding that

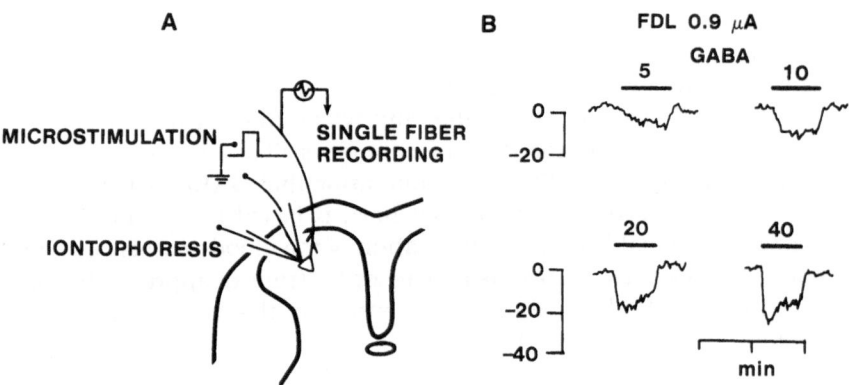

Figure 3. GABA and the excitability of afferent fibers. (A) Schematic diagram of the method of excitability testing of afferent terminals. Afferent fiber terminals are stimulated antidromically in the dorsal horn and the antidromic action potentials of single afferent fibers are recorded from a nerve filament. GABA and other compounds are applied in the vicinity of the terminals via an iontophoretic electrode. (B) Effects of iontophoretically applied GABA on the threshold of the terminals of a flexor digitorum longus (FDL) nerve fiber of the cat. The terminal was stimulated to threshold with 0.9 μA of current, and GABA was ejected with 5, 10, 20, and 40 nA of current passed through the microiontophoretic pipette. Ordinate: percentage decrease in threshold of afferent terminals induced by the applications of GABA. (Modified from Curtis and Lodge, 1982.)

suggests that the density of GABA receptors is higher on the terminal regions than on the nonterminal regions of afferent fibers.

7.2. The Isolated Spinal Cord

Because known concentrations of drugs and transmitters can be added to a superfusing solution, use of isolated frog and newborn rat spinal cords maintained in a bath of oxygenated Ringer's or Krebs' solution (Tebēcis and Phillis, 1969; Otsuka and Konishi, 1974; Kudo, 1978) has permitted quantitative studies of the effects of amino acids. Appropriate ionic substitutions are also possible, and the membrane potential of afferent fibers can be measured in a stable and high resolution fashion by means of the sucrose gap technique (Fig. 4A).

GABA and a number of closely related amino acids rapidly and reversibly depolarize amphibian dorsal roots (Fig. 4B,C). Because the addition of Mg^{2+} or other divalent cations or tetrodotoxin to the solution in concentrations sufficient to fully suppress synaptic activity does not alter the ability of the fibers to respond to GABA (Davidoff, 1972; Barker and Nicoll, 1973), it is clear that this depolarization is caused by the direct action of the amino acids on afferent fibers rather than by an indirect action mediated by interneurons. The effect of GABA appears to take place at, or near, the afferent terminals, since sectioning the cord at the dorsal root entrance to the cord abolishes the depolarization recorded from the root.

Agreement is still lacking about the ionic mechanism of the PAD induced by GABA in the isolated cord. Some data indicate that the GABA response on the terminals is abolished in Na^+-free medium (e.g., Barker and Nicoll, 1973; Constanti and Nistri, 1976)—a finding expected if an increased Na^+ conductance with an inward flux of the cation is responsible for the potential change. However, other experiments with Na^+ substitution have indicated that the GABA-evoked depolarization is depressed only when the extracellular Na^+ concentration is substantially reduced (10% of normal) and that at intermediate levels of the cation, the response can actually be augmented (Nishi et al., 1974; Otsuka and Konishi, 1976). On the other hand, most studies have shown that superfusing the cord with solutions containing low concentrations of Cl^- depresses GABA-induced PAD (e.g., Nishi et al., 1974; Otsuka and Konishi, 1976). If an outward flux of Cl^- ions produces the depolarizing GABA response, one would expect that reduction of the external Cl^- level would augment the response by transiently increasing the Cl^- gradient. Therefore, it is unclear if the process involves an increased permeability to Na^+ or to Cl^- ions, or to both ions. Furthermore, analysis is complicated by a number of limitations inherent in extracellular recording from a population of fibers. On the other hand, it has been concluded that GABA acts postsynaptically on most vertebrate neurons by increasing Cl^- conductance (Krnjevíc, 1974).

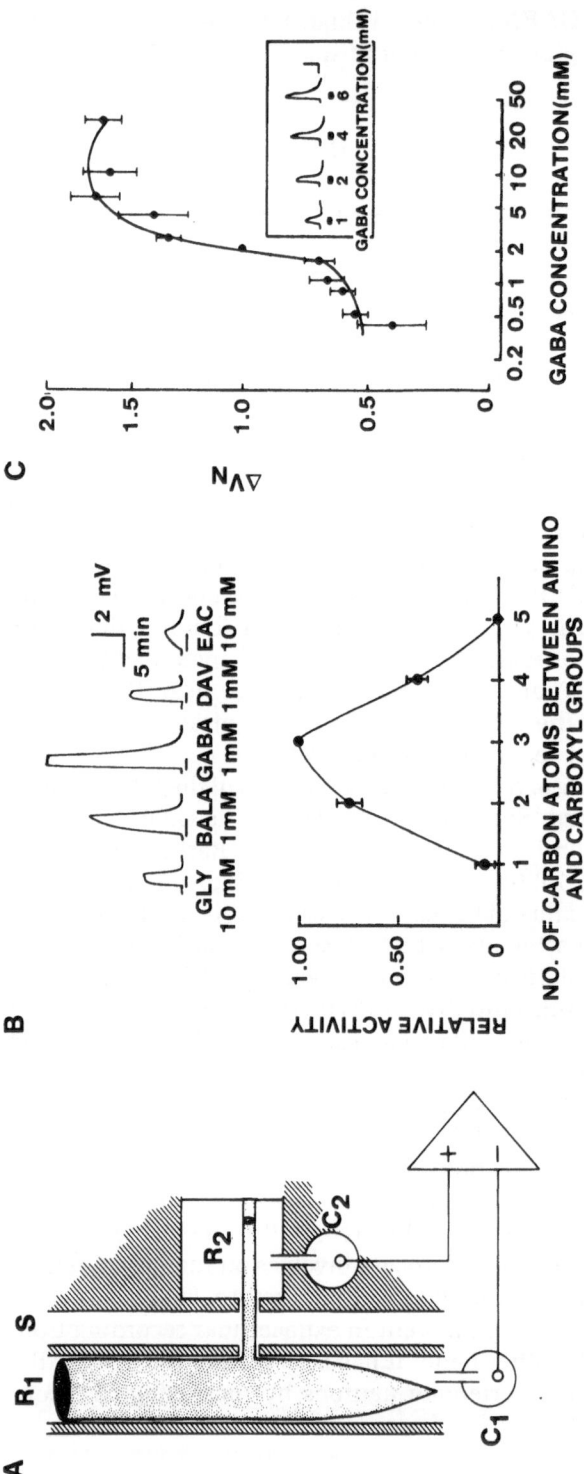

Figure 4. Effect of GABA and related amino acids on the dorsal root of the frog spinal cord. (A) Schematic diagram of the isolated frog spinal cord placed in a sucrose gap apparatus. R_1, cord bath perfused with Ringer's solution; S, sucrose compartment perfused with Ringer's solution; C_1, calomel electrode in contact with cord bath via agar-Ringer's bridge; C_2, second calomel electrode in contact with pool R_2, pool of Ringer's solution; C_1, calomel electrode in contact with cord bath via agar-Ringer's bridge; C_2, second calomel electrode in contact with pool R_2. Both electrodes are connected to a differential amplifier. (B) Neutral amino acids and afferent terminal depolarization. Records of depolarizations produced by application of different amino acids to frog spinal cord bathed in Ringer's solution containing 20 mM Mg^{2+} to eliminate synaptic transmission. GLY, glycine; BALA, β-alanine; DAV, δ-aminovaleric acid; EAC, ε-aminocaproic acid. Below: graphic representation of the effect of the number of carbon atoms separating amino and carboxyl groups and the depolarizing potency of the neutral amino acids applied in sample records. (From Barker et al., 1975a, with permission.) (C) Log dose—response curve for GABA applied to isolated frog cord. Experiment performed on cord treated with tetrodotoxin to block synaptic activity. Abscissa, GABA concentration; ordinate, normalized depolarizations obtained in nine experiments. (ΔV_N was calculated by dividing all GABA depolarizations in one experiment by the response to 2 mM GABA in that cord). Inset shows examples of GABA-evoked depolarizations. Calibration: 1.0 mV, 1.0 min. (From Constanti and Nistri, 1976, with permission.)

7.3. The Dorsal Root Ganglion

GABA depolarizes the somata of mammalian and amphibian primary afferent neurons (Nishi et al., 1974; Deschenes et al., 1976). Although there are no GABAergic synapses in dorsal root ganglia, it has been assumed that the membrane of the cell body has GABA receptors similar to those on the afferent terminals. Intracellular investigations on dorsal root ganglion neurons have clearly indicated that the depolarization is caused by an increased conductance to Cl^- ions (Fig. 5A) (Nishi et al., 1974; Gallagher et al., 1978). Thus, the reversal potential of the depolarization is related to the logarithmic concentration of extracellular Cl^- (Fig. 5B) and is unaffected by changing the external Na^+, K^+, or Ca^{2+} concentrations.

Attempts have been made by the intracellular injection of foreign anions to define the properties of the ionic permeability mechanism of the soma membrane activated by GABA. Anions smaller in hydrated size than ClO_3^- and ClO_3^- ions themselves augment the amplitude of the depolarization produced by GABA and shift the reversal potential for the response in a positive direction (Fig. 5C). In contrast, injection of larger anions and cations do not alter the GABA response. These results are consistent with the idea that the membrane activated by GABA becomes permeable to anions having a hydrated size equal to or less than that of the ClO_3^- ion (2.85 Å). It is not known if the ionic channels have any chemical specificity for anions or if the activated membrane behaves as a sieve with pores or channels of a precisely standardized size.

Different investigators using ganglion cells from different species have reported a variety of measurements of the reversal potential of the GABA response, but despite the differences, all reported values are more positive than the resting membrane potential. Since it seems that the GABA response of dorsal root ganglion cells is entirely dependent upon a conductance change to Cl^- ions, the electrochemical gradient for Cl^- ions across the membrane is directed outward. In other words, the Cl^- equilibrium potential is positive with respect to the resting membrane potential. Therefore, one would expect a "high" concentration of the anion in dorsal root ganglion cells and probably also in afferent terminals. Such a concentration gradient for Cl^- could only be explained if an *inwardly* directed Cl^- pump maintained the intracellular level of Cl^- ions.

Attempts have been made to depress the Cl^- pump with agents that interfere with Cl^- pumps present in other systems. Use of such agents—including NH_4^+, furosemide, and $CuSO_4$—applied to the frog cord and to the frog dorsal root ganglion have been unsuccessful in interfering with the Cl^- gradient. On the other hand, the Cl^--transport inhibitor piretanide reduces the GABA depolarization (Fig. 5D) and does produce a small shift of the reversal potential for GABA toward the resting membrane potential—a finding consistent with a reduction of the inward pumping of Cl^- ions. However, the major effect of piretanide on GABA responses appears to be a

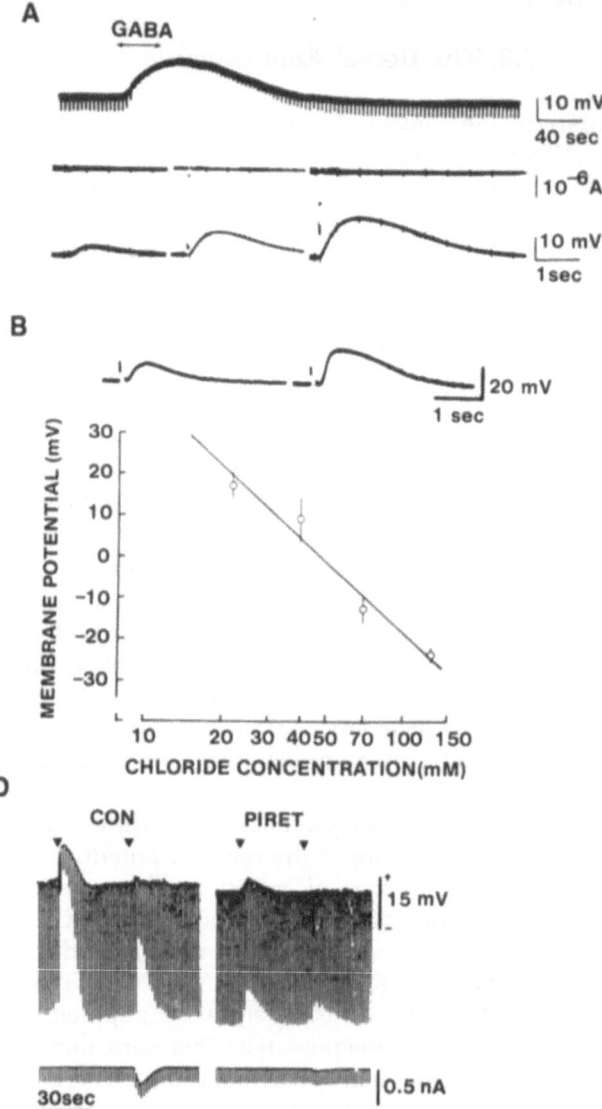

Figure 5. Effects of GABA on dorsal root ganglion cells. (A) GABA-induced depolarization of single ganglion cells. Upper trace: GABA (10^{-4} M) applied to frog ganglion cell for 40 sec (between arrows). Note attenuation of electrotonic potentials produced by passing current pulses (0.5 nA, 50 msec) through recording electrode. Lower traces: recordings from another cell depolarized by iontophoretic applications of GABA. Middle traces: current records from iontophoretic electrode (downward deflections). (From Nishi et al., 1974.) (B) Effect of low external Cl^- concentration on GABA depolarizations of cat dorsal root ganglion cells. Upper left record: response in normal Krebs' solution. Upper right record: response in solution containing 40 mM Cl^- demonstrating an increased amplitude and rate of rise of potential change. The graph shows that changing the Cl^- concentration shifts the equilibrium potential (ordinate) of the GABA depolarization. (From Gallagher et al., 1978, with permission.) (C) Diagram of the correlation between the size of anions in aqueous solution and their ability to pass through the activated GABA receptor membrane of cat dorsal root ganglion cells. The length of the bands indicates

C

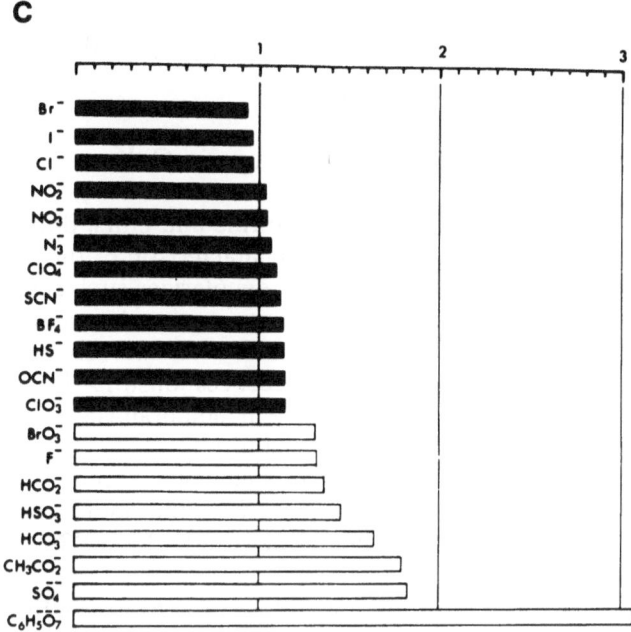

E

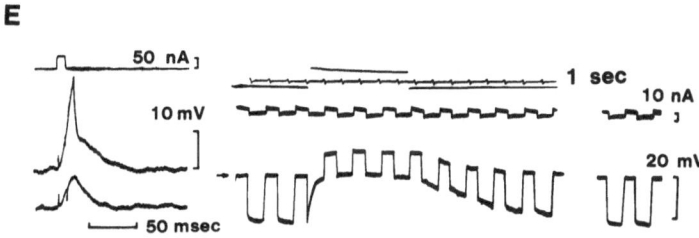

ionic radii. The black bands are for intracellularly injected anions able to augment the depolarization produced by the application of GABA (i.e., permeable anions). The white bands are for anions without effect (i.e., impermeable anions). Hydrated radius of K^+ is unity on the horizontal scale. (From Gallagher et al., 1978, with permission.) (D) Depression of GABA responses produced by piretanide. Intracellular recording from a frog dorsal root ganglion cell. GABA was iontophoretically applied (300-msec pulses at arrows). GABA depolarized the cell (11 mV in control record) and increased the membrane conductance as shown by the decrease in the size of the voltage change produced by the passage of short constant hyperpolarizing current pulses (lower traces). The second response to GABA was "clamped" at the resting membrane potential by the passage of hyperpolarizing current. Exposure to piretanide (10^{-3} M) reduced the potential and conductance changes induced by GABA. (From Wojtowicz and Nicoll, 1982, with permission.) (E) Effects of GABA on cultured rat dorsal root ganglion cells. Left traces: iontophoretic application of GABA to two different spots (upper and middle traces) on the same cell. Note action potential produced by GABA-induced depolarization. Iontophoretic current shown in top trace. Middle traces: increased conductance produced by GABA administered iontophoretically during the time indicated in the second trace. Hyperpolarizing constant current pulses (shown in third trace) given through intracellular electrode. The arrow on the left indicates the resting membrane potential. Right traces: obtained 5 sec after end of middle records. (After Obata, 1974.)

block of the conductance increase elicited by GABA (Wojtowicz and Nicoll, 1982).

7.4. Sensory Neurons in Culture

There is evidence that cultured murine and chick dorsal root ganglion cells possess many of the properties characteristic of the same nerve cells *in vivo*. As expected, GABA reversibly depolarizes such cells and decreases their membrane resistance in a concentration-related manner (Fig. 5E). When dorsal root ganglion cells are penetrated with microelectrodes filled with KCl, the reversal potential for the GABA response is shifted in a positive direction, an indication that the change in membrane conductance is caused at least in part by an increased permeability to Cl^- ions. Furthermore, preliminary analyses of the fluctuations in membrane current in voltage-clamped dorsal root ganglion cells are consistent with the notion that GABA affects a single population of two-state (open and closed) Cl^- channels (see Chapter 3).

GABA may also affect other membrane properties of cultured dorsal root ganglion cells. For example, in some cells application of the amino acid is reported to decrease the Ca^{2+} component of the action potential in the soma (Dunlap and Fischbach, 1981). The reduction in the inward Ca^{2+} current appears to result from a selective suppression of the voltage-sensitive Ca^{2+} conductance in these cells. Such effects are produced by concentrations of GABA that do not cause a change in resting membrane potential or conductance and may be produced by activation of GABA receptors which differ in their pharmacology from the usual GABA receptors (GABA$_B$ sites, *vide infra*).

7.5. The Dorsal Column Nuclei

In addition to sending collaterals into the spinal cord, primary afferent fibers bifurcate and project long ascending axons rostrally to terminate in the dorsal column nuclei. As in the spinal cord, axo-axonic synapses are present on the terminals of these primary afferent collaterals in the dorsal column nuclei. Such terminals (either isolated *in vitro* or superfused in *in vivo*) are depolarized by GABA and their excitability is increased (Simmonds, 1978; Davidson and Southwick, 1971). This depolarization appears to be caused by a change in Cl^- permeability and in many ways resembles the process of PAD in the spinal cord.

7.6. Characteristics of the GABA Receptor on Afferent Neurons

In general, the transmitter function of GABA is thought to involve the interaction of the amino acid with a specific receptor that when activated opens a channel (pore or ionophore) permeable to Cl^- ions. There is evidence that the properties of GABA receptors vary among different CNS neurons and that there are a multiplicity of receptors on different neurons and possibly even on the same neuron.

The properties of the GABA receptor can be studied in different ways (for review see Olsen, 1981; Davidoff, 1982). For example, determination of the electrophysiological effects of structurally related compounds can be used to draw inferences about the mode of interaction between GABA and its receptor and thereby to delineate the dimensions of the site. In the past, this type of study has been limited by the flexibility of the GABA molecule and the molecules of related amino acids—flexibility that allows rotation around single bonds. For example, GABA can exist in several energetically favorable conformations. Recently, a variety of relatively rigid GABA agonists of restricted conformation have been synthesized that allow study of the conformations of GABA on afferent neurons. This information can be supplemented with use of specific antagonist substances.

Attempts have been made to investigate the stoichiometry of the GABA interaction with its receptor on afferent neurons (see Nistri and Constanti, 1979, for references). Such attempts using the terminals of the isolated cord are complicated by two factors. First, the measurements consist of electrotonically conducted potential changes of a population of neurons and, second, fading ("desensitization") of GABA effects makes estimates of concentration difficult. However, when concentration–response curves of dorsal root depolarizations are transformed into log-log plots (Werman, 1969), measurements of the limiting slopes (an estimate of the number of transmitter molecules that interact with a single receptor site) suggest that one GABA molecule interacts with one receptor (Fig. 4C). Analysis of the problem on single neurons of isolated cat dorsal root ganglion indicates that at least two molecules of GABA are required to activate the receptor, but again the phenomena of desensitization precludes accurate calculation of the number of GABA molecules necessary to produce receptor activation (Gallagher et al., 1978).

7.6.1. GABA Agonists

Structure–activity studies have been performed on the intramedullary portion of primary afferent fibers in both frog and mammalian spinal cords (Nistri and Constanti, 1979). As shown in Fig. 4B, a variety of ω-aminoalkanecarboxylic acids related to GABA depolarize frog afferent terminals. The figure also indicates that there is a clear correlation between the distance between the two charged ends of the molecules (the carboxyl and amino groups) and potency. The most effective molecule is GABA with a chain of three methylene groups and potency falls off rapidly with a shorter or longer chain length. Investigations of the depolarizing effects of conformationally restricted analogues of GABA indicate that those molecules that have a spatial geometric separation of charged groups closest to that of the GABA molecule in its fully extended conformation are the most potent in depolarizing afferent terminals (Nicoll, 1977; Allan et al., 1980).

Charged groups at both the amino and carboxyl ends of the molecule are required for a compound to possess significant depolarizing activity. Removal of either charged group from the GABA molecule drastically reduces the ability of the substance to depolarize frog dorsal roots. However, these groups may be replaced by other active groups of the same charge (e.g., sulphonate for carboxyl, as in taurine; guanidino for amino, as in β-guaninopropionic acid), an indication that the charges carried by these groups are of importance in determining potency (Curtis and Watkins, 1960). In the series of ω-aminoalkanesulfonic acids, the peak effect is produced by 3-aminopropane sulfonic acid, in which the sulfone group is separated from the amino group by a three-carbon atom chain.

Studies of structure–activity relationships have also been performed on the cell bodies in the dorsal root ganglion of the cat and rat. In ganglia, chain length is an important variable—GABA is the most active compound and β-alanine is almost devoid of activity. Furthermore, taurine is inactive, an indication that on the receptors located on cell bodies, the more strongly acidic sulfonic group cannot be substituted for the carboxyl group. However, the presence of an amino group may not be as essential to activity since substitution of the guanidino moiety for the amino group only reduces activity by a third (Gallagher et al., 1978); however, in other respects the receptor on dorsal root ganglion cells appears very similar to that located on afferent terminals.

7.6.2. Pharmacological Antagonists

Several compounds (e.g., bicuculline, picrotoxin, penicillin) are potent and relatively specific GABA antagonists on various vertebrate and invertebrate neurons. Although these compounds have the ability to antagonize the depolarizing effects of GABA on primary afferent neurons, the nature of the antagonism of GABA responses on afferent neurons is not well understood. In large measure, this reflects an inability to record intracellularly from afferent terminals.

Picrotoxin, bicuculline, and penicillin antagonize the GABA-produced depolarization of primary afferent terminals and cell bodies (Figs. 6A,B,C). This is a relatively specific action when compared with the ability of these antagonists to affect the responses evoked by other putative amino acid transmitters (e.g., glycine, glutamate) (Figs. 6A,B), but all of the antagonists do attenuate the depolarizing responses produced by amino acids closely related to GABA (Fig. 6A).

An important question concerns the mechanism of the GABA antagonism produced by picrotoxin, bicuculline, and penicillin. For the sake of simplicity, it is now usually stated that bicuculline acts at, or very close to, the recognition site for GABA and that picrotoxin and penicillin influence the associated Cl^- channel. Indeed, the action of picrotoxin on frog dorsal root terminals, on isolated cat spinal ganglia, and on afferent terminals in the isolated cuneate nucleus is reported to be noncompetitive (Constanti and Nistri, 1976; Gallagher et al., 1978; Simmonds, 1980) (Fig. 6D). The noncompetitive antagonism indicates that picrotoxin acts at a site other than the GABA recognition site. Since in other preparations, picrotoxin does not interfere with the binding of tritiated GABA to membranes and does not appear to alter the kinetics of the single Cl^- channel opened by GABA, it is reasonable to hypothesize that the compound acts to decrease the probability of opening of transmitter-activated ion channels. Bicuculline, in contrast, is reported to act at most vertebrate GABAergic synapses as a competitive antagonist, and this hypothesis is by and large supported by data from binding studies. But although bicuculline competitively antagonizes the effects of GABA on afferent fibers of the rat cuneate nucleus (Simmonds, 1978), it acts noncompetitively on isolated cat dorsal root ganglion cells (Gallagher et al., 1978). These discrepancies may reflect methodological differences (e.g., differences in duration of amino acid application in different experiments) or may mean that there are dissimilarities in the organization of the GABA receptor complex on different parts of the same neuron or that there are differences in the GABA receptor in different species. The mechanism of the GABA antagonism by penicillin has not been intensively investigated, but it is known that the antibiotic acts as a noncompetitive GABA antagonist on presynaptic fibers in the cuneate nucleus. Work performed with invertebrate preparations has indicated that the antibiotic interferes either with the Cl^- conductance change produced by interaction of GABA with its receptor or with the electrochemical gradient for Cl^- ions. Sufficient data is not available to distinguish between these explanations.

7.6.3. Antagonists and PAD

If GABA is the transmitter responsible for generating PAD, then agents such as picrotoxin, bicuculline, and penicillin should reduce PAD in the same concentrations that decrease the ability of GABA to depolarize afferent terminals. Early investigations convincingly demonstrated such a parallel suppression of PAD and GABA depolarizations (Fig. 7A,B). Most workers, however, used an AC-coupled recording system that artifactually and significantly shortened the DRP by filtering out the slower components of the potential. More recent studies have utilized sucrose gap DC recordings from dorsal roots of the isolated frog cord. These recordings show that GABA antagonists abolish the DRP evoked by electrically stimulating the ventral root (Fig. 7C). However, the action of these compounds on the DRP elicited by stimulating an adjacent dorsal root is quite complex. The peak amplitude of the DRP is reduced, but this reflects only a decrease in the size of an early phase of the DRP—the initial 150–200 msec of the potential. The latter portion of the potential is enlarged and prolonged even during the peak action of the antagonists (Fig. 7C) (Barker et al., 1975b; Davidoff et al., 1980).

Since picrotoxin and bicuculline antagonize the effects of GABA at a

A

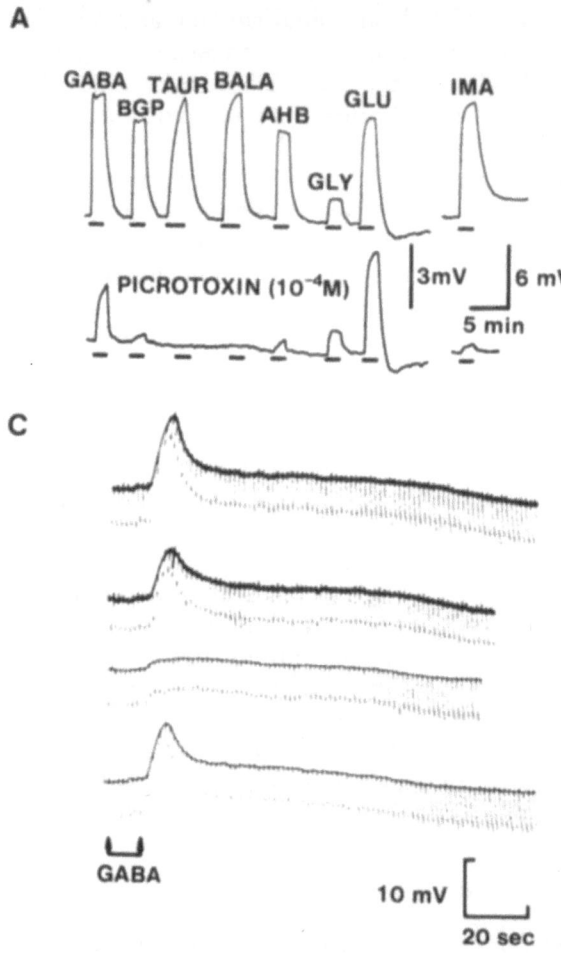

Figure 6. Effects of GABA antagonists. (A) Picrotoxin antagonism of depolarizations of afferent terminals produced by amino acids. Sucrose gap recordings from isolated frog cord superfused with Mg^{2+}-containing Ringer's solution. Upper record: control responses. BGP, β-guanidino-propionic acid; TAUR, taurine; BALA, β-alanine; AHB, β-amino-γ-hydroxybutyric acid; GLY, glycine; GLU, glutamate; IMA, imidazoleacetic acid. Bars indicate duration of application of amino acids at a concentration of 10^{-3} M. Lower record: responses obtained 20 min after beginning superfusion with solution containing picrotoxin (10^{-4} M). (From Barker et al., 1975a, with permission.) (B) Reduction of GABA depolarization by bicuculline. Upper traces: amino acid depolarizations (10^{-3} M) of frog afferent terminals. Cord bathed in Mn^{2+}-containing Ringer's solution. Lower trace: responses obtained 30 min after exposure to bicuculline (10^{-5} M)

number of synaptic sites, the most likely explanation of their ability to block the early phase of PAD rests with the capacity of these compounds to exert the same antagonistic activity at GABAergic (presumably axo-axonic) synapses located on afferent terminals. In other words, there is good reason to believe that the early component of PAD is mediated by the action of the amino acid.

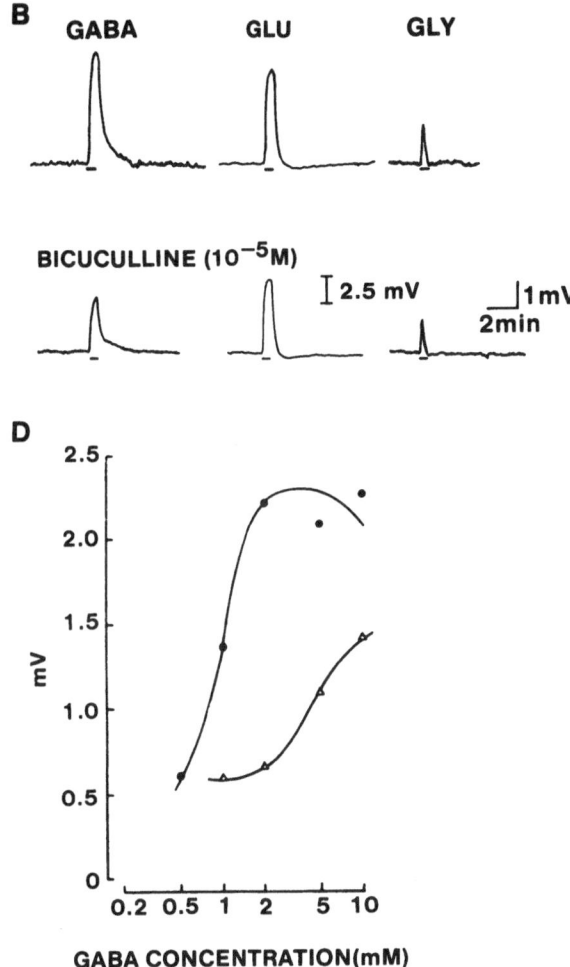

(J. C. Hackman and R. A. Davidoff, unpublished observations). (C) Effect of penicillin. Intra-cellular records obtained from cat dorsal root ganglion cell. The vertical deflections were produced by the passage of constant hyperpolarizing current pulses. Upper trace: control produced by superfusion with solution containing GABA (1.0 mM; 10 sec, arrows). Second and third traces: obtained after exposure to penicillin (0.08 mM and 2.0 mM, respectively). Fourth trace: after washing. (From Kinnes et al., 1980, with permission.) (D) Effect of picrotoxin. Log-dose response curve of GABA depolarizations of frog afferent terminals in tetrodotoxin-containing Ringer's solution before ($\bullet$) and after ($\triangle$) superfusion with picrotoxin (10^{-6} M, 20 min). (From Constanti and Nistri, 1976, with permission.)

The finding that a late part of the DRP is augmented by picrotoxin and bicuculline suggests that the major component of this potential (at least in the presence of the two GABA antagonists) is not mediated by GABA. It may be that accumulation of interstitial K^+ accounts for the slow component of PAD since concentrations of picrotoxin and bicuculline that increase the amplitude of the slow phase of the DRP substantially enhance the evoked

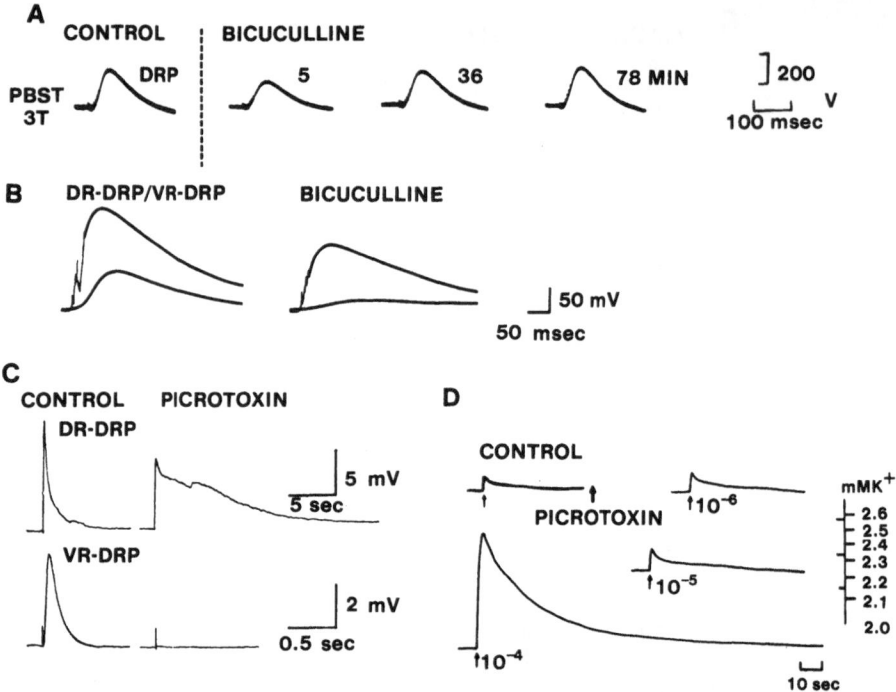

Figure 7. Effects of GABA antagonists on primary afferent depolarization. (A) Effect of bicuculline on DRPs evoked by stimulation at $3 \times$ threshold (3T) of hamstrings nerve (PBST) in cat. Bicuculline (0.5 mg/kg) was administered intravenously at time indicated by dashed line and records obtained at various times after drug administration. (From Curtis et al., 1971, with permission.) (B) Action of bicuculline on DRPs in isolated frog cord. Left traces: control DR-DRP (large potential) and VR-DRP (small potential). Right traces: DRPs recorded after exposure of the cord to bicuculline methiodide (2×10^{-5} M̃, 12 min). (From Davidoff et al., 1973, with permission.) (C) Effects of picrotoxin on DRPs in isolated frog cord. Picrotoxin was applied in a concentration of 5×10^{-5} M for 20 min. (From Barker et al., 1975b, with permission.) (D) Effects of various concentrations of picrotoxin on extracellular K^+ activity. Responses were recorded by means of a K^+-sensitive microelectrode placed in the intermediate gray matter of an isolated frog spinal cord. The dorsal root was supramaximally stimulated once in each record. Left upper trace: control record. Other traces obtained after the cord was exposed to increasing concentrations of picrotoxin (10^{-6} M, 10^{-5} M, 10^{-4} M). (Modified from Syková and Vyklický, 1978.)

release of K^+ in the frog spinal cord (Syková and Vyklický, 1978) (Fig. 7D); an augmented local level of K^+ ions could be the main factor in the convulsant-induced enhancement of the slow phase of PAD. Alternatively, a transmitter resistant to the blocking actions of picrotoxin and bicuculline may be involved in the production of the late part of PAD. Substance P or an acidic amino acid such as L-glutamate are possibilities, but further data is needed to clarify this.

7.6.4. GABA Antagonists, Strychnine, and Other Amino Acids

The identity of the transmitter responsible for the type of PAD elicited in the amphibian by stimulation of the ventral roots is disputed. Evidence points to GABA as the mediator of the process since picrotoxin, bicuculline, and penicillin abolish this potential and also reduce GABA depolarizations. But other pharmacological data have indicated that either β-alanine or taurine may be responsible (Barker et al., 1975a,b). The DRP produced by ventral root stimulation is blocked by strychnine which also depresses the direct depolarizing effects of β-alanine and taurine—but not of GABA—on primary afferent terminals. The specificity of strychnine's effects suggests that primary afferent terminals may have receptors sensitive to β-alanine and/or taurine. It should also be noted that both picrotoxin and bicuculline readily antagonize the depolarizations produced by β-alanine and taurine.

Neurochemical data, however, provide little support for a transmitter role for either of these amino acids. Frog spinal tissue contains only very low concentrations of these compounds. There is no uptake system for taurine in frog cord, and β-alanine appears to be taken up and released from glial cells (Davidoff, 1978). In sum, uncertainty remains about the function of primary afferent terminal receptors that are activated by these latter amino acids.

7.6.5. "Classical" and "Nonclassical" GABA Receptors

Recent work has indicated that there may be at least two types of GABA receptors: "classical" receptors (GABA$_A$ type), which can be activated by GABA and by some GABA agonists (e.g., 3-aminopropane sulfonic acid, muscimol, isoguvacine), and which are blocked by bicuculline, and "nonclassical" receptors (GABA$_B$ type), which are activated by GABA, but not by the majority of recognized GABA mimetics, and which are not affected by bicuculline (Bowery et al., 1983). Baclofen, a β-p-chlorophenyl derivative of GABA used in the treatment of spasticity, is stereospecifically active at the latter sites.

It has been hypothesized that GABA$_A$ receptor sites are linked to Cl^- channels and that their activation results in the increased permeability to Cl^- ions expected when GABA occupies its recognition sites. On the other hand, it is now thought unlikely that activation of GABA$_B$ receptors increases the opening of Cl^- channels. Instead, present information would favor the hypothesis that GABA$_B$ sites on sensory neurons exert their effects by reducing the movement of Ca^{2+} ions. In other words, GABA$_B$ sites may be associated with Ca^{2+} channels in neuronal membranes on afferent neurons (Bowery et al., 1984).

The levorotatory form of baclofen [$(-)$-baclofen] produces a potent and prolonged depression of synaptic activity in both mono- and polysynaptic spinal pathways that reflects a reduction in the amplitude of EPSPs. The drug hyperpolarizes spinal afferent terminals, but it does not produce consistent effects on the postsynaptic membranes of motoneurons and inter-neurons. These findings have led to the hypothesis that baclofen exerts its depressant action on spinal neurotransmission mainly through reduction of the release of excitatory amino acids from afferent terminals (Davidoff and Sears, 1974). A similar hypothesis has emerged from biochemical studies that show that baclofen suppresses the release of endogenous excitatory amino acids from neural tissue (Potashner, 1979). It may be that baclofen reduces EPSPs by an effect on $GABA_B$ receptors located on primary afferent nerve terminals. Although definitive data to support this idea in the spinal cord is still unavailable (Davidoff and Hackman, 1983), it is of interest that $GABA_B$ sites are present in the spinal cord. Moreover, it appears that the site responsible for the ability of GABA to reduce Ca^{2+} conductance in dorsal root ganglion neurons has the characteristics of a $GABA_B$ receptor. On the other hand, preliminary data (Bowery et al., 1984) indicates that $GABA_B$ receptors appear distinctly concentrated in the dorsal horn—the site of ter-mination of cutaneous afferent fibers and the effects of baclofen appear to be exerted on both muscle and cutaneous afferents.

8. GABA METABOLISM AND PAD

The formation of GABA in neural tissue is catalyzed by the enzyme L-glutamic acid decarboxylase (GAD). If GABA is responsible for PAD, exper-imental reduction of GAD activity should lead to reduced PAD. Depletion of GABA levels by administration of either semicarbazide (which is thought to act by trapping the carbonyl group of pyridoxal phosphate thereby block-ing its function as a coenzyme for GAD), or 3-mercaptopropionic acid (which competitively inhibits GAD) reduces GAD activity, GABA levels, and PAD in the spinal cord (Bell and Anderson, 1972) (Fig. 8A) and cuneate nucleus (Roberts et al., 1978) (Fig. 8B). It is not known if these compounds affect both the early and late components of the DRP, and, in addition, it has recently been shown that 3-mercaptopropionic acid blocks the release of GABA, as well as its synthesis.

Inhibition of GABA-transaminase, the enzyme responsible for the ca-tabolism of the amino acid, by amino oxyacetic acid or hydroxylamine results in increased levels of GABA in the spinal cord and increases PAD in the frog (Davidoff et al., 1973), but the results in the cat are inconsistent (cf. Bell and Anderson, 1974; Larson and Anderson, 1979).

9. GABA DESENSITIZATION

Chemically transmitting synapses appear to have mechanisms to remove or inactivate transmitters released from presynaptic terminals. At GABAergic

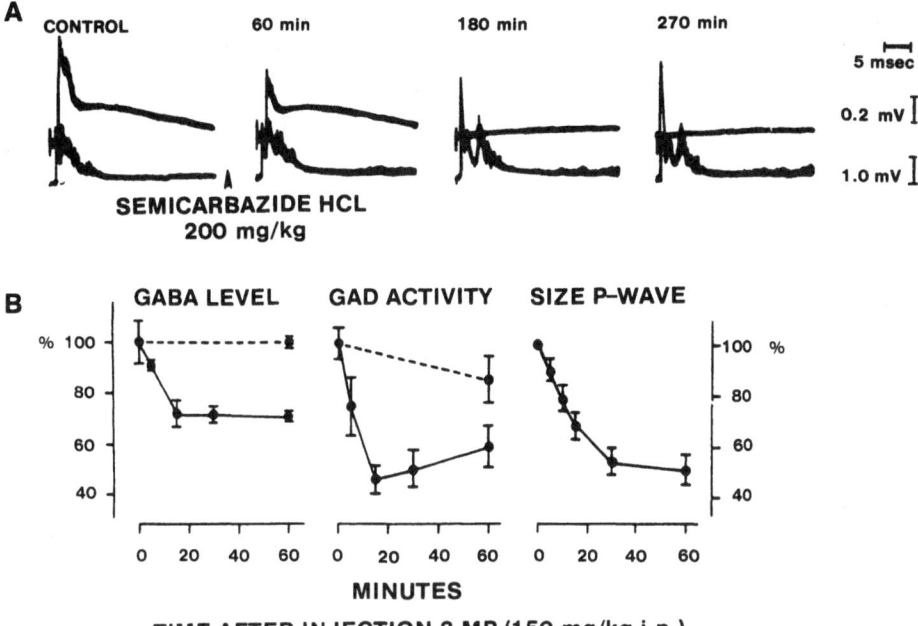

Figure 8. Effects of glutamic acid decarboxylase inhibitors on primary afferent depolarization and GABA levels. (A) Effects of semicarbazide on cat cord. Control records: upper trace is a DRP recorded from a dorsal root and bottom trace is reflex recorded simultaneously from a ventral root in response to a dorsal root volley. Each trace represents three superimposed oscilloscope sweeps. The time above subsequent traces indicates the duration after the injection of semicarbazide HCl (200 mg/kg). (From Bell and Anderson, 1972, with permission.) (B) Comparison of GABA levels, glutamic acid decarboxylase (GAD) activity, and PAD in the rat cuneate nucleus during the 60 min following administration of 3-mercaptopropionic acid (3-MP). PAD was measured by the size of the P (positive) wave recorded from the surface of the cuneate in response to electrical stimulation of the ipsilateral forepaw. Values are means ± S.E.M. (n = 6). The dashed lines indicate the changes expected in the absence of 3-MP. (From Roberts et al., 1978, with permission.)

synapses, GABA is removed by uptake into perisynaptic structures, presumably presynaptic terminals and glial cells (Iversen and Kelly, 1975). In spinal tissue this function is served by a specific, high-affinity, energy-requiring, Na^+-dependent uptake system (Balcar and Johnston, 1973). This GABA uptake system can affect the responses of primary afferent terminals to GABA.

During sustained or repetitive application of GABA to afferent terminals, the amplitude of the depolarization is characterized by a rapid and exponential decline (fade) to a steady plateau level ("desensitization") (Fig. 9A). Such fading of GABA responses may in part be caused by receptor desensitization. In the frog spinal cord, however, procedures that interfere with GABA uptake (e.g., reduction of Na^+ and temperature, addition of ouabain or dinitrophenol) reduce the fading of GABA responses (Hackman et al., 1982) (Fig. 9B). Similar effects were produced by the application of specific

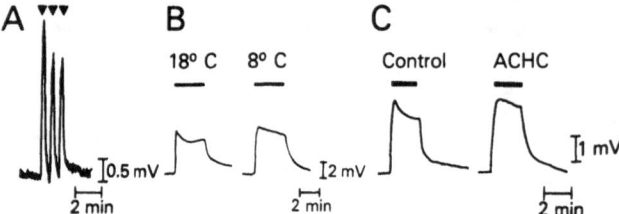

Figure 9. GABA "desensitization." All records in this figure were obtained from the dorsal root of the isolated frog cord superfused with Mn^{2+}-containing Ringer's solution. (A) GABA (5 $\times$ 10^{-4} M) applied in short (10 sec) pulses every 30 sec. (B) Effects of change of temperature on GABA depolarizations of frog dorsal root. GABA (5 $\times$ 10^{-4} M) was applied for 3 min (bars). Right-hand trace was obtained at a temperature of 18°C and left-hand trace after the temperature was lowered to 8°C. (C) Effect of GABA uptake blocker. Depolarizations produced by applications of GABA (5 $\times$ 10^{-5} M, 2 min) before (control) and after exposure to cis-1,3-aminocyclohexane carboxylic acid (ACHC, 10^{-4} M, 10 min). (From Hackman et al., 1982, with permission.)

antagonists of high-affinity GABA uptake (e.g., nipecotic acid, cis-1,3-aminocyclohexane carboxylic acid). These results suggest that cellular transport processes can influence the form of GABA responses on afferent terminals; the results also indicate that removal of GABA is responsible in part for GABA desensitization.

10. GABA AND OTHER PRESYNAPTIC TERMINALS

10.1. Sympathetic Ganglia

Even though GABAergic synapses are *not* present in sympathetic ganglia, application of the amino acid produces two effects referable to presynaptic nerve terminals—depolarization (Fig. 10A) and inhibition of nicotinic transmission (Fig. 10B). The latter appears caused by reduction of the evoked release of acetylcholine from preganglionic nerve terminals. Thus, data obtained from frog sympathetic ganglia demonstrated a decreased quantal content of the EPSP without a concomitant change in miniature EPSP size or postsynaptic sensitivity to acetylcholine (Fig. 10C) (Kato and Kuba, 1980).

These two effects—depolarization and decreased transmitter release—are the result of activation of two independent populations of receptors. $GABA_A$ receptors appear responsible for the depolarizing action of the amino acid. Picrotoxin diminishes this effect and eliminates the preganglionic depolarization produced by GABA without altering the block of nicotinic transmission. For this reason it is thought that the depolarizing action of GABA on preganglionic terminals is not essential to its inhibitory action on synaptic transmission. The receptor responsible for the "presynaptic inhibition" of acetylcholine release, although insensitive to bicuculline and picrotoxin, is activated by baclofen. The mechanism of this inhibition is not understood, but an increase in Cl^- conductance may play a part because the inhibitory concentration is lowered (Fig. 10C). The physiological role of GABA in sympathetic ganglia is unknown, although it is possible that there is a sufficient concentration of GABA in blood (at least in frogs) to affect presynaptic terminals.

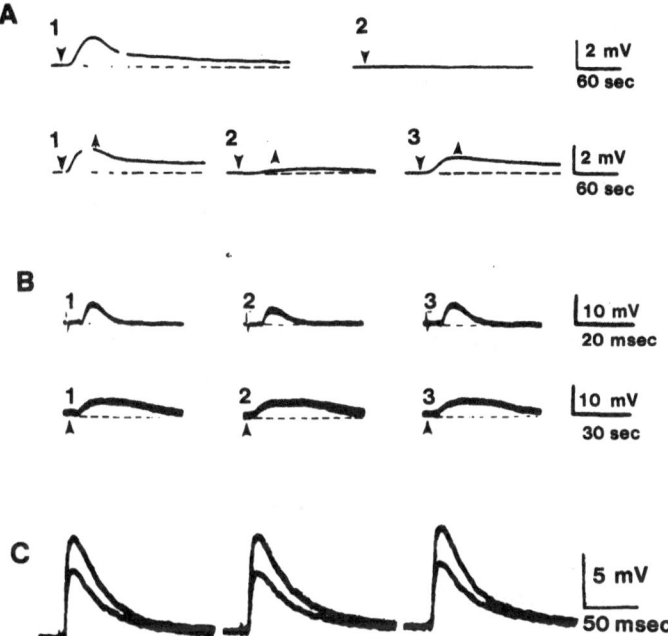

Figure 10. Effect of GABA on bullfrog sympathetic ganglia. (A) Sucrose gap records showing depolarization of preganglionic nerve terminals by GABA (0.1 mM). Upper traces: record 1 obtained from preganglionic terminals; record 2 from preganglionic nerve. Lower traces: record 1 is control exposure to GABA; record 2 is after superfusion with picrotoxin (10^{-5} M, 20 min); and record 3 is after washing (30 min). (From Koketsu et al., 1974, with permission.) (B) Upper traces: effect of GABA on fast EPSPs recorded intracellularly from a ganglion cell. Recordings of EPSPs before (1), 1 min after application of GABA (2), and 5 min after washing (3). Note the reduction in EPSP unaccompanied by change in membrane potential during GABA application. Lower traces: sucrose gap record of the effect of GABA on nicotinic acetylcholine response. Acetylcholine superfused before (1), 1 min after GABA (2), and 5 min after washing (3). Note that the postsynaptic acetylcholine response remains unchanged. (From Koketsu et al., 1974, with permission.) (C) Effect of GABA on fast EPSP. Intracellular recordings from a ganglion cell in Cl^--deficient (15.6 mM) solution before (left records), 5 min after application of GABA (middle records), and after washing (right records). Superimposed traces represent EPSPs of different quantal size and demonstrate the lack of a response to GABA in low-Cl^- solution. All solutions contained low-Ca^{2+} and high-Mg^{2+} concentrations. (From Kato and Kuba, 1980, with permission.)

10.2. Olfactory Cortex

The lateral olfactory tract is a bundle of fibers that originates in the olfactory bulb and runs to the olfactory cortex. The fibers make excitatory synapses with distal dendrites of neurons located in the olfactory cortex. The terminals of the lateral olfactory tract are depolarized by appropriate stimuli applied to the tract and the process appears mediated by GABA receptors of the $GABA_A$ type (Pickles, 1979). However, the process does not appear analogous to PAD in the spinal cord since GABA receptors are not exclusively located on nerve terminals, but may be present on the entire axonal membrane and there is some data that indicate that GABA has different actions on different portions of the axons of the lateral olfactory tract. The amino acid may decrease the excitability of terminals and increase the excitability of unmyelinated portions of the tract (Simmonds, 1984). Interpretation of the functional significance of the data is complicated since appropriate axo-axonic synapses are not present. However, antidromic impulses in lateral olfactory tract fibers can be elicited by conditioning stimuli to the tract, and these stimuli also increase the excitability of the terminal regions of lateral olfactory tract fibers. These phenomena, which resemble PAD in the spinal cord, can be tentatively attributed to an action of GABA since they are reduced by GABA antagonists (Cain and Simmonds, 1982). It is possible that GABA diffuses to olfactory tract terminals from neighboring synapses.

11. AUTORECEPTORS

There is neurochemical (but no physiological) evidence that GABA exerts at least one other type of presynaptic effect—that of reducing the release of GABA released from GABAergic nerve terminals. This process is thought to be mediated by so-called autoreceptors. The pharmacological properties of the autoreceptors appears to be very similar to that of $GABA_A$ sites. The significance of such sites is presently unknown, but in other systems autoreceptors are activated by transmitter released from the presynaptic terminal releasing the transmitter and act in a feedback mechanism to regulate the output of transmitter from a particular terminal or population of terminals.

12. SUMMARY

There is a great deal of evidence that GABA affects the properties of presynaptic terminals in the spinal cord and in other neural structures. In addition, there is firm evidence that GABA fulfills many of the criteria required of a transmitter responsible for spinal PAD—at least the early part of the terminal depolarization. Nevertheless, the function of PAD is still controversial. The major question concerns the relationship between PAD and presynaptic inhibition. There is still no direct evidence that GABA inhibits release of transmitter from spinal presynaptic terminals. Eccles and his colleagues postulated a causal relationship between PAD and inhibition; the depolarization of afferent terminals (produced by the action of GABA) was hypothesized to diminish the amplitude of the action potential in the terminals; this change in the action potential was hypothesized to reduce the output of excitatory transmitter (Eccles, 1964). The possible mechanism by which a smaller action potential reduced transmitter release was left unspecified.

Several processes are possible. Depolarization may decrease transmitter release by reducing the amplitude of the action potential in afferent fibers or by producing a block of conduction of the action potential at a branch point in preterminal arborizations conveying the afferent volley. Alternatively, the depolarization per se may be unimportant, and a conductance change induced by GABA in the afferent terminals may be the important phenomenon responsible for decreasing the presynaptic spike (Padjen and Hashiguchi, 1983) or for reduction of Ca^{2+} influx into terminals. A decreased Ca^{2+} influx would result in a decreased release of transmitter. A GABA-evoked reduction in Ca^{2+} current has recently been demonstrated in cultured chick dorsal root ganglion cells (Dunlap and Fischbach, 1981). In fact, there may be two GABA receptors on such cells—a conventional type ($GABA_A$), blocked by GABA antagonists, and an unconventional type ($GABA_B$), unresponsive to the blocking actions of bicuculline and picrotoxin, but activated by baclofen (Dunlap, 1981). There is an obvious analogy to the situation at frog sympathetic ganglionic presynaptic terminals (Kato and Kuba, 1980), but information is needed as to whether or not these effects occur on the terminals of spinal afferent fibers in mature mammals.

Understanding of the basic physiological processes responsible for presynaptic inhibition is thus still quite incomplete. Further information is needed about the role of GABA in affecting transmitter release, the types of GABA receptors present on afferent terminals, and the role of K^+ and presynaptic inhibition.

ACKNOWLEDGMENTS. Preparation of this chapter was supported by Veterans Administration Medical Center Funds (MRIS 1769) and by U.S. Public Health Service Grant # NS 17577-02.

REFERENCES

Allan, R. D., Evans, R. H., and Johnston, G. A. R., 1980, γ-aminobutyric acid agonists: An in vitro comparison between depression of spinal synaptic activity and depolarization of spinal root fibres in the rat, Br. J. Pharmacol. 70:609–615.

Balcar, V. J., and Johnston, G. A. R., 1973, High affinity uptake of transmitters: Studies on the uptake of L-aspartate, GABA, L-glutamate, and glycine in cat spinal cord, *J. Neurochem.* **20:**529–539.

Barker, J. L., and Nicoll, R. A., 1973, The pharmacology and ionic dependency of amino acid responses in the frog spinal cord, *J. Physiol. (Lond.)* **228:**259–277.

Barker, J. L., Nicoll, R. A., and Padjen, A., 1975a, Studies on convulsants in the isolated frog spinal cord. I. Antagonism of amino acid responses, *J. Physiol. (Lond.)* **245:**521–536.

Barker, J. L., Nicoll, R. A., and Padjen, A., 1975b, Studies on convulsants in the isolated frog spinal cord. II. Effects on root potentials, *J. Physiol. (Lond.)* **245:**537–548.

Bell, J. A., and Anderson, E. G., 1972, The influence of semicarbazide-induced depletion of γ-aminobutyric acid on presynaptic inhibition, *Brain Res.* **43:**161–169.

Bell, J. A., and Anderson, E. G., 1974, Dissociation between amino-oxyacetic acid-induced depression of spinal reflexes and the rise in cord GABA levels, *Neuropharmacology* **13:**885–894.

Bowery, N. G., Hill, D. R., and Hudson, A. L., 1983, Characteristics of GABA$_B$ receptor binding sites on rat whole brain synaptic membranes, *Br. J. Pharmacol.* **78:**191–206.

Bowery, N. G., Hill, D. R., Hudson, A. L., Price, G. W., Turnbull, M. J., and Wilkin, G. P., 1984, Heterogeneity of mammalian GABA receptors, in: *Actions and Interactions of GABA and Benzodiazepines* (N. G. Bowery, ed.), Raven Press, New York, pp. 81–108.

Burke, R. E., and Rudomín, P., 1977, Spinal neurons and synapses, in: *Handbook of Physiology,* Section 1, *The Nervous System,* Volume 1, *Cellular Biology of Neurons, Part 2* (E. R. Kandel, ed.), American Physiological Society, Bethesda, pp. 877–944.

Cain, C. R., and Simmonds, M. A., 1982, GABA-mediated changes in excitability of the rat lateral olfactory tract *in vitro, J. Physiol. (Lond.)* **332:**487–499.

Carlson, C. B., 1964, Sodium and the dorsal root potential, *J. Physiol. (Lond.)* **172:**295–304.

Conradi, S., 1969, On motoneuron synaptology in adult cats, *Acta Physiol. Scand.* [Suppl.] 332.

Constanti, A., and Nistri, A., 1976, A comparative study of the action of γ-aminobutyric acid and piperazine on the lobster muscle fibre and the frog spinal cord, *Br. J. Pharmacol.* **57:**347–358.

Curtis, D. R., and Lodge, D., 1982, The depolarization of feline ventral horn group Ia spinal afferent terminations by GABA, *Exp. Brain Res.* **46:**215–233.

Curtis, D. R., and Watkins, J. C., 1960, The excitation and depression of spinal neurones by structurally related amino acids, *J. Neurochem.* **6:**117–141.

Curtis, D. R., Duggan, A. W., Felix, D., and Johnston, G. A. R., 1971, Bicuculline, an antagonist of GABA and synaptic inhibition in the spinal cord, *Brain Res.* **32:**69–96.

Curtis, D. R., Lodge, D., and Brand, S., 1977, GABA and spinal afferent terminal excitability in the cat, *Brain Res.* **130:**360–363, 1977.

Davidoff, R. A., 1972, Gamma-aminobutyric acid antagonism and presynaptic inhibition in the frog spinal cord, *Science* **175:**331–333.

Davidoff, R. A., 1978, Identification of the presynaptic inhibitory transmitter, in: *Iontophoresis and Transmitter Mechanisms in the Mammalian Central Nervous System* (R. W. Ryall and J. S. Kelly, eds.), Raven Press, New York, pp. 261–263.

Davidoff, R. A., 1982, Studies of neurotransmitter actions (GABA, glycine, and convulsants), in: *Epilepsy* (A. A. Ward, ed.), Raven Press, New York, pp. 53–85.

Davidoff, R. A., and Hackman, J. C., 1978, Pentylenetetrazol and reflex activity of isolated frog spinal cord, *Neurology (Minneap.)* **28:**488–494.

Davidoff, R. A., and Hackman, J. C., 1983, Drugs, chemicals, and toxins: Their effects on the spinal cord, in: *Handbook of the Spinal Cord,* Volume 1, *Spinal Cord Pharmacology* (R. A. Davidoff, ed.), Marcel Dekker, New York, pp. 409–476.

Davidoff, R. A., and Hackman, J. C., 1984, Spinal inhibition, in: *Handbook of the Spinal Cord,* Volume 2, *Anatomy and Physiology of the Spinal Cord* (R. A. Davidoff, ed.), Marcel Dekker, New York, pp. 385–459.

Davidoff, R. A., and Sears, E. S., 1974, The effects of Lioresal on synaptic activity in the isolated spinal cord, *Neurology (Minneap.)* **24:**957–963.

Davidoff, R. A., Grayson, V., and Adair, R., 1973, GABA-transaminase inhibitors and presynaptic inhibition in the amphibian spinal cord, Am. J. Physiol. **224:**1230–1234.

Davidoff, R. A., Hackman, J. C., and Osorio, I., 1980, Amino acid antagonists do not block the depolarizing effects of potassium ions on frog primary afferents, Neuroscience **5:**117–126.

Davidson, N., and Southwick, C. A. P., 1971, Amino acids and presynaptic inhibition in the rat cuneate nucleus, J. Physiol. (Lond.) **219:**689–708.

Deschenes, M., Feltz, P., and Lamour, Y., 1976, A model for an estimate in vivo of the ionic basis of presynaptic inhibition: an intracellular analysis of the GABA-induced depolarization in rat dorsal root ganglia, Brain Res. **118:**486–493.

Dunlap, K., 1981, Two types of γ-aminobutyric acid receptors on embryonic sensory neurones, Br. J. Pharmacol. **74:**579–585.

Dunlap, K., and Fischbach, G. D., 1981, Neurotransmitters decrease the calcium conductance activated by depolarizing embryonic chick sensory neurones, J. Physiol. (Lond.) **317:**519–535.

Eccles, J. C., 1964, Presynaptic inhibition in the spinal cord, Prog. Brain Res. **12:**65–89.

Eccles, J. C., Eccles, R. M., and Magni, F., 1961, Central inhibitory action attributable to presynaptic depolarization produced by muscle afferent volleys, J. Physiol. (Lond.) **159:**147–166.

Eccles, J. C., Schmidt, R., and Willis, W. D., 1963, Pharmacological studies on presynaptic inhibition, J. Physiol. (Lond.) **168:**500–530.

Frank, K., and Fuortes, M. G. F., 1957, Presynaptic and postsynaptic inhibition of monosynaptic reflexes, Fed. Proc. **16:**39–40.

Gallagher, J. P., Higashi, H., and Nishi, S., 1978, Characterization and ionic basis of GABA-induced depolarizations recorded in vitro from cat primary afferent neurones, J. Physiol. (Lond.) **275:**263–282.

Hackman, J. C., Auslander, D., Grayson, V., and Davidoff, R. A., 1982, GABA "desensitization" of frog primary afferent fibers, Brain Res. **253:**143–152.

Iversen, L. L., and Kelly, J. S., 1975, Uptake and metabolism of γ-aminobutyric acid by neurones and glial cells, Biochem. Pharmacol. **24:**933–938.

Jankowska, E., McCrea, D., Rudomín, P., and Syková, E., 1981, Observations on neuronal pathways subserving primary afferent depolarization, J. Neurophysiol. **46:**506–516.

Kato, E., and Kuba, K., 1980, Inhibition of transmitter release in bullfrog sympathetic ganglia induced by γ-aminobutyric acid, J. Physiol. (Lond.) **298:**271–283.

Kinnes, C. G., Connors, B., and Somjen, G., 1980, The effects of convulsant doses of penicillin on primary afferents, dorsal root ganglion cells, and on 'presynaptic' inhibition in the spinal cord, Brain Res. **192:**495–512.

Koketsu, K., Shoji, T., and Yamamoto, K., 1974, Effects of GABA on presynaptic terminals in bullfrog (Rana catesbiana) sympathetic ganglia, Experientia **30:**382–383.

Kříž, N., Syková, E., Ujec, E., and Vyklický, L., 1974, Changes of extracellular potassium concentration induced by neuronal activity in the spinal cord of the cat, J. Physiol. (Lond.) **238:**1–15.

Krnjević, K., 1974, Chemical nature of synaptic transmission in vertebrates, Physiol. Rev. **54:**418–540.

Kudo, Y., 1978, The pharmacology of the amphibian spinal cord, Prog. Neurobiol. **11:**1–76.

Larson, A. A., and Anderson, E. G., 1979, Changes in primary afferent depolarization after administration of γ-acetylenic γ-aminobutyric acid (GAG), a γ-aminobutyric acid (GABA) transaminase inhibitor, J. Pharmacol. Exp. Ther. **211:**326–330.

Levy, R. A., 1977, The role of GABA in primary afferent depolarization, Prog. Neurobiol. **9:**211–267.

Miyata, Y., and Otsuka, M., 1975, Quantitative histochemistry of γ-aminobutyric acid in cat spinal cord with special reference to presynaptic inhibition, J. Neurochem. **25:**239–244.

Nicoll, R. A., 1977, The effect of conformationally restricted amino acid analogues on the frog spinal cord in vitro, Br. J. Pharmacol. **59:**303–309.

Nicoll, R. A., and Alger, B. E., 1979, Presynaptic inhibition: Transmitter and ionic mechanisms, Int. Rev. Neurobiol. **21:**217–258.

Nishi, S., Minota, S., and Karczmar, A. G., 1974, Primary afferent neurones: The ionic mechanism of GABA-mediated depolarization, Neuropharmacology **13:**215–219.

Nistri, A., 1983, Spinal cord pharmacology of GABA and chemically related amino acids, in: *Handbook of the Spinal Cord*, Volume 1, *Spinal Cord Pharmacology* (R. A. Davidoff, ed.), Marcel Dekker, New York, pp. 45–104.

Nistri, A., and Constanti, A., 1979, Pharmacological characterization of different types of GABA and glutamate receptors in vertebrates and invertebrates, *Prog. Neurobiol.* **13**:117–235.

Obata, K., 1974, Transmitter sensitivities of some nerve and muscle cells in culture, *Brain Res.* **73**:71–88.

Olsen, R. W., 1981, GABA-benzodiazepine-barbiturate receptor interactions, *J. Neurochem.* **37**:1–13.

Otsuka, M., and Konishi, S., 1974, Electrophysiology of mammalian spinal cord in vitro, *Nature* **252**:733–734.

Otsuka, M., and Konishi, S., 1976, GABA in the spinal cord, in: *GABA in Nervous System Function* (E. Roberts, T. N. Chase, and D. B. Tower, eds.), Raven Press, New York, pp. 197–202.

Padjen, A. L., and Hashiguchi, T., 1983, Primary afferent depolarization in frog spinal cord is associated with an increase in membrane conductance, *Can. J. Physiol. Pharmacol.* **61**:626–631.

Pickles, H. G., 1979, Presynaptic γ-aminobutyric acid responses in the olfactory cortex, *Br. J. Pharmacol.* **65**:223–228.

Potashner, S. J., 1979, Baclofen: Effects on amino acid release, *J. Neurochem.* **32**:103–109.

Roberts, F., Taberner, P. V., and Hill, R. G., 1978, The effect of 3-aminopropionate, an inhibitor of glutamate decarboxylase, on the levels of GABA and other amino acids and on presynaptic inhibition in the rat cuneate nucleus, *Neuropharmacology* **17**:715–720.

Schmidt, R. F., 1971, Presynaptic Inhibition in the vertebrate nervous system, *Ergeb. Physiol.* **63**:20–101.

Simmonds, M. A., 1978, Presynaptic actions of γ-aminobutyric acid and some antagonists in a slice preparation of cuneate nucleus, *Br. J. Pharmacol.* **63**:495–502.

Simmonds, M. A., 1980, Evidence that bicuculline and picrotoxin act at separate sites to antagonize γ-aminobutyric acid in rat cuneate nucleus, *Neuropharmacology* **19**:39–45.

Simmonds, M. A., 1984, Physiological and pharmacological characterization of the actions of GABA, in: *Actions and Interactions of GABA and Benzodiazepines* (N. G. Bowery, ed.), Raven Press, New York, pp. 27–41.

Somjen, G. G., 1983, Spinal fluids and ions, in: *Handbook of the Spinal Cord*, Volume 1, *Spinal Cord Pharmacology* (R. A. Davidoff, ed.), Marcel Dekker, New York, pp. 329–380.

Syková, E., and Vyklický, L., 1978, Effects of picrotoxin on potassium accumulation and dorsal root potentials in the frog spinal cord, *Neuroscience* **3**:1061–1067.

Tebēcis, A. K., and Phillis, J. W., 1969, The pharmacology of the isolated toad spinal cord, in: *Experiments in Physiology and Biochemistry*, Volume 2 (G. A. Kerkut, ed.), Academic Press, London, pp. 361–395.

Wall, P. D., 1958, Excitability changes in afferent fibre terminations and their relation to slow potentials, *J. Physiol. (Lond.)* **142**:1–21.

Werman, R., 1969, An electrophysiological approach to drug-receptor mechanisms, *Comp. Biochem. Physiol.* **30**:997–1017.

Wojtowicz, J. M., and Nicoll, R. A., 1982, Selective action of piretanide on primary afferent GABA responses in the frog spinal cord. *Brain Res.* **236**:173–181.

GABA and Glycine: Postsynaptic Actions

B. E. ALGER

1. BACKGROUND

γ-Aminobutyric acid (GABA) was known to exist in plants and bacteria long before it was discovered to be a major constituent of brain tissue in mammals. Its primary metabolic pathway

$$\text{L-glutamate} \xrightarrow{\text{glutamic acid decarboxylase (GAD)}} \text{GABA} + CO_2$$

$$\text{GABA} + \alpha\text{-ketoglutarate} \xrightarrow{\text{GABA-transaminase (GABA-T)}}$$
$$\text{succinic semialdehyde} + \text{L-glutamate}$$

$$\text{Succinic semialdehyde} + \text{NAD} + H_2O \xrightarrow{\text{succinic semialdehyde dehydrogenase}}$$
$$\text{succinate} + \text{NADH} + H^+$$

results in the net oxidative decarboxylation of α-ketoglutarate to succinate and can thus serve as an alternate for the production of succinate in the Krebs cycle. This, plus the very high concentrations of GABA found in brain, suggested for a time that GABA might serve simply a metabolic role. Clues to its function came from demonstrations that it was the major "factor" in mammalian brain extract that inhibited activity of the crayfish stretch receptor, although, at the time, GABA was not known to exist in significant concentrations in invertebrate nervous systems.

In the vertebrate central nervous system (CNS), hyperpolarizing inhibitory potentials had been known since the study of spinal motoneurons by Brock et al. (1952) and were found at both spinal and supraspinal levels to be chemical in nature and chloride (Cl^-)-dependent. However, acceptance of GABA as the endogenous substance responsible for these inhibitory potentials in mammals was delayed following demonstrations that, in spinal cord, the effects of exogenously applied GABA were not identical to the effects of the synaptically released transmitter. Thus, the case for GABA's role as a neurotransmitter was unclear, since, on the one hand, its potent inhibitory effects occurred in systems in which it did not seem to be present, while, on the other hand, GABA did not mimic the natural transmitter where it was present in high concentrations.

In the 1960s Kravitz and his colleagues (Kravitz et al., 1963; Otsuka et al., 1967) decisively established the presence of GABA in lobster inhibitory nerves. This, in conjunction with demonstrations of potent inhibitory action, contributed to the acceptance of GABA as a neurotransmitter. The issues in mammalian CNS were largely resolved with the recognition that glycine, rather than GABA, is the predominant transmitter of postsynaptic inhibition in the spinal cord, whereas GABA is the major inhibitory neurotransmitter at supraspinal levels (see reviews by Kelly and Beart, 1975; Ryall, 1975; Nicoll, 1978). This resolution was greatly aided by the discovery of specific antagonists for both glycine and GABA. Strychnine blocked both the action of glycine and spinal inhibition, whereas picrotoxin and bicuculline blocked GABA actions and supraspinal inhibition. Neither glycine nor GABA have been proven to be neurotransmitters in the peripheral nervous systems, although GABA does affect peripheral ganglion cells and is a putative transmitter in the myenteric plexus.

This chapter highlights some features of synaptic inhibition mediated by GABA and glycine in vertebrate nervous systems. No attempt has been made to be comprehensive, and, throughout the chapter, the reader is referred to more complete reviews for details regarding specific topics.

1.1. GABA in the Invertebrate Nervous System

Of the *in vitro* invertebrate preparations used in the study of GABA, perhaps the most complete story has been developed on the neuromuscular junctions of crayfish and lobster (Atwood, 1976; Obata, 1977). Invertebrate muscle fibers are innervated by both inhibitory (I) and excitatory (E) axons. Biochemical studies on single neurons showed that GABA, GAD, and GABA-T are found in concentrations at least 100 times higher in I than in E neurons and that, within the I neurons, these substances are concentrated in the axons, rather than the cell bodies. GABA release is evoked by stimulation of the I axons and is dependent on the frequency of stimulation and on extracellular calcium (Ca^{2+}). Exogenous GABA mimics the effects of nerve stimulation. Picrotoxin and bicuculline block inhibitory synaptic potentials and the action of GABA on invertebrate muscle fibers. GABA is released in a quantal fashion from the I axon, although its association with synaptic vesicles is not yet completely established. A number of EM studies have shown that, depending on the fixation conditions, one type of synaptic vesicle appears flat, whereas another type is round. Evidence linking GABA with flat vesicles was first obtained at the crayfish neuromuscular junction, where one class of nerve terminals was known to contain flat vesicles. Stimulating the physiologically identified I nerve to exhaustion resulted in depletion of flat vesicles from terminals, whereas stimulation of the E nerve depleted other terminals of round vesicles (see review by Atwood, 1976).

In lobster inhibitory neurons, intracellular GABA levels may reach concentrations as high as 100 mM. GABA accumulation to these levels occurs because the biosynthetic enzyme GAD has a relatively faster turnover rate than the metabolic enzyme GABA-T. However, when intracellular GABA reaches high levels, there is direct feedback inhibition of GABA on GAD activity, so that steady state GABA levels are maintained by an interaction of several factors.

Following its release at the neuromuscular junctions, GABA is inactivated by uptake, largely into connective tissue and Schwann cells. The uptake mechanism is saturable, Na^+-dependent and has a high specific affinity for GABA. In *Aplysia* high concentrations of a number of neutral amino acids including glycine, cause pronounced Na^+-dependent depolarizations that differ from ordinary neurotransmitter effects (Kehoe, 1976). In addition to requiring very high concentrations, these responses do not desensitize and are blocked by metabolic inhibitors, whereas synaptic potentials are not. These characteristics suggest that the depolarizations are due to the operation of a metabolically-dependent, electrogenic, amino acid uptake mechanism.

At both crayfish and lobster neuromuscular junctions, GABA causes inhibitory effects by increasing Cl^- conductance. In contrast, the response of invertebrate neurons to GABA is highly complex and individual neurons can respond in multiple ways. GABA produces six different permeability changes when applied to *Aplysia* neurons, including conductance increases for Cl^-, Na^+, Na^+ plus Cl^-, and K^+. Nevertheless, all of these responses are blocked by the same GABA antagonist, thus suggesting that ionic channels and recognition sites can be linked in a number of combinations (Yarowsky and Carpenter, 1978).

Glycine is apparently not a neurotransmitter in invertebrates.

1.2. GABA in the Vertebrate CNS

While not as complete as that developed in invertebrates, the evidence supporting the identification of GABA and glycine as neurotransmitters in vertebrates is extensive (Kelly and Beart, 1975; Ryall, 1975; Obata, 1977). GABA is found in large quantities in the CNS. The highest concentrations are in gray matter, especially in regions known to receive dense inhibitory projections. For example, cerebellar Purkinje cells are inhibitory and GABA is present in high concentration in the nuclei to which the Purkinje cells project. Microchemical analyses of single Purkinje cells reveal high levels of GABA. Okada (1981) microdissected Deiter's nucleus cells and showed that much of the GABA, and almost all of the GAD, associated with these cells is actually present in the Purkinje cell terminals which continue to adhere to the cells. As expected, the GABA content of the Deiter's cells decreases following ablation of the cerebellar cortex containing Purkinje cells.

The cerebellum is atypical, however. Most GABAergic cells in vertebrate CNS are interneurons (or "local circuit" neurons) whose axons remain within a small, restricted region. Study of the morphology and localization of likely GABAergic neurons is commonly carried out using an immunocytochemical technique in which horseradish-peroxidase (HRP) is coupled to an antibody which binds specifically to GAD. GAD is considered a good marker for GABAergic neurons. The HRP reaction product stains darkly and can be visualized at both the light and electronmicroscopic levels (Barber and Saito, 1976). In cortical areas GABAergic neurons are frequently basket cells, whose axons ramify in dense plexi about the somata of principal projection neurons. A very interesting type of GABAergic interneuron is the "axo-axonic cell" (Somogyi et al., 1983). Its axonal terminals form quite specific connections on the initial axon segments of cortical cells. Other GABA neurons are stellate in form. In some cases, e.g., the olfactory cortex, GABAergic cells may lack an axon and participate in local circuits via dendritic interactions (see Section 3.3).

Immunocytochemical studies indicate GAD staining in a punctate pattern around cells receiving GABAergic projections. Ultrastructural studies confirm that the HRP-staining is contained within synaptic terminal boutons which have the characteristic electronmicrographic profiles associated with inhibitory nerve terminals: symmetrical pre- and postsynaptic densities and flat synaptic vesicles. GABA and GAD are found in the cytoplasm, and GAD antibody staining has been associated with the outside (but not the inside) of vesicle membranes. Some GABAergic inhibitory cell bodies, such as hippocampal basket cells, may also stain for GAD. A large increase in the apparent number of GAD-staining cell bodies occurs if the tissue is pretreated with the axonal transport blocker colchicine. Evidently GAD is transported from the soma to the terminal regions so rapidly that, in many cells, an undetectable amount remains in the soma unless it is artificially caused to accumulate there. The degradative enzyme GABA-T has also been localized in Purkinje cells with immunocytochemical techniques (Barber and Saito, 1976).

Recent immunocytochemical studies have revealed an important complication to the concept of a "GABAergic" neuron. Neurons in mammalian CNS have been found which contain both GABA (or GAD) and a neuropeptide suspected of playing a role in synaptic transmission. Indeed, in both cat visual cortex and hippocampus, there are three groups of interneurons: those staining only for GABA, those staining for GABA plus cholecystokinin (CCK), and those staining for GABA plus somatostatin (SST) (Somogyi, et al., 1984). The crucial questions, as yet unanswered, are whether or not two neurotransmitters can be released from the same neuron and, if so, what, if any, interactions might they have.

Release of GABA has been demonstrated in a number of systems. Following stimulation of the cerebellum, GABA can be collected in the fourth ventricle. Stimulation of the neocortical surface also releases GABA which can be collected in perfusion cups. Finally depolarization caused by high potassium concentrations can induce Ca^{2+}-dependent GABA release.

Specific high-affinity uptake systems for GABA are found in vertebrate CNS associated with the synaptosomal fraction. Glial cells also possess high-affinity uptake sites. Blockers which are relatively selective for neuronal, or for glial, transport systems are available (Schousboe, et al., 1981).

1.3. Glycine in the Vertebrate CNS

Glycine is distributed in highest concentration in the gray matter of the ventral spinal cord (see reviews by Aprison, 1978; Johnston, 1975; Ryall, 1975; Obata, 1977). The next highest glycine levels are in brainstem centers and concentrations are lowest in the cerebrum and cerebellum. The actual metabolic pathway for glycine in the CNS remains obscure. It may derive from serine, via serine transhydroxy-methylase, although there are other possibilities. A minor but important pathway of glycine metabolism is its incorporation into peptides in CNS neurons.

High-affinity uptake systems for glycine exist in spinal cord, but not cerebrum or cerebellum. Glycine is taken up into synaptosomes by a Na^+-dependent mechanism, however, like GABA, it is also taken up into glial cells. Nicoll (1978) has shown that glycine (and other neutral amino acids) in high concentrations produces strychnine-resistant, Na^+-dependent depolarizations in frog spinal cord. These responses are probably due to an electrogenic uptake process coupled to Na^+. Stimulation of rat spinal cord elicits Ca^{2+}-dependent release of glycine.

Strychnine blocks synaptic inhibition and the action of glycine on motoneurons in spinal cord, but at comparable doses does not affect synaptic inhibition or GABA action in supraspinal regions. Tetanus toxin irreversibly blocks both glycinergic and GABAergic synaptic inhibition in cultured spinal neurons, probably by preventing transmitter release. Responses to directly-applied GABA are unaffected by toxin. The effects of tetanus toxin are initially quite selective for inhibitory potentials and only affect excitatory potentials after a long delay (Bergey et al., 1983).

Glycinergic cells are probably also chiefly interneurons. In the spinal cord hypoxic destruction of small interneurons results in a concomitant decrease in the amount of glycine present. No system of glycinergic projection neurons has been described.

Thus a great deal of evidence supports the inference that GABA is the predominant inhibitory transmitter in supraspinal regions and that glycine serves a similar role in spinal regions.

1.4. GABA Receptor Complexes

The GABA recognition molecule and its associated functional units make up the "GABA receptor complex." At the minimum, in addition to the recognition site, this consists of an ion channel, such that GABA, binding to the recognition site, controls the permeability of the channel. The resulting ionic movements determine the biological response. Other elements of the complex are GABA reuptake sites and binding sites for benzodiazepines, barbiturates and, perhaps, an endogenous GABA receptor inhibitor. Among the receptor complexes which have been studied, differences in every aspect of this generalized structure seem to have been found. Various classification schemes have been devised.

Figure 1 suggests that GABA receptor complexes are distinguished by their location (pre- or postsynaptic; somatic, dendritic and axonal), pharmacological properties (bicuculline-sensitive and insensitive), ion selectivity (Cl^--dependent, a mixed dependence on Cl^- and probably a cation, and Ca^{2+}-dependent), and function (electrophysiological response versus uptake). GABA uptake sites may be neuronal or glial, and may occur on pre-

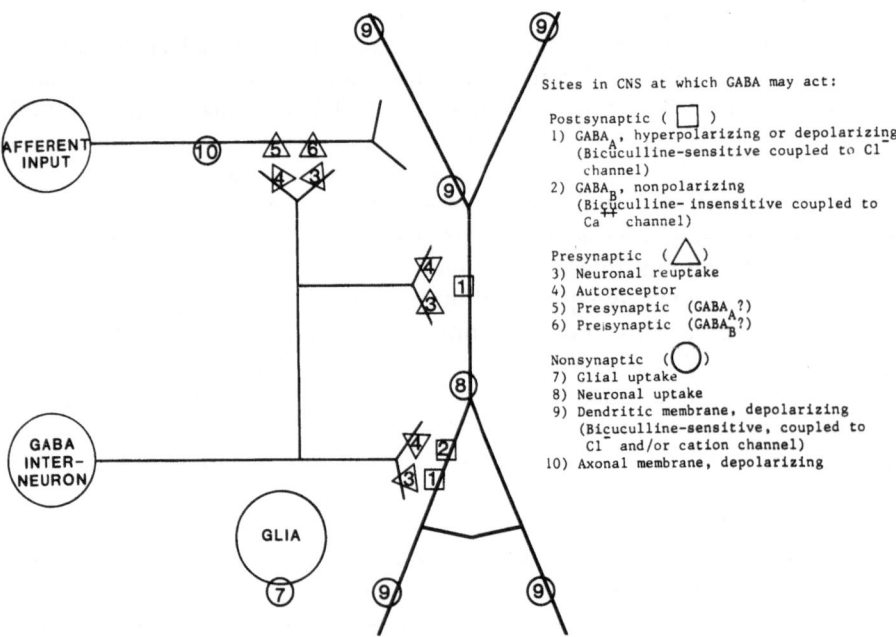

Figure 1. Possible sites of GABA action in vertebrate CNS. The large cell diagrammed at the right represents a typical principal neuron. It is invested with many different GABA binding sites that subserve a variety of functions. The cells on the left represent either GABA-releasing interneuron systems, various afferent input systems, or glial cells. (Modified from Gallagher and Shinnick-Gallagher, 1983, with permission.)

synaptic GABA releasing terminals. In addition, recent data have indicated that GABA, acting at a bicuculline-insensitive receptor, can increase a K^+-conductance on hippocampal pyramidal cells (Newberry and Nicoll, 1984). Almost all of these sites of action have been defined with biochemical and pharmacological techniques, however. With the exception of a postsynaptic Cl^--dependent, bicuculline-sensitive action there is very little evidence demonstrating the involvement of any of these sites in the course of synaptic transmission. Glycine receptor complexes are presumably constructed along similar lines, with agonist, and antagonist binding sites coupled to an ion channel.

An unresolved issue concerns the number of GABA molecules necessary to activate a single conductance event. The Hill plot of the relationship between the concentration of the transmitter applied and the resulting response can suggest whether one, or more than one, transmitter molecule is involved. Usually more than one GABA molecule seems to be required and, hence, some form of cooperativity is implied. Whether the actual number is two or more is not clear (e.g., Barker and Ransom, 1978). The problems in analyzing dose-response relationships include receptor desensitization, which may decrease either binding to the recognition site, or the ability of the bound site to activate the channel. Transmitter uptake can cause the maximal response to be underestimated and an overestimate of the effective drug concentration at the receptors.

Picrotoxin and bicuculline are two potent and reasonably selective GABA antagonists. Their exact interaction with GABA receptors is somewhat unclear and may be different in different tissues. Generally bicuculline is found to be a competitive antagonist, whereas picrotoxin is noncompetitive, but exceptions exist. Strychnine is a fairly selective noncompetitive antagonist of glycine actions, although in very high concentrations it will inhibit GABA as well.

Discussion of the electrophysiological properties of GABA receptor complexes can be found in recent reviews by Gallagher and Shinnick-Gallagher (1983), and by Enna and Gallagher (1983); of the binding assays of GABA receptors by Johnston (1981) and of pharmacological properties of GABA receptors by Nistri and Constanti (1979).

2. PHYSIOLOGICAL ACTIONS IN THE CENTRAL NERVOUS SYSTEM

In vivo studies have been instrumental in revealing the actions of GABA and glycine in vertebrate systems. GABA inhibits virtually all cells to which it is applied in the CNS. Glycine is potent in the spinal cord, but is largely ineffective at levels above the brainstem. Neurochemical studies on the intact CNS lent support to the putative neurotransmitter roles of both of these amino acids. However, detailed experiments on synaptic transmissions requires greater control over the neuronal environment than is possible in studies on vertebrate central neurons *in vivo*. Therefore, a variety of *in vitro* preparations utilizing organ and tissue cultures and slices from different areas of the brain have been widely used. Among the brain slice preparations, cortical structures (such as the hippocampus, olfactory and neocortex, and cerebellum) have been most useful because their orderly architecture greatly facilitates intracellular recording. The hippocampal slice has a further advantage in that a variety of afferent synaptic inputs to the pyramidal cells are preserved and can be stimulated (Andersen, 1975; Schwartzkroin, 1975, 1977).

Once released from presynaptic nerve terminals, GABA and glycine cause inhibitory postsynaptic potentials (IPSPs) in target cells. In view of the complexity of synaptic organization in the vertebrate CNS, it is useful to distinguish different forms of IPSPs according to the presynaptic element involved in producing them (Burke and Rudomin, 1977). An IPSP resulting from the activation of many inhibitory interneurons of the same type is a "composite" IPSP. An IPSP resulting from the activation of a single cell is a "single-cell" IPSP and is probably composed of several "single-terminal" IPSPs. The smallest unit is the "quantal" IPSP. In the vertebrate CNS these distinctions remain largely hypothetical. For example, single-cell and single-terminal IPSPs have not been clearly differentiated in most systems. It is also possible, as discussed below, that the quantal and single-terminal IPSPs are identical in some instances. IPSPs in any of the categories may be either "evoked" by electrical stimulation, or "spontaneous," meaning not explicitly due to an experimental manipulation.

2.1. Release Mechanisms

2.1.1. Spontaneous IPSPs

As expected for a chemical synaptic transmitter, GABA release and IPSPs are Ca^{2+}-dependent and are blocked by antagonists of Ca^{2+} currents. Some evidence suggests that GABA may be released in vertebrate CNS in preformed quantal packets. For example, a population of small spontaneous IPSPs recorded in pyramidal cells in the hippocampal slice preparation (Brown and Johnston, 1980) and in tissue-cultured spinal neurons (Mathers and Barker, 1981) is resistant to bath perfusion with tetrodotoxin (TTX), as is quantal ACh release at the frog neuromuscular junction. These TTX-resistant IPSPs may be quantal IPSPs.

However, in hippocampal pyramidal cells a much larger population of small spontaneous IPSPs is blocked by TTX perfusion (Fig. 2; Alger and Nicoll, 1980). It is usually possible to detect these small IPSPs when recording intracellularly with 3 M KCl-filled electrodes, although they can sometimes be seen under other conditions. When intracellular Cl^- is increased as a result of Cl^- leaking out of a recording electrode, IPSPs are reversed into depolarizations due to the shift in the electrochemical gradient for Cl^- (see Section 2.2.2). Since EPSPs are also depolarizing, it is necessary to use pharmacological tests in order to confirm that depolarizing potentials

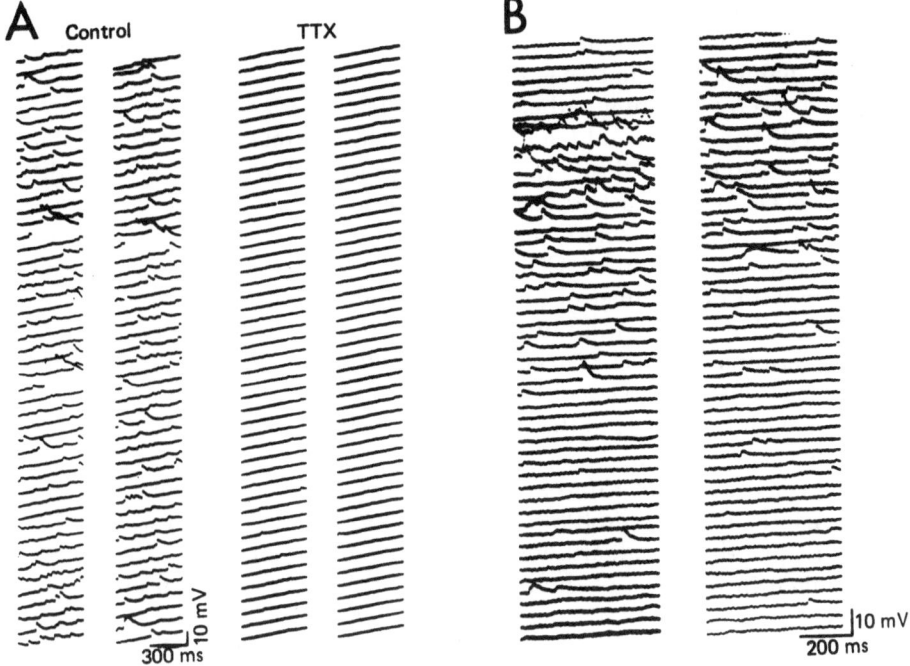

Figure 2. Spontaneous IPSPs in hippocampal CA_1 pyramidal cells recorded with 3M KCl-filled electrodes. These are continuous moving film records of the membrane potentials of two cells. In (A) numerous spontaneous reversed IPSPs were recorded in a control saline before a saline containing 10^{-6} M TTX was perfused. Nearly all of the spontaneous activity was blocked by TTX and could also be abolished by picrotoxin (not shown). The few small depolarizing events visible in some of the traces in the left-hand column in TTX could be "quantal" IPSPs. The cell shown in (B) illustrates the tendency of the spontaneous IPSPs to occur in clusters, alternating with periods of relative quiet. The total time of recording is about 50 sec for each condition in (A) and 20 sec in (B). (Alger and Nicoll, unpublished observations.)

are reversed IPSPs. Spontaneous IPSPs in hippocampal CA_1 pyramidal cells are blocked by picrotoxin and are prolonged by pentobarbital.

The occurrence of spontaneous IPSPs indicates that the pyramidal cells are subject to a constant inhibitory bombardment; however, the IPSPs tend to occur in clusters, i.e., nonrandomly (Fig. 2). This, in conjunction with their sensitivity to TTX, suggests that these potentials are the result of activity in the presynaptic GABA-releasing interneurons and are probably either single-cell or single-terminal IPSPs.

2.1.2. Quantal Analysis

Faber, Korn and their colleagues (Faber and Korn, 1982; Korn et al., 1982; Triller and Korn, 1982) studied inhibitory transmitter release using simultaneous intracellular impalements of the goldfish Mauthner cell and a glycinergic inhibitory interneuron that projects to the Mauthner cell. This arrangement provides good control over the pre- and postsynaptic side of an inhibitory synapse. When the interneuron was stimulated directly to fire an action potential, a single-cell IPSP was recorded in the Mauthner cell. Quantal analysis revealed that fluctuations in single-cell IPSPs could be described best by binomial, rather than by Poisson statistics. Agreement with a Poisson distribution would suggest that a large number of events (n) contributed to a single-cell IPSP and that a given event had a small probability of occurrence. In contrast, the binomial fit suggested that the number of contributing events was small, and that each had a relatively high probability of occurrence. In the goldfish CNS the statistically determined n was closely correlated with the number of histologically identified synapses made on a Mauthner cell by a given inhibitory interneuron. The implication is that each synaptic terminal releases transmitter in an all-or-none way and that statistical fluctuations in the size of the single-cell IPSP from trial to trial can be identified with variations in the number of terminals that do, in fact, release transmitter on any trial.

The conclusions of Kuno and Weakly (1972) regarding the apparently monosynaptic, glycinergic IPSPs in motoneurons in cat spinal cord resembled those just discussed, although control over the synaptic input was less precise than in the case of the Mauthner cell IPSPs. Statistical analysis of the fluctuation of the IPSPs indicated that they were composed of "unit" potentials each having a high probability of occurrence. The release process was described by a binomial distribution that gave an estimate of the "quantal" content of about 2 with a probability of occurrence of a unit potential of 0.5. The number available for release was estimated to be about 4.

GABAergic IPSPs in guinea pig hippocampal pyramidal cells have very similar properties. By making simultaneous intracellular recordings from a pyramidal cell and an inhibitory interneuron, Miles and Wong (1984) were able to study monosynaptic IPSPs in the pyramidal cell. The single-cell IPSPs were composed of units, the amplitude distribution of which was best described by a binomial process. The mean unit potential amplitude was about 0.5 mV, and the probability of release was about 0.6. It is interesting that release from these, and other (e.g., Edwards et al., 1976), central synapses appears to differ fundamentally from that at the frog neuromuscular junction, where large numbers of "units" are releaseable at every instant. Perhaps this is a reflection of the more complex synaptic integration performed in the central nervous system, as compared to the periphery.

2.1.3. Effects of a Quantum of GABA

These studies raise the question as to the influence of a single synaptic vesicle, i.e., a true quantal IPSP. If a single-terminal IPSP is "all-or-none," then it would seem that either a vesicle has such a tiny effect that small, statistical fluctuations in a large number of them released simultaneously cannot be resolved, or that a single vesicle has a large effect and that only one is released from a terminal at any given time. Triller and Korn (1982) found that only one releasing site was present on each terminal bouton and favor the hypothesis that only one vesicle at a time is released. Hence in the Mauthner cell each vesicle may have a relatively large effect. The similarity of the results discussed in Section 2.1.2 suggests this conclusion may be generally applicable.

At the lobster neuromuscular junction, the quantity of GABA released per impulse onto a muscle fiber has been estimated to be on the order of 10^{-16}–10^{-17} mole (Obata, 1977; Takeuchi, 1977). From iontophoresis experiments a comparable, but somewhat higher, value was found necessary to mimic a given evoked IPSP in CNS. Pressure ejection of small amounts of GABA yielded estimates of 5×10^{-16} mole for GABA responses comparable to small IPSPs in hippocampal pyramidal cells (Wong and Watkins, 1982).

Assuming a single channel conductance of 25 pS (see Chapter 3), Faber and Korn (1982) estimated that approximately 6800 Cl^- channels could account for the conductance of the single-cell IPSP in the Mauthner cell. If fluctuations of the Mauthner cell IPSP were indeed due to fluctuations in the number of terminals releasing transmitter, then it could be estimated that the released contents of a vesicle opens about 1500–2000 channels.

In a study of lamprey Muller cells Gold and Martin (1983a,b) combined quantal analysis of IPSCs with fluctuation analysis of single glycine channel conductance. As in other systems discussed above, the spontaneous IPSCs were TTX-sensitive and appeared to be due, typically, to the action of only one quantum of transmitter. The quantal IPSC could be accounted for by the opening of about 1500 Cl^- channels.

In contrast, unitary IPSPs in hippocampus are associated with a conductance of about 6 nS. Assuming a "quantal content" of about 5 (Miles and Wong, 1984) and a mean GABA-channel conductance of 20 pS (Segal and Barker, 1984) gives a value of about 60 channels activated by a single quantum in guinea pig hippocampal pyramidal cells. This value is comparable to the recent estimate of 40–240 ion channels opened by the excitatory transmitter released from a single Ia synaptic bouton in cat spinal cord (Finkel and Redman, 1983).

2.1.4. Evoked IPSPs

The physiological actions of GABA or glycine are usually characterized by studying the properties of the intracellularly recorded composite IPSPs elicited by stimulation of various fiber tracks. This approach is most useful when there is reasonable evidence that the stimulated systems are homogeneous and monosynaptic. These criteria are frequently hard to achieve in studies of the mammalian CNS, where typically the transmitters are released from small interneurons and the evoked IPSP is, therefore, usually secondary to activation of excitatory synapses. Thus, apparent properties of inhibitory synapses must be distinguished from properties of the excitatory synapses and from the response properties of the inhibitory cells themselves. There are other complications as well.

In mammalian hippocampal cortex, evoked GABAergic IPSPs were found in initial studies to be enormous, reaching amplitudes of 15–20 mV and durations of 600 msec. It now seems that the great difficulties in recording intracellularly in intact cortex resulted in membrane potentials that were artificially low and hence IPSP amplitudes that were artificially high. In addition, the anesthetics used in most animal surgery, e.g., pentobarbital (Nembutal) markedly enhances GABAergic IPSPs (Nicoll et al., 1975). Nevertheless, even when the effects of anesthetics could be ruled out, it was usually found that the evoked IPSP was much longer in duration than EPSPs. This is due in part to the tendency of inhibitory interneurons to fire repetitively in response to stimulation. However, motoneuronal IPSPs, which are primarily glycinergic, are much briefer than GABAergic IPSPs and Renshaw cells clearly fire repetitively. Probably the slow time course of the GABAergic IPSP resides in part in interaction of GABA with its receptors, since iontophoretically applied glycine has a faster time course than applied GABA (Diamond and Roper, 1973), and the lifetime of GABA channels is longer than that of glycine channels (see Chapter 3). In the goldfish Mauthner cell, spontaneous glycinergic IPSPs decay with an exponential time constant which is the same as the duration of the mean glycine channel open time (Faber and Korn, 1982). The same is true for glycinergic IPSCs in the lamprey Muller cell (Gold and Martin, 1983). This suggests that, in these cases, most channels open and close only once during the IPSP and that the time course of the IPSP is determined by channel kinetics, and not by concentration of transmitter in the cleft or by passive membrane properties. It is not yet known what factors prevent the released glycine molecules from repeatedly binding to receptors, but diffusion or uptake are likely candidates. In contrast, the time course of the GABAergic IPSP in hippocampal pyramidal cells is significantly influenced by the neuronal membrane properties. Another distinction between glycinergic and GABAergic IPSCs is that the duration of the latter is voltage-sensitive, being prolonged by membrane depolarization and vice versa (Collingridge et al., 1984), whereas the former is voltage-independent.

Voltage clamp analysis of small evoked GABAergic IPSCs in hippocampal pyramidal cells yields a value of about 100 nS for the peak conductance (Brown and Johnston, 1983). If the single GABA channel conductance is about 20 pS (Segal and Barker, 1984; Gray et al., 1983) then about 5000 single channel events would contribute to a single small evoked IPSP and about 15 inhibitory interneurons participate (Miles and Wong, 1984).

2.2. Membrane Mechanisms

2.2.1. Effects on Conductance

In most CNS cells GABAergic and glycinergic IPSPs are recorded by an intracellular microelectrode as hyperpolarizing potentials that are associated with a decrease in neuronal input resistance.

2.2.2. Ionic Mechanisms

The increase in membrane conductance associated with GABA and gly-cinergic IPSPs implies that the transmitter causes a change in the permea-bility of the membrane to some ionic species. Since the IPSPs are usually hyperpolarizing, the relevant ions must have net reversal potentials that are hyperpolarized with respect to the resting membrane potential. To discover which ions are involved, the ideal experiment would be to change, instan-taneously, the transmembrane ionic gradient for an individual ion, thus changing its Nernst potential.

Until the advent of in vitro preparations, it was not possible to change the extracellular ionic concentrations precisely in most vertebrate systems. Furthermore, even with in vitro preparations it is difficult to change the gradients quickly enough.

Coombs et al. (1955) originally investigated the ionic mechanisms of the IPSP in spinal motoneurons by increasing the intracellular concentrations of different anions. Injections of small anions into cells via the recording electrode reversed the IPSP into a depolarizing potential. Injections of larger anions did not, and, in fact, shifted the reversal potential to a more hyper-polarized level. These experiments suggested that a "pore" (channel) was opened by the inhibitory transmitter, and anions of the right size could pass through it. When the electrochemical gradient was inward, small anions entered and hyperpolarized the cell, and vice versa when the electrochemical gradient was outward, they left the cell and depolarized it. Injection of large impermeant anions led to a hyperpolarizing shift in the reversal potential for the IPSP (E_{IPSP}) because the injecting current itself was partially carried across the membrane by Cl^-, which reduced $[Cl^-]_i$ and shifted E_{Cl} in the hyperpolarizing direction. The effect of a given anion on E_{IPSP} indicated, therefore, whether the anion was permeant or impermeant. Knowing the hydrated size of the permeant anions allowed an estimate of the size of the channel to be made: it was about 20% larger than the hydrated radius of the potassium ion (K^+). Since Cl^- is the only permeant anion normally present in the extracellular space in appreciable amounts, these results strongly suggested that an increase in Cl^- permeability was involved in the IPSP. With the in vitro brain slice technique $[Cl^-]_o$ can also be changed and such experiments further strengthen the hypothesis that Cl^- is involved in the IPSP.

However, the question of whether Cl^- is the only ion involved remains open. The K^+ equilibrium potential (E_K) is hyperpolarized with respect to the resting membrane potential. However, because the resting neuronal permeability to K^+ is quite high, it is not possible to alter intracellular K^+ substantially by injecting it into cells; K^+ simply passes across the membrane and $[K^+]_i$ is unchanged. Using the brain slice technique it is possible to alter $[K^+]_o$, but not fast enough to prevent concomitant changes in $[K^+]_i$. Changes in $[K^+]_o$ can also result in changes in $[Cl^-]_i$ through quasi-Donnan equilib-rium effects. In a simple Donnan cell equally permeable to Cl^- and K^+

$$[Cl^-]_i = ([Cl^-]_o \times [K^+]_o)/[K^+]_i \tag{1}$$

i.e., $[Cl^-]_i$ is a function of $[K^+]_i$ and $[K^+]_o$ as well as of $[Cl^-]_o$. Slow changes in $[K^+]_o$ will alter both $[K^+]_i$ and $[Cl^-]_i$. Because of this indirect effect a purely Cl^--dependent IPSP will be affected by changes in $[K^+]_o$. A simple Donnan equilibrium expression does not strictly apply to neurons because of unequal ionic permeabilities and transport processes. Nevertheless, Martin (1979), using a derivation based on the constant field equation, deduced that under nonequilibrium conditions for the ionic species

$$[Cl^-]_i = ([Cl^-]_o \times [K^+]_o)/[K^+]_i + \theta[Na^+]_o \{([Cl^-]_o/[K^+]_i) - 1/\phi\} \tag{2}$$

This equation consists of two terms: one is identical to the simple Donnan expression (equation 1), and the other is a factor dependent on the transport processes, which adds or subtracts an increment to, or from, the equilibrium concentrations represented by the Donnan quantity. The impact of this modification can be seen in the graph of Fig. 3, which demonstrates that even under the nonequilibrium conditions that apply in cells, $[Cl^-]_i$ still depends directly on $[K^+]_o$.

This dependence would not cause a problem if changes in $[K^+]_o$ could be made so fast that no changes in intracellular ionic concentrations could occur. In such cases shifts in E_K would immediately parallel changes in $[K^+]_o$ while E_{Cl} would not change. A qualitative approach to this problem can be made by iontophoretically applying K^+ to a cell from an extracellular K^+-containing microelectrode. Barker and Ransom (1978) found that the reversal potential for the iontophoretic GABA response on cultured spinal cord neurons did not change immediately after $[K^+]_o$ increased. This suggested that the effects of K^+ were indirect, and presumably the GABA reversal potential was affected by an increase in $[Cl^-]_i$. McCarren and Alger (1985) found that pressure ejection of small amounts of K^+ did have immediate effects on the GABAergic IPSP of hippocampal pyramidal cells. Whether this was due to a K^+-component of the IPSP, or to some other factor, was not clear. Because of the difficulties in controlling and measuring $[K^+]_o$ direct application techniques do not yield exact quantitative results.

In addition to uncertainty regarding the cation specificity of GABA-activated conductances, recordings of IPSPs in mammalian neocortex suggested that the channels opened during these potentials could pass anions larger than Cl^- (Kelly et al., 1969). These IPSPs were reversed by intracellular injection of large, as well as small, anions; however, various complicating factors could account for these effects. For example, acetate causes a shift in the IPSP reversal potential in hippocampal cells, and other large anions may be able to affect the IPSP as well (Eccles et al., 1977; Allen et al., 1977). These effects could be due to a weak permeability of the membrane to acetate anion; alternatively, an effect on the Cl^- pump or on intracellular pH, which then affects $[Cl^-]_i$, could be responsible for the reversal potential shift.

Another unresolved issue in the CNS is the dependence of GABA chan-

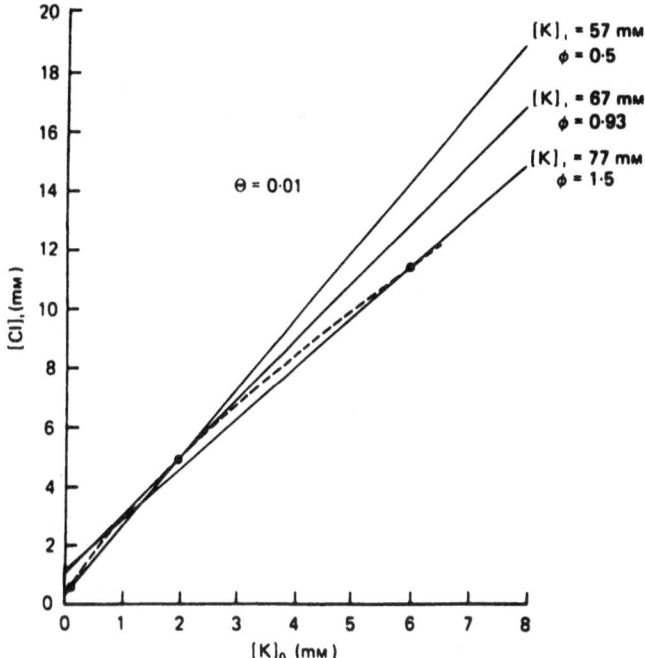

Figure 3. The effects predicted by the constant field equation of $[K^+]_o$ on $[Cl^-]_i$. The graph plots the theoretical relationship between $[K^+]_o$ and $[Cl^-]_i$ according to the equation

$$[Cl^-]_i = ([Cl^-]_o \times [K^+]_o)/[K^+]_i + \theta\,[Na^+]_o\,\{([Cl^-]_o/[K^+]_i) - 1/\phi\}$$

(see text). $\theta = -p_{Na}i'_K/p_K i'_{Na}$, and $\phi = p_{Cl}i'_K/p_K i'_{Cl}$, where p_{Na}, p_K and p_{Cl} are permeability constants for Na^+, K^+, and Cl^-, respectively and i'_{Na}, i'_K, and i'_{Cl} are the currents due to the active transport of Na^+, K^+, and Cl^-, respectively. θ was assumed to be 0.01 and ϕ to have values from 0.5 to 1.5. A nonlinear dependence of $[Cl^-]_i$ on $[K^+]_o$ arises if ϕ and $[K^+]_i$ are dependent on $[K^+]_o$, and this is represented by the dashed curved line. Notice that although different assumed values for the variable parameters produce slight differences in the slope and curvature of the function, in all cases there is a strong dependence of $[Cl^-]_i$ on $[K^+]_o$, even though all transmembrane distributions were assumed to be dependent on active processes. (Reprinted from Appendix by A. R. Martin in Matthews and Wickelgren, 1979, with permission.)

nel conductance on Cl^-. This relationship might take one of several forms. According to the constant field equations, the conductance of a chloride channel will be directly related to $[Cl^-]_o$, provided that the membrane potential and the transmembrane chloride gradient have been allowed to come into equilibrium following establishment of new levels of $[Cl^-]_o$. This relationship has been observed at the crayfish neuromuscular junction (Takeuchi and Takeuchi, 1967). A simple linear conductance model predicts that channel conductance would be independent of permeant ion concentration. This relationship was originally determined by Takeuchi and Takeuchi (1960) to describe the acetylcholine channels at the frog neuromuscular junction, although its adequacy has recently been questioned (Lewis, 1979). However, Gold and Martin (1983b) have documented that the conductance of the glycine channel on lamprey Muller cells *decreases* with increases in intracellular Cl   (see Section 2.4). This effect is not predicted by any previous models of the interactions between channel conductance and permeant ion concentration and is opposite to that predicted by the constant field equation. The depression of Cl^- channel conductance by increased $[Cl^-]_i$ may have functional implications (see Section 2.4).

2.2.3. Chloride Pump Hypothesis

Indirect evidence regarding the ionic mechanisms of the IPSP comes from investigations of the transport processes that maintain the ionic gradients of the IPSP. If the IPSP were exclusively Cl^--dependent, then the hyperpolarization would result from Cl^- entering the cell, and a concentration gradient, from the outside to the inside of the cell, would have to exist. This would require a mechanism for transporting Cl^- out of the cells, as first postulated by Dreifuss et al. (1969). In some cases there is evidence for such a Cl^- "pump." Perfusion of spinal motoneurons with ammonia abolishes the hyperpolarization of the glycinergic IPSP without affecting the inhibitory conductance change (Lux, 1971). Thus ammonia does not prevent release of the neurotransmitter, binding of the transmitter to receptors, or the opening of ionic channels. The interpretation of these results was that ammonia blocked an outwardly directed Cl^- pump with a consequent passive redistribution of Cl^-. Ammonia also slowed the rate at which the IPSP became hyperpolarizing again after an intracellular Cl^- injection had inverted it to a depolarization. In most neurons the maintenance of the IPSP polarity has not been investigated. It is clear that some active process must be involved in maintaining the relevant ionic gradients or else it would not be possible to maintain stable IPSPs during impalements lasting hours.

Besides revealing an important mechanism in the maintenance of this IPSP, the ammonia experiments also indirectly eliminated a role for K^+, since ammonia did not change K^+-dependent potentials such as the resting potential or the equilibrium potential for the action potential afterhyperpolarization. Similar data suggest that a GABAergic IPSP recorded in neocortical cells may be abolished by ammonia (Raabe and Gumnit, 1975). However, in hippocampal pyramidal cells, Alger and Nicoll (1983) could not find any effects of NH_4^+ on E_{IPSP} that could not be explained as simple univalent cation effects, such as the effects of K^+ on Cl^- discussed in Section 2.2.1. NH_4^+ can substitute for K^+ in many neurophysiological processes.

2.2.4. Hyperpolarizing IPSPs

An interesting, and not fully resolved issue concerns the nature of the IPSP in the unimpaled cell. Inserting a microelectrode into a cell creates two major problems. First, the leak resistance caused by the electrode effectively shunts the membrane creating a "voltage-divider" effect. Even if the ionic batteries for the membrane and synaptic potentials are not affected per

se, values other than the true values will be recorded by the intracellular
electrode.

The second problem is that impaling a cell with a microelectrode may
alter the ionic gradients. Measurements of $[K^+]_i$ and $[Cl^-]_i$ with ion-sensitive
electrodes show that these values change after impaling a cell and low, steady
values of $[K^+]_i$ are recorded in conjunction with lower membrane potentials
(Buhrle and Sonnhof, 1983). Hence, intracellular recording techniques produce
erroneous values for E_{IPSP}. Thus the question arises as to whether the IPSP
in the unimpaled cell is truly hyperpolarizing.

An approach to this problem can be made by extracellular measurements
of the current that accompanies transmembrane ionic fluxes. The flow of
current through the extracellular resistance creates a voltage drop that can
be measured with two electrodes positioned along the path of the current.
Since the cell is not penetrated, the problems with electrode impalements
are avoided. Such measurements suggest that glycinergic IPSPs in unimpaled
motoneurons are in fact hyperpolarizing (see review by Takeuchi, 1977).
Extracellular measurements also formed the basis of the reasoning used by
Andersen et al. (1964) to deduce that IPSPs in hippocampal pyramidal cells
are initiated principally on the soma. While conceptually this technique
might seem ideal, the drawback is that the measurements are difficult to
make and interpret precisely. They cannot give precise quantitative data on
the polarity, magnitude, or duration of the intracellular potential changes
and are subject to complications due to summation of currents from different
sources.

2.2.5. Depolarizing IPSPs

Although most IPSPs are probably hyperpolarizing, this is not always
the case. In the olfactory cortex, Scholfield (1978) found that, while cells
with resting potentials of about -55 mV had hyperpolarizing GABAergic
IPSPs, in cells with resting potentials near -75 mV, the IPSPs were depolarizing. Besides underscoring the importance of determining the polarity
of IPSPs in unimpaled cells, this observation raises questions regarding the
transport process involved. Would, e.g., the direction of ion transport depend
on membrane potential, or can a unidirectional mechanism explain IPSPs
of different polarity? The polarity of the IPSP depends on the relationship
between the resting membrane potential and E_{IPSP}. Extracellular measurements suggest that the IPSPs may, in fact, be depolarizing in unimpaled
olfactory cortex cells (Pickles and Simmonds, 1978).

A related, but different, issue is the observation in mammalian CNS
neurons that GABA (Andersen et al., 1980; Alger and Nicoll, 1982b; Barker
and Ransom, 1978) and glycine (Barker and Ransom, 1978) produce depolarizing, as well as hyperpolarizing, responses. GABA applied to cells near
their soma predominantly causes a Cl^--dependent hyperpolarizing (H) response that has the same reversal potential as the IPSP. Application of GABA
to the dendrites, however, results primarily in depolarizing (D) responses,

although H responses can also be detected. The D GABA response is due to the activation of receptors with different pharmacological properties than those of H receptors. D responses are more readily blocked by antagonists, such as picrotoxin and bicuculline, than H responses. (This rules out the possibilities that GABA-induced depolarizations are artifacts of pH or represent ion transport phenomena [Section 1.1], since those effects are not blocked by GABA antagonists.) The D GABA responses are also enhanced more by potentiators of GABA, such as pentobarbital, than the H responses. On the other hand, receptors mediating H responses (H receptors) are more readily activated than those mediating D responses (D receptors) by the GABA agonist THIP. Given the relative paucity of GABAergic synapses on pyramidal cell dendrites, the lack of depolarizing GABAergic IPSPs, and the apparent ubiquity of D GABA responses in the dendritic field, it has been proposed that most of the D GABA receptors are not associated with the immediate subsynaptic region; i.e., that they are extrasynaptic (Alger and Nicoll, 1982a).

Two questions which immediately arise are: (1) What is the ionic mechanism of the D response? and (2) Can the D receptors ordinarily be activated by synaptically released GABA? The first question has not been answered. One possibility would be that, as in other cells in which GABA produces D responses, the dendritic Cl^- gradient is outward. However, dendritic Cl^--dependent H responses have been observed. This strongly suggests that some other ion is involved in the D GABA responses. While Na^+ or Ca^{2+} are the most likely candidates, their involvement has not yet been demonstrated. It is even conceivable that part of the D response is not associated with a conductance increase at all, and could, for example, be due to a K^+-conductance decrease.

Although depolarizing IPSPs are not ordinarily seen in hippocampal pyramidal cells D GABA receptors must be accessible to activation by synaptically released GABA since, in the presence of pentobarbital, a biphasic IPSP (hyperpolarizing-depolarizing IPSP) is produced by orthodromic stimulation (Fig. 4B). Because the synaptically activated D response is only seen in the presence of barbiturates and is blocked by GABA antagonists, it is evidently a GABA-mediated potential. (Notice that this discussion only applies to cells in which both hyperpolarizing and depolarizing responses are seen. IPSPs in dentate granule cells [Assaf et al., 1981], like those in olfactory cortical cells and peripheral ganglia, are purely depolarizing, and this is explained by an outwardly directed Cl^- gradient.)

Pentobarbital does not simply transform all H GABA receptors into biphasic (H–D) ones, because GABAergic antidromic IPSPs remain exclusively hyperpolarizing in pentobarbital. The reason for the difference between ortho- and antidromic responses was partly elucidated using small localized injections of either GABA antagonists or TTX into somatic and dendritic regions (Fig. 4B, top). The D phase of the orthodromic response was blocked by local application of TTX or bicuculline methiodide (BMI) to the dendrites, while the H phase was more sensitive to the drugs applied somatically. Since

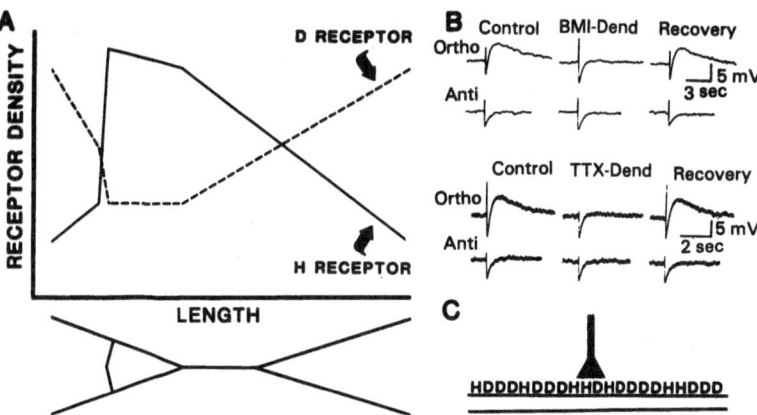

Figure 4. Distribution of hyperpolarizing (H) and depolarizing (D) GABA receptors on hippocampal pyramidal cells. (A) plots the hypothetical receptor density distributions relative to the schematic drawing of the pyramidal cell beneath the abscissa. These distributions were determined on the basis of experiments such as the two illustrated in (B). Intracellular recordings were made from hippocampal pyramidal neurons in the presence of pentobarbital. Stimulation of the orthodromic pathway produced an action potential (fast upstroke) followed by a biphasic IPSP, whereas stimulation of the antidromic pathway produced an action potential followed by a monophasic hyperpolarizing IPSP. In the experiment shown in the top two series of traces, bicuculline methiodide (BMI) was injected into the dendritic region after a period of control recording. In this case the D phase of the response was blocked, while the H phases of both ortho- and antidromic responses were unaffected. The D phases recovered with washing. In the converse experiment (not shown) injection of BMI into the somatic region blocked the H, but not the D, phase of the responses. Thus, the D receptors activated by synaptically released GABA are primarily located in the dendritic region. The experiment illustrated in the lower two traces of (B) was the same as the previous one except that TTX rather than BMI was injected into the dendritic region. TTX also blocked the D phase of the orthodromic response, presumably by blocking the activity of GABA releasing neuronal elements in the dendritic region. (C) Schematic representation of the H and D receptor distribution at the level of a single dendrite, suggested by these and other experiments with iontophoretically applied GABA. The dendrite (two solid lines) is assumed to be densely covered with H and D receptors. Immediately under the presynaptic element (heavy black structure above the dendrite) H receptors predominate, whereas away from the synaptic region D receptors are in relatively greater number. The diagram makes the point that the classification of H and D receptors as "synaptic" and "extrasynaptic" refers to their relative density of distribution rather than to an absolute property. (From Alger and Nicoll, 1982a, with permission.)

TTX is not a GABA antagonist, its effect was probably due to interruption of a neuronal pathway in the dendritic region. The effects of BMI indicated that the D receptors are more prevalent on the dendrites of the cells, while H receptors are more heavily distributed on the cell somata. Undoubtedly, this separation is not an absolute one, and probably both receptor types populate both regions (Figs. 4A and 4C). Since synaptic activation of D receptors can be revealed in pentobarbital, synaptically released GABA must reach them. The hypothesis put forward to account for these findings was that of transmitter "spillover," i.e., transmitter released from the synaptic bouton primarily reaches the immediate subsynaptic receptors, but an ordinarily undetectably small proportion "spills over" to nearby extrasynaptic D receptors. In the presence of a potentiator of D-receptor action, such as pentobarbital, activation of D receptors becomes visible. D receptors have been identified with extrasynaptic sites because direct application of GABA produces prominent D responses everywhere in the dendritic field, but only secondarily in the somatic region. It is also possible that a small proportion of the synaptic receptors are actually D receptors, and a small proportion of extrasynaptic receptors are H receptors (Fig. 4C). This would provide an explanation of large D responses in pentobarbital without requiring the hypothesis that GABA actually diffuses from the synaptic cleft and reaches extrasynaptic receptors. On the other hand, if there were true spillover, then the GABA uptake into glial cells might protect cells from excessive activation of extrasynaptic receptors (Brown, 1979). The function of extrasynaptic GABA receptors is unknown. It is interesting that such receptors may not exist for glycine or other amino acids (Brown, 1979).

2.3. Termination of Transmitter Action

Biochemical evidence indicates that GABA is taken up into neurons and glia by a Na^+-dependent mechanism (see reviews by Kelly and Beart, 1975; Obata, 1977). In the hippocampal slice, depletion of Na^+, application of nipecotic acid (a rigid conformational analog of muscimol that blocks neuronal GABA uptake), and low temperatures prolong the action of iontophoretically applied GABA, presumably by blocking uptake (Alger and Nicoll, 1982b). On the other hand, blockade of the degradative enzymes GABA-T and AOAA do not prolong GABA action (see Cooper et al., 1982). Thus Na^+-dependent reuptake, rather than enzymatic degradation, may be the primary means by which the action of GABA is terminated. Nevertheless it has not yet been demonstrated that responses to synaptically, as well as to iontophoretically, applied GABA are affected by uptake blocking treatments.

In general, in neuronal amino acid transport systems uptake is accompanied by Na^+ influx into the cell. This effect can be electrogenic. Amino acid-induced depolarizations, which are produced in the spinal cord and which are not blocked by antagonists (Nicoll, 1978), may reflect such an electrogenic effect. A characteristic of Na^+-dependent transport systems is that they can be made to run backwards. Constanti et al. (1980) iontophoresed GABA or glycine into spinal motoneurons and measured the resulting effects on membrane potential. Injection of GABA, but not glycine, caused a slight membrane hyperpolarization that outlasted the duration of the injection. The hyperpolarization due to intracellular GABA injection was insensitive to Cl^-, did not decrease the membrane resistance, and was not potentiated by application of benzodiazepines. Hence, GABA was probably not leaking out of the cell and activating extracellular GABA receptors. Constanti et al. (1980) argued that the high intracellular GABA concentrations caused GABA to be transported out of the cells in conjunction with Na^+, and this outward current hyperpolarized the cells.

2.4. Use-Dependence of IPSPs

Repetitive activation causes many alterations in excitatory synaptic transmission, and it is important to ask whether or not inhibitory potentials also undergo use-dependent modifications. In general, the efficacy of synaptic transmission might be either increased (facilitation, posttetanic potentiation, etc.) or decreased (homosynaptic depression, habituation, etc.) as a result of prior activation, and the mechanisms for these changes might be either pre- or postsynaptic.

However, an interesting difference between inhibitory and excitatory synaptic transmission in vertebrate CNS seems to be the relative stability of inhibitory synaptic transmission. Although potentiation of IPSPs was reported at the glycinergic synapse between Renshaw cells and spinal motoneurons in cat (Spencer and April, 1970), only small effects were seen and those could not unambiguously be attributed to increased inhibitory synaptic transmission. There is less evidence that GABAergic synapses in the vertebrate CNS can show facilitation, although there is clear facilitation of GABAergic transmission at the crayfish neuromuscular junction (e.g., Dudel and Kuffler, 1961).

Repetitive stimulation at low to moderate frequencies results in either no change or depression of inhibitory synaptic transmission. An interesting aspect of the studies of Faber and Korn (1982) on monosynaptic glycinergic IPSPs in goldfish Mauthner cells was that very little plasticity of inhibitory transmission was found. Monosynaptic IPSP amplitudes only decreased at frequencies above 5 Hz, whereas IPSPs evoked via collateral (disynaptic) stimulation were nearly abolished at 5 Hz (see Fig. 5). The more pronounced sensitivity of the disynaptic collateral IPSP was apparently due to depression at some point in the pathway leading to excitation of the interneuron. Thus, in this system, the inhibitory synapse per se did not potentiate and was resistant to depression.

Disynaptic IPSPs in other neuronal systems, however, are reduced by repetitive stimulation, and this may be functionally important, since deficiency in inhibition is associated with various pathophysiological states (see Section 5). Various mechanisms could account for IPSP plasticity at different loci. For example, possible presynaptic causes are transmitter depletion or inhibition of inhibitory interneurons, whereas at postsynaptic sites there could be receptor desensitization, a shift in E_{IPSP}, or multiple transmitter effects. At extrasynaptic sites, enhancement of transmitter uptake or effects of extracellular K^+ accumulation are possibilities.

Responses produced by prolonged application of a neurotransmitter to its receptors typically decrease with time, and this has sometimes been attributed to receptor desensitization. "True" receptor desensitization would

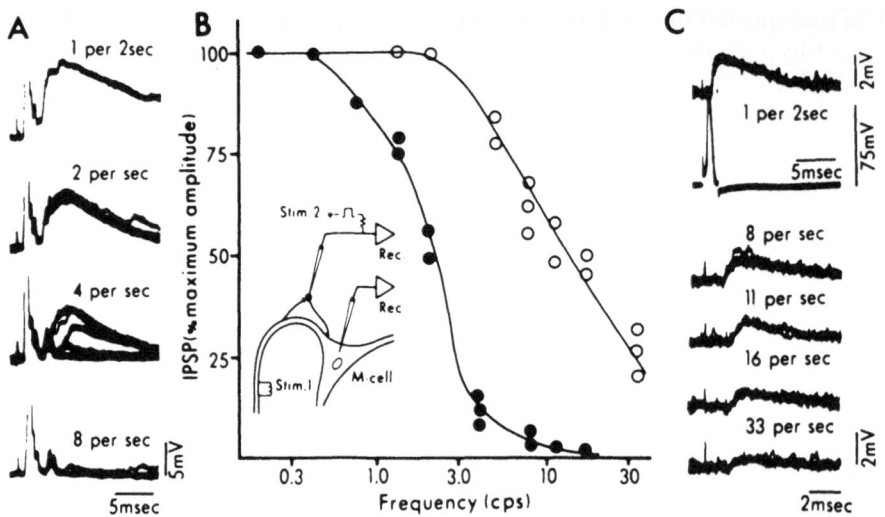

Figure 5. Comparison of the "collateral" and single-cell IPSPs in the goldfish Mauthner cell. The experimental arrangement is illustrated in the small schematic drawing in the inset of (B). An interneuron (small black circle) could be activated either by: (1) stimulation of a Mauthner cell axon collateral (Stim. 1), which produced the collateral IPSP (e.g., top trace in [A]); or (2) direct stimulation via depolarizing current pulses passed through a microelectrode impaling it (Stim. 2), which produced the single cell IPSP in the Mauthner cell (e.g., top trace in [C]). IPSPs are inverted due to Cl⁻ leakage from the recording electrode. As the frequency of stimulation was gradually raised the collateral IPSP (filled circles) was quickly reduced and was essentially abolished by 8 Hz. The single cell IPSP (open circles) was only about 50% depressed at 16 Hz and was still present at 33 Hz. (From Faber and Korn, 1982, with permission.)

involve a decreased ability of a given amount of transmitter to produce a given conductance change when applied repeatedly to a given set of receptors. This could be due either to a reduced capacity of the receptor to bind transmitter or a reduced ability of the bound receptor to induce a given change in the conductance state of the channel. Fading of GABA responses during prolonged application has frequently been seen in vertebrate CNS (Kelly and Beart, 1975). To what extent this fading is attributable to true desensitization is not clear.

To demonstrate desensitization, it is essential to show that not only the potential change, but also the conductance change caused by the transmitter, has been reduced (Fig. 6). Reduction in response amplitude may be explained by a shift in the reversal potential for the transmitter resulting from changes in transmembrane ionic gradients, and this may not be accompanied by a marked change in the conductance increase (see Section 4.1). If the conductance change produced by the transmitter is depressed, however, then either binding to the receptor or activation of the channel must have been reduced.

Nevertheless, decreased transmitter-activated conductance is not a sufficient criterion for identifying desensitization. GABA uptake mechanisms

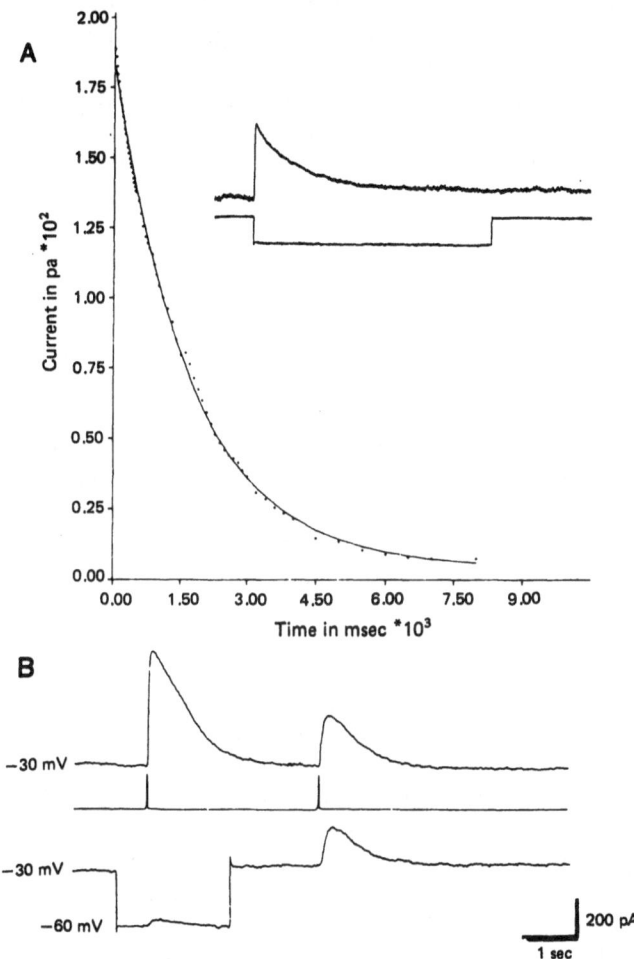

Figure 6. Desensitization of GABA responses on an isolated hippocampal cell. (A) The outward ionic current response (top trace) to a long pulse of GABA (indicated by the lower trace) is shown under voltage clamp. The decline of this outward current is plotted in the graph. (B) In the top traces, two identical pulses of GABA were given at an interval of several seconds at a holding potential of −30 mV. The current induced by the second pulse is markedly depressed. The holding potential for the lowest trace was also −30 mV, but the membrane was stepped to −60 mV during the duration of the first GABA response. Notice there is only a very slight outward current at this membrane potential. The membrane was then returned to −30 mV and the second pulse of GABA delivered. The response to the second pulse was also depressed relative to the control response (first response in the top trace of [B]). (From Numann and Wong, 1984, with permission.)

could cause the response to fade, but this would not be desensitization. For example, uptake, rather than desensitization, may account for the "inactivation" of bath-applied GABA responses at the crayfish stretch receptor, since stirring the bath restores the responses (Kuffler and Edwards, 1958). Other factors may cause GABA responses on CNS neurons to decline. A high dose of directly applied GABA will activate not only the H receptors that are most obviously involved in synaptic transmission but also the D receptors that have been identified with an extrasynaptic location (see Section 2.2.4). Enhancement of a depolarizing potential could contribute to a decline in a hyperpolarizing potential and could also affect the measured conductance change.

Presynaptic factors complicate attempts to decide if decreases in GABAergic IPSPs are due to desensitization. If less transmitter were released due to depletion, or to depression of the interneuron pathway, then IPSPs would decline, but again this would not be desensitization. Certain endogenous compounds, including acetylcholine (Haas, 1982) and enkephalin (Nicoll et al., 1980), depress interneuron activity in the hippocampus and reduce GABAergic IPSPs. In these cases GABA receptor desensitization can probably be eliminated as a cause of the IPSP depression, since iontophoretically applied GABA responses are not affected. Nevertheless, it should be kept in mind that receptors actually activated by released transmitter probably comprise a small proportion of the total number of receptors on a cell. Small alterations in the responsiveness of receptors in the synaptic cleft would not necessarily be detectable by direct application techniques.

A possible example of receptor desensitization in the hippocampus is based on observations that repetitive stimulation of afferent pathways depressed IPSPs and responses to iontophoretically applied GABA on pyramidal cells (Ben-Ari et al., 1979). Numann and Wong (1984), using acutely isolated single hippocampal cells *in vitro*, voltage-clamped these neurons and studied GABA-activated currents. Application of two brief pulses of GABA separated by intervals of a few seconds led to a reduction in the amplitude of the second response. To reduce any contribution of the D GABA response (see Section 2.2.4) they delivered both pulses with the cell clamped near the reversal potential for the inward current which mediates the D response. As at the resting potential, the second response was depressed when it occurred within a few seconds of the first. To test the possibility that the second response was depressed due to intracellular Cl^- accumulation caused by the first response, they also repeated the two-pulse protocol with the first pulse delivered when the membrane was held near E_{Cl} (Fig. 6B). Depression of the second response still occurred, suggesting accumulation of Cl^- was not responsible. These data strongly support the idea that GABA receptors on hippocampal pyramidal cells desensitize. This is true in other neuronal membranes as well. For example, Mauthner cell responses to both GABA and glycine become depressed with prolonged application. Interestingly, on Mauthner cells, application of glycine may influence the GABA response, but the reverse is not found (Diamond and Roper, 1973).

Despite clear evidence that exogenously applied GABA can cause receptor desensitization, the important physiological question remains whether or not responses to synaptically released GABA also desensitize. McCarren and Alger (1985) were able to account for most of the IPSP depression recorded in hippocampal pyramidal cells *in vitro* by presynaptic (depression of GABA release) and postsynaptic factors (shift in IPSP and GABA reversal potential). In these studies, receptor desensitization appeared to play only a minor role in IPSP depression.

Decreased responsiveness to GABA or glycine may be due to factors related to the ionic channel rather than the binding site of the receptor complex. In their study of the large glycine-activated Cl^- channels of lamprey CNS, Gold and Martin (1983b) noted that the channel conductance was markedly dependent on $[Cl^-]_i$. As $[Cl^-]_i$ increased, the channel conductance decreased, although the mechanism by which this occurs is unknown. Gold and Martin suggest that during repetitive activity, especially during concurrent excitatory activity, increases in $[Cl^-]_i$ will occur (Section 2.2.3), and this will lead to decreased Cl^- conductance. Such effects would clearly alter the efficacy of IPSPs.

3. MODES OF INHIBITORY ACTION

Ultimately, synaptic inhibition reduces the ability of a cell to communicate with other cells. However, the variety of inhibitory synaptic arrangements suggests that there are many nuances of this general function.

3.1. Prevention of Impulse Generation

In vertebrate CNS, a large proportion of inhibitory synapses is found on the somata and initial axon segments of principal cells. Prevention of impulse generation is probably a major function of these synapses.

Since many IPSPs in vertebrate CNS are associated with both an increase in membrane conductance and a hyperpolarization of the membrane potential, the question arises as to which is the more important for inhibition. In spinal motoneurons, injection of depolarizing current pulses of different intensities and durations was used to bring motoneurons to threshold (see review by Eccles, 1964). These pulses were then applied at successive times after the elicitation of a Ia IPSP. It was found that inhibition was due to both potential change and conductance increase and that the degree to which each contributed was dependent, in part, on the intensity and duration of the depolarizing current injected. Inhibition of firing during long current pulses was more pronounced than that during brief intense pulses. It was argued that, in the latter case, inhibitory current could not effectively antagonize the powerful stimulating current. Therefore, inhibition of firing caused by brief intense pulses must have been due to the level of hyper-polarization present when the pulse occurred. During the longer, weaker excitatory current pulses, the inhibitory current would have an appreciable effect.

In trochlear motoneurons, an ammonia-sensitive Cl^- pump maintains an inward Cl^- gradient. Ammonium ions result in a dissipation of the gradient so that E_{IPSP} becomes equal to the resting potential, and the inhibitory transmitter no longer hyperpolarizes the membrane although the conductance change is unaffected (Section 3.2). Ammonia reduces the inhibitory effectiveness of the IPSP by 90%, suggesting that hyperpolarization *per se*, rather than the conductance increase, is of primary importance for inhibition in these cells.

Apart from these types of experiments there is little direct information regarding details of inhibitory actions in vertebrate CNS. Analyses of mathematical models have been used to provide insights into the effects of inhibition of cells with elaborate dendritic trees (Jack et al., 1975). Some of the questions that can be addressed are:

1. What aspects of the inhibitory input are the most important for causing inhibition?
2. Where should inhibitory synapses be located in order to produce maximal effects?
3. What determines the optimal location of inhibitory synapses on a neuron?

3.2. Dendritic Inhibition

Certain principle neurons such as cerebellar Purkinje cells (Llinas and Nicolson, 1971) and hippocampal pyramidal cells (Wong and Prince, 1979; Alger and Nicoll, 1982a, Somogyi et al., 1983) have inhibitory synapses on their dendrites, as well as their somata. There are at least three specific functions of dendritic inhibition: (1) local depression of EPSPs, (2) prevention of the development and spread of dendritic action potentials, and (3) inhibition of transmitter release from dendrites.

Assuming that excitatory synapses are made principally on dendrites, there are two major theoretical considerations regarding the placement of inhibitory synapses: (1) the maximal reduction of the somatic depolarization caused by the EPSPs and (2) the optimal means of achieving selective inhibition of certain EPSPs. In general, the greatest reduction in the somatic depolarization occurs when the inhibitory synapses are located on the soma. The reason for this is that the IPSP hyperpolarization is also attenuated when spreading electrotonically. Thus, maximal somatic hyperpolarization, and somatic inhibition, are produced by inhibitory synapses on the soma. An exception is that if the dendrites are long and branching, then maximal reduction of the somatic voltage response resulting from depolarization near the ends of the dendrites can be effected by nearby dendritic inhibitory input. In this case, the closer the excitatory and inhibitory synapses to the tips of the dendrites, the more substantial the effect. This is because, near the dendritic tip, the excitatory current is "reflected" back to the dendritic trunk; i.e., the current reaching the tip does not fully leak across the tip but continues to spread along the dendritic membrane back to the soma. It is the reflected current that is inhibited by the distal inhibitory synapse (see Jack et al., 1975).

The optimal location for an inhibitory synapse may be determined by a need for selective, rather than maximal, inhibition. The conductance increase caused by an inhibitory synaptic input on one dendrite will have essentially no effect on an excitatory input on another dendrite, although an associated inhibitory membrane hyperpolarization could sum with and reduce an EPSP at branch points. Thus, the most specific block of a particular excitatory input will occur when inhibitory and excitatory synapses are located on the same dendrite. The maximal effect results when the inhibitory synapse is on the somatic side of the excitatory synapse and close to it. Indeed, inhibitory synapses on the distal side of excitatory synapses may not affect EPSP amplitudes at all, unless they are both near the dendritic tips.

The dendrites of certain cells support action potential generation (Llinas and Nicholson, 1971; Wong et al., 1979) and another function of dendritic inhibition is to block these potentials (see review by Spencer, 1977). Usually action potential propagation in dendrites is decremental; i.e., the action potentials are fully developed at dendritic trigger zones but only affect the soma through electrotonic spread, presumably because the membrane between the trigger zone and the soma cannot support regenerative propagation. If dendritic action potentials are necessary to communicate distal excitatory influences to the soma, then a few well-placed dendritic inhibitory synapses could, by blocking propagation, cause a "functional amputation" of entire branches of a dendritic tree (Llinas and Nicholson, 1971).

Finally, some dendrites are specialized to form synaptic contacts and to release transmitter. As discussed in the next section, dendritic inhibition can block dendritic transmitter release.

3.3. Dendrodendritic Inhibition

Morphological specializations identical to those present in presynaptic axon terminals have been found within dendrites and somata of cells in various parts of the vertebrate CNS, suggesting these may function as presynaptic elements and release neurotransmitters (see Shepherd, 1979). The most detailed information regarding the morphology and functional role of these specializations has been obtained from the olfactory bulb. In the external plexiform layer of the bulb, there are reciprocal connections between dendrites of mitral and granule cells (Fig. 7A). The mitral (M) cell dendrite

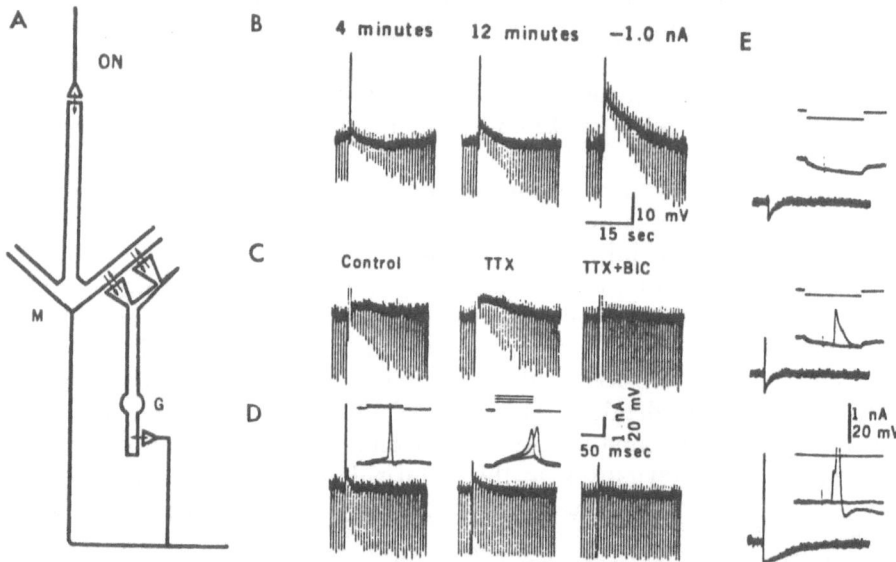

Figure 7. Demonstration of dendrodendritic inhibition in the olfactory bulb using intracellular recording. (A) Schematic drawing of the circuit (ON, olfactory nerve; M, mitral cell; G, granule cell). The opposing arrows at the site of dendritic contact indicate the reciprocal nature of the interaction between the cells. The responses in (B–D) are pen recorder traces of the membrane potential of a mitral cell recorded with a 3 M KCl-filled electrode; the downward deflections are responses to hyperpolarizing constant current pulses. (B) Orthodromic responses are recorded 4 and 12 min after impalement and during injection of − 1.0 nA hyperpolarizing current. The IPSPs became increasingly depolarizing as the cell filled with Cl⁻ or during hyperpolarization with current. The responses in (C) were produced by direct depolarization of the cell by current injection. In the control solution, the direct depolarization was followed by a slower depolarization associated with a large decrease in resistance. After 15 min of perfusion with 10^{-6} M TTX, the same depolarizing pulse produced a larger depolarization and resistance decrease. Bicuculline methiodide (BIC) was then added to the perfusion and the response following the pulse was blocked, indicating it was a reversed GABA IPSP. The first response in (D) was recorded under control conditions. The second response in (D) was recorded in TTX, which blocked the fast action potential. A slow Ca^{2+}-dependent action potential continued to occur, as did the reversed IPSP, which could be blocked by BIC (third trace in [D]). (E) Antidromic responses were recorded from a mitral cell with a potassium methylsulfate-filled electrode. In the top records, a strong hyperpolarizing current pulse injected during antidromic stimulation entirely blocked action potential invasion of the soma. In the middle traces, a reduction in the hyperpolarization permitted the action potential to invade the initial segment, but not the soma-dendritic membrane. In the lower traces invasion of the soma-dendritic membrane was allowed. Note the IPSP became larger only in the last case. (From Jahr and Nicoll, 1980, with permission.)

makes synaptic contact on the granule (G) cell dendrite at specialized dendritic spines called gemmules. Adjacent to the mitral-to-granule-cell-synapse, on the same gemmule, the granule cell makes a synapse on the mitral cell. Ultrastructural serial reconstruction of these regions indicates that the mitral cell side is specialized to excite the granule cell, while the granule cell side is specialized to inhibit the mitral cell. The gemmule stains heavily for GAD (Ribak et al., 1977). Despite a wealth of indirect evidence based on field potential recordings, the physiological effect of this apparent reciprocal dendrodendritic interaction has only recently been demonstrated conclusively by Jahr and Nicoll (1980, 1982).

Using intracellular recording from turtle olfactory bulb in vitro, Jahr and Nicoll showed that a single, directly-activated action potential in a mitral cell resulted in the immediate production of a Cl^--dependent IPSP in the same cell. Apparently the mitral cell excited the granule cell, which then produced an IPSP in the mitral cell. Two types of evidence supported the conclusion that this IPSP was not generated by a recurrent inhibitory circuit, i.e., did not depend on an action potential traveling out the mitral cell axon.

First, the IPSP was not blocked by bath perfusion of TTX sufficient to block axonal conduction (Figs. 7C and 7D). In this instance, large Ca^{2+}-dependent action potentials occurred in the mitral cell and these were sufficient to permit synaptic transmission to take place (Fig. 7D). Ca^{2+}-dependent action potentials cannot propagate in these cells.

Second, antidromic stimulation was applied to mitral cell axons and the degree of antidromic invasion of the mitral cell soma/dendritic (SD) membrane was controlled by hyperpolarization of its membrane. When action potential invasion of the SD membrane was prevented, only a small IPSP was recorded (Fig. 7E, top and middle). Only when the antidromic action potential was allowed to invade the SD membrane was a full-sized IPSP produced (Fig. 7E, bottom trace). Since the same antidromic stimulus was used throughout, the increment in IPSP size must have been related to depolarization of the SD membrane.

These experiments indicate that the mitral cell soma dendritic membrane has properties similar to a presynaptic terminal, including voltage-dependent Ca^{2+} channels and the capability of releasing excitatory transmitter in the absence of voltage-dependent Na^+ current.

Depolarization of the granule cell gemmules by the mitral cell excitatory transmitter resulted in their releasing GABA onto the mitral cells. While granule cells can produce action potentials, it is not clear whether an action potential is necessary to cause transmitter release from these cells. Since the reciprocal pathway functions in the presence of TTX, it is apparent that Na^+-dependent action potentials in the granule cell are not required, but whether Ca^{2+} spikes are evoked or whether subthreshold depolarizations in the gemmules can release transmitter, is unknown.

From the point of view of the mitral cell, reciprocal dendrodendritic inhibition provides a pronounced "self-inhibition"; i.e., an action potential in a mitral cell is invariably followed by an IPSP. This coupling is much tighter than is typically found in local inhibitory circuits. For example, "recurrent" axon collateral inhibition does not usually result in an IPSP following a single action potential in cortical pyramidal cells. A considerably lower threshold for IPSP production exists in the reciprocal dendrodendritic inhibition arrangement where only a gemmule, and not an entire cell, must be excited. This synaptic arrangement is ideal for the transformation of prolonged tonic excitatory input to the mitral cells into a spike train output, such as probably occurs in olfactory processing (Shepherd, 1979).

4. PHYSIOLOGICAL ACTIONS OF GABA IN PERIPHERAL SYSTEMS

Neurons in peripheral ganglia, including dorsal root ganglia, sympathetic ganglia and ganglia of the myenteric plexus are richly invested with GABA receptors. These cells all respond to GABA with a Cl^--dependent depolarization (DeGroat, 1970). Nevertheless, with the possible exception of myenteric plexus neurons, cells in peripheral ganglia do not seem to have GABA synapses on their somata. The physiological role of the somatic GABA receptors is unclear, although they have been studied intensively.

4.1. Sympathetic Ganglia

Adams and Brown (1975) used an *in vitro* preparation to analyze the responses of rat superior cervical ganglion (SCG) cells to bath-applied GABA. GABA caused a conductance increase and a depolarization that reversed at about -40 to -50 mV. Nevertheless, GABA had only slight effects on ganglionic transmission, even though it reduced the amplitude and prolonged the duration of the action potentials. The GABA response was affected by $[Cl^-]_o$, but not by $[Na^+]_o$. To account for the GABA-induced depolarizations due to Cl^- movements, it is necessary to postulate that the Cl^- concentration gradient is directed outward, i.e., that the internal Cl^- concentration is higher than can be accounted for on the basis of passive diffusion. Increasing Cl^- conductance would lead to an efflux, with a consequent depolarization, of the membrane. A high internal Cl^- concentration suggests the existence of a mechanism for establishing and maintaining such a Cl^- gradient, i.e., an inward, rather than an outward, Cl^- pump (cf. Section 2.2.3).

GABA receptors on sympathetic ganglion cells appear pharmacologically similar to hyperpolarizing GABA receptors in the brain in their sensitivity to picrotoxin and bicuculline. The ganglionic GABA response amplitude and conductance increase attenuate markedly over the course of GABA applications prolonged beyond 20 sec. Depletion of intracellular Cl^-, which, theoretically, could produce a diminution of both the maximal depolarization and conductance increase (see Section 2.2), was eliminated as a possible cause for these effects. Thus receptor desensitization, or another process unrelated to $[Cl^-]_i$, was implicated. Subsequently, in fact, Brown and Galvan (1977) found that depression of responses to low concentrations of GABA are due to uptake of GABA. In sympathetic ganglia GABA is taken up into glial cells by a high-affinity, Na^+-dependent system. This system has a low velocity, but a high capacity, and may thus provide a long-term buffering capability. Therefore, uptake could, in part, account for the decreases in conductance increase which occur during prolonged GABA application.

The function of the GABA receptors on SCG cells remains unclear. As noted earlier there is no neural GABAergic input to the sympathetic ganglia. Indeed, in view of the relatively slight inhibitory effects of GABA on ganglionic transmission, Adams and Brown suggest that the high internal Cl^- renders the action of any circulating GABA virtually harmless. The glial uptake system would provide further protection.

4.2. Parasympathetic Ganglia

In the cat parasympathetic vesical ganglion, bath-applied GABA produces a biphasic response (Mayer et al., 1983). The early phase is a depolarization due to the outward movement of Cl^-, which is apparently identical to the responses in other peripheral ganglia. The late phase of the response is associated with a membrane resistance decrease and, thus far, appears unique to this system. The late phase has a reversal potential near E_{Cl} and is dependent on a high intracellular permeant anion concentration. Mayer et al. (1983) suggested that GABA caused first an increase and then a decrease in a resting Cl^- conductance. However the details and functional implications of this unusual response remain unknown.

4.3. Myenteric Plexus

A growing body of evidence supports the hypothesis that GABA is a neurotransmitter in the enteric nervous system. The best established data are that GABA, GABA receptors, and GAD are found within the tissues of the gut, and moreover that high concentrations of these markers are specifically localized to layers containing the myenteric plexus (see review by Jessen, 1981). Intracellular recordings from neurons in guinea pig myenteric plexus have shown that GABA depolarizes the cells, apparently by a Cl^--sensitive mechanism. Unlike the sympathetic and dorsal root ganglia, the myenteric plexus contains neurons, about 5% of the total, which can accumulate GABA by uptake mechanisms that are sensitive to neuronal uptake blockers and are resistant to glial uptake blockers. In addition, GABA is released in a Ca^{2+}-dependent fashion from cat colon, although it is not certain that this release is from neurons.

It has been suggested that GABA might function in the enteric nervous system to modulate the release of transmitters from intestinal nerves presynaptically. Application of GABA causes either contractions or relaxations of the mammalian ileum, but these actions are blocked by both atropine and TTX, as well as by picrotoxin, suggesting an indirect action mediated ultimately by interposed cholinergic neurons. GABA does not affect nerve-free preparations of longitudinal muscle from the guinea pig ileum; to date neither the site of contact nor the target cells of GABAergic enteric nerves have been directly identified.

5. CONCLUSIONS AND FUNCTIONAL CONSIDERATIONS

It is now well accepted that GABA and glycine are inhibitory neurotransmitters in the vertebrate CNS; their roles in the peripheral nervous system are less certain. Although the precise function of inhibition in the CNS is unclear in most cases, its importance is emphasized by studies on cellular mechanisms in epilepsy. It is well known that agents whose major action is interference with GABA or glycine neurotransmission cause convulsions in animals and man. Moreover, it appears that repetitive action potential firing (epileptiform "burst" activity) is to a large extent an intrinsic characteristic of certain CNS neurons but that the tendency to burst is normally under the control of GABA-mediated inhibition. For example, in hippocampus, pyramidal cells fire bursts of action potentials when exposed to GABA antagonists. Thus, pyramidal cells are normally prevented from firing burst responses by GABA inhibition (Schwartzkroin and Prince, 1980; Wong and Prince, 1979). This insight, from studies on epilepsy, may be useful in interpreting normal physiological states as well. For example, under some normal conditions individual cells fire burst potentials, such as during sleep (Ranck, 1975). It is tempting to speculate that the transition from the awake firing pattern to the sleeping pattern may be controlled by GABAergic IPSPs.

A similar argument may be made with regard to neuronal synchronization in normal and pathological situations. Extreme synchronization of firing is a characteristic of the epileptic state and can be induced in a number of model systems by blocking GABA synapses (Wong and Traub, 1983). However, synchronized neuronal firing also occurs in normal conditions, such as during sleep or certain voluntary behaviors. Again the implication may be that the transition between synchronized and asynchronized brain states involves modulation at sites along inhibitory pathways.

A major area for future research will be to specify the functions of synaptic inhibition from the point of view of the behaving organism. At present it remains difficult to go beyond the idea expressed by Eccles that inhibition is a sculpturing process that "chisels away at the diffuse and rather amorphous mass of excitatory action and gives a more specific form to the neuronal process at every stage of synaptic relay" (Eccles, 1977).

ACKNOWLEDGMENTS. This work was supported by NIH Grant NS 17539 and a McKnight Foundation Scholar's Award.

REFERENCES

Adams, P. R., and Brown, D. A., 1975, Actions of gamma-aminobutyric acid on sympathetic ganglion cells, *J. Physiol. (Lond.)* **250:**85–120.

Alger, B. E., and Nicoll, R. A., 1980, Spontaneous inhibitory post-synaptic potentials in hippocampus: Mechanism for tonic inhibition, *Brain Res.* **200:**195–200.

Alger, B. E., and Nicoll, R. A., 1982a, Feed-forward dendritic inhibition in rat hippocampal pyramidal cells studied in vitro, *J. Physiol. (Lond.)* **328:**105–123.

Alger, B. E., and Nicoll, R. A., 1982b, Pharmacological evidence for two kinds of GABA receptor on rat hippocampal pyramidal cells studied in vitro, *J. Physiol. (Lond.)* **328:**125–141.

Alger, B. E., and Nicoll, R. A., 1983, Ammonia does not selectively block IPSPs in rat hippocampal pyramidal cells, *J. Neurophysiol.* **49:**1381–1391.

Allen, G. I., Eccles, J. C., Nicoll, R. A., Oshima, T., and Rubia, F. J., 1977, The ionic mechanisms concerned in generating the i.p.s.p.s of hippocampal pyramidal cells, *Proc. R. Soc. Lond.* B **198:**363–384.

Andersen, P., 1975, Organization of hippocampal neurons and their interconnections, in: *The Hippocampus*, Volume 1 (R. L. Isaacson and K. H. Pribram, eds.), Plenum Press, New York, pp. 155–175.

Andersen, P., Eccles, J. C., and Loyning, Y., 1964, Location of postsynaptic inhibitory synapses on hippocampal pyramidal cells, *J. Neurophysiol.* **27:**592–607.

Andersen, P., Dingledine, R., Gjerstad, L., Langmoen, I. A., and Mosfeldt-Laursen, A., 1980, Two different responses of hippocampal pyramidal cells to application of gamma-amino butyric acid, *J. Physiol. (Lond.)* **305:**279–296.

Aprison, M. H., 1978, Glycine as a neurotransmitter, in: *Psychopharmacology: A Generation of Progress* (M. A. Lipton, A. DiMascio, and K. F. Killam, eds.), Raven Press, New York, pp. 333–346.

Assaf, S. Y., Crunelli, V., and Kelly, J. S., 1981, Electrophysiology of the rat dentate gyrus *in vitro*, in: *Electrophysiology of Isolated Mammalian CNS Preparations* (G. A. Kerkut and H. V. Wheal, eds.), Academic Press, London, pp. 153–188.

Atwood, H. L., 1976, Synaptic physiology of crustacean neuromuscular systems, *Progr. Neurobiol.* **7:**291–391.

Barber, R. P., and Saito, K., 1976, Light microscopic visualization of GAD and GABA-T in immunocytochemical preparations of rodent CNS, in: *GABA in Nervous System Function* (E. Roberts, T. N. Chase, and D. B. Tower, eds.), Raven Press, New York, pp. 113–132.

Barker, J. L., and Ransom, B. R., 1978, Amino acid pharmacology of mammalian central neurones grown in tissue culture, *J. Physiol. (Lond.)* **280:**331–354.

Ben-Ari, Y., Krnjevic, K., and Reinhardt, W., 1979, Hippocampal seizures and failure of inhibition, *Can. J. Physiol. Pharmacol.* **57:**1462–1466.

Bergey, G. K., MacDonald, R. L., Habig, W. H., Hargegree, M. C., and Nelson, P. G., 1983, Tetanus toxin: Convulsant action on mouse spinal neurons in culture, *J. Neurosci.* **3:**2310–2324.

Brock, L. G., Coombs, J. S., and Eccles, J. C., 1952, The recording of potentials from motoneurons with an intracellular electrode, *J. Physiol. (Lond.)* **117:**431–460.

Brown, D. A., 1979, Extrasynaptic GABA systems, *Trends Neurosci.* **2:**271–273.

Brown, D. A., and Galvan, M., 1977, Influences of neuroglial transport on the action of gamma aminobutyric acid on mammalian ganglion cells, *Br. J. Pharmacol.* **59:**373–378.

Brown, T. H., and Johnston, D., 1980, Two classes of spontaneous miniature synaptic potentials in CA3 hippocampal neurons, *Soc. Neurosci. Abst.* **6:**10.

Brown, T. H., and Johnston, D., 1983, Voltage-clamp analysis of mossy fiber synaptic input to hippocampal neurons, *J. Neurophysiol.* **50:**487–507.

Buhrle, C. P., and Sonnhof, U., 1983, Intracellular ion activities and equilibrium potentials in motoneurones and glia cells of the frog spinal cord, *Pflügers Arch.* **396**:144–153.

Burke, R. E., and Rudomin, P., 1977, Spinal neurons and synapses, in: *The Nervous System*, Vol. 1, *Cellular Biology of Neurons*, (J. M. Brookhart, V. B. Mountcastle, and E. R. Kandel, eds.), American Physiological Society, Bethesda, pp. 877–944.

Collingridge, G. L., Gage, P. W., and Robertson, B., 1984, Inhibitory post-synaptic currents in rat hippocampal CA1 neurones, *J. Physiol. (Lond.)* **356**:551–564.

Constanti, A., Krnjevic, K., and Nistri, A., 1980, Intraneuronal effects of inhibitory amino acids, *Can. J. Physiol. Pharmacol.* **58**:193–204.

Coombs, J. S., Eccles, J. C., and Fatt, P., 1955, The specific ionic conductances and the ionic movements across the motoneuronal membrane that produce the inhibitory post-synaptic potential, *J. Physiol. (Lond.)* **130**:326–373.

Cooper, J. R., Bloom, F. E., and Roth, R. H., 1982, *The Biochemical Basis of Neuropharmacology*, Oxford University Press, New York.

DeGroat, W. D., 1970, The actions of gamma-aminobutyric acid and related amino acids on mammalian autonomic ganglia, *J. Pharmacol. Exp. Ther.* **172**:384–396.

Diamond, J., and Roper, S., 1973, Analysis of Mauthner cell responses to iontophoretically delivered pulses of GABA, glycine and L-glutamate, *J. Physiol. (Lond.)* **232**:113–128.

Dreifuss, J. J., Kelly, J. S., and Krnjević, K. K., 1969, The effects of copper on cortical neurons, *Brain Res.* **13**:607–611.

Dudel, J., and Kuffler, S. W., 1961, Presynaptic inhibition at the crayfish neuromuscular junction, *J. Physiol. (Lond.)* **155**:543–562.

Eccles, J. C., 1964, *The Physiology of Synapses*, Springer-Verlag, New York.

Eccles, J. C., 1977, *The Understanding of the Brain*, McGraw-Hill, New York.

Eccles, J., Nicoll, R. A., Oshima, T., and Rubia, F. J., 1977, The anionic permeability of the inhibitory postsynaptic membrane of hippocampal cells, *Proc. R. Soc. Lond. B* **198**:345–361.

Edwards, F. R., Redman, S. J., and Walmsley, Y. B., 1976, Non-quantal fluctuations and transmission failures in charge transfer at Ia synapse in spinal motoneurons, *J. Physiol. (Lond.)* **259**:689–704.

Enna, S. J., and Gallagher, J. P., 1983, Biochemical and electrophysiological characteristics of mammalian GABA receptors, *Int. Rev. Neurobiol.* **24**:181–212.

Faber, D. S., and Korn, H., 1982, Transmission at a central inhibitory synapse. I. Magnitude of unitary postsynaptic conductance change and kinetics of channel activation, *J. Neurophysiol.* **48**:654–678.

Finkel, A. S., and Redman, S. J., 1983, The synaptic current evoked in cat spinal motoneurones by impulses in single group Ia axons, *J. Physiol. (Lond.)* **342**:615–632.

Gallagher, J. P., and Shinnick-Gallagher, P., 1983, Electrophysiological characteristics of GABA receptor complexes, in: *The GABA Receptors* (S. J. Enna, ed.), Humana Press, New York.

Gold, M. R., and Martin, A. R., 1983a, Characteristics of inhibitory post-synaptic currents in brain-stem neurones of the lamprey, *J. Physiol. (Lond.)* **342**:85–98.

Gold, M. R., and Martin, A. R., 1983b, Analysis of glycine-activated inhibitory post-synaptic channels in brain-stem neurones of the lamprey, *J. Physiol. (Lond.)* **342**:99–117.

Gray, R., Kellaway, J., and Johnston, D. J., 1983, Recordings of GABA-activated channels from acutely isolated hippocampal neurons, *Soc. Neurosci. Abst.* **9**:1189.

Haas, H. L., 1982, Cholinergic disinhibition in hippocampal slices of the rat, *Brain Res.* **233**:200–204.

Jack, J. J. B., Noble, D., and Tsien, R. W., 1975, *Electric Current Flow in Excitable Cells*, Clarendon Press, Oxford.

Jahr, C. E., and Nicoll, R. A., 1980, Dendrodendritic inhibition: Demonstration with intracellular recording, *Science* **207**:1473–1475.

Jahr, C. E., and Nicoll, R. A., 1982, An intracellular analysis of dendrodendritic inhibition in the turtle *in vitro* olfactory bulb, *J. Physiol.* **326**:213–234.

Jessen, K. R., 1981, GABA and the enteric nervous system, *Mol. Cell. Biochem.* **38**:69–76.

Johnston, D., and Brown, T. H., 1981, Giant synaptic potential hypothesis for epileptiform activity, *Science* **211**:294–297.

Johnston, G. A. R., 1975, Biochemistry of glycine, taurine, glutamate and aspartate, in: *Handbook of Psychopharmacology*, Volume 4 (L. L. Iversen, S. D. Iversen, and S. H. Snyder, eds.), Plenum Press, New York, pp. 59–82.

Johnston, G. A. R., 1981, GABA receptors, in: *Progress in Clinical and Biological Research*, Volume 68 (J. B. Lombardini and A. D. Kenny, eds.), Liss, New York, pp. 1–18.

Kehoe, J. S., 1976, Electrogenic effects of neutral amino acids on neurons of Aplysia californica, *Cold Spring Harbor Symp. Quant. Biol.* **40**:145–156.

Kelly, J. S., and Beart, P. M., 1975, Amino acid receptors in CNS. II. GABA in supraspinal regions, in: *Handbook of Psychopharmacology*, Volume 4 (L. L. Iversen, S. D. Iversen, and S. H. Snyder, eds.), Plenum Press, New York, pp. 129–210.

Kelly, J. S., Krnjević, K., Morris, M. E., and Yim, G. K. W., 1969, Anionic permeability of cortical neurones, *Exp. Brain Res.* **7**:11–31.

Korn, H., Mallet, A., Triller, A., and Faber, D. S., 1982, Transmission at a central inhibitory synapse. II. Quantal description of release, with a physical correlate for binomial n, *J. Neurophysiol.* **48**:679–707.

Kravitz, E. A., Kuffler, S. W., and Potter, D. D., 1963, Gamma-aminobutyric acid and other blocking compounds in Crustacea. Their relative concentrations in separated motor and inhibitory axons, *J. Neurophysiol.* **26**:739–751.

Kuffler, S. W., and Edwards, C., 1958, Mechanism of gamma aminobutyric acid (GABA) action and its relation to synaptic inhibition, *J. Neurophysiol.* **21**:589–610.

Kuno, M., and Weakly, J. N., 1972, Quantal components of the inhibitory synaptic potential in spinal motoneurones of the cat, *J. Physiol. (Lond.)* **224**:282–303.

Lewis, C. A., 1979, Ion-concentration dependence of the reversal potential and the single channel conductance of ion channels at the frog neuromuscular junction, *J. Physiol. (Lond.)* **286**:417–445.

Llinas, R., and Nicholson, C., 1971, Electrophysiological properties of dendrites and somata in Alligator Purkinje cells, *J. Neurophysiol.* **34**:532–551.

Lux, H. D., 1971, Ammonium and chloride extrusion: Hyperpolarizing synaptic inhibition in spinal motoneurons, *Science* **173**:555–557.

Martin, A. R., 1979, in an Appendix to Matthews, G., and Wickelgren, W. O., Glycine, GABA and synaptic inhibition of reticulospinal neurones of lamprey, *J. Physiol.* **293**:393–415.

Mathers, D. A., and Barker, J. L., 1981, Spontaneous hyperpolarizations at the membrane of cultured mouse dorsal root ganglion cells, *Brain Res.* **211**:451–455.

Mayer, M. L., Higashi, H., Gallagher, J. P., and Shinnick-Gallagher, P., 1983, On the mechanism of action of GABA in pelvic vesical ganglia: Biphasic responses evoked by two opposing actions on membrane conductance, *Brain Res.* **260**:233–248.

McCarren, M., and Alger, B. E., 1985, Use-dependent depression of IPSPs in rat hippocampal pyramidal cells in vitro, *J. Neurophysiol.* **53**:557–571.

Miles, R., and Wong, R. K. S., 1984, Unitary synaptic inhibitory potentials in the guinea pig hippocampus in vitro, *J. Physiol. (Lond.)* **356**:97–113.

Newberry, N. R., and Nicoll, R. A., 1984, Direct hyperpolarizing action baclofen on hippocampal pyramidal cells, *Nature (Lond.)* **308**:450–452.

Nicoll, R. A., 1978, Physiological studies on amino acids and peptides as prospective transmitters in the CNS, in: *Psychopharmacology: A generation of Progress* (M. A. Lipton, A. DiMascio, and K. F. Killam, eds.), Raven Press, New York, pp. 103–118.

Nicoll, R. A., Eccles, J. C., Oshima, T., and Rubia, F., 1975, Prolongation of hippocampal inhibitory postsynaptic potentials by barbiturates *Nature (Lond.)* **258**:625–627.

Nicoll, R. A., Alger, B. E., and Jahr, C. E., 1980, Enkephalin blocks inhibitory pathways in the vertebrate CNS, *Nature (Lond.)* **287**:22–25.

Nistri, A., and Constanti, A., 1979, Pharmacological characterization of different types of GABA and glutamate receptors in vertebrates and invertebrates, *Prog. Neurobiol.* **13**:117–235.

Numann, R. E., and Wong, R. K. S., 1984, Electrophysiology of single pyramidal cells dissociated from the hippocampus of adult guinea pigs: GABA desensitization, *Neurosci. Lett.*, **47**:289–294.

Obata, K., 1977, Biochemistry and physiology of amino acid transmitters, in: *Handbook of*

Physiology, Section 1, *The Nervous System*, Volume 1, *Cellular Biology of Neurons* (J. M. Brookhart, V. B. Mountcastle, and E. R. Kandel, eds.), American Physiological Society, Bethesda, pp. 625–650.

Okada, Y., 1981, Fine localizations of GABA (gamma-aminobutyric acid) and GAD (glutamate decarboxylase) in a single Deiter's neuron—significance of the uneven distribution of GABA and GAD in the CNS, in: *Problems in GABA Research* (Y. Okada and E. Roberts, eds.), Excerpta Medica, Amsterdam, pp. 23–29.

Otsuka, M., Kravitz, E. A., and Potter, D. D., 1967, Physiological and chemical architecture of a lobster ganglion with particular reference to gamma-aminobutyrate and glutamate, *J. Neurophysiol.* **30:**725–752.

Pickles, H. G., and Simmonds, M. A., 1978, Field potentials, inhibition and the effect of pentobarbitone in the rat olfactory cortex slice, *J. Physiol.* **275:**135–148.

Raabe, W., and Gumnit, R. J., 1975, Disinhibition in cat motor cortex by ammonia, *J. Neurophysiol.* **38:**347–355.

Ranck, Jr., J. B., 1975, Behavioral correlates and firing repertoiries of neurons in the dorsal hippocampal formation and septum of unrestrained rats, in: *The Hippocampus*, Volume 2 (R. L. Isaacson and K. H. Pribram, eds.), Plenum Press, New York, pp. 207–247.

Ribak, C. E., Vaughn, J. E., Saito, K., Barber, B., and Roberts, E., 1977, Glutamate decarboxylase localization in neurons of the olfactory bulb, *Brain Res.* **126:**1–18.

Ryall, R. W., 1975, Amino acid receptors in CNS. I. GABA and glycine in spinal cord, in: *Handbook of Psychopharmacology*, Volume 4 (L. L. Iversen, S. D. Iversen, and S. H. Snyder), Plenum Press, New York, pp. 83–128.

Scholfield, C. N., 1978, A depolarizing inhibitory potential in neurones of the olfactory cortex in vitro, *J. Physiol. (Lond.)* **275:**547–557.

Schousboe, A., Larsson, O. M., Hertz, L., and Krogsgaard-Larsen, P., 1981, Heterocyclic GABA analogues as new selective inhibitors of astroglial GABA transport, *Drug Devel. Res.* **1:**115–127.

Schwartzkroin, P. A., 1975, Characteristics of CA1 neurons recorded intracellularly in the hippocampal slice, *Brain Res.* **85:**423–435.

Schwartzkroin, P. A., 1977, Further characteristics of CA1 cells in vitro, *Brain Res.* **128:**53–68.

Schwartzkroin, P. A., and Prince, D. A., 1980, Changes in excitatory and inhibitory synaptic potentials leading to epileptogenic activity, *Brain Res.* **183:**61–76.

Segal, M., and Barker, J. L., 1984, Rat hippocampal neurons in culture: Properties of GABA-activated Cl ion conductance, *J. Neurophysiol.* **51:**500–515.

Shepherd, G. M., 1977, The olfactory bulb: A simple system in the mammalian brain, in: *Handbook of Physiology*, Section 1, *The Nervous System* Volume 1, *Cellular Biology of Neurons* (J. M. Brookhart, V. B. Mountcastle, and E. R. Kandel, eds.), American Physiological Society, Bethesda, pp. 945–968.

Shepherd, G. M., 1979, *The Synaptic Organization of the Brain*, Oxford University Press, New York.

Somogyi, P., Smith, A. D., Nunzi, M. G., Gorio, A., Takagi, H., and Wu, J. Y., 1983, Glutamate decarboxylase immunoreactivity in the hippocampus of the cat: Distribution of immunoreactive synaptic terminals with special reference to the axon initial segment of pyramidal neurons, *J. Neurosci.* **3:**1450–1468.

Somogyi, P., Hodgson, A. J., Smith, A. D., Nunzi, M. G., Gorio, A., and Wu, J.-Y., 1984, Different populations of GABAergic neurons in the visual cortex and hippocampus of cat contain somatostatin—or cholecystokinin—immunoreactive material, *J. Neurosci.* **4:**2590–2603.

Spencer, W. A., 1977, The physiology of supraspinal neurons in mammals, in: *Handbook of Physiology*, Section 1, *The Nervous System*, Volume 1, *Cellular Biology of Neurons* (J. M. Brookhart, V. B. Mountcastle, and E. R. Kandel, eds.), American Physiological Society, Bethesda, pp. 969–1022.

Spencer, W. A., and April, R. S., 1970, Plastic properties of monosynaptic pathways in mammals, in: *Short-Term Changes in Neural Activity and Behavior* (G. Horn and R. A. Hinde, eds.), Cambridge University Press, Cambridge, pp. 433–475.

Takeuchi, A., 1977, Junctional transmission. I. Postsynaptic mechanisms, in: *Handbook of Physiology*, Section 1, *The Nervous System*, Volume 1, *Cellular Biology of Neurons* (J. M.

Brookhart, V. B. Mountcastle, and E. R. Kandel, eds.), American Physiological Society, Bethesda, pp. 295–324.

Takeuchi, A., and Takeuchi, N., 1960, On the permeability of end-plate membrane during the action of transmitter, *J. Physiol. (Lond.)* **154**:52–67.

Takeuchi, A., and Takeuchi, N., 1967, Anion permeability of the inhibitory postsynaptic membrane of the crayfish neuromuscular junction, *J. Physiol. (Lond.)* **191**:575–590.

Triller, A., and Korn, H., 1982, Transmission at a central inhibitory synapse. III. Ultrastructure of physiologically identified and stained terminals, *J. Neurophysiol.* **48**:708–736.

Wong, R. K. S., and Prince, D. A., 1979, Dendritic mechanisms underlying penicillin induced epileptiform activity, *Science* **204**:1228–1231.

Wong, R. K. S., and Traub, R. D., 1983, Synchronized burst discharge in disinhibited hippocampal slice. I. Initiation in CA2-CA3 region, *J. Neurophysiol.* **49**:442–457.

Wong, R. K. S., and Watkins, D. J., 1982, Cellular factors influencing GABA response in hippocampal pyramidal cells, *J. Neurophysiol.* **48**:938–951.

Wong, R. K. S., Prince, D. A., and Basbaum, A. I., 1979, Intradendritic recordings from hippocampal neurons, *Proc. Natl. Acad. Sci. USA* **76**:986–990.

Yarowsky, P. J., and Carpenter, D. O., 1978, Receptors for gamma-aminobutyric acid (GABA) on Aplysia neurons, *Brain Res.* **144**:75–94.

3

GABA and Glycine:
Ion Channel Mechanisms

JEFFERY L. BARKER

1. INTRODUCTION

It is now evident that the naturally occurring neutral amino acids γ-aminobutyric acid (GABA) and glycine are present in many, if not all, nervous systems and that these substances mediate specific types of intercellular communication. Although their actions in the mammalian central nervous system (CNS) have been studied for 30 years, it is only recently that some understanding of the membrane mechanisms underlying the transmitter actions of these substances has been achieved. Chapter 2 reviews the cellular physiology of GABA and glycine based upon studies in vivo, in acutely prepared slices of CNS tissue, and in peripheral ganglia.

This chapter summarizes the contemporary view of the microscopic (i.e., channel) mechanisms thought to underlie the macroscopic inhibitory signals recorded at postsynaptic sites. For several reasons, quantitative investigations into the membrane actions of these amino acids have relied almost exclusively upon electrical recordings from embryonic central neurons maintained in vitro using cell culture techniques. The exceptional visibility of the monolayer culture allows precise placement of one or more recording electrodes within individual neurons (Fig. 1). In addition, pipettes used to apply pharmacological agents by pressure ejection or iontophoresis can be accurately situated at any point along the cell membrane. Finally, because the membrane of cultured neurons is exposed without a layer of supporting glial cells or surrounding neurons, patch-clamp recordings can easily be carried out (see below). As with other in vitro recording techniques, impalements can be maintained for long periods due to the stability of the preparation. However, the insights gained from examining amino acid ac-

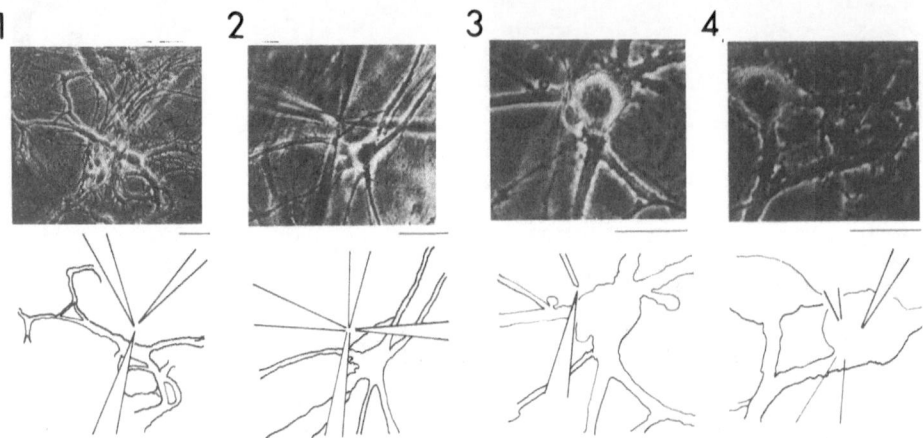

Figure 1. Light micrographs of mouse spinal cord neurons growing in monolayer culture. The four photomicrographs were taken on the stage of an inverted microscopic using phase contrast optics. The shanks of the microelectrodes and micropipettes used to make recordings and apply substances are visible in the first and second panels. The tips of two microelectrodes can clearly be seen just outside the cell body in panel 3. In panel 4 two tips can be detected inside the right-hand cell body. Schematic diagrams of the arrangements are shown below each of the micrographs. The bars indicate 50 μm.

tions in this preparation of embryonic CNS tissue are somewhat attenuated by our incomplete knowledge of the development and differentiation of the mammalian CNS either *in vivo* or *ex vivo*. Despite this, all of the electro-physiological observations made *in vitro* are consistent with effects recorded *in vivo* or in acutely prepared slices of CNS tissue.

2. ELECTROPHARMACOLOGY OF Cl⁻ CONDUCTANCE MECHANISMS

2.1. Current-Clamp Observations

Pharmacological applications of GABA to cultured spinal and supra-spinal neurons causes an electrical response that closely approximates the response to GABA observed in recordings *in vivo* or in tissue slices (see Chapter 2). When GABA is applied discretely at the cell body of a cultured neuron by iontophoresis or pressure ejection, there is a rapid hyperpolarization associated with an increase in conductance (Fig. 2). Applications at distal parts of cell processes of spinal cord neurons are often more complex, consisting of a rapidly desensitizing, depolarizing phase superimposed on the hyperpolarizing responses (Barker and Ransom, 1978). The depolarizing effect of GABA on distal processes differs from the depolarization recorded with applications to dendrites of hippocampal neurons in the *in vitro* slice (see Chapter 2) in that the former are rapidly desensitizing. The dual-response character of the complex response is superficially similar to that

Figure 2. Electrical responses activated by brief applications of GABA to cultured mouse spinal neurons. An intracellular recording was made using a 4 M potassium acetate-filled microelectrode placed in the cell body. GABA was applied by microiontophoresis with 100-msec pulses (marked by upward-downward deflections in all traces) at sites indicated by the arrows. Three of the voltage traces also exhibit repeated hyperpolarizing responses to 50-msec current pulses, which are used to measure membrane resistance before, during, and after the GABA-evoked membrane response. When GABA is applied at sites on the cell body a simple, monophasic hyperpolarizing response is typical, while delivery of GABA to sites distant from the cell body evokes a dual response, consisting of depolarizing and hyperpolarizing phases. The voltage responses to constant-current stimuli decrease during the membrane potential response evoked by GABA, suggesting that the response is accompanied by a transient increase in conductance. (Modified from Barker and Ransom, 1978.)

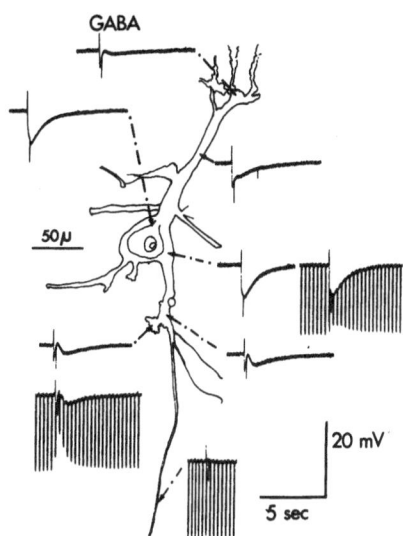

evoked pharmacologically or elaborated physiologically in various invertebrate ganglia by acetylcholine (Wachtel and Kandel, 1971; Blankenship et al., 1971; Levitan and Tauc, 1972), as well as that recorded in cultured spinal neurons following pharmacological application of opioid peptides (Barker et al., 1980a). When responses to discrete applications of GABA at different sites on the same cell are compared, the most intense hyperpolarizing responses arise at spots close to the cell body.

The hyperpolarizing nature of the voltage responses and the increase in membrane conductance are sensitive to the Cl^- ion gradient across the cell (Fig. 3). Indeed, the electrical response appears to be due primarily, if not

Figure 3. The electrical properties of GABA-evoked responses are dependent on the Cl^- ion gradient across the cell. The experimental arrangements are schematized in the insert. Membrane potential has been recorded with a potassium acetate-filled microelectrode, while the cell is bathed in media containing low $[Cl^-]_o$ (9 mM). Under these conditions the Cl^- gradient across the cell is such that the voltage response to an iontophoretic pulse of GABA is depolarizing at the resting potential (-50 mV). Furthermore, there is only a 30% increase in membrane conductance. When the immediate vicinity of the cell is flooded with Cl^- ions from a blunt pipette containing a relatively high $[Cl^-]_o$ (159 mM), the voltage response to GABA becomes markedly hyperpolarizing and there is an associated 600% increase in membrane conductance. Arrowheads mark the time constant of decay of the conductance increases. (From Barker and Ransom, 1978, with permission.)

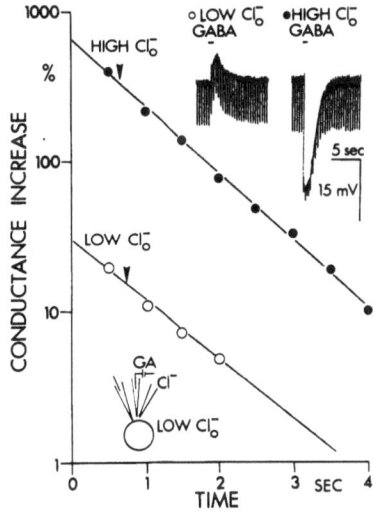

exclusively, to changes in the membrane's permeability to Cl^- ions. The direction of the gradient is critical to the functional effects of GABA's action as can readily be seen when the gradient is altered. Under physiological conditions, the potential at which responses to GABA invert in polarity, i.e., the "reversal potential", is commonly hyperpolarized to the resting potential. When the Cl^- gradient is altered by injecting Cl^- ions intracellularly, the reversal potential invariably shifts in such a way that it usually is depolarized not only to the level of the resting potential but also to that required for triggering action potentials. Thus, rapid activation of Cl^- conductance can effectively excite, rather than inhibit a neuron when the Cl^- ion gradient is altered (see insert in Fig. 4B).

2.2. Voltage-Clamp Observations

The mechanisms underlying the Cl^--dependent actions of GABA and glycine have been studied using the voltage-clamp technique, which allows direct examination of the membrane's conductance to Cl^- ions. Electronic circuitry is employed to hold the cell's membrane potential constant during the conductance response. Thus, the driving force, V_D, which is the difference between the reversal potential and the potential at which the response is measured, stays constant throughout the response. Since, by Ohms's law, the ionic current is related to the product of the ionic conductance and V_D, the conductance is directly proportional to the current when V_D is held constant. Control, or "clamping" of membrane potential, also eliminates current generated when membrane potential changes rapidly enough that the product of membrane capacitance, C, and dV/dt becomes significant. Furthermore, ion conductances whose activation and inactivation are sensitive to membrane potential can be isolated, or subtracted from the amino acid-induced current. The fidelity with which the potential is controlled determines the accuracy with which the conductance can be resolved, and is limited both by the properties of the electronic circuitry and the physical distribution of the ion channels in the membrane with respect to the location of the measuring electrode.

2.2.1. Two-Electrode Measurements of Cl^- Conductance

Two-electrode measurements using feedback circuitry to voltage-clamp cells have been employed to study the Cl^--dependent conductance responses of cultured central neurons induced by GABA and glycine. Repeated applications of these substances while clamping the cell at different membrane potentials reveals the reversal potential which is the potential where the electrical and chemical gradients involved are precisely balanced so that the membrane current response disappears (Fig. 4). Under physiological conditions the reversal potential for Cl^- ion movements (about -60 mV in Fig. 4A) is usually hyperpolarized relative to the resting membrane potential

(Fig. 4A, insert). When the ion gradient is altered by injecting Cl^- ions into the cell, the Cl^- ion currents reverse at a new potential (about -15 mV in Fig. 4B), depolarized relative to that usually observed under physiological conditions. The relationship between the current response evoked at different potentials and the membrane potential is not constant, as can be seen

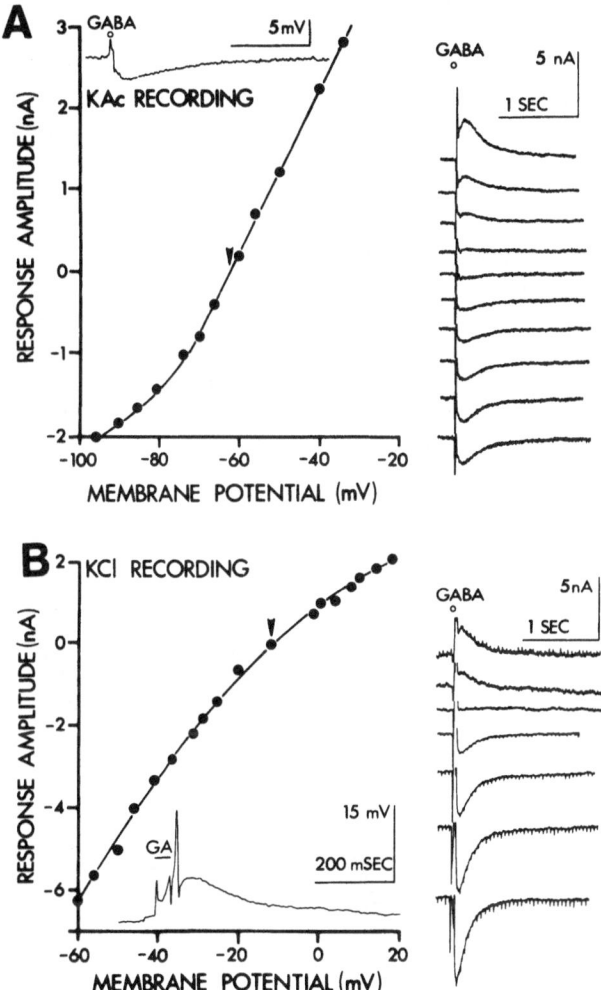

Figure 4. The reversal potential of GABA-evoked current responses is dependent on the Cl^- ion gradient across the cell. (A) The cell was recorded with two intracellular microelectrodes containing potassium acetate and GABA was applied by identical iontophoretic pulse at different potentials. The inset shows the cell recorded in current-clamp mode with GABA eliciting a transient hyperpolarization. When the cell is voltage-clamped GABA evokes membrane current responses which invert in polarity at about -63 mV (arrowhead in current response-membrane potential plot). (B) The cell was recorded with two KCl-filled microelectrodes. Under current clamp the cell depolarizes in response to GABA, triggering an action potential (inset). Under these conditions the current responses invert in amplitude at about -20 mV.

in the nonlinear plots shown in Fig. 4. Some of the nonlinearity is derived from changes in the Cl^- ion gradient that occur as the cell is conditioned at different potentials prior to evoking the current response. However, some of the nonlinearity reflects membrane potential-sensitive aspects of the conductance response. Systematic study of the conductance over a wide range of potential reveals that GABA and glycine invariably evoke relatively more conductance at depolarized levels of membrane potential. The mechanism underlying this phenomenon involves changes in the kinetics of elementary ion channel activation (*vide infra*). This relationship contrasts with that of nicotinic cholinergic-receptor-activated conductances in sympathetic ganglia and muscle membranes, where the kinetics of the conductance at the microscopic level change so that the cholinergic action effectively *diminishes* at depolarized potentials (Dionne and Stevens, 1975). Functionally, then, the inhibitory actions of GABA and glycine are enhanced, and the excitatory actions of acetylcholine reduced when the cell is depolarized, or excited, relative to when it is hyperpolarized, or at rest.

Dose–response curves of brief GABA- and glycine-evoked conductance responses evoked on spinal (Barker and Ransom, 1978) and cortical neurons (Dichter, 1980) invariably have nonlinear portions and log-log plots whose limiting slopes are consistently greater than 1 (Fig. 5). The nonlinearity in

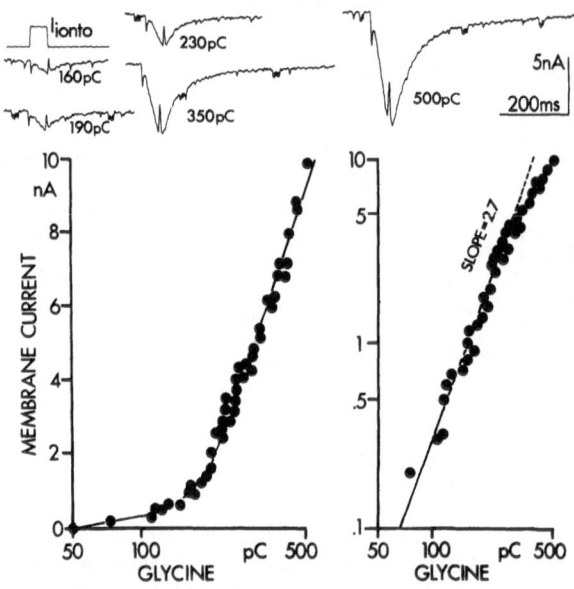

Figure 5. Dose–response curve for glycine-induced membrane currents evoked at −70 mV in a cultured spinal cord neuron. Glycine was applied by microiontophoresis (I_{ionto}) using 50-msec pulses of current. Membrane current responses to increasing iontophoretic charge [indicated in picocoulombs (pc) next to each current trace] are illustrated above semi-log (left) and log-log (right) plots of membrane current as a function of iontophoretic charge. The relationship between response and dose is exponential with a slope of about 2.7. (J. L. Barker, unpublished observations.)

the dose–response relationship reflects a positive cooperativity in the agonist–receptor interaction. The limiting slope of the log-log dose–response curve has been interpreted to reflect the number of agonist molecules involved in the pharmacological response. Dose–response curves for both GABA and glycine (Fig. 5) indicate that binding of two or more transmitter molecules to each receptor site are likely to underlie the pharmacological response.

2.2.2. Fluctuation Analysis of Membrane Current Responses

The mechanisms underlying the conductance responses evoked by GABA and glycine in whole-cell recordings of cultured CNS neurons have been studied using a rather simple model of agonist-receptor activation first applied by Katz and Miledi (1972) to cholinergic activation of cationic conductance in muscle membranes. Katz and Miledi conceptualized that the macroscopic conductance was comprised of many microscopic conductance steps of similar amplitude but variable duration. They analyzed the rapid fluctuations ("noise") in membrane voltage recorded during cholinergic responses as if the fluctuations actually reflected changes in the number of successful agonist–receptor interactions. Their statistical analysis of cholinergic responses and subsequent predictions of the electrical dimensions for the unitary conductance have been confirmed and extended by many other investigators studying agonist responses at muscle and other membranes.

The simple model that has been utilized to analyze macroscopic conductance responses evoked by GABA, glycine, and other agonists involves the following assumptions: (1) that the probability of a successful agonist–receptor interaction is low; (2) that when successful, the interaction leads to an all-or-none, virtually instantaneous transition in membrane conductance to a new constant level; (3) that these transitions occur by Poisson or random processes; and (4) that the duration of the new conductance state is variable in duration. These assumptions are schematically represented in Fig. 6A.

The macroscopic conductance (G) induced by the agonist is thus thought to reflect the summed activities of many independent, microscopic conductance steps. The instantaneous average value of G varies according to N number of channels conducting ions, as depicted in the lowermost trace of Fig. 6A. Activating conductance at a membrane potential where substantial driving force exists leads to detectable current flow, i, through open, conducting ion channels. The macroscopic current response, I, shown in Fig. 6B, thus represents the summed average of N i-sized currents and the average value of I can be equated to Npi, where p is the probability of the conductance mechanism being activated and current flowing.

Inspection of Fig. 6B shows that the current trace during the peak of the agonist-induced response is apparently noisier than that before or following the response. The "noise" associated with the agonist-induced response is quite evident when the response is amplified and AC-coupled to eliminate the slow DC components of the response. Membrane current variance, σ^2,

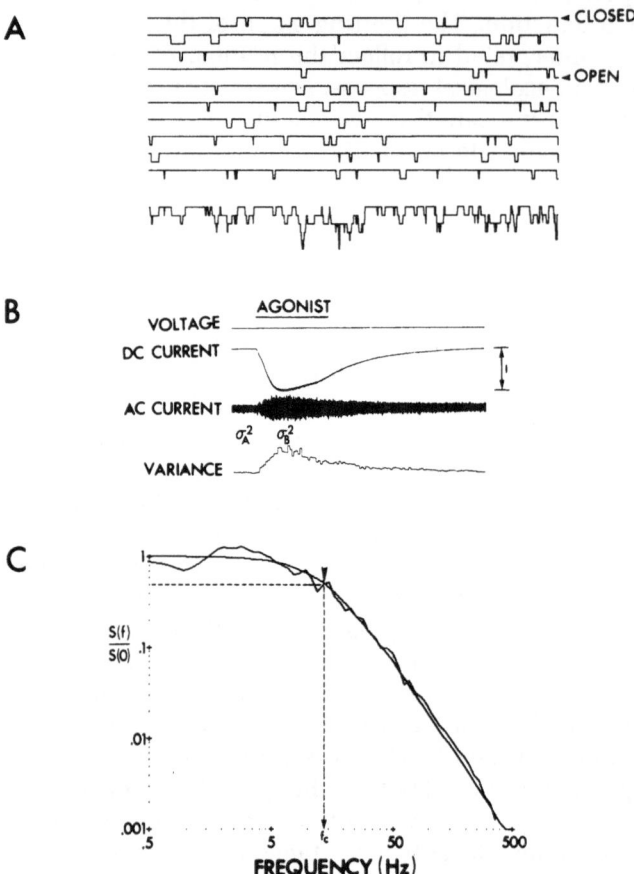

Figure 6. Analysis of agonist-induced fluctuations in membrane conductance. (A) The model at a microscopic level. Computer simulation of agonist-activated microscopic transitions in membrane conductance hypothesized to underlie the agonist-induced current response shown in panel B. The transitions proceed almost instantaneously from a closed (ground) state to an open (conducting) state in a random, all-or-none manner. The activities of 10 independently occurring transitions are schematized individually over the same observation period and then when summed together (lowest trace). The latter shows that the number of open, conducting states fluctuates about an average value. (B) The macroscopic response. Agonist-induced current response in a cell whose membrane potential has been held constant under voltage-clamp. Application of the agonist (indicated by bar) evokes a DC-current response, I, that, when amplified and filtered, is associated with a considerable increase in "noise," as shown in the AC-current trace. Continuous integration of membrane current variance shows that variance changes from a baseline level (σ_A^2) in direct proportion to the evoked current response so that at the peak of the current response the associated variance (σ_B^2) is considerably increased. (C) Spectral analysis of the macroscopic response. Normalized spectrum of agonist-induced current fluctuations (jagged line) plotted in log-log coordinates and fit by a single Lorentzian equation (smooth line). The corner frequency, f_c, of the spectrum (arrowhead) or frequency at which spectral power fails by 50 percent, is 12.7 Hz. Assuming the simple model of microscopic conductance activity outlined above, the calculated f_c yields an estimate for the mean open time of agonist-induced microscopic conductance, τ, from $\tau = (2\pi f_c)^{-1}$.

calculated and displayed at 1 sec intervals, shows that σ^2 increases in direct proportion to the amplitude of the current response. The variance is equal to $Npi^2(1 - p)$. Hence, if $I = Npi$ and $\sigma^2 = Npi^2(1 - p)$, then $\sigma^2/I = i(1 - p)$ and, when $p << 1$, $\sigma^2/I = i$.

Since I and σ^2 can be measured, i can be calculated, and, by knowing the driving force, V_D, the unitary microscopic conductance, γ, can be derived according to the relation $\gamma = I/V_D$. The current variance directly attributable to the agonist can be calculated by measuring the average current variance present before or after the response (σ_A^2) and, assuming this remains constant during the response, subtracting σ_A^2 from the average variance measured during the response, σ_B^2. In this way γ can be derived from I, σ^2, and V_D:

$$\gamma = [(\sigma_B^2 - \sigma_A^2)/I]/V_D$$

The kinetics of fluctuations in microscopic conductance have been studied using statistical techniques that are detailed in recent review articles (Neher and Stevens, 1977; Mathers and Barker, 1982). Much of the statistical analysis utilized in studying unitary conductance kinetics involves calculating the Fourier transform of the autocorrelation function, the power spectrum, which reflects the variance contributed at different frequencies of fluctuation. The power spectrum predicted for the simple model of all-or-none fluctuations in membrane conductance outlined above is the Fourier transform of an exponential. As shown in Fig. 5C, the predicted spectrum can be fit by a Lorentzian curve of the following form

$$S(f) = S(0)/[1 + (f/f_c)^2]$$

where $S(f)$ is the spectral intensity at frequency f, $S(0)$ is the intensity at zero frequency, and f_c is the frequency at which $S(f) = S(0)/2$, or the half-power frequency. If the spectrum of agonist-induced fluctuations can be adequately described by a Lorentzian equation of this form, then the average duration, τ, of γ can be derived from the relationship $\tau = (2 \pi f_c)^{-1}$ (Neher and Stevens, 1977).

In sum, "fluctuation analysis" is the statistical study of what superficially appears to be noise but is really a complex biological signal induced in the membrane by the agonist. From such study, one can estimate the elementary electrical properties of the ion conductance. These quantitative estimates allow hypotheses to be formulated regarding underlying molecular mechanisms and can be used to compare the conductance systems in different biological membranes in a more rigorous manner.

2.2.3. GABA- and Glycine-Induced Conductance Fluctuations are Different

Sustained applications of GABA or glycine to the cell body and processes of cultured spinal neurons invariably evoke current responses that are associated with increases in membrane current variance (Barker et al., 1982). Substantial current and variance responses can be recorded with consistency when GABA is applied to membrane sites up to 100 μm from the cell body, where the intracellular recording microelectrodes are located (Fig. 7). At the level of the cell body, GABA and glycine evoke membrane current responses in a dose-dependent manner (Fig. 8). From cursory inspection it is evident that the variance increase is directly proportional to the amplitude of the current response, as would be expected if more and more of the same microscopic conductance elements were recruited at increasing concentrations of agonist.

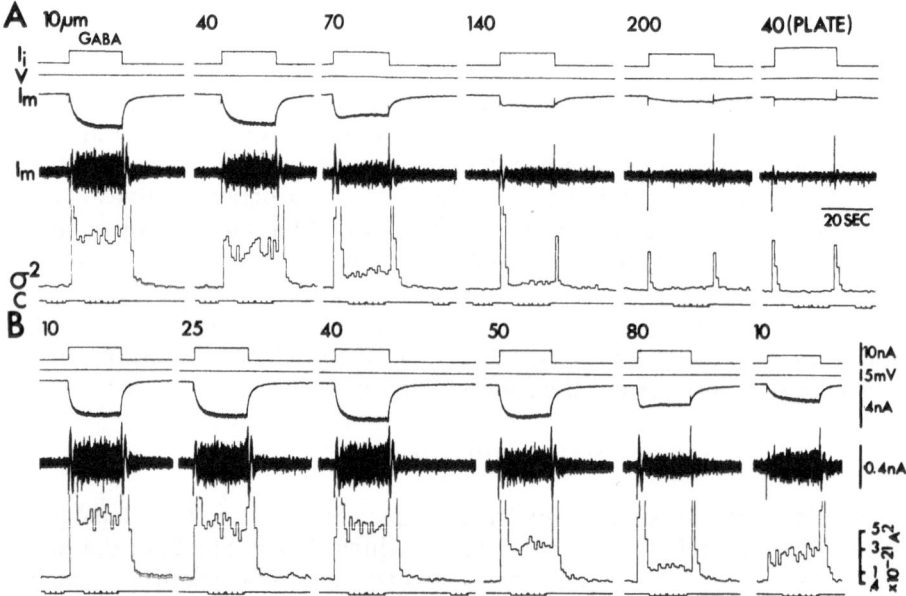

Figure 7. GABA induces current responses at many sites on a cultured spinal neuron. The cell was voltage-clamped at -60 mV and GABA was applied to two processes (A and B) with 30-sec iontophoretic current pulses (I_i) at different distances from the two microelectrodes in the cell body. The iontophoretic pipette was always placed within 2 or 3 μm of the membrane surface. The charge used to pass GABA was such that for most of the applications, no effect could be detected when the pipette was 10 μm above the cell surface. From these results GABA is presumed to be activating membrane conductance within 10 μm of the application site. Current responses obtained within 50 μm of the cell body are similar in amplitude and time course, while those elicited at 70–140 μm have a relatively rapid phase and subsequent sag in the response. A current response is just detectable when GABA is applied at 200 μm, while no response can be obtained when significantly more charge than normally employed is used to iontophorese GABA onto the plate 40 μm from the microelectrodes. All responses elicited at sites closer than 50 μm are associated with microscopic fluctuations, which are obvious in the high-gain, AC-coupled record, and membrane current variance, which is plotted on-line in the trace labeled σ^2. When current responses of the same amplitude are evoked near and far from the recording electrodes, the closer response has considerably more variance. (From Barker et al., 1982, with permission.)

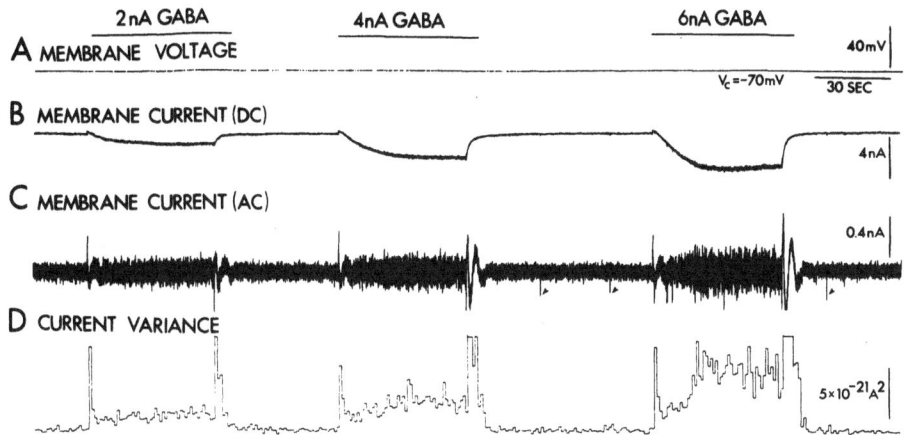

Figure 8. GABA applied to the cell body evokes membrane current responses in a dose-dependent manner. Increasing iontophoretic applications of 2, 4, and 6 nA elicit membrane current responses of increasing amplitude (B), which are associated with progressively more fluctuations (C) and variance (D). The arrowheads mark inward-going spontaneous synaptic currents (shown in Figs. 18, 19). (From Barker et al., 1982, with permission.)

Spectral analysis of the current fluctuations in the baseline current trace reveals that the power in particular fluctuation frequencies decreases monotonically over the range of frequencies studied (Fig. 9A). Spectral analysis of the fluctuations associated with current responses induced by GABA demonstrates that the power inherent in the spectrum is substantially greater over the entire range of frequencies studied relative to that associated with the baseline variance and, further, that the spectrum "rolls off" as frequency increases such that power is distributed exponentially across the range of frequencies analyzed (Fig. 9A). Subtracting the variance of the baseline current from the GABA-induced variance gives the variance attributable to GABA's actions, the spectrum of which is well fitted by a Lorentzian equation of the form expected from exponentially distributed power (Fig. 9B). Spectral analysis of the variance thus indicates that, *as a first approximation*, the membrane current response evoked by GABA can be interpreted as resulting from the summed activities of many similarly sized, all-or-none microscopic currents whose durations are exponentially distributed. Estimates of the microscopic conductance and average duration of pharmacological responses to GABA are schematized in Fig. 10B.

Analysis of membrane current responses induced by glycine has led to a similar conclusion, namely, that glycine's macroscopic actions can be characterized as arising from the summed activities of all-or-none transitions in unitary-sized microscopic conductances whose durations are exponentially distributed. However, when compared to current responses evoked by GABA in the same cell, it is apparent that the variance associated with a current response of about the same amplitude induced by glycine is appreciably

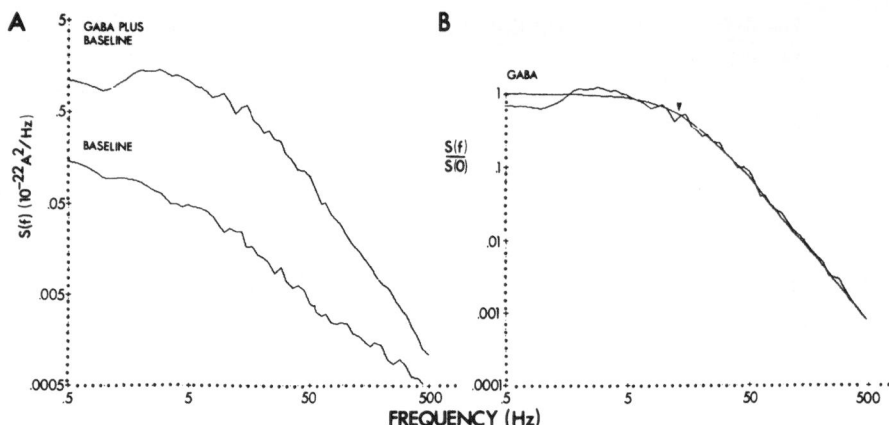

Figure 9. Spectral analysis of GABA-induced fluctuations in membrane current. Shown are two normalized spectra similar to that illustrated in Fig. 5C. (A) The spectrum of fluctuations in membrane current obtained at the level of resting membrane potential before delivery of GABA (baseline) shows that power decreases monotonically with increasing frequency. After application of GABA sufficient to sustain a current response of several nA, the power in the spectrum is greater at all frequencies sampled relative to that derived from analysis of baseline fluctuations (GABA plus baseline). (B) The spectrum calculated from the difference between the spectrum obtained before and during the GABA-induced response is closely fit by a Lorentzian equation. The corner-frequency, f_c (marked by an arrowhead), is 12.7 Hz, corresponding to an estimated channel lifetime of 12.5 msec. (From Barker et al., 1982, with permission.)

greater than that induced by GABA (Fig. 10A). Spectral analysis of the variance has led to estimates of the average duration of the microscopic conductance that are significantly shorter than that estimated for ion channels activated by GABA (Fig. 10B). β-Alanine, another endogenous neutral amino acid, activates ion channels whose electrical properties appear to be consistently different from those estimated for either GABA or glycine (Fig. 10B).

2.2.4. Direct Recording of Ion Channels Activated by GABA and Glycine

Direct recordings of the electrical activities of ion channels activated by GABA and glycine have recently been obtained by several groups of investigators using an innovative electrophysiological approach called the "patch clamp" (Hamill et al., 1981). The technique involves fashioning a tight mechanical and electrical seal between a micron-sized patch of surface membrane and a smooth-edged glass microelectrode, which is connected to a fast, low-noise current-amplifying system. By electrically isolating the patch of membrane, it becomes possible to detect ion channel currents resulting from individual agonist–receptor interactions (see Sakmann and Neher, 1983). In this way pharmacological actions of agonists in the patch can be resolved directly at an elementary level.

The results thus far demonstrate that, as predicted from fluctuation analysis, the microscopic conductances of Cl^- ion channels activated by GABA

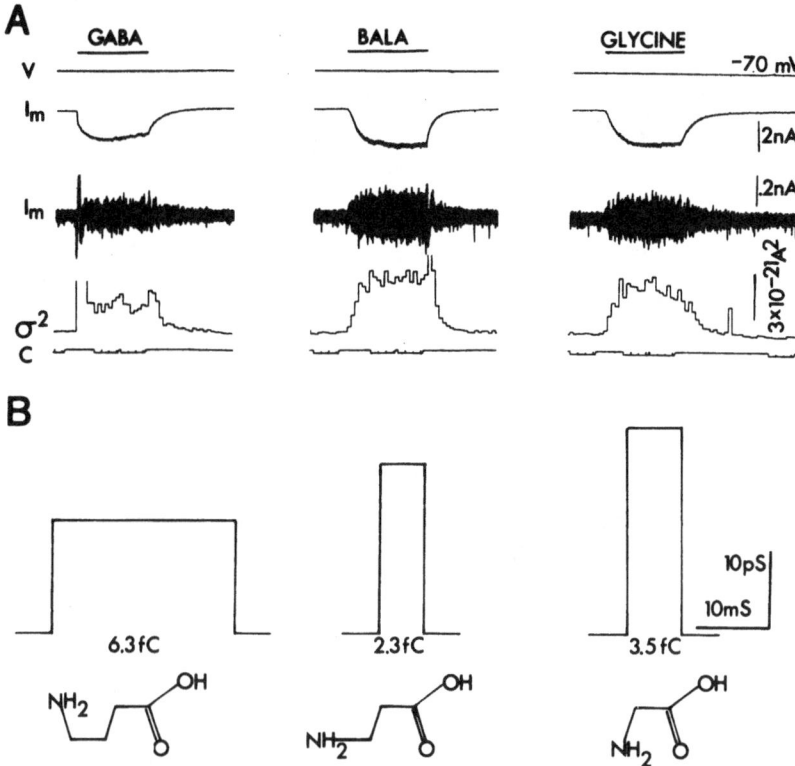

Figure 10. Fluctuation analysis of membrane current responses to GABA, glycine, and β-alanine (BALA) yields estimates of different ion channel properties. (A) The spinal cord cell was voltage-clamped at −70 mV (V) and the three amino acids applied to the cell body by pressure. Each evokes an inward current response of about the same amplitude (upper traces marked I_m). Each response is associated with an increase both in current fluctuations (shown in the AC-coupled, 10× amplified lower traces marked I_m) and in current variance (trace labeled σ^2). Disproportionately more variance is observed during the glycine- and β-alanine-evoked responses. Traces marked C indicate periods when baseline and response were sampled for computer-assisted analysis. (B) Schematic representations of the estimated average electrical properties underlying the amino acid-elicited responses. The charge estimated for each average-sized microscopic event is indicated in femtocoulombs (fC). The chemical structures of each amino acid are shown at the bottom. The results reveal that for these particular responses, and for all others studied thus far in otherwise "unidentified" spinal neurons, the estimated electrical properties of ion channels are unique to each amino acid transmitter.

and glycine are indeed significantly different (Fig. 11). In fact, in "on-cell" patch-clamp recordings, which are similar in their ionic conditions to those used in fluctuation analysis experiments, direct measurements of the unitary conductance are in excellent agreement with estimates derived from fluctuation analysis (Jackson et al., 1982). The resolution afforded by patch-clamp measurements has also revealed the existence of secondary, and, in the case of glycine, tertiary conductance states that occur about one-sixth as often as the primary, or "main-state" conductance event. Two of the con-

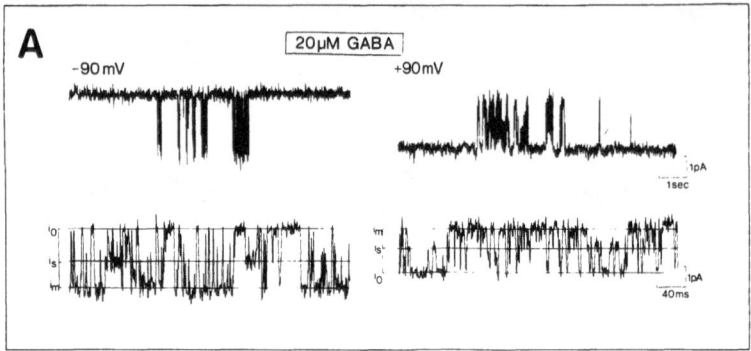

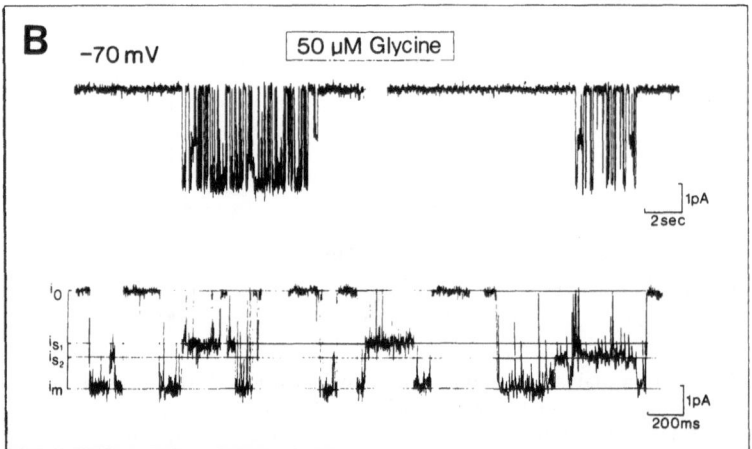

Figure 11. Elementary ion channel behavior recorded in a microscopic patch of somal membrane excised from a cultured mouse spinal cord neuron. The direct recording of channel activity has been made under conditions designed to isolate Cl⁻ ion conductances from all others. Using ultra-sensitive amplifiers, the single channel currents developing in response to GABA (A) and glycine (B) can readily be detected and their electrical properties studied at high resolution. Both amino acids cause virtually instantaneous transitions in membrane conductance at a microscopic level, resulting in the sudden appearance of picoampere (pA)-sized currents. The amplitude of the current flow is dependent on the potential at which the currents are recorded, and the current steps reverse in polarity when the transmembrane potential is brought past the equilibrium potential level where the electrical and ionic gradients are equal and opposite. In panel (A), GABA evokes mostly 2-pA-sized events that are downward-going at -90 mV and upward-going at $+70$ mV. Expanded versions of the activity in these recordings (lower traces) reveals three distinct current levels, corresponding to baseline (i_o), a secondary state accounting for 3% of the activity (i_s) and a main level (i_m), which is obtained 97% of the time. Panel (B) shows glycine-activated channel events [recorded at -70 mV and displayed at slow (upper traces) and fast time bases (lower traces)]. There are three distinct levels evident during current flow. The primary state (i_m) occurs 80% of the time, while the secondary is seen 15% (i_{s2}) and the tertiary 5% (i_{s1}). (From Hamill et al., 1983, with permission.)

ductance states activated by GABA and glycine are identical, as if certain aspects of the molecular actions of these transmitters are quite similar. Indeed, occlusion rather than addition of macroscopic conductance responses at the whole cell level (Barker and McBurney, 1979a; Fig. 12) and activation of channels by both transmitters within the same patch have both been observed (Hamill et al., 1983), suggesting that certain steps in the process of Cl^- conductance activation by GABA and glycine may well be shared. However, some patches exhibit only GABA-activatable ion channels and others express only glycine-inducible events, indicating that, at the microscopic level, not all Cl^- channels are necessarily operated by both transmitters. Whether the two receptors can physically couple to and operate the same Cl^- ion channel has not yet been resolved.

The kinetics of GABA-activated ion channels have been studied in detail with the single-channel recording technique. The transitions between open, conducting and closed, nonconducting states occur with kinetics more complex than can be detected when the population of ion channels is activated

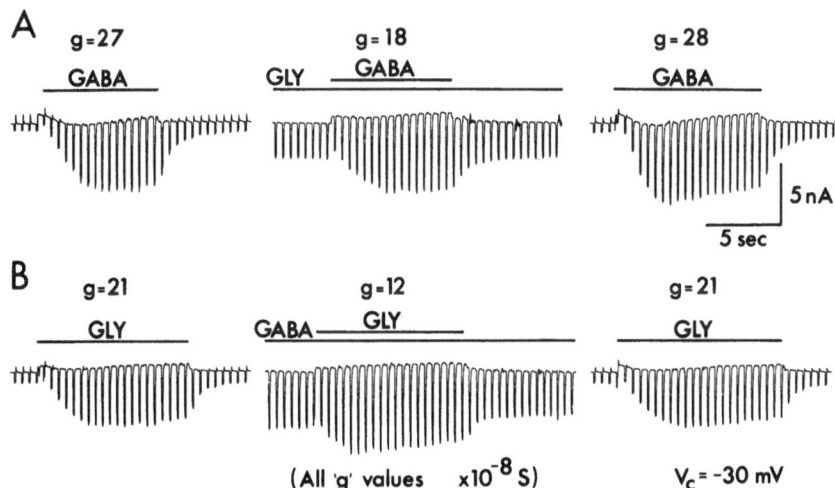

Figure 12. GABA- and glycine-evoked conductance responses occlude rather than add. A spinal cord neuron was clamped at -30 mV using two KCl-filled microelectrodes. GABA and glycine were iontophoresed independently or together during periods indicated by the bars above the current traces. The downward-going deflections are current responses to 20 nA, 100-msec voltage commands. The amplitude of these responses directly reflects membrane conductance. GABA activates peak, sustained-conductance responses of 270 and 280 nS and glycine evokes responses of 210 nS. If the two independent responses were simply additive, then one might expect a total conductance increase amounting to 470 or 480 nS. However, when the substances are applied coincidentally, the total conductance amounts to less than 300 nS, and subtracting the conductance activated by one from that activated by both gives values that, in each case, are significantly less than "control" values obtained before and after coincident application. This, as well as other data, have led to the notion that the amino acids may share a common step at some point in the reaction that culminates in membrane conductance. (J. L. Barker and R. N. McBurney, unpublished observations.)

for fluctuation analysis. At the single-channel level, two distinct phases of ion channel kinetics can be resolved in the majority of patches (Jackson et al., 1982; Sakmann et al., 1983; Redmann et al., 1983, 1984). Both phases can be adequately described by exponential kinetics. The slower of the two phases has a time constant that closely approximates estimates derived from spectral analysis and accounts for about 95% of the current signal. The faster component readily seen in patch-clamp recordings has been detected, albeit infrequently, in spectra of macroscopic conductance responses. Unfortunately, its insignificant contribution to the conductance response and its inconsistent expression in spectral analyses of fluctuations have obviated detailed study and, at present, it is not clear how the fast and slow kinetic phases of Cl^- ion conductance activity at the level of the single-channel are related to each other. Thus, at equilibrium, the distribution of GABA-activated conducting periods recorded in patches of membrane can be described by two exponential processes, the slower of which accounts for most of the signal and corresponds closely to that detectable at the level of the whole cell.

Kinetic analysis of the nonconducting periods in patch-clamp recordings shows that this aspect of ion channel activity can also be described by fast and slow exponentials as if there might be several distinct moments in the binding and unbinding reactions associated with all-or-none triggering of Cl^- ion movement (Redmann et al., 1984).

These results with patch-clamp assays confirm and extend estimates of ion channel properties derived from fluctuation analysis. Taken together, the results obtained with the two strategies indicate that, in neurons cultured from the mammalian spinal cord, the elementary mechanisms underlying the Cl^- conductance responses induced by pharmacological applications of GABA and glycine involve essentially all-or-none, microscopic transitions to different levels of conductance, each lasting for a variable time. Essentially similar conclusions have been drawn from the results obtained in experiments carried out in lamprey brainstem neurons, which are sensitive to both GABA and glycine (Gold and Martin, 1983a,b). Fluctuation analysis of current responses induced by GABA in cultured mouse sensory neurons, where the Cl^- ion gradient is such that the action is typically depolarizing, and in cultured hippocampal neurons, where the effect is invariably hyperpolarizing, strongly suggest that the electrical properties of the activated Cl^- ion channels are quite similar in functionally distinct cell types. Since some of the data is likely to be derived from extrasynaptic as well as synaptic ion channels, it also appears that, in contrast to cholinergically operated cation channels at synaptic and extrasynaptic sites in muscle membranes, the properties of anion channels closely overlap at the two sites. Similar results have been reported for GABA-evoked responses in invertebrate *muscle* membranes (Dudel et al., 1980; Cull-Candy, 1983) where the estimated duration is shorter but the conductance values predicted are close to those observed in cultured neuronal membranes. The electrical properties of pharmacologically operated channels in several invertebrate and vertebrate membranes

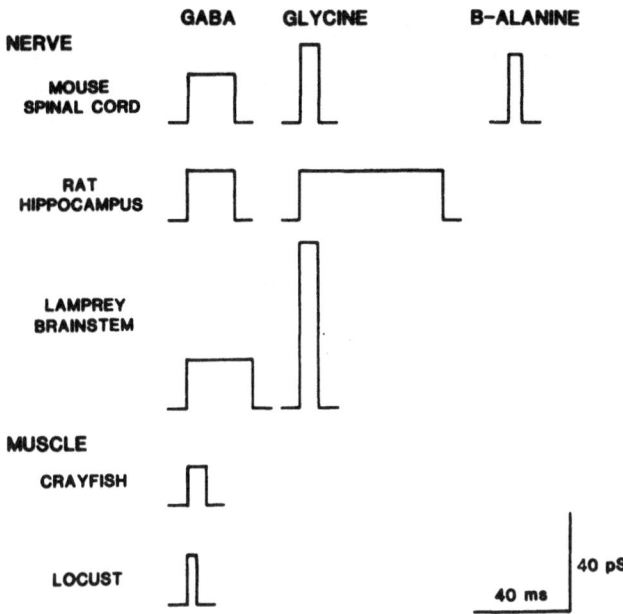

Figure 13. Schematic representations of the estimated electrical properties of GABA, glycine, and β-alanine activated Cl⁻ channels in different nerve and muscle membranes. In each case the properties, which are estimates derived from fluctuation analysis, are those reported for −60 mV and a temperature of 24°C, or extrapolated to these parameters. GABA-activated conductance is relatively constant, while elementary duration is longer in nerve than muscle. In neuronal membranes these properties appear independent of functional synaptic innervation. Glycine-evoked channels have significantly different electrical dimensions in those membranes whose functional physiological innervation by both transmitters is either quite likely or considered to be established. The effects of glycine recorded in hippocampus may reflect GABA-mimetic properties of high concentrations of glycine. (Data derived for Onodera and Takeuchi, 1979; Cull-Candy, 1983; Gold and Martin, 1983a,b).

are summarized in Fig. 13. They should serve as useful reference for considering Cl⁻-dependent conductance mechanisms physiologically elaborated at synapses (*vide infra*).

2.2.5. Pharmacological Modulation of Transmitter-Activated Cl⁻ Channels

A variety of clinically important drugs alter Cl⁻ ion conductance responses evoked by GABA and glycine. For example, CNS depressants potentiate these pharmacological responses, while other drugs that stimulate CNS excitability (e.g., convulsants) depress the responses. Although the results strongly implicate transmitter-activated Cl⁻ conductances as an important site for these drug actions *in vivo*, causality has not been established between the modulation of GABA-induced responses and the gross behavioral state induced by the drugs.

The drug effects have been examined by applying fluctuation analysis to GABA-induced responses under control conditions and in the presence of modulating concentrations of drug. GABA-evoked responses potentiated by the benzodiazepine diazepam and the anesthetic barbiturate pentobarbital are shown in Fig. 14. At the level of resolution afforded by fluctuation analysis, it is apparent that these (and related) drugs all affect the *kinetics* rather than the conductance associated with ion channel activity (Study and Barker, 1981; Barker et al., 1983). For example, diazepam potentiates GABA-evoked responses primarily by increasing the rate of ion channel activation and secondarily by decreasing the rate at which channels close so that more channel openings occur per unit time and, on average, somewhat more charge is transferred per opening. The effects of increasing doses of diazepam on estimated ion channel properties are summarized in Fig. 15. In contrast, pentobarbital potentiates GABA-evoked responses primarily by decreasing the rate of channel closure so that once open, channels conduct for a substantially longer period, as if the drug cooperates with the transmitter to stabilize the open, conducting state of the channel.

The depressant effects of strychnine on glycine-induced responses, and of bicuculline and picrotoxin on GABA-evoked responses, all appear to result from a dose-dependent decrease in the rate of ion channel activation. A summary of the results of fluctuation analysis applied to strychnine-depressed glycine-evoked responses is shown in Fig. 16.

These results have led to the tentative conclusion that some clinically important drugs can modulate the rate of channel opening and/or the rate of channel closing. These modulatory actions effectively change the flux of

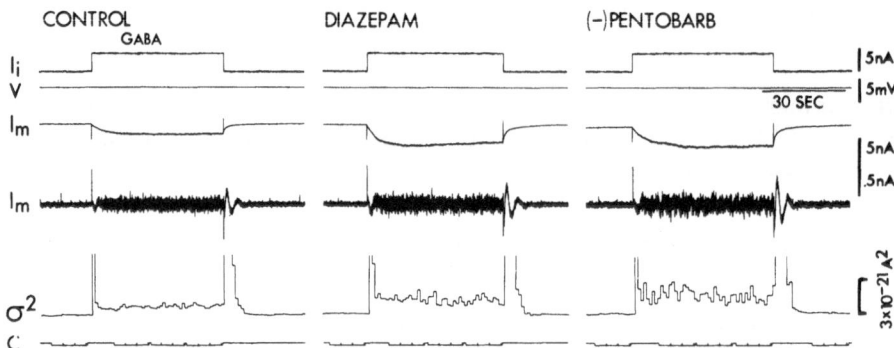

Figure 14. Clinically important drugs potentiate GABA-evoked responses. GABA was iontophoresed with identical current pulses (I_i) onto a cell held at -60 mV (V) under control conditions or in the presence of clinically relevant concentrations of diazepam (10 μM) or ($-$)pentobarbital (100 μM). The DC-coupled current response evoked by GABA (upper row of traces marked I_m) is nearly doubled in amplitude in the presence of the drugs. There is a corresponding increase in membrane current fluctuations (lower row of traces marked I_m) and 1-sec integrations of current variance (σ^2). (From Study and Barker, 1981, with permission.)

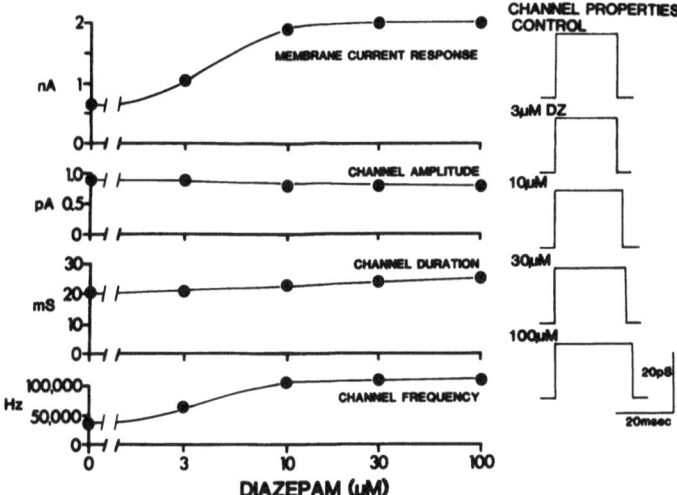

Figure 15. Fluctuation analysis of dose-dependent potentiation of GABA-evoked responses by diazepam. Changes in the amplitude of the macroscopic membrane current response evoked by identical applications of GABA are plotted in the topmost graph as a function of the logarithim of diazepam concentration. The response increases from 0.6 nA to about 2.0 nA over the 3–30 μM range. Estimates of elementary ion channel properties derived from analyses of macroscopic current responses are plotted as a function of drug concentration in the lower three graphs. Elementary current amplitude, a direct reflection of unitary conductance, does not change, while the duration of the unitary conductance and the rate of its activation are both increased. Since the macroscopic current is equal to the product of the number of channels conducting at any moment and the microscopic current flowing through each channel, it is evident that one can account, in a quantitative manner, for the potentiation of macroscopic responses in terms of changes in microscopic kinetics. The estimated average electrical properties of the GABA-activated channels under control conditions and at the different drug concentrations are shown in schematic fashion on the right. (R. E. Study and J. L. Barker, unpublished observations.)

Cl^- ions induced by these transmitters in characteristic ways that are consistent with their clinical pharmacology.

3. SYNAPTICALLY ACTIVATED Cl^- CONDUCTANCE MECHANISMS

Physiologically activated Cl^- conductances during "inhibitory" postsynaptic potentials (IPSPs) have been studied in a variety of experimental preparations of invertebrate and vertebrate tissue, including cells cultured from the embryonic CNS. It is clear that some of the functional contacts between cultured neurons involve activation of Cl^- conductances that serve to momentarily depress action potential generation in target cells. Cells cultured from the embryonic vertebrate spinal cord exhibit presumed Cl^--me-

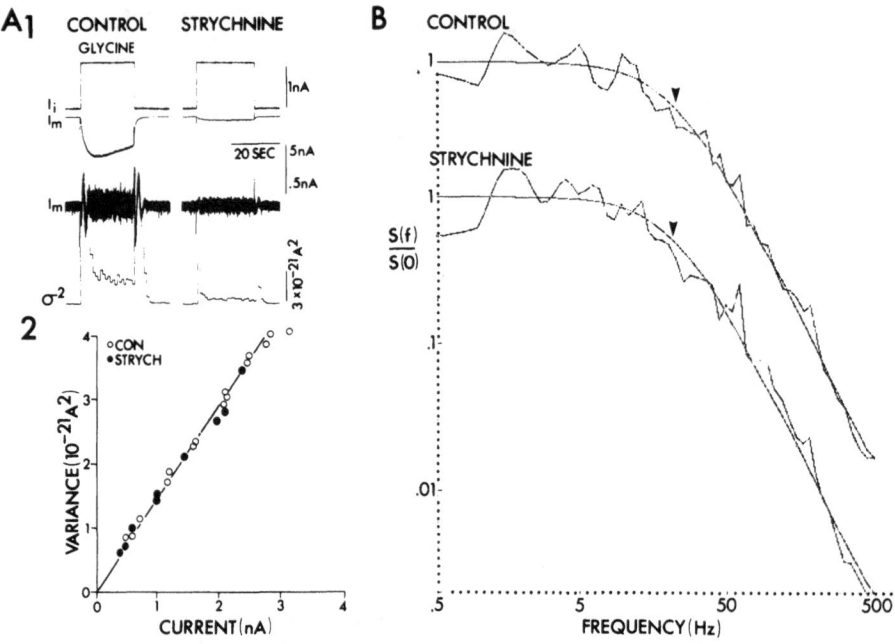

Figure 16. Fluctuation analysis of strychnine-induced depression of glycine-evoked membrane current responses. The recording was made with two KCl-filled microelectrodes and the cell was held at -60 mV while different amounts of glycine were iontophoresed under control conditions or in the presence of strychnine. (A1) Representative examples of control and strychnine-depressed current responses (I_m) evoked by identical iontophoretic pulses (I_i) of glycine. The fluctuations apparent on the lower I_m trace during the control response and the corresponding variance (σ^2) are virtually eliminated by strychnine. (A2) Plot of σ^2 as a function of current response amplitude for a range of responses evoked under control conditions and in the presence of strychnine, showing that the linear relationship between σ^2 and current amplitude is not changed by the drug. (B) Normalized power spectra of the type illustrated in Fig. 8B reflecting the distribution of log (power) as a function of log (frequency) for spectra calculated from fluctuations generated under control conditions and in the presence of strychnine. The jagged line is the experimental data, while the smooth curve shows the best-fitting Lorentzian equation that accounts for the data. In each spectra the arrowhead indicates the corner frequency, f_c, at which power falls by 50%. This is unchanged in strychnine, indicating no apparent difference in the estimated average open-time for channels activated under control and during experimental conditions. (From Barker et al., 1983, with permission.)

diated synaptic potentials that are heterogenous with respect to time courses and pharmacological sensitivities. Those events decaying in less than 10 msec are consistently blocked by strychnine and are insensitive to both picrotoxin and diazepam (Choi et al., 1981; Fig. 17). Those decaying in more than 10 msec (Fig. 18) are sensitive to picrotoxin (Barker et al., 1980b; Choi et al., 1981; Fig. 19). Superficially, the different time courses and drug sensitivities of these naturally occurring signals appear to be related to the pharmacological actions of GABA and glycine discussed above and suggest that the faster and slower signals may be mediated by glycine and GABA,

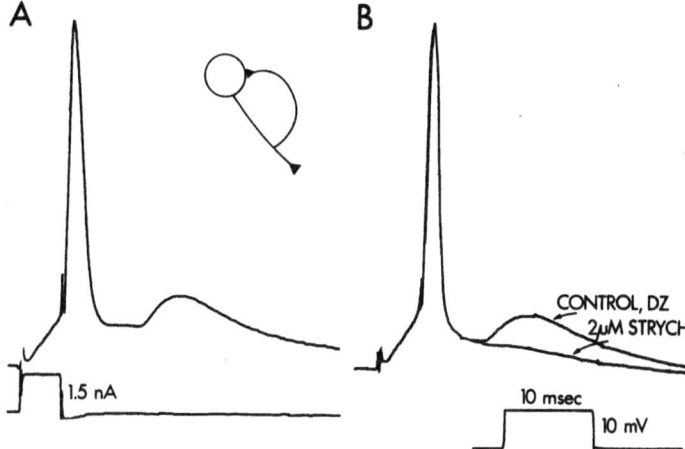

Figure 17. Strychnine-sensitive synaptic potential evoked in a cultured spinal neuron is short-lasting. An intracellular recording was made with a single KCl-filled microelectrode. (A) A brief depolarizing 1.5 nA current stimulus triggers an action potential, which is followed after several msec delay by a depolarizing event that decays in less than 10 msec. This event probably reflects a recurrent synaptic circuit (schematized in the inset since the event could be elicited with both minimal delay and little failure at 10-Hz stimulation rate. Its amplitude was dependent on Ca_o^{2+} and it disappeared in low concentrations of Co^{2+}. (B) Strychnine applied in the vicinity of the recorded cell, blocked the synaptic event without affecting the presynaptic action potential, while diazepam (DZ) was altogether ineffective. (J. L. Barker and M. A. Rogawski, unpublished observations.)

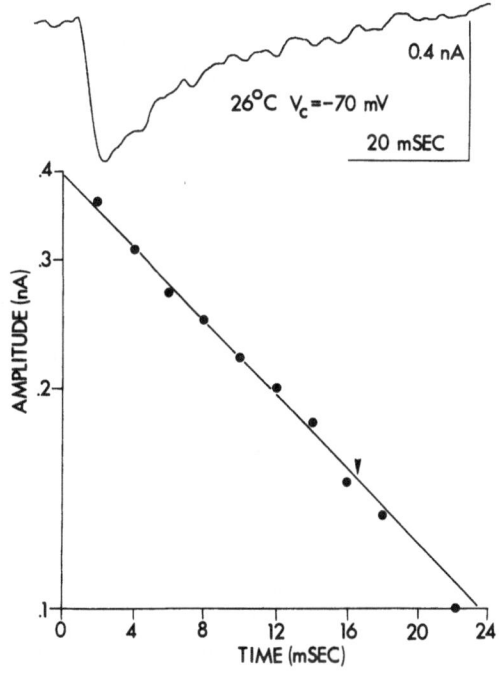

Figure 18. Long-lasting spontaneous postsynaptic current recorded in a cultured spinal neuron. The cell was voltage-clamped at −70 mV with two KCl-filled microelectrodes. Spontaneously occurring, rapidly rising, slowly decaying currents that inverted at the same membrane potential as pharmacological responses to GABA were recorded in this cell. The top trace shows a pen-recorder tracing derived off-line from a digital oscilloscope recording of a representative event recorded at −70 mV. Below is plotted in semilogarithmic fashion the time course of current decay. The arrowhead indicates a time constant of decay of about 16 msec. (Modified from Barker and McBurney, 1979b.)

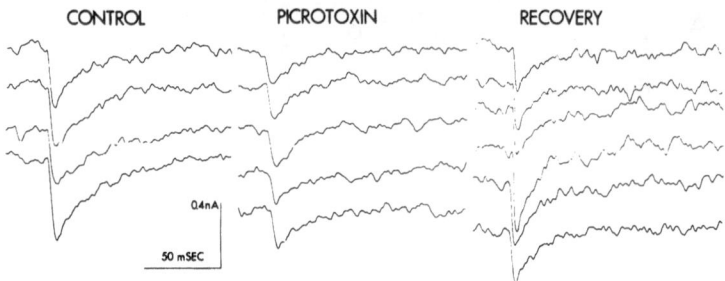

`Figure 19.` Picrotoxin attenuates long-lasting spontaneous synaptic currents in a cultured spinal neuron. The synaptic events were recorded at -70 mV in the same cell shown in Fig. 18. Representative currents are shown before, during, and after application of picrotoxin in the vicinity of the recorded cell. (J. L. Barker and R. N. McBurney, unpublished observations.)

respectively. The variable expression of specific synaptic potentials in cultured spinal neurons has thus far precluded little more than superficial identification of the transmitters and associated ionic conductances. However, detailed comparisons of postsynaptic physiology with the pharmacological actions of GABA have been made using cultured hippocampal cells, in which long-lasting, Cl^--dependent synaptic events have been frequently recorded.

3.1. Long-Lasting Synaptic Conductance in Cultured Hippocampal Neurons

About half of the synaptic potentials recorded in cultured hippocampal cells are hyperpolarizing and reverse in polarity at -60 mV, like GABA-evoked responses (Fig. 20A–D) (Segal and Barker, 1984a). Under current clamp, the IPSP decay lasts many tens of milliseconds. Changes in the Cl^- gradient alter the reversal potentials of the synaptic response and the GABA-evoked response in an identical, Nernstian manner, indicating that they both primarily involve activation of Cl^- conductance. Functionally, the hyperpolarizing property of the synaptic conductance and the shunting of membrane resistance effectively decrease the probability of action potential generation so the synaptic events are considered IPSPs. High-frequency electrical stimulation of the presynaptic neuron evokes a succession of IPSPs that fade in amplitude yet summate sufficiently to hold the cell hyperpolarized (Fig. 20E,F). For at least brief periods inhibitory signals can be repeated at rates up to 20 Hz with little, if any decrement in functional effect. At rates of ~1 Hz the signal remains constant for long periods.

Voltage clamp of the postsynaptic cell using two intracellular electrodes in the cell body reveals the Cl^- ion currents activated during synaptic transmission (Fig. 21). When the cell is clamped within the normally observed range of resting membrane potential and a sizable driving force is sustained with Cl -filled microelectrodes, the evoked synaptic currents typically peak at about 2 nA and decay with single exponential kinetics. The time constant of inhibitory postsynaptic current decay, τ_{IPSC}, averages about 20 msec, which is not significantly different from the mean duration of ion channels activated by GABA, τ_{GABA}, in the same neuron at the same potential as determined by fluctuation analysis (Segal and Barker, 1984b). When the cell is depolarized to positive membrane potentials, τ_{IPSC} usually increases slightly as does τ_{GABA}. Thus, the kinetics of both the pharmacological response and the physiological event appear similar at resting and depolarized potentials. The one-to-one correspondence between τ_{GABA} and τ_{IPSC} strongly suggests that the synaptically driven event is mediated by GABA. If so, then the kinetics of pharmacologically activated conductances in CNS neurons may serve as useful reference in identifying specific synaptic signals in these cells.

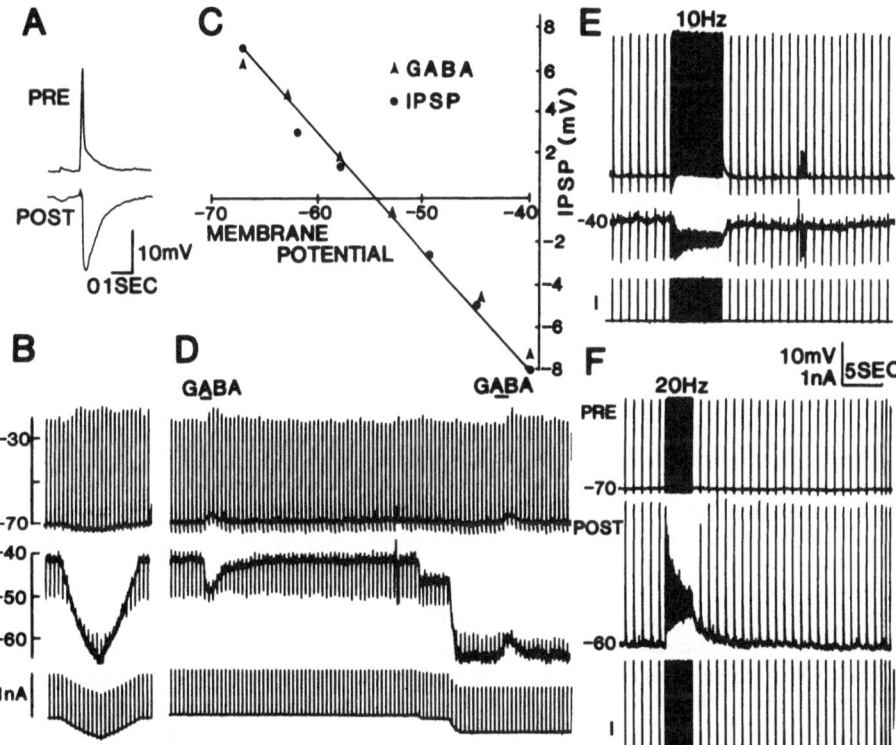

Figure 20. Evoked synaptic potentials invert at the same potential as GABA-induced responses in a cultured hippocampal neuron. Simultaneous intracellular recordings were made in two cells, the postsynaptic element being recorded with a potassium acetate-filled microelectrode. (A) Depolarizing current injected in the presynaptic element triggers an action potential and evokes a hyperpolarizing synaptic potential in the postsynaptic cell. (B) Current injected postsynaptically polarizes the cell and inverts the synaptic event. (C) Both synaptic potentials and GABA-evoked responses (several of which are illustrated in panel D) invert at the same potential (−55 mV). (E) Repetitive synaptic stimulation at 1 Hz elicits a constant-amplitude signal, while at higher stimulation frequency, the signal summates and then declines in amplitude. (F) Similar effects of increasing stimulation frequency occur when the cell is recorded with a KCl-filled microelectrode. (From M. Segal and J. L. Barker, 1984b, with permission.)

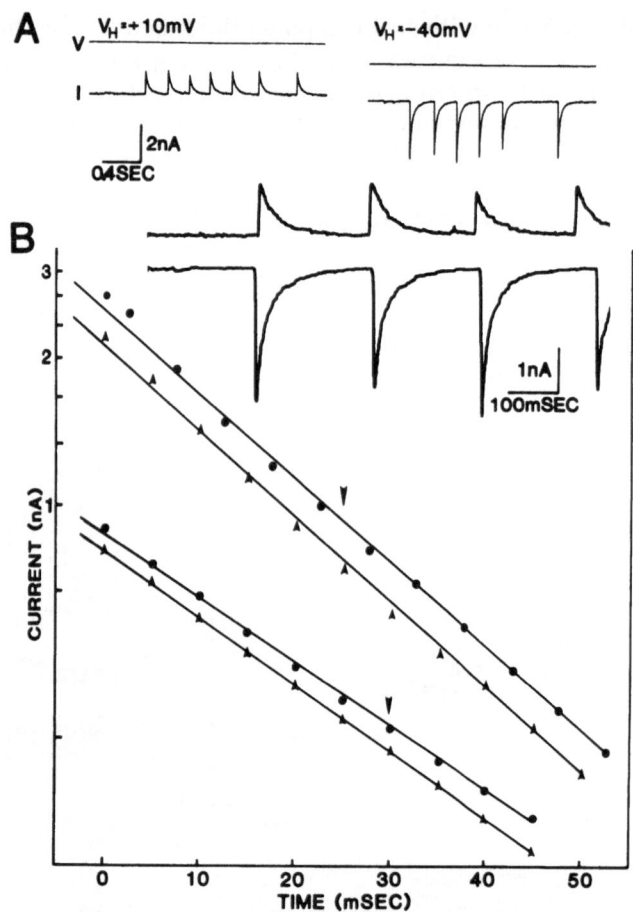

Figure 21. Long-lasting synaptic currents recorded in a cultured hippocampal neuron. The cell was voltage-clamped with two KCl-filled microelectrodes and synaptic currents were evoked by applying brief pulses of glutamate to a presumed presynaptic neuron. (A) Since under these recording conditions the synaptic responses invert at -15 mV, inwardly directed currents (I) are observed at -40 mV and outwardly directed currents are seen at $+10$ mV. (B) Semilogarithmic plots of synaptic current decay as a function of time shows that at both potentials the currents decay as single exponentials and that the time constant of decay (arrowheads) is about 25 msec at -40 mV and 30 msec at $+10$ mV. (From Segal and Barker, 1984b, with permission.)

A comparison between the kinetics of IPSC decay and GABA-activated channel open time estimated from fluctuation analysis of macroscopic current responses obtained in cultured hippocampal neurons under various experimental conditions is summarized in Table 1. The ratio between τ_{IPSC} and τ_{GABA} is close to unity for most of these comparisons indicating that at the postsynaptic membrane the time course of the physiologically evoked conductance corresponds quite closely to the average duration of channels activated by GABA for a variety of experimental conditions. These results, coupled with immunocytochemical evidence for the presence of glutamic

Table 1. Comparison of τ_{IPSC} and τ_{GABA} in Rat Hippocampal Neurons

	τ_{IPSC}(ms)	τ_{GABA}(ms)	Ratio	Reference [a]
Culture				
−60 mV	20	20	1.0	A
+10 mV	30	30	1.0	A
Picrotoxin	18	21	0.8	A
Pentobarbital	70	50	1.4	A
Diazepam	30	26	1.1	A
Slice				
−60 mV	10–18	—	—	B
Pentobarbital	(increased)	—	—	B

[a](A) Segal and Barker, 1984b; (B) Collingridge, Gage, and Robertson, 1983.

acid decarboxylase-positive terminals investing cultured hippocampal neurons (Caserta and Barker, 1983), lead to the logical conclusion that the IPSCs are mediated by GABA.

Assuming this to be true, then from knowledge of the average unitary conductance activated by GABA (~16 pS), one can estimate that during the peak of the synaptic conductance about 1700 channels are active. Moreover, the open-time distribution of the individual channels seems to account for the exponential time course of IPSC decay. Thus, one might consider the time course of the evoked synaptic current to reflect the rapid diffusion of GABA across the synaptic cleft followed by near simultaneous activation of several thousand receptor-coupled ion channel complexes that conduct Cl^- ions at more-or-less the same rate, but for variable periods. The time course of synaptic current decay, then, may be a histogram of the number of channels conducting Cl^- ions for various durations. Most of the channels activated are open for only brief periods with fewer and fewer numbers open for longer and longer times. There is little, if any, convincing evidence that the synaptic current decays in two, kinetically distinct phases. Thus, the fast phase of ion channel activity observed in patch-clamp recordings cannot clearly be detected in whole-cell recordings of macroscopic pharmacologic responses or synaptic signals.

3.2. Pharmacological Modulation of IPSCs in Cultured Hippocampal Neurons

Further evidence that these inhibitory synaptic conductances are indeed mediated by GABA comes from pharmacological experiments involving modulation of IPSCs by clinically important drugs that affect GABA-evoked Cl^- conductance (*vide supra*). At clinically relevant concentrations, benzodiazepines and barbiturates like diazepam and pentobarbital, which potentiate GABA-induced conductance by modulating the kinetics of channel activity, alter the amplitude and/or decay kinetics of IPSCs evoked in cultured hippocampal neurons (Segal and Barker, 1984b; Fig. 22). Each drug

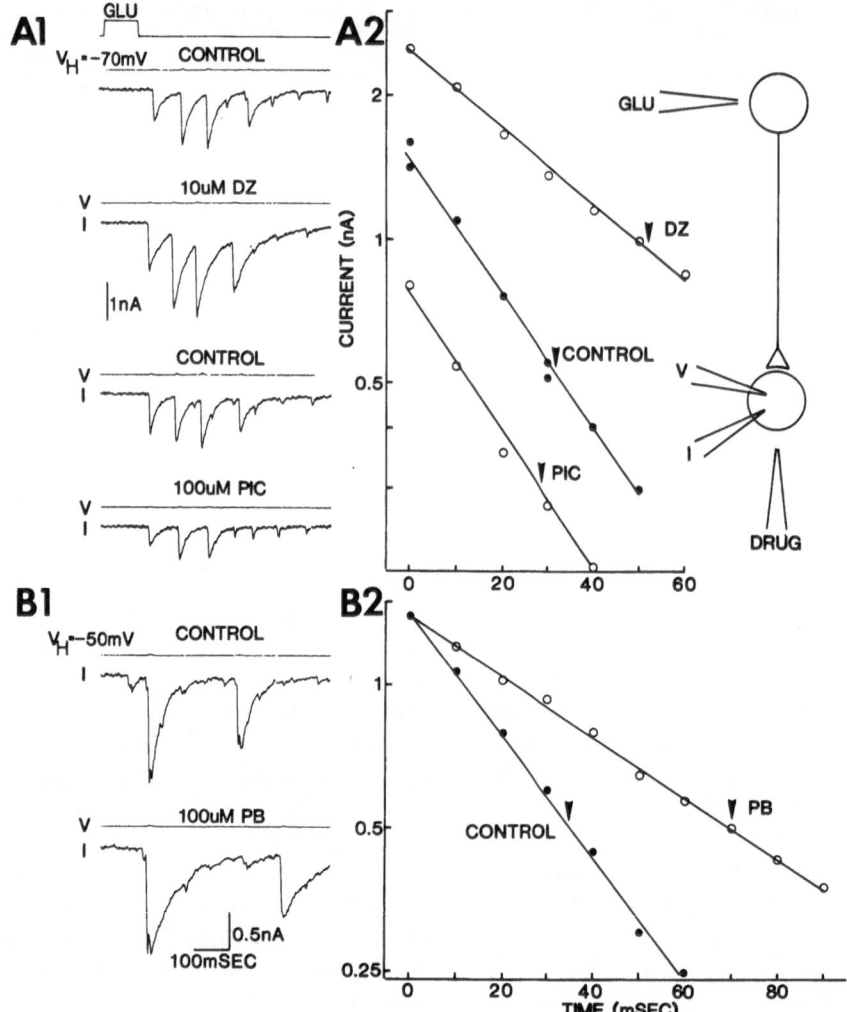

Figure 22. Clinically important drugs modulate long-lasting synaptic currents evoked in cultured hippocampal neurons. The experimental arrangements are schematized in the inset of panel A2. The post-synaptic target cells were recorded with KCl-filled current (I) and voltage (V) microelectrodes, while glutamate was applied to the presynaptic element to trigger synaptic events. Diazepam (DZ), picrotoxin (PIC), and pentobarbital (PB) were delivered in the vicinity of the recorded cell. (A1) With the cell held at −70 mV, a brief pulse of glutamate evokes long-lasting inwardly directed synaptic currents that are enhanced by DA and depressed by PIC. (A2) Semilogarithmic plots of current decay show that the time constant of decay (arrowheads) is about 30 msec both under control conditions and in the presence of PIC, but increases to about 50 msec with DZ. (B1) With the cell held at −50 mV, application of PB leads to a marked prolongation in the synaptic currents. (B2) Semi-logarithmic plots of current decay shows that the time constant increases from about 33 msec to about 70 msec in the presence of the drug. (Modified from Segal and Barker, 1984b.)

has a distinctive effect. Diazepam consistently enhances the amplitude of IPSCs and increases τ_{IPSC} so that in the presence of the drug the IPSC is both greater in amplitude and longer-lasting (Fig. 22A). On the other hand pentobarbital, while having little, if any effect on IPSC amplitude, markedly enhances τ_{IPSC} (Fig. 22B). The net effect of these pharmacological actions is to facilitate the intensity and/or duration of the physiologically triggered conductance. In contrast, picrotoxin, which reduces GABA-evoked Cl^- conductance ostensibly by eliminating activation of ion channels in an all-or-none manner (Barker et al., 1983), depresses IPSC amplitude with little effects on τ_{IPSC} (Fig. 22A).

One can account for the drug actions on hippocampal IPSCs in terms of the drug interactions with the kinetics of GABA-activated channels described above. Diazepam increases the rate of channel activation and decreases the rate of channel closing. In the presence of the drug, a physiological pulse of GABA activates more channels that effectively reopen more often and remain conducting, on average, for a somewhat longer time. Pentobarbital does not increase the rate of channel activation but rather acts by markedly decreasing the rate of channel closing. Therefore, in the presence of this drug, IPSC current amplitude does not increase, but once activated the channels remain effectively open for significantly longer times. Picrotoxin, which eliminates GABA-triggered channel activation in an all-or-none manner, depresses IPSCs without changing their time course, as if the drug effectively blocked a proportion of the channels normally opened while leaving the remainder to conduct in a physiological manner.

4. CONCLUSIONS

The results summarized in this chapter indicate that monolayers of central neurons cultured from different regions of the CNS are a useful preparation to study some of the molecular details underlying activation of Cl^- conductances by neutral amino acids. All of the evidence obtained thus far shows that these transmitter substances act in a manner quite similar to certain other transmitters, such as acetylcholine at the neuromuscular junction (see Chapter 5), in that they activate all-or-none, microscopic transitions in membrane conductance to specific ions through channel-like mechanisms. The primary electrical properties of the ion channels pharmacologically activated by the different amino acids are significantly different, yet results from whole-cell and single-channel recording suggest that the amino acids may utilize a similar channel complex in the membrane to trigger ion movement. The differences in primary elementary electrical properties observed for responses activated by GABA and glycine have also been recorded in normally developed vertebrate CNS, indicating that these results are not simply a consequence of differentiation in vitro.

Physiologically elaborated, Cl^--dependent synaptic potentials whose time course and pharmacological sensitivity suggest mediation by neutral amino acid transmitter substances have been observed in cultures of neurons dissociated from the embryonic spinal cord. If these synaptic signals do indeed reflect neutral amino acid transmitter actions, then GABA mediates a relatively longer lasting form of inhibition than glycine. Cl^--dependent synaptic events have been examined in more detail using monolayers of neurons cultured from the rat hippocampus, where many cells are invested with GAD-positive terminals and where all cells express GABA-activated channels with electrical properties similar to those observed in cultured spinal neurons. The time course of the synaptically activated Cl^- conductance is virtually identical to that associated with the average duration of GABA-activated channels. Furthermore, the effects of clinically important drugs on the synaptic conductance parallel their actions on the kinetics of ion channels activated by GABA. From this we may conclude that pharmacologically and physiologically operated channels behave in almost identical manner, that several thousand ion channels open at the peak of the synaptic event, and that drugs modulate the synaptic signal by altering channel kinetics. That the physiologically activated conductance has been preserved in the cultures is strongly implied by the close correspondence between its time course in cultured hippocampal neurons and in acutely prepared slices of hippocampal tissue (Table 1).

In conclusion, the strategy outlined in this chapter has allowed quantitative analysis of some neutral amino acid transmitter actions. *The close correspondence between pharmacological and physiological properties observed in electrophysiological recordings from embryonic cultured neurons under a variety of experimental conditions indicates that such quantitative analysis of transmitter action may provide a useful and precise reference for identifying specific synaptic signals.* This strategy may be generalizable to other transmitters as well as to other transmitter actions that alter the excitability of CNS neurons. From these quantitative methods and comparisons, it should be possible to gain some insight into the "transmitter code" as it applies to intercellular signals mediating changes in the excitability of target cells.

REFERENCES

Barker, J. L., and McBurney, R. N., 1979a, GABA and glycine may share the same conductance channel on cultured mammalian neurones, *Nature* **277**:234–236.

Barker, J. L., and McBurney, R. N., 1979b, Phenobarbitone modulation of post-synaptic GABA receptor function on cultured mammalian neurons, *Proc. R. Soc. Lond. B* **206**:318–326.

Barker, J. L., and Ransom, B. R., 1978, Amino acid pharmacology of mammalian central neurones grown in tissue culture, *J. Physiol. (Lond.)* **280**:331–354.

Barker, J. L., Gruol, D. L., Huang, L. M., MacDonald, J. F., and Smith, T. G., 1980a, Peptides: Three forms of chemical excitability on cultured mouse spinal neurons, *Neuropeptides* **1**:63–82.

Barker, J. L., MacDonald, J. F., Mathers, D. A., McBurney, R. N., and Oertel, W., 1980b, GABA receptor functions in cultured mouse spinal neurons, in: *Amino Acid Neurotransmitters* (F. V. DeFeudis and P. Mandel, eds.), Raven Press, New York, pp. 281–293.

Barker, J. L., McBurney, R. N., and MacDonald, J. F., 1982, Fluctuation analysis of neutral amino acid responses in cultured mouse spinal neurons, *J. Physiol. (Lond.)* 322:365–387.

Barker, J. L., McBurney, R. N., and Mathers, D. A., 1983, Convulsant-induced depression of amino acid responses in cultured mouse spinal neurons studied under voltage clamp, *Br. J. Pharmacol.* 80:619–629.

Blankenship, J. E., Wachtel, H., and Kandel, E. R., 1971, Ionic mechanisms of excitatory, inhibitory, and dual-synaptic actions mediated by an identified interneuron in the abdominal ganglion of *Aplysia, J. Neurophysiol.* 34:76–92.

Caserta, M. T., and Barker, J. L., 1983, Development of glutamic acid decarboxylase immunoreactivity in mouse spinal cord cultures, *Soc. Neurosci. Abstr.* 9:7.

Choi, D. W., Farb, D. H., and Fischbach, G. D., 1981, Chlordiazeperoxide selectively potentiates GABA conductance of spinal cord and sensory neurons in cell culture, *J. Neurophysiol.* 45:621–631.

Collingridge, G., Gage, P. W., and Robertson, B., 1984, Inhibitory postsynaptic currents in rat hippocampal neurons, *J. Physiol. (Lond.)* 356:551–564.

Cull-Candy, S., 1983, Glutamate- and GABA-receptor channels at the locust nerve-muscle junction: noise analysis and single-channel recording, *Cold Spring Harbor Symp. Quant. Biol.* 48:269–278.

Dichter, M., 1980, Physiological identification of GABA as the inhibitory transmitter for mammalian cortical neurons in cell culture, *Brain Res.* 190:111–121.

Dionne, V., and Stevens, C. F., 1975, Voltage dependance of agonist effectiveness at the frog neuromuscular function: Resolution of a paradox, *J. Physiol.* 251:245–270.

Dudel, J., Finger, W., and Stettmeier, H., 1980, Inhibitory synaptic channels activated by GABA in crayfish muscle, *Pflügers Arch.* 387:143–151.

Gold, M. R., and Martin, A. R., 1983a, Analysis of glycine-activated inhibitory post-synaptic channels in brainstem neurons of the lamprey, *J. Physiol. (Lond.)* 342:88–98.

Gold, M. R., and Martin, A. R., 1983b, Characteristics of inhibitory postsynaptic currents in brainstem neurons of the lamprey, *J. Physiol. (Lond.)* 342:99–117.

Hamill, O. P., Marty, A., Neher, E., Sakmann, B., and Sigworth, F. J., 1981, Improved patch-clamp techniques for high resolution current recording from cells and cell-free membrane patches, *Pflügers Arch.* 391:85–100.

Hamill, O. P., Bormann, J., and Sakmann, B., 1983, Activation of multiple-conductance state chloride channels in spinal neurons by glycine and GABA, *Nature* 305:805–808.

Jackson, M. B., Lecar, H., Mathers, D. A., and Barker, J. L., 1982, Single channel currents activated by GABA, muscimol, and (−)pentobarbital in cultured mouse spinal neurons, *J. Neurosci.* 2:889–894.

Katz, B., and Miledi, R., 1972, The statistical nature of the acetylcholine potential and its molecular components, *J. Physiol.* 224:665–699.

Levitan, H., and Tauc, L., 1972, Acetylcholine receptors: Topographic distribution and pharmacological properties of two receptor types on a single molluscan neuron, *J. Physiol. (Lond.)* 222:537–558.

Levitan, H., and Tauc, L., 1975, Polyphasic synaptic potentials in the ganglion of the mollusc, *Navanax, J. Physiol. (Lond.)* 248:35–44.

Mathers, D. A., and Barker, J. L., 1982, Chemically induced ion channels in nerve cell membranes. *Int. Rev. Neurobiol.* 23:1–34.

Neher, E., and Stevens, C. F., 1977, Conductance fluctuations and ionic pores in membranes. *Annu. Rev. Biophys. Bioeng.* 6:345–381.

Onodera, K., and Takeuchi, A., 1979, An analysis of the inhibitory post-synaptic current in the voltage-clamped crayfish muscle, *J. Physiol. (Lond.)* 286:265–282.

Redmann, G. A., Lecar, H., and Barker, J. L., 1983, Single muscimol-activated ion channels show voltage-sensitive kinetics in cultured mouse spinal neurons, *Soc. Neurosci. Abst.* 9:507.

Redmann, G., Lecar, H., and Barker, J. L., 1984, Diazepam increases GABA-activated single channel burst duration in cultured mouse spinal neurons, *Biophys. J.* **45**:386a.

Sakmann, B., and Neher, E., 1983, *Single-Channel Recording*, Plenum Press, New York.

Sakmann, B., Hamill, O. P., and Borman, J., 1983, Patch-clamp measurements of elementary chloride currents activated by the putative inhibitory transmitters GABA and glycine in mammalian spinal neurons, *J. Neural Transm. (Suppl.)* **1**:83–95.

Segal, M., and Barker, J. L., 1984a, Rat hippocampal neurons in culture: properties of GABA-activated Cl^- ion conductance, *J. Neurophysiol.* **52**:500–515.

Segal, M., and Barker, J. L., 1984b, Rat hippocampal neurons in culture: Voltage clamp analysis of inhibitory connections, *J. Neurophysiol.* **52**:469–487.

Study, R. E., and Barker, J. L., 1981, Diazepam and (−)pentobarbital: Fluctuation analysis reveals different mechanisms for potentiation of GABA responses in cultured central neurons, *Proc. Natl. Acad. Sci. USA* **78**:7180–7184.

Wachtel, H., and Kandel, E. R., 1971, Conversion of synaptic excitation to inhibition at a dual chemical synapse, *J. Neurophysiol.* **34**:56–68.

4

Glutamate

ANDREA NISTRI

1. INTRODUCTION

1.1. Overview and Synaptic Pathways

The first study of the actions of the excitatory amino acid L-glutamate* on the brain was carried out more than 30 years ago. In 1954, Hayashi found that application of glutamate to the surface of the cerebral cortex evoked strong convulsive activity. A few years later Curtis et al. (1960) demonstrated that microiontophoretic administration of glutamate in the vicinity of spinal neurons of the cat produced intense discharges of action potentials recorded extracellularly.

Further studies have shown that excitatory amino acids, including glutamate and also aspartate, may act as transmitters in the CNS. The identification of neuronal pathways utilizing excitatory amino acids as transmitters has required a combined multidisciplinary approach based on neurochemical, electrophysiological, and anatomical techniques. Figure 1 schematically illustrates those pathways which have been proposed. One of the best described pathways is the corticostriatal projections (Divac et al., 1977; Kim et al., 1977; McGeer et al., 1977); other cortical fiber pathways utilizing excitatory amino acids have also been proposed (Fonnum et al., 1981). In the hippocampus, an excitatory amino acid is thought to be a transmitter of the Schaffer collateral-commissural pathway and of the hippocampal perforant path (Crawford and Connor, 1973; Nadler et al., 1978). The lateral olfactory tract pathway to the olfactory cortex may also utilize

---

*Throughout this chapter isomers of glutamate and related compounds are assigned the conventional (L or D) rather than the Cahn-Ingold-Prelog (S or R) nomenclature. Unless otherwise indicated in the text, amino acids are assumed to have L configuration.

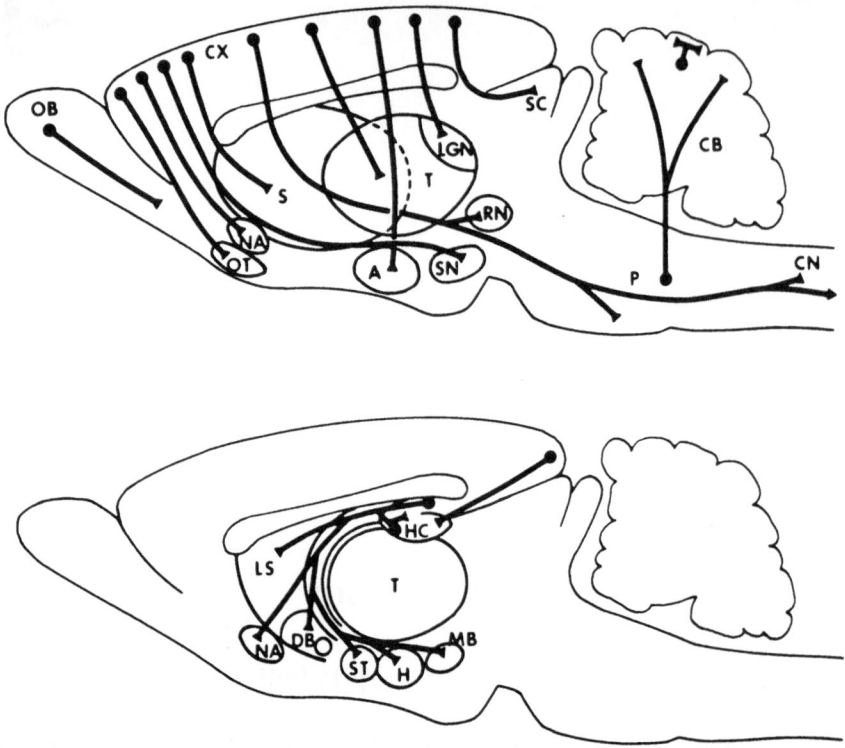

Figure 1. Some pathways proposed to use acidic amino acid transmitters in the mammalian brain. Few studies are able to discriminate between glutamate and aspartate systems. The identification of these pathways is based upon a variety of criteria including evoked release, amino acid uptake or content (in some instances in conjunction with neural lesions), and physiological studies showing identity of action or pharmacological antagonism. *Abbreviations:* A, amygdala; CB, cerebellum; CN, cuneate nucleus; CX, cerebral cortex; DB, nucleus of the diagonal band; GP, globus pallidus; HC, hippocampus; H, hypothalamus; LGN, lateral geniculate nucleus; LS, lateral septum; LVN, lateral vestibular nuclei; MB, mammillary body; NA, nucleus accumbens; OB, olfactory bulb; OT, olfactory tubercle; P, pons; RN, red nucleus; S, striatum; SC, superior colliculus; SN, substantia nigra; ST, bed nucleus of the stria terminalis; T, thalamus. (From Fagg and Foster, 1983, with permission.)

an excitatory amino acid as transmitter (Collins, 1979; Collins and Probett, 1981). In some species, an excitatory amino acid may be released by retinotectal (Cuénod et al., 1981) and auditory nerve terminals (Wenthold, 1981). In the cerebellum, glutamate may be the transmitter of parallel fibers (Sandoval and Cotman, 1978; Hackett et al., 1979) while aspartate might be used by climbing fibers (Nadi et al., 1977). In some brain regions, N-methyl-D-aspartate (NMDA) antagonists have been shown to block synaptic transmission (Watkins and Evans, 1981); this is also the case of the spinal cord where NMDA receptors are supposed to be involved in the polysynaptic excitatory pathways on motoneurons (Padjen and Smith, 1980; Evans et al., 1982).

Unfortunately the lack of identification of the endogenous substance acting on NMDA sites makes a full characterization of these neurotransmitter systems impossible.

1.2. Distribution and Release

Glutamate is present in high concentration in the central nervous system; for example, levels in the human cerebral cortex are 9–11 μmoles/g (Perry et al., 1971).

Brain concentrations of L-aspartate, another acidic amino acid structurally similar to glutamate and often implicated in synaptic transmission, are 4–5 times lower than those of glutamate. It is, however, difficult to establish if these levels are indeed indicative of a neurotransmitter function or if they more generally reflect a metabolic role. An approach to solving this problem may be provided by monitoring the release of glutamate (and aspartate) from specific neuronal pathways and by studying the turnover of this amino acid, i.e., the quantity of transmitter liberated from known endogenous stores in a given period of time. The first investigation into the release of endogenous glutamate from the cat cerebral cortex in vivo was carried out by Jasper et al. (1965) who noted that such release was higher during wakefulness than during sleep, although no associated change in cortical glutamate concentrations was found (Pepeu et al., 1970).

In broad terms, the release of glutamate and aspartate, if it is relevant to neurotransmission, ought to be evoked by depolarizing stimuli and be dependent on the extracellular Ca^{2+} concentration. So far the most convincing demonstration of physiologically relevant glutamate release comes from a correlation between Ca^{2+}-dependent efflux of endogenous glutamate and excitatory synaptic potentials elegantly demonstrated by Takeuchi and his collaborators using relatively simple synaptic systems. At the crustacean neuromuscular junction, 0.05–0.075 fmoles of glutamate were released by each excitatory fiber in order to elicit the excitatory junctional potential (Kawagoe et al., 1981). In later studies using the isolated frog spinal cord of the frog about 16–30 pmoles of glutamate were released by afferent fiber stimulation, which elicited motoneuronal discharges recorded as ventral root potentials (Takeuchi et al., 1983).

In the mammalian cerebral cortex, Ca^{2+}-dependent glutamate release has been measured in several areas (see review by Fonnum, 1984). In the visual cortex, local electrical stimulation at the site of amino acid collection increased glutamate release (Iversen et al., 1971; Clark and Collins, 1976); a similar phenomenon was observed by Dodd and Bradford (1974) following weak photic stimuli. Rather unexpectedly, electrical pulses applied to the cortical tissue immediately outside the collecting area or to the contralateral cortex depressed glutamate release (Clark and Collins, 1976). This finding remains unexplained although in other brain areas electrical stimuli have also been reported to diminish glutamate release (see Moroni et al., 1981 a,b).

It is uncertain whether this diminution is caused by activation of inhibitory inputs, accelerated conversion of glutamate to GABA, or other causes.

Other cortical areas, including the sensorimotor cortex, liberated more glutamate during stimulation of the controlateral brachial plexus (Abdul-Ghani et al., 1979), topical application of the excitatory scorpion neurotoxin tityustoxin (Coutinho-Netto et al., 1980), intravenous administration of amphetamine (Moroni et al., 1981a) or EEG wakefulness (Jasper and Koyama, 1969) than under "resting" conditions. Parallel experiments on in vitro cortical slices of the guinea pig brain suggest that glutamate (and aspartate) release is predominantly from nerve terminals (Potashner, 1978 a,b). The exact location and function of these releasing structures is not known.

Two cortical regions, the hippocampus and the olfactory cortex, have received special attention because of their relatively simple and well-defined anatomical organization and the large number of electrophysiological studies characterizing their function. In keeping with the proposal that glutamate (and perhaps aspartate) are transmitters in the hippocampus (Cotman and Nadler, 1981), release of this substance has been demonstrated in vitro (Nadler et al., 1977) and in vivo (Crawford and Connor, 1973).

Release of excitatory amino from the olfactory cortex has repeatedly been demonstrated: glutamate and aspartate were liberated in a Ca^{2+}-dependent fashion following application of depolarizing stimuli (Bradford and Richards, 1976; Collins et al., 1981), particularly after blockade of glutamate uptake systems with L-cysteate (Yamamoto and Matsui, 1975). Using in vitro slice preparations, Collins has provided evidence that aspartate rather than glutamate is the transmitter of the lateral olfactory tract fibers (Collins 1979; 1980; Collins et al., 1981; Collins and Probett, 1981); however, other studies have suggested that a different substance, perhaps N-acetylaspartylglutamate (ffrench-Mullen et al., 1985), is the actual transmitter.

Interest in the release of glutamate from the striatum stems from the proposal that this amino acid may be the transmitter of corticostriatal neurons. Although there is good evidence for the localization and uptake of glutamate in this system, release studies are somewhat inconclusive. For instance, Friedle et al. (1978) reported that high-K^+ solutions, but not the neuroexcitant kainate (however, see conflicting data of Ferkany et al., 1982), stimulated glutamate release, whereas Moroni et al. (1981b) found that these conditions diminished glutamate release and caused a dramatic fall in tissue concentrations of the amino acid.

In the cerebellum, where glutamate may be the transmitter liberated from the granule cell parallel fibers, Levi et al. (1982) have shown that glutamate, rather than aspartate, is preferentially released in a Ca^{2+}-dependent manner. Their study also revealed that 1-week old rats (lacking full maturation of the parallel fiber system) did not possess a Ca^{2+}-dependent release of this amino acid. Ferkany et al. (1982) described how kainate can enhance, in a tetrodotoxin-insensitive fashion, the release of endogenous glutamate and aspartate apparently through activation of excitatory receptors located on presynaptic terminals. This conclusion differs from that of McBean and Roberts (1981), who suggested that increased release of glutamate would *reduce* further efflux of excitatory amino acids in hippocampal slices by a presynaptic mechanism. The release patterns of glutamate and aspartate from *in vitro* slices of cochlear nucleus have been reviewed by Wenthold (1981).

In summary, the release experiments strongly suggest that glutamate is a transmitter for some neocortical, striatal, and cerebellar neurons. Conversely, the role of aspartate appears to be a relatively minor one with the possible exception of the synapses between lateral olfactory fibers and olfactory cortex neurons, cerebellar climbing fibers and Purkinje neurons, and in the spinal cord. It is now possible to demonstrate glutamate like immunoreactivity in nerve terminals using antibodies raised against the amino acid coupled to bovine serum albumin (Storm–Mathisen et al., 1983). Binding of these antibodies is localized to nerve terminals in regions believed to have glutamate synapses, such as the hippocampal mossy fibers, where the amino acid seems to be concentrated in synaptic vesicles.

2. PHYSIOLOGICAL ACTIONS OF GLUTAMATE

2.1. Invertebrate Preparations

An important contribution to understanding the membrane mechanisms underlying the action of excitatory amino acids stems from work on invertebrate preparations such as insect and crustacean neuromuscular junctions.

In the locust, glutamate is believed to be the excitatory transmitter at the synapse between the terminals of motor nerve fibers and the extensor tibiae muscle (see review by Usherwood, 1981). The reversal potential for the excitatory junction potential (EJP) and the membrane response evoked by iontophoretically applied glutamate was close to O mV; these findings suggested that several ionic species (Na^+, K^+, and Ca^{2+}) might be involved in the generation of the EJP. Studies using patch-clamp techniques have shown that the glutamate-activated membrane channels had a large unitary conductance (120 pS) and a relatively short lifetime (2 msec) (Cull-Candy et al., 1980). Like vertebrate skeletal muscle (where acetylcholine is the transmitter), insect muscles develop receptor supersensitivity following denervation (Usherwood, 1969). Interestingly, the glutamate receptor population of the locust neuromuscular junction is heterogenous: the synaptic receptors ("D receptors") mediating membrane depolarization are distinct from extrasynaptic receptors mediating hyperpolarization ("H receptors") (Cull-Candy and Usherwood, 1973). The hyperpolarizing H receptors seem to act by increasing Cl^- permeability. Extrajunctional areas also possess D receptors whose density is actually increased by denervation. Furthermore, the presynaptic nerve terminals have glutamate receptors modulating the release of endogenous glutamate. Hence, the complex receptor pharmacology of the locust neuromuscular junction represents a useful test system reminiscent of the different excitatory amino acid receptor classes found on vertebrate neurons (see below). However, the invertebrate system provides little insight into the specific details of the vertebrate receptors because of major differences in receptor pharmacology and presumed underlying channel mechanisms. For example, glutamate responses rapidly desensitize on insect muscle but not on central neurons. Furthermore, the locust muscle unlike most mammalian neurons, is comparatively insensitive to the powerful excitant kainate or to N-methly-D-aspartate.

Electrophysiological studies on crustacean preparations have mainly focused on the crayfish neuromuscular junction. Like the locust neuromuscular junction, the crayfish synapse appears to use glutamate as excitatory transmitter (Nistri and Constanti, 1979), although some discrepancies between the receptor characteristics of the EJP and of the glutamate-evoked responses have been noted (Shinozaki, 1980). On crayfish muscle the glutamate-evoked response and the EJP had a positive reversal potential and involved membrane permeability increase mainly to Na^+ and partly to Ca^{2+} (Onodera and Takeuchi, 1976). Noise analysis showed that at resting membrane potential the glutamate-operated channels had a mean conductance of 32 pS and a lifetime of about 1 msec (Stettmeir et al., 1983). Under control conditions, extrasynaptic glutamate receptors on crayfish muscle have a rather sparse distribution, although there are depolarizing responses to exogenous glutamate (Onodera and Takeuchi, 1980). Similar to insect muscle, the crayfish neuromuscular synapse displays desensitization to glutamate and relatively low sensitivity to kainate (Shinozaki, 1980).

2.2. The Lamprey, a Lower Vertebrate

The action of glutamate has been well characterized by intracellular recording in the lamprey brain. *In vitro* experiments on giant reticulospinal neurons (Müller cells) have shown that glutamate depolarized neuronal cell bodies and evoked a modest fall in their input resistance (Matthews and Wickelgren, 1979). A small depolarization, but no conductance change, was also noted in axons, and this was attributed to passive current flow from the nearby cells. The lack of physiological receptors for glutamate on Müller cell axons corresponds with the absence of morphologically identifiable synaptic inputs and the inability to record synaptic potentials in these structures. On the other hand, the soma and dendrites are studded with synaptic endings and have fast depolarizing synaptic potentials. The reversal potential for excitatory synaptic potentials in Müller cell bodies was identical with that of the depolarization produced by glutamate. Ion substitution experiments suggested that both the natural excitatory transmitter and glutamate cause membrane depolarization by increasing membrane conductance to Na^+ and K^+. Thus glutamate seems to act on these lamprey neurons in a manner similar to that of acetylcholine at the skeletal neuromuscular junction. Although glutamate is able to precisely mimic the actions of the transmitter for the excitatory synaptic response in Müller cells, positive identification of the actual endogenous transmitter cannot be achieved from physiological experiments alone.

2.3. Amphibia and Mammals

The early work of Curtis and his associates (1960) showed that acidic amino acids such as glutamate and aspartate had a powerful excitatory effect on cat spinal neurons *in vivo*. The excitation was often studied in terms of enhanced firing of action potentials and had a rapid onset and offset following iontophoretic applications of these compounds. Systematic studies with the same amino acids applied to cortical cells (Krnjević and Phillis, 1963) revealed similar actions. Indeed, most, if not all, central neurons are readily excited by glutamate and chemically related drugs (see reviews by Krnjević, 1974; Curtis and Johnston, 1974; Nistri and Constanti, 1979; Puil, 1981).

Shortly after their initial iontophoretic work on feline neurons, Curtis et al. (1961) reported that another spinal preparation, the *in vitro* spinal cord of the toad, showed great sensitivity to bath-applied amino acids. Thereafter the *in vitro* amphibian spinal cord has been proven to be a very useful preparation for receptor studies aimed at classifying excitatory amino acid receptors (see review by Watkins and Evans, 1981).

Despite the powerful excitatory actions of glutamate on virtually all amphibian and mammalian central neurons, an understanding of the membrane mechanisms underlying this effect has been elusive. This has been in part due to the difficulty in manipulating the ionic environment of neurons *in vivo* or exposing them to pharmacological agents that block ion channels. This problem can be overcome to some extent through the use of *in vitro* slice preparations.

In at least one series of experiments using such a slice preparation, it has been possible to demonstrate a clear reversal of both the depolarizing response to glutamate and the synaptic excitatory response (Hablitz and Langmoen, 1982). However, this simple situation, which is similar to that obtained in the lamprey, does not often apply in other vertebrate neurons (see Chapter 5).

The experiments showing a clear reversal of glutamate depolarizations were carried out on CA_1 neurons in the *in vitro* hippocampal slice (Hablitz and Langmoen, 1982; Fig. 2). In order to block voltage-sensitive potassium conductances that cause severe membrane rectification and make polarization of the cell difficult, neurons were injected with cesium, a potassium channel blocker, and recordings were effected with a switching circuit that minimizes the artefacts associated with conventional bridge systems. The average value for the glutamate reversal potential was near zero and not significantly different from that of the EPSP produced by stimulation of the striatum radiatum. It was therefore suggested that glutamate and the natural EPSP acted via a simultaneous increase in membrane permeability to Na^+

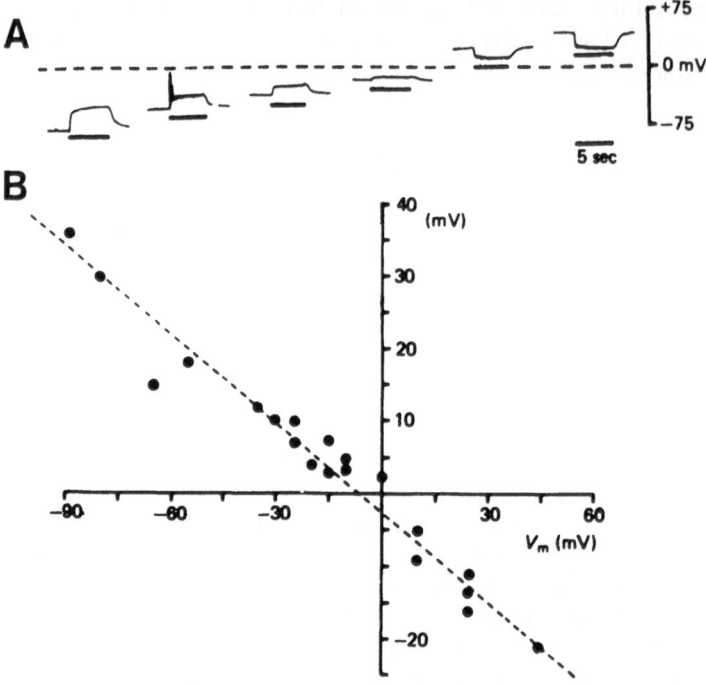

Figure 2. Reversal potential for the glutamate response in a Cs$^+$-loaded hippocampal neuron. (A) Effect of an 80-nA glutamate pulse at different membrane potentials. (B) Relationship between glutamate response (ordinate) and membrane potential (abscissa). The regression line indicates glutamate reversal potential of -6.2 mV. (From Hablitz and Langmoen, 1982, with permission.)

and K$^+$ through similar conductance channels. These data are consistent with but do not prove that the amino acid serves as neurotransmitter in this synaptic pathway.

In other brain slice preparations, notably the olfactory cortex of the guinea pig, glutamate and aspartate evoked quite complex neuronal responses beside a conventional membrane depolarization (Constanti et al., 1980). In fact, apparent reversals of depolarizing effects into hyperpolarizations were noted spontaneously even at levels near resting potential. This phenomenon was interpreted as activation of two separate conductances, one presumably involving Na$^+$ influx (responsible for the depolarization) and the other perhaps involving K$^+$ outflux (responsible for the hyperpolarization). Other actions of excitatory amino acids were also revealed during recordings from olfactory cortex neurons. One of these effects consisted of a slow hyperpolarization during washout of excitatory amino acids that perhaps involved activation of either the Na$^+$–K$^+$ membrane pump or a Ca^{2+}-dependent K$^+$ conductance (Constanti et al., 1980).

In the rat cerebellar slice, iontophoretic application of glutamate or aspartate elicited large depolarizations of Purkinje neurons with little conductance change (Crepel et al., 1982). These responses appeared to be mediated by receptor sites mainly on dendrites. At times bicuculline-sensitive inhibitory responses to glutamate were also noted and these were thought to be due to the release of endogenous GABA from nearby cells that were excited by the amino acids. One distinctive feature of this study was the short latency (down to 7 msec) of neuronal excitatory responses to brief (5 msec) pulses of excitatory amino acids. It was suggested that glutamate and/or aspartate may be the transmitter for the fast excitation of Purkinje cells by parallel and climbing fibers.

In search for a simple in vitro preparation of vertebrate CNS, some investigators have focused their attention on motoneurons in the frog spinal cord. Using this tissue, Shapovalov et al. (1978) and Sonnhof and Bührle (1980) examined the depolarizing action of glutamate and found it to be associated with rather small conductance changes. Two possible interpretations were advanced, namely, that glutamate could increase Na^+ permeability while decreasing K^+ permeability or that glutamate enhanced Na^+ and K^+ permeabilities, but these conductance changes were not easily detected by conventional intracellular recording. This is not surprising since Puil (1981) has calculated that on spinal motoneurons large membrane depolarizations could be produced by glutamate with only small conductance changes. The current view as to how this might be resolved is discussed in Chapter 5.

Based on recordings of ion activities with ion-sensitive microelectrodes Bührle and Sonnhoff (1983) have shown that, although Na^+ conductance was the main mechanism activated by glutamate, Ca^{2+} permeability was also stimulated by the amino acid. Hence the divalent cation may be involved in the glutamate response together with Na^+ and K^+ (see below).

Although glutamate produced similar depolarizations in frog motoneurons and spinal interneurons, this response was accompanied by a large conductance increase in interneurons, but not in motoneurons (Nistri and Arenson, 1983a); moreover, in the presence of glutamate, spontaneous repetitive firing was usually elicited from interneurons but very rarely from motoneurons. This suggests a possible difference in the significance of a glutamate-mediated signal depending on the target cell type and suggests that central neurons may not be uniformly sensitive to the amino acid.

Frog motoneurons also displayed hyperpolarizations preceding the depolarization evoked by glutamate (Fig. 3). Notable features of this hyperpolarization were its fast onset, the large conductance rise, and the powerful inhibition of spike activity, which amounted to an effective inhibitory mechanism for motoneurons (see bottom, Fig. 3). Fast inhibitory effects of excitatory amino acids were also found in the hippocampus by Segal (1981) and in the cerebellum as noted above. It seems unlikely that the inhibitory action of glutamate on frog motoneurons is due to activation of interneurons as it remained (or was even more noticeable) in Mn^{2+}-containing solutions, which fully blocked synaptic transmission and hence presynaptic, Ca^{2+}-dependent release of inhibitory transmitters (see bottom of Fig. 3). A powerful glutamate

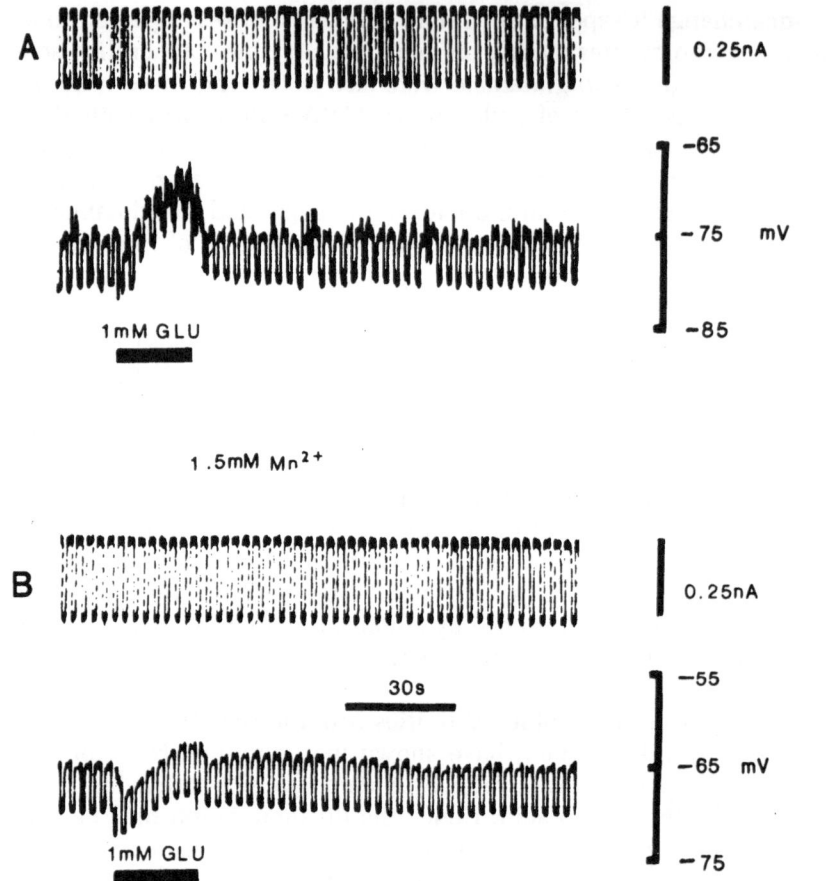

Figure 3. Effect of glutamate superfusion on a frog motoneuron. Chart record of membrane potential (bottom) and injected current (top) in control Ringer (A) and in 1.5 Mn^{2+}/1 mM Ca^{2+}-containing solution (B). Downward deflections are hyperpolarizing electrotonic potentials used to monitor input conductance. Note in (B) that the tracing is less "noisy," indicating the synaptic transmission has been blocked and that the depolarizing effect of glutamate is reduced and now clearly preceded by a hyperpolarizing response. (From Nistri and Arenson, 1983b, with permission.)

analog, D,L-homocysteic acid, could also produce similar hyperpolarizing responses. Since these hyperpolarizations were not reduced by intracellularly applied Cs^{+} and had the same polarity of Cl^{-}-mediated GABA responses, it has been proposed that they were generated by a Cl^{-} permeability increase (Arenson and Nistri, 1982). It would therefore appear that on some neurons glutamate may exert a dual action, inhibitory and excitatory; the balance of the two components will determine the overall response in terms of neuronal behavior following the application of this amino acid.

In all electrophysiological experiments described so far, one should be aware that excitatory amino acids may also affect glial cells which are depolarized with virtually no change in input conductance (see Hösli et al., 1979). This might be caused by extracellular K^+ accumulation due to neuronal activity or operation of the glutamate transport system. In fact, both neurons and glia possess an avid uptake system for most excitatory amino acids (Hösli and Hösli, 1978). Since this uptake process is Na^+ dependent and might be electrogenic (Wheeler, 1980), that is concentrating Na^+ inside cells and producing a depolarization (again with little conductance change), active transport of glutamate or aspartate across neuronal or glial membrane may elicit an electrical response that is independent of the activation of specific excitatory amino acid receptors. Note also that, in addition to its Na^+ dependence, the glutamate uptake system may be influenced by extracellular levels of chloride ions (Kuhar and Zarbin, 1978). In many in vitro or in vivo experiments, it is difficult to ascertain how important any electrogenic uptake of glutamate and aspartate might be for the recorded neuronal depolarizations. Moreover, any glutamate response elicited by this mechanism would not change polarity even with very large shifts in membrane potential.

It has previously been mentioned that glutamate may raise frog motoneuronal permeability to Ca^{2+}, which, by allowing influx of positively charged cations, would contribute to the depolarization elicited by the amino acid. Of course, this is not the only possible role or Ca^{2+} in glutamate responses. For instance, glutamate could excite cells partly through activation of afferent neurons with consequent release of endogenous transmitters. This releasing action may not require propagated action potentials in presynaptic cells. Rather, the effect may be induced by direct depolarization of the nerve terminals and consequent Ca^{2+} entry. In support of this concept is the fact that glutamate can enhance radiolabeled Ca^{2+} uptake by brain slices and synaptosomes (Harris and Stokes, 1982; Ichida et al., 1982).

3. GLUTAMATE AGONISTS

Intracellular recording of glutamate responses from mammalian neurons in vivo is technically difficult and plagued with problems of interpretation, such as the possible selective interactions of anesthetics with amino acid responses (Engberg et al, 1979; Lambert and Flatman, 1981). Hence, in vivo studies have not yielded conclusive data on the membrane mechanisms responsible for the action of glutamate and aspartate. On the other hand, in vivo studies are very useful for comparing the action of glutamate with that of related excitants.

N-Methyl-D-aspartate (NMDA) is more powerful than glutamate in producing membrane depolarization and its effect is usually characterized by a conductance decrease (provided that the applied doses are not excessively large) and by comparatively slow onset/offset rates (see for hippocampal neurones: Hablitz, 1982; Dingledine, 1983; cat motoneurons: Lambert et al.,

1981; mouse cultured neurons: MacDonald and Wojtowicz, 1982; cortical slice neurons: Flatman et al., 1983). An interesting feature of NMDA action is the appearance of sustained burst firing throughout its application and often outlasting it. This phenomenon was well described on a population of cat striatal neurons (Herrling et al., 1983). The possible mechanisms underlying this effect are discussed in Chapter 5. The effects of homocysteate (see Lambert et al., 1981) are very similar to those of NMDA (Hablitz, 1982) on CA_1 neurons of the hippocampus, although the homocysteate conductance mechanism was more comparable to that evoked by glutamate in CA_3 hippocampal cells (Sawada et al., 1982). The D isomers of glutamate and aspartate are also capable of depolarizing cortical neurons in vitro, although less potently than the L compounds (Constanti et al., 1980; Yamamoto and Sawada, 1982). Another glutamate analog characterized by powerful depolarizing activity is quisqualate (cf. Lambert et al., 1981): bath-applied quisqualate was over 50 times more powerful than glutamate on intracellularly recorded frog motoneurons (A. Nistri and M.S. Arenson, unpublished).

Kainic acid is one of the most powerful excitatory substances known. This glutamate–related agent has spectacular depolarizing actions on most central neurons, which are eventually killed by its prolonged application (see review by Nistri and Constanti, 1979). Figure 4 shows an example of kainate effects on olfactory cortex neurons in vitro (Constanti et al., 1980). In Fig. 4A glutamate evoked a slow and reversible depolarization with a comparatively modest conductance increase, while kainate produced a dramatic conductance rise with complete shunting of cell resistance and irreversible depolarization. In Fig. 4B (different cell from A), after test doses of glutamate and aspartate, application of kainate evoked a much larger depolarization and conductance rise from which the cell recovered only poorly. Similar phenomena have also been noted on cultured neurons (MacDonald and Wojtowicz, 1982). Not all central neurons are equally sensitive to kainate: For example, hippocampal CA_1 (unlike CA_3) cells are less susceptible to the neurotoxicity of this substance of (de Montigny and Tardif, 1981). Mesencephalic trigeminal neurons are also strikingly resistant to it (Colonnier et al., 1979). On the basis of the available data, it seems that kainate has a different mode of action from glutamate, although one should note that large and prolonged applications of most excitatory amino acids will also destroy nerve cells (cell bodies and dendrites) while sparing axons en passage (Kizer et al., 1978; Olney, 1981). Kainate also stimulates release of endogenous glutamate and aspartate from several brain areas (Ferkany et al., 1982; Potashner and Gerard, 1982). It is therefore possible that neuronal destruction is brought about via a direct action of kainate as well as via sustained presynaptic release of excitatory transmitters.

Another glutamate analog, the naturally occurring ibotenate, unlike most other excitatory amino acids, produced mixed excitation and inhibition of central neurons (MacDonald and Nistri, 1978). The inhibitory action of ibotenate has been postulated, but never demonstrated, to be caused by tissue conversion of this compound into muscimol, a potent GABA-mimetic analog

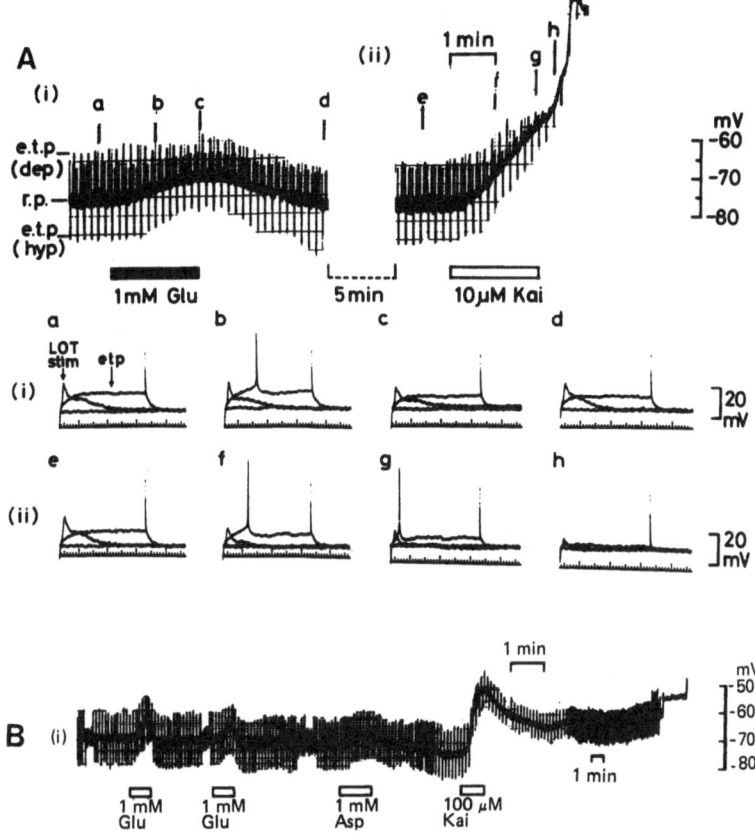

Figure 4. Depolarizing responses to L-glutamate, L-aspartate, and kainate recorded in two different olfactory cortex neurons. (A) Upper trace shows chart record of membrane potential. Upward deflections are depolarizing electrotonic potentials (etp) and truncated spikes, followed by lateral olfactory tract (LOT) stimuli; downward deflections are hyperpolarizing electrotonic potentials. Current pulses were ± 0.2 nA; 300 msec; 0.2 Hz. (i) Response to 1 mM glutamate (filled bar); (ii) response to 10 μM kainate (open bar). Note the large depolarization and eventual loss of membrane potential at peak of response. Oscilloscope traces (a–h) below were taken at corresponding times indicated on chart record. Records show superimposed responses to the depolarizing current pulse (hyperpolarizing pulse not shown) and to LOT stimulation. Note that LOT stimulus produced synaptic response but no spike. Small time marks show 10-msec divisions. (B) Continuous DC chart record from a different neuron (current pulses ± 0.1 nA; 100 msec; 0.3 Hz) showing responses to 1 mM glutamate, 1 mM aspartate, and 100 μM kainate; again note loss of neuron after kainate response. Temperature = 30°C. (From Constanti et al., 1980, with permission.)

(Curtis et al., 1979). Further studies have instead suggested that the rather unusual excitatory-inhibitory effect of ibotenate was not the result of chemical transformation of this agent (MacDonald and Barker, 1980; Nistri, 1981). This left open the possibility that ibotenate-evoked inhibitions were caused either by its interaction with a special type of inhibitory glutamate receptor (analogous to the type found on invertebrate muscle; Nistri and Constanti 1979) or by sustained release of endogenous inhibitory substances.

A recently synthesized ibotenate analog, α-amino-3-hydroxy-5-methyl-4-isoxazolepropionic acid (AMPA), is a powerful excitant of cat spinal interneurons (Krogsgaard-Larsen et al., 1980). A particularly attractive feature of AMPA is its lack of interference with glutamate uptake systems and with kainate binding sites, suggesting that AMPA might be a selective agonist for some glutamate receptors.

4. EXCITATORY AMINO ACID RECEPTORS

While early work might have suggested that excitatory amino acids could act via a common receptor system, this view has been gradually modified by observations of different neuronal sensitivities to amino acid agonists and, later, to various receptor antagonists (see review by Nistri and Constanti, 1979). Important contributions to theories of different classes of excitatory amino acid receptors were first provided by experiments on invertebrate preparations. For instance, molluscan neurons seem to possess a variety of receptors for glutamate (for references, see Nistri and Constanti, 1979); similarly, locust muscle fibers display depolarizing and hyperpolarizing responses (mediated by D and H receptors, respectively) to glutamate (reviewed by Usherwood, 1981). The locust H receptor recognizes as a selective agonist ibotenate, while the D receptor accepts quisqualate as a very powerful agonist. Interestingly, invertebrate cells are usually insensitive to NMDA (Nistri and Constanti, 1979). These studies have led to the concept of distinct receptor sites (coupled to various ionic channels) recognizing as agonists selected conformationally restricted glutamate analogs.

One important finding provided by experiments on locust muscle fibers is the explanation, in molecular terms, of receptor agonist potency. By using the patch-clamp technique adapted for microperfusion of relevant compounds, Cull-Candy et al. (1980) have shown that on D receptors agonist potency can be expressed in terms of channel lifetime. In particular, single channels opened by quisqualate, a more powerful depolarizing agent than glutamate, have a lifetime about 3 times longer than glutamate-activated channels. The weaker excitant fluoroglutamate opened channels whose lifetime was only 60% that of those activated by glutamate. No significant difference in the single channel conductance operated by the various agonists was found. Similar data were also obtained by Gration et al. (1981).

In recent years, great progress has been made toward characterizing excitatory amino acid receptors in the vertebrate CNS. While excitatory receptors may be easily studied in view of the widespread depolarizing properties of these amino acids, the inhibitory receptor class is more elusive and the only agent that so far has shown some potential value for their identification is ibotenate (but see also recent binding data on "inhibitory" glutamate receptors; Fagg et al., 1982). It is therefore no surprise that many investigations have been centered on the classification of excitatory receptors (see Chapter 5, and Watkins and Evans, 1981).

The current view is that there are at least three distinct receptor classes, those activated preferentially by NMDA, quisqualate, and kainate. At present, the pharmacology of NMDA-selective receptors is the most advanced, and there are potent antagonists available such as 2-amino-5-phosphonovalerate (APV) and 2-amino-7-phosphonoheptanoate (APH). Studies on mammalian cortical neurons in vivo for example, have confirmed that APV [particularly the (−)-isomer] is a selective antagonist of NMDA responses versus glutamate or kainate responses (Stone et al., 1981). No specific antagonists are known for quisqualate and kainate receptors. Glutamic acid diethylester (GDEE) is rather nonselective and seems to have nonspecific effects on neuronal activity (MacDonald et al., 1977; Nistri and Constanti, 1975). γ-D-Gutamylglycine (γ–DGG) may preferentially block kainate (and NMDA) responses over those to quisqualate.

With presently available antagonists, therefore, it is possible to distinguish pharmacologically between NMDA and non-NMDA (quisqualate and kainate) responses, but further classification is difficult. It seems that the endogenously occurring glutamate and aspartate may be mixed agonists with affinity for both receptor types. Should these different receptors be spatially well separated, then local application of glutamate to restricted cell areas could activate one receptor type. However, such an arrangement is probably unusual in vertebrate neurons. Hence, in many vertebrate preparations, glutamate may act on multiple receptors unless selective antagonists for a given set of receptors also applied.

Although the pharmacology of excitatory amino acid receptors has been defined to some extent, the identity of the receptors stimulated during excitatory synaptic transmission is unclear (see Chapter 5). Intracellular recording from hippocampal granule cells has shown that (±)APV antagonized responses to NMDA, but not to quisqualate or kainate (Crunelli et al., 1983). Since the neurally evoked EPSP was blocked by γ–DGG, and not by APV, it was proposed that the receptor involved in this excitatory neurotransmission was of quisqualate/kainate type. Similar suggestions were put forward by Collingridge et al. (1983), who recorded extracellularly the population EPSP of hippocampal pyramidal cells. It will be of interest to ascertain if in this mammalian brain area the NMDA-type receptors, so powerfully blocked by APV, might be involved in physiological synaptic transmission or whether they might have a mainly extrasynaptic location.

McLennan and collaborators (McLennan et al. 1981, 1982) have examined the structural requirements of the excitatory amino acid receptors with two main objectives: to study whether extended or folded agonist molecules might be preferentially recognized by different receptor types and to look at the possibility that glutamate and aspartate act in different spatial conformations on separate receptors. As to the first issue, McLennan et al. suggest that the NMDA receptors preferentially bound the extended conformation of excitatory amino acids, while the quisqualate and kainate receptors preferred folded agonist molecules (McLennan et al., 1981; McLennan et al., 1982). Second, since the rigid glutamate analog cis-1-aminocyclopentane-1,3-dicarboxylic acid had an intercharge distance longer than that of L-aspartate and was also a potent excitant, it seems that this compound could interact with glutamate receptors not usually accessible to aspartate (McLennan and Wheal, 1978). One should however bear in mind that these conclusions have not been fully accepted by other workers (Watkins and Evans, 1981).

In summary, then, several classes of receptors for excitatory amino acids have been proposed on the basis of recent pharmacological studies. Unfortunately, a systematic biochemical analysis of these ligand sites is still lagging behind the pharmacology based on extracellular recording because of the highly polar nature of these compounds. Hence, we do not know yet if neurons possess various receptors of different molecular structure to accommodate different ligands or if the neuronal receptors are structurally similar but capable of large conformational changes in order to bind different ligands (a model, as noted by Puil [1981], similar to the "glove fitting a hand" theory).

5. IMPLICATIONS FOR CLINICAL MEDICINE AND NEUROTOXICOLOGY

Studies of glutamate transmitter actions have provided possible insights into the pathophysiology of some neurological diseases. Since glutamate is a potent excitant of cortical neurons, its role in epilepsy has often been investigated. For instance, in experimental models of epilepsy with established chronic cobalt foci, there is a clear and selective increase in glutamate release from these areas during convulsive activity (Dodd and Bradford, 1976). Moreover, the synthetic antagonist of NMDA receptors, 2-amino-7-phosphonoheptanoic acid is a very potent anticonvulsant in mice (Croucher et al., 1982), raising the possibility that NMDA-like compounds may be implicated in the genesis or maintenance of seizures (Coutinho-Netto et al., 1981).

An interesting topic for basic and clinical research is represented by the observations that ketamine and phencyclidine, two dissociative anaesthetics with good analgesic activity, can preferentially and reversibly block NMDA-induced responses of feline neurons in vivo (Anis et al., 1983). The (+) isomer of ketamine was more potent than the (−) form as an NMDA antagonist and its potency was similar to that of APV (Lodge et al., 1982). It has been suggested that if adequate brain levels of NMDA antagonists (ketamine or dicarboxylic amino acid derivatives) can be achieved, this might account for the dissociative anaesthetic state.

Another area of research concerns the neuronal destruction produced by excitatory amino acids. Indeed, application of kainate to the striatum in animals produces a neurological deficit resembling Huntington's chorea (Coyle and Schwarcz, 1976). It has been suggested that local accumulation of endogenous glutamate (or related compounds) in discrete brain regions might determine at least part of the neuronal degeneration found in this condition (Coyle et al., 1977). Although there is no apparent reduction in glutamate and aspartate uptake mechanisms in choreic patients (Mangano and Schwarcz, 1981), it appears that some cells from these patients (for example, fibroblasts) might be unusually sensitive to glutamate (Gray et al., 1980; Wong et al., 1982). Furthermore, the glial metabolic inactivation process for glutamate is found decreased in several areas of the choreic brain (Carter, 1982).

Olivopontocerebellar atrophy is a genetic condition characterized by partial deficiency in glutamate dehydrogenase activity with resulting rise in free glutamate concentrations in plasma and possibly in brain (Plaitakis et al., 1982). Again increased amounts of glutamate at neuronal level may well trigger the nerve cell degeneration. The overall importance of deranged glutamate metabolism for brain pathology has recently been discussed (Prusiner, 1981).

There has also been interest in the potential neurotoxic effects of glutamate in the diet. When given systemically to infant animals, glutamate produces lesions of those brain areas (e.g., the arcuate hypothalamic nucleus) not protected by the blood brain barrier (see Olney, 1978). These findings have raised concern about using monosodium glutamate as a baby food additive. In the adult it is known that ingestion of large amounts of monosodium glutamate can produce the so-called "Chinese Restaurant Syndrome" characterized by facial and chest pain and cardiovascular disturbances.

6. CONCLUSION

Excitatory amino acids appear to act as neurotransmitters in several CNS regions. Glutamate and aspartate, the parent compounds of this group, can influence neuronal activity in a variety of ways. Pharmacological studies suggest the existence of heterogenous populations of excitatory amino acid receptors, particularly on the basis of the differential antagonism of amino acid responses by selected organic compounds. Although structurally related to glutamate, other chemical analogs such as N-methyl-D-aspartate (NMDA), kainate, and quisqualate probably excite central neurons through separate receptors. The role of aspartate and glutamate as neurotransmitters per se is gradually receiving more attention. Further impetus to current research on the mode of action of excitatory amino acids comes from the realization that glutamate and aspartate may be involved in the pathophysiology of neuropsychiatric diseases or in the genesis of neurotoxic brain lesions, and a variety of clinically important sensory-motor conditions.

ACKNOWLEDGMENTS. I wish to thank Miss Carol Brown for her patient typing and Mr. John Gomersall for photography. This work was supported by a grant from the Joint Research Board of St. Bartholomew's Hospital, London.

REFERENCES

Abdul-Ghani, A.-S., Bradford, H. F., Cox, D. W. G., and Dodd, P. R., 1979, Peripheral sensory stimulation and the release of transmitter amino acids in vivo from specific regions of cerebral cortex, Brain Res. **171**:55–66.

Anis, N. A., Berry, S. C., Burton, N. R., and Lodge, D., 1983, The dissociative anaesthetics, ketamine and phencyclidine, selectively reduce excitation of central mammalian neurones by N-methyl-aspartate, Br. J. Pharmacol. **79**:565–575.

Arenson, M. S., and Nistri, A., 1982, A novel inhibitory-excitatory response of frog motoneurones in vitro to glutamate, J. Physiol. (Lond.) **328**:9P.

Bradford, H. F., and Richards, C. D., 1976, Specific release of endogenous glutamate from piriform cortex stimulated in vitro, Brain Res. **105**:168–172.

Bührle, C. P., and Sonnhof, U., 1983, The ionic mechanism of the excitatory action of glutamate upon the membranes of motoneurones of the frog, Pflüger's Arch. **396**:154–162.

Carter, C. J., 1982, Glutamine synthetase activity in Huntington's disease Life Sci. **31**:1151–1159.

Clark, R. M., and Collins, G. G. S., 1976, The release of endogenous amino acids from the rat visual cortex, J. Physiol. (Lond.) **262**:383–400.

Collingridge, G. L., Kehl, S. J., and McLennan, H., 1983, Excitatory amino acids in synaptic transmission in the Schaffer collateral-commissural pathway of the rat hippocampus, J. Physiol. (Lond.) **334**:33–46.

Collins, G. G. S., 1979, Evidence of a neurotransmitter role for aspartate and γ-aminobutyric acid in the rat olfactory cortex, J. Physiol. (Lond.) **291**:51–60.

Collins, G. G. S., 1980, Release of endogenous amino acid neurotransmitter candidates from rat olfactory cortex slices: Possible regulatory mechanisms and the effects of pentobarbitone, Brain Res. **190**:517–528.

Collins, G. G. S., and Probett, G. A., 1981, Aspartate and not glutamate is the likely transmitter of the rat lateral olfactory tract fibres, Brain Res. **209**:231–234.

Collins, G. G. S., Anson, J., and Probett, G. A., 1981, Patterns of endogenous amino acid release from slices of rat and guinea-pig olfactory cortex, Brain Res. **204**:103–120.

Colonnier, M., Steriade, M., and Landry, P., 1979, Selective resistance of sensory cells of the mesencephalic trigeminal nucleus to kainic acid-induced lesions, Brain Res. **172**:552–556.

Constanti, A., Connor, J. D., Galvan, M., and Nistri, A., 1980, Intracellularly recorded effects of glutamate and aspartate on neurones in the guinea-pig olfactory cortex slice, Brain Res. **195**:403–420.

Cotman, C. W., and Nadler, J V., 1981, Glutamate and aspartate as hippocampal transmitters: Biochemical and pharmacological evidence, in: Glutamate: Transmitter in the Central Nervous System (P. J. Roberts, J. Storm-Mathisen, and G. A. R. Johnston, eds.), Wiley, New York, pp. 117–154.

Coutinho-Netto, J., Abdul-Ghani, A.-S., Norris, P. J., Thomas, A. J., and Bradford, H. F., 1980, The effects of scorpion venom toxin on the release of amino acid neurotransmitters from cerebral cortex in vivo and in vitro, J. Neurochem. **35**:558–565.

Coutinho-Netto, J., Abdul-Ghani, A. S., Collins, J. F., and Bradford, H. F., 1981, Is glutamate a trigger factor in epileptic hyperactivity? Epilepsia **22**:289–296.

Coyle, J. T., and Schwarcz, R., 1976, Lesion of striatal neurones with kainic acid provides a model for Huntington's chorea, Nature **263**:244–246.

Coyle, J. T., Schwarcz, R., Bennett, J. P., and Campochiaro, P., 1977, Clinical, neuropathological and pharmacological aspects of Huntington's disease: Correlates with a new animal model, Prog. Neuropsychopharmacol. **1**:13–30.

Crawford, I. L., and Connor, J. D., 1973, Localization and release of glutamic acid in relation to the hippocampal mossy fibre pathway, Nature **244**:442–443.

Crepel, F., Dhanjal, S. S., and Sears, T. A., 1982, Effect of glutamate, aspartate and related derivatives on cerebellar Purkinje cell dendrites in the rat: An in vitro study, J. Physiol. (Lond.) **329**:297–317.

Croucher, M. J., Collins, J. F., and Meldrum, B. S., 1982, Anticonvulsant action of excitatory amino acid antagonists, Science **216**:899–901.

Crunelli, V., Forda, S., and Kelly, J. S., 1983, Blockade of amino acid-induced depolarizations and inhibition of excitatory post-synaptic potentials in rat dentate gyrus, *J. Physiol. (Lond.)* **341**:627–640.

Cuénod, M., Beaudet, A., Canzek, V., Streit, P., and Reubi, J. C., 1981, Glutamatergic pathways in the pigeon and the rat brain, in: *Glutamate as a Neurotransmitter* (G. DiChiara and G. L. Gessa, eds.), Raven Press, New York, pp. 57–68.

Cull-Candy, S. G., and Usherwood, P. N. R., 1973, Two populations of L-glutamate receptors in locust muscle fibres, *Nature New Biol.* **246**:62–64.

Cull-Candy, S. G., Miledi, R., and Parker, I., 1980, Single glutamate-activated channels recorded from locust muscle fibres with perfused patch-clamp electrodes, *J. Physiol. (Lond.)* **321**:195–210.

Curtis, D. R., and Johnston, G. A. R., 1974, Amino acid transmitters in the mammalian central nervous system, *Ergebn. Physiol.* **69**:97–188.

Curtis, D. F., Phillis, J. W., and Watkins, J. C., 1960, The chemical excitation of spinal neurones by certain acidic amino acids, *J. Physiol. (Lond.)* **150**:656–682.

Curtis, D. R., Phillis, J. W., and Watkins, J. C., 1961, Actions of amino-acids on the isolated hemisected spinal cord of the toad, *Br. J. Pharmacol.* **16**:262–283.

Curtis, D. R., Lodge, D., and McLennan, H., 1979, The excitation and depression of spinal neurones by ibotenic acid, *J. Physiol. (Lond.)* **291**:19–28.

de Montigny, C., and Tardif, D., 1981, Differential excitatory effects of kainic acid on CA_3 and CA_1 hippocampal pyramidal neurons: Further evidence for the excitotoxic hypothesis and for a receptor-mediated action, *Life Sci.* **29**:2103–2111.

Dingledine, R., 1983, N-Methyl-D-aspartate activates voltage-dependent calcium conductance in rat hippocampal pyramidal cells, *J. Physiol. (Lond.)* **343**:385–405.

Divac, I., Fonnum, F., and Storm-Mathisen, J., 1977, High affinity uptake of glutamate in terminals of corticostriatal axons, *Nature* **266**:377–378.

Dodd, P. R., and Bradford, H. F., 1974, Release of amino acids from the chronically superfused mammalian cerebral cortex, *J. Neurochem.* **23**:289–292.

Dodd, P. R., and Bradford, H. F., 1976, Release of amino acids from the maturing cobalt-induced epileptic focus, *Brain Res.* **111**:377–388.

Engberg, I., Flatman, J. A., and Lambert, J. D. C., 1979, The actions of excitatory amino acids on motoneurones in the feline spinal cord, *J. Physiol. (Lond.)* **288**:227–261.

Evans, R. H., Francis, A. A., Jones, A. W., Smith D. A. S., and Watkins, J. C., 1982, The effects of a series of ω-phosphonic α-carboxylic amino acids on electrically evoked and excitant amino acid-induced responses in isolated spinal cord preparations, *Br. J. Pharmacol.* **75**:65–75.

Fagg, G. E., and Foster, A. C., 1983, Amino acid neurotransmitters and their pathways in the mammalian central nervous system, *Neuroscience* **9**:701–719.

Fagg, G. E., Foster, A. C., Mena, E. E., and Cotman, C. W., 1982, Chloride and calcium ions reveal a pharmacologically distinct population of L-glutamate binding sites in synaptic membranes: correspondence between biochemical and electrophysiological data, *J. Neurosci.* **2**:958–965.

Ferkany, J. W., Zaczek, R., and Coyle, J. T., 1982, Kainic acid stimulates excitatory amino acid neurotransmitter release at presynaptic receptors, *Nature* **298**:757–759.

ffrench-Mullen, J. M. H., Koller, K., Zaczek, R., Coyle, J. T., Hori, N., and Carpenter, D. O., 1985, N-Acetylaspartylglutamate: Possible role as the neurotransmitter of the lateral olfactory tract, *Proc. Natl. Acad. Sci. USA* (in press).

Flatman, J. A., Schwindt, P. C., Crill, W. E., and Stafstrom, C. E., 1983, Multiple actions of N-methyl-D-aspartate on cat neocortical neurons in vitro, *Brain Res.* **266**:169–173.

Fonnum, F., 1984, Glutamate: A neurotransmitter in mammalian brain, *J. Neurochem.* **42**:1–11.

Fonnum, F., Søreide, A., Kvale, I., Walter, J., and Walaas, I., 1981, Glutamate in cortical fibers, in: *Glutamate as a Neurotransmitter* (G. DiChiara and G. L. Gessa, eds.), Raven Press, New York, pp. 29–41.

Friedle, N. M., Kelly, P. H., and Moore, K. E., 1978, Regional brain atrophy and reductions in glutamate release and uptake after intrastriatal kainic acid, *Br. J. Pharmacol.* **63**:151–158.

Gration, K. A. F., Lambert, J. J., Ramsey, R., and Usherwood, P. N. R., 1981, Potency of glutamate and agonists determined by patch clamp analysis of individual receptors on locust muscle, *J. Physiol. (Lond.)* **317**:34–35P.

Gray, P. N., May, P. C., Munday, L., and Elins, J., 1980, L-Glutamate toxicity in Huntington's disease fibroblasts. *Biochem. Biophys. Res. Comm.* **95**:707–714.

Hablitz, J. J., 1982, Conductance changes induced by DL-homocysteic acid and N-methyl-DL-aspartic acid in hippocampal neurons, *Brain Res.* **247**:149–153.

Hablitz, J. J., and Langmoen, I. A., 1982, Excitation of hippocampal pyramidal cells by glutamate in the guinea-pig and rat, *J. Physiol. (Lond.)* **325**:317–331.

Hackett, J. T., Hou, S.-M., and Cochran, S. L., 1979, Glutamate and synaptic depolarization of Purkinje cells evoked by parallel fibers and by climbing fibers, *Brain Res.* **170**:377–380.

Harris, R. A., and Stokes, J. A., 1982, Effects of a sedative and a convulsant barbiturate on synaptosomal calcium transport, *Brain Res.* **242**:157–163.

Hayashi, T., 1954, Effects of sodium glutamate on the nervous system, *Keio J. Med.* **3**:183–192.

Herrling, P. L., Morris, R., and Salt, T. E., 1983, Effects of excitatory amino acids and their antagonists on membrane and action potentials of cat caudate neurones, *J. Physiol. (Lond.)* **339**:207–222.

Hösli, L., and Hösli, E., 1978, Action and uptake of neurotransmitters in CNS tissue culture, *Rev. Physiol. Biochem. Pharmacol.* **81**:135–188.

Hösli, L., Andrés, P. F., and Hösli, E., 1979, Depolarization of cultured astrocytes by glutamate and aspartate, *Neuroscience* **4**:1593–1598.

Ichida, S., Tokumaga, H., Moriyama, M., Oda, T., Tanaka, S., and Kita, T., 1982, Effects of neurotransmitter candidates on ^{45}Ca uptake by cortical slices of rat brain: Stimulatory effect of L-glutamic acid, *Brain Res.* **248**:305–311.

Iversen, L. L., Mitchell, J. F., and Srinivasan, V., 1971, The release of GABA during inhibition in the cat visual cortex, *J. Physiol. (Lond.)* **212**:519–534.

Jasper, H. H., and Koyama, I., 1969, Rate of release of amino acids from the cerebral cortex in the cat as affected by brain stem and thalamic stimulation, *Can. J. Physiol. Pharmacol.* **47**:889–905.

Jasper, H. H., Khan, R. T., and Elliott, K. A. C., 1965, Amino acids released from cerebral cortex in relation to its state of activation, *Science* **147**:1448–1449.

Kawagoe, R., Onodera, K., and Takeuchi, A., 1981, Release of glutamate from the crayfish neuromuscular junction, *J. Physiol. (Lond.)* **312**:225–236.

Kim, J.-S., Hassler, R., Hang, P., and Paik, K.-S., 1977, Effect of frontal cortex ablation on striatal glutamic acid level in rat, *Brain Res.* **132**:370–374.

Kizer, J. S., Nemeroff, C. B., and Youngblood, W. W., 1978, Neurotoxic amino acids and structurally related analogs, *Pharmacol. Rev.* **29**:301–318.

Krnjević K., 1974, Chemical nature of synaptic transmission in vertebrates, *Physiol. Rev.* **54**:418–540.

Krnjević, K., and Phillis, J. W., 1963, Iontophoretic studies of neurones in the mammalian cerebral cortex, *J. Physiol. (Lond.)* **165**:274–304.

Krogsgaard-Larsen, P., Honoré, T., Hansen, J. J., Curtis, D. R., and Lodge, D., 1980, New class of glutamate agonist structurally related to ibotenic acid, *Nature* **284**:64–66.

Kuhar, M. J., and Zarbin, M. A., 1978, Synaptosomal transport: A chloride dependence for choline, GABA, glycine and several other compounds, *J. Neurochem.* **31**:251–256.

Lambert, J. D. C., and Flatman, J. A., 1981, The interaction between barbiturate anaesthetics and excitatory amino acid responses on cat spinal neurones, *Neuropharmacology* **20**:227–240.

Lambert, J. D. C., Flatman, J. A., and Engberg, I., 1981, Actions of excitatory amino acids on membrane conductance and potential in motoneurones, in: *Glutamate as a Neurotransmitter* (G. DiChiara and G. L. Gessa, eds.), Raven Press, New York, pp. 205–216.

Levi, G., Gordon, R. D., Gallo, V., Wilkin, G. P., and Balázs, R., 1982, Putative acidic amino acid transmitters in the cerebellum. I. Depolarization-induced release, *Brain Res.* **239**:425–445.

Lodge, D., Anis, N. A., and Burton, N. R., 1982, Effects of optical isomers of ketamine on excitation of cat and rat spinal neurones by amino acids and acetylcholine, *Neurosci. Lett.* **29**:281–286.

MacDonald, J. F., and Barker, J. L., 1980, Two distinct inhibitory responses of cultured, mammalian spinal neurones to ibotenic acid, *Can. J. Physiol. Pharmacol.* **58**:1135–1137.

MacDonald, J. F., and Nistri, A., 1978, A comparison of the action of glutamate, ibotenate and other related amino acids on feline spinal interneurones, *J. Physiol. (Lond.)* **275**:449–465.

MacDonald, J. F., and Wojtowicz, J. M., 1982, The effects of L-glutamate and its analogues upon the membrane conductance of central murine neurones in culture, *Can. J. Physiol. Pharmacol.* **60**:282–296.

MacDonald, J. F., Nistri, A., and Padjen, A. L., 1977, Neuronal depressant effects of diethylester derivatives of excitatory amino acids, *Can. J. Physiol. Pharmacol.* **55**:1387–1390.

Mangano, R. M., and Schwarcz, R., 1981, Platelet glutamate and aspartate uptake in Huntington's disease, *J. Neurochem.* **37**:1072–1074.

Matthews, G., and Wickelgren, W. C., 1979, Glutamate and synaptic excitation of reticulospinal neurones of lamprey, *J. Physiol. (Lond.)* **293**:417–433.

McBean, G. J., and Roberts, P. J., 1981, Glutamate-preferring receptors regulate the release of D-[³H] aspartate from rat hippocampal slices, *Nature* **291**:593–594.

McGeer, P. L., McGeer, E. G., Scherer, U., and Singh, K., 1977, A glutamatergic corticostriatal path? *Brain Res.* **128**:369–373.

McLennan, H., and Wheal, H. V., 178, A synthetic, conformationally restricted analogue of L-glutamic acid which acts as a powerful neuronal excitant, *Neurosci. Lett.* **8**:51–54.

McLennan, H., Hicks, T. P., and Hall, J. G., 1981, Receptors for excitatory amino acids, in: *Amino Acid Neurotransmitters* (F. V. DeFeudis and P. Mandel, eds.), Raven Press, New York, pp. 213–221.

McLennan, H., Hicks, T. P., and Liu, J. R., 1982, On the configuration of the receptors for excitatory amino acids, *Neuropharmacology* **21**:549–554.

Moroni, F., Corradetti, R., Casamenti, F., Moneti, G., and Pepeu, G., 1981a, The release of endogenous GABA and glutamate from the cerebral cortex in the rat, *Naunyn Schmiedebergs Arch. Pharmacol.* **316**:235–239.

Moroni, F., Bianchi, C., Tanganelli, S., Moneti, G., and Beani, L., 1981b, The release of γ-aminobutyric acid, glutamate, and acetylcholine from striatal slices: A mass fragmentographic study, *J. Neurochem.* **36**:1691–1697.

Nadi, N. S., Kanter, D., McBride, W. J., and Aprison, M. H., 1977, Effects of 3-acetylpyridine on several putative neurotransmitter amino acids in the cerebellum and medulla of the rat, *J. Neurochem.* **28**:661–662.

Nadler, J. V., White, W. F., Vaca, K. W., Redburn, D. A., and Cotman, C. W., 1977, Characterization of putative amino acid transmitter release from slices of rat dentate gyrus, *J. Neurochem.* **29**:279–290.

Nadler, J. V., White, W. F., Vaca., K. W., Perry, B. W., and Cotman, C. W., 1978, Biochemical correlates of transmission mediated by glutamate and aspartate, *J. Neurochem.* **31**:147–155.

Nistri, A., 1981, Excitatory and inhibitory actions of ibotenic acid on frog spinal motoneurones in vitro, *Brain Res.* **208**:397–408.

Nistri, A., and Arenson, M. S., 1983a, Differential sensitivity of spinal neurones to amino acids: An intracellular study on the frog spinal cord, *Neuroscience* **8**:115–122.

Nistri, A., and Arenson, M. S., 1983b, Multiple postsynaptic responses evoked by glutamate on in vitro spinal motoneurones, in: *CNS Receptors: From Molecular Pharmacology to Behavior* (P. Mandel and F. V. DeFundis, Eds.) Raven Press, New York, pp. 229–236.

Nistri, A., and Constanti, A., 1975, Effect of glutamate and glutamic acid diethyl ester on the lobster muscle fiber and the frog spinal cord, *Eur. J. Pharmacol.* **31**:377–379.

Nistri, A., and Constanti, A., 1979, Pharmacological characterization of different types of GABA and glutamate receptors in vertebrates and invertebrates, *Prog. Neurobiol.* **13**:117–235.

Olney, J. W., 1981, Kainic acid and other excitotoxins: A comparative analysis, in: *Glutamate as a Neurotransmitter* (G. DiChiara, and G. L. Gessa, eds.), Raven Press, New York, pp. 375–384.

Onodera, K., and Takeuchi, A., 1976, Permeability changes produced by L-glutamate at the excitatory post-synaptic membrane of the crayfish muscle, *J. Physiol. (Lond.)* **255**:669–685.

Onodera, K., and Takeuchi, A., 1980, Distribution and pharmacological properties of synaptic and extrasynaptic glutamate receptors on crayfish muscle, *J. Physiol. (Lond.)* **306**:233–250.

Onodera, K., and Takeuchi, A., 1980, Distribution and pharmacological properties of synaptic and extrasynaptic glutamate receptors on crayfish muscle, *J. Physiol. (Lond.)* **306**:233–250.

Padjen, A. L., and Smith, P. A., 1980, Specific effects of α-D,L-aminoadipic acid on synaptic transmission in frog spinal cord, *Can J. Physiol. Pharmacol.* **58**:692–698.

Pepeu, G., Bartolini, A., and Bartolini, R., 1970, Differences of GABA content in the cerebral cortex of cats transected at various midbrain levels, *Biochem. Pharmacol.* **19**:1007–1013.

Perry, T. L., Berry, K., Diamond, S. and Mok, C., 1971, Regional distribution of amino acids in human brain obtained at autopsy, *J. Neurochem.* **18**:513–519.

Plaitakis, A., Berl, S., and Yahr, M. D., 1982, Abnormal glutamate metabolism in an adult-onset degenerative neurological disorder, *Science* **216**:193–196.

Potashner, S. J., 1978a, The spontaneous and electrically evoked release, from slices of guinea-pig cerebral cortex, of endogenous amino acids labelled via metabolism of D-[U-^{14}C] glucose, *J. Neurochem.* **31**:177–186.

Potashner, S. J., 1978b, Effects of tetrodotoxin, calcium and magnesium on the release of amino acids from slices of guinea-pig cerebral cortex, *J. Neurochem.* **31**:187–195.

Potashner, S. J., and Gerard, D., 1982, Actions of kainic acid and depressant drugs on the release of D-[^{3}H] aspartate in brain slices, *Soc. Neurosci. Abstr.* **8**:882.

Prusiner, S. B., 1981, Disorders of glutamate metabolism and neurological dysfunction, *Annu. Rev. Med.* **32**:521–542.

Puil, E., 1981, S-Glutamate: Its interactions with spinal neurons, *Brain Res. Rev.* **3**:229–322.

Sandoval, M. E., and Cotman, C. W., 1978, Evaluation of glutamate as a neurotransmitter of cerebellar parallel fibers, *Neuroscience* **3**:199–206.

Sawada, S., Takada, S. and Yamamoto, C., 1982, Excitatory actions of homocysteic acid on hippocampal neurons, *Brain Res.* **238**:282–285.

Segal, M., 1981, The actions of glutamic acid on neurons in the rat hippocampal slice, in: *Glutamate as a Neurotransmitter* (G. DiChiara and G. L. Gessa, eds.), Raven Press, New York, pp. 217–225.

Shapovalov, A. I., Shiriaev, B. I., and Velumian, A. A., 1978, Mechanisms of post-synaptic excitation in amphibian motoneurones, *J. Physiol. (Lond.)* **279**:437–455.

Shinozaki, H., 1980, The pharmacology of the excitatory neuromuscular junction in the crayfish, *Prog. Neurobiol.* **14**:121–155.

Sonnhof, U., and Bührle, C. P., 1980, On the postsynaptic action of glutamate in frog spinal motoneurons, *Pflügers Arch.* **388**:101–109.

Stettmeier, H., Finger, W., and Dudel, J., 1983, Glutamate activated postsynaptic channels in crayfish muscle investigated by noise analysis, *Pflügers Arch.* **397**:13–19.

Stone, T. W., Perkins, M. N., Collins, J. F., and Curry, K., 1981, Activity of the enantiomers of 2-amino-5-phosphono-valeric acid as stereospecific antagonists of excitatory amino acids, *Neuroscience* **6**:2249–2252.

Storm-Mathisen, J., Leknes, A. K., Bore, A. T., Vaaland, J. L., Edminson, P., Hang, F. M.-S., and Ottersen, O. P., 1983, Glutamate and GABA: First visualization in neurones by immuno-cytochemistry, *Nature* **301**:517–520.

Takeuchi, A., Onodera, K., and Kawagoe, R., 1983, The effects of dorsal root stimulation on the release of endogenous glutamate from the frog spinal cord, *Proc. Jpn. Acad. ser.* B **59**:88–92.

Usherwood, P. N. R., 1969, Glutamate sensitivity of denervated insect muscle fibers, *Nature* **223**:411–413.

Usherwood, P. N. R, 1981, Glutamate synapses and receptors on insect muscle, in: *Glutamate as a Neurotransmitter* (G. DiChiara and G. L. Gessa, eds.), Raven Press, New York, pp. 183–193.

Watkins, J. C., and Evans, R. H., 1981, Excitatory amino acid transmitters, *Annu. Rev. Pharmacol.* **21**:165–204.

Wenthold, R. J., 1981, Glutamate and aspartate as neurotransmitters for the auditory nerve, in: *Glutamate as a Neurotransmitter* (G. DiChiara and G. L. Gessa, eds.), Raven Press, New York, pp. 69–78.

Wheeler, D. D., 1980, A model for GABA and glutamic acid transport by cortical synaptosomes, *Pharmacology* **21**:141–152.

Wong, P. T.-H., Singh, V. K., and McGeer, E. G., 1982, Glutamic acid binding in fibroblasts from patients with Huntington's disease, *Soc. Neurosci Abstr.* **8:**152.

Yamamoto, C., and Matsui, S., 1976, Effect of stimulation of excitatory nerve tract on release of glutamic acid from olfactory cortex slices *in vitro, J. Neurochem.* **26:**487–491.

Yamamoto, C., and Sawada, S., 1982, Sensitivity of hippocampal neurons to glutamic acid and its analogues, *Brain Res.* **225:**358–362.

Excitatory Amino Acids: Membrane Physiology

MARK L. MAYER and GARY L. WESTBROOK

1. INTRODUCTION

1.1. Receptor Pharmacology

The excitatory action of acidic amino acids on neuronal membranes was first revealed in electrophysiological studies on cortical neurons (Hayashi, 1954) and, subsequently, on spinal neurons (Curtis et al., 1960). Amino acids such as L-glutamate and L-aspartate excite neurons in virtually every area of the vertebrate nervous system with the exception of those in sensory and autonomic ganglia. A large number of other acidic amino acids, including the sulphur-containing analogs cysteic and homocysteic acids, are also potent excitatory substances, and since the optical isomers of aspartate, glutamate and homocysteate show relatively little difference in potency it is easy, in retrospect, to appreciate the disappointment this lack of specificity must have generated. This ubiquitous excitatory action of acidic amino acids initially led Curtis and Watkins (1960) to suggest that these substances were unlikely to act as synaptic transmitters.

However, Watkins and his colleagues have recently developed selective antagonists that clearly reveal the presence of three populations of receptors for acidic amino acids on vertebrate neurons, and L-glutamate and L-aspartate are now favored excitatory transmitter candidates. Amino acid receptors are classified by their most selective and potent agonists (an analogous classification would be the separation of cholinergic receptors into those selectively activated by nicotine or by muscarine). Thus, excitatory amino acid receptors are distinguished using the following three selective agonists:

N-methyl-D-aspartate (NMDA), kainate, and quisqualate. Selective and quite potent NMDA receptor antagonists have been developed; of these D($-$)-2-amino-5-phosphonopentanoic acid (2-APV) is the most useful with a K_i of 0.62 μM (Olverman et al., 1984). Antagonists for kainate and quisqualate receptors have also been developed, but these are less well characterized. γ-D-glutamylglycine blocks responses to NMDA, kainate and to a lesser degree quisqualate, but is less potent and selective than 2-APV (Watkins, 1981).

1.2. Physiology

Intracellular recording techniques revealed that, as expected, the excitatory action of acidic amino acids is produced by membrane potential depolarization presumably due to an increase in permeability to Na^+ and perhaps Ca^{2+}. Attempts to further analyze the mechanism of action of excitatory amino acids on vertebrate neurons have been disappointing. Briefly, the following difficulties were encountered:

1. The depolarizing action of amino acids frequently occurs with little or no change in membrane resistance (this is especially true for L-glutamate).
2. The use of a single intracellular electrode for both recording membrane potential and injecting current, using "bridge" amplifiers, has limited the membrane potential range over which the current-voltage relationship of amino acid responses may be examined and hindered attempts to depolarize the membrane potential towards the reversal potential for amino acid responses.
3. Most vertebrate neurons exhibit both inward and outward rectification reflecting activation of voltage-sensitive membrane conductances that results in subtle nonlinearities in the resting membrane current–voltage relationship upon which the depolarizing response to acidic amino acids is superimposed.

Much of the early work on vertebrate neurons with L-aspartate and L-glutamate was performed before the pharmacology of amino acid receptors was described by Watkins and his colleagues; consequently, since selective agonists were not used, it is difficult to interpret the results obtained as reflecting activation of any particular receptor species. In addition, studies of the membrane physiology of vertebrate neurons were then in their infancy and the great complexity of the conductance mechanisms present was not fully appreciated. Despite these limitations, a number of important results were obtained. Zieglgänsberger and Puil (1972) showed that tetrodotoxin, at concentrations which block the generation of action potentials, does not interfere with the depolarizing action of L-glutamate. Using a tour de force of microelectrode technology to accurately record the membrane resistance of feline motoneurons *in vivo*, Engberg et al (1979) found complex actions of iontophoretically applied L-glutamate and D,L-homocysteate, which produce voltage-dependent responses associated with biphasic changes in membrane resistance. Engberg et al. (1978) found that NMDA selectively evokes membrane resistance *increases*, while kainate behaves classically to *decrease* membrane resistance (i.e., kainate acts by opening ion channels). Although the excitatory action of other transmitters had been shown to occur via a mechanism involving a membrane resistance increase (e.g., the muscarinic excitatory action of acetylcholine), the apparently similar action of NMDA was unexpected.

2. INTRACELLULAR RECORDING, VOLTAGE CLAMP AND PATCH CLAMP

Due to the technical difficulties encountered with intracellular recording *in vivo* and the demonstration by many investigators that mammalian neurons in cell culture respond to excitatory amino acids, two-electrode voltage-clamp and patch-clamp experiments on cultured neurons have been used to study the membrane physiology of excitatory amino acids. This has greatly facilitated study of the mechanisms underlying the excitatory action of acidic amino acids.

2.1. *N*-Methyl-D-aspartic Acid (NMDA)

The depolarizing response of agonists acting at NMDA receptors is usually accompanied by an increase in the amplitude of electrotonic potentials used to measure membrane resistance. This response was first described by Engberg et al. (1978) and also occurs in neurons in culture (MacDonald and Wojtowicz, 1982). Initially it was suggested that NMDA closed potassium channels open at the resting potential, hence increasing the membrane resistance and producing depolarization by reduction of a steady outward potassium current. Since the NMDA response decreases with hyperpolarization, but does not reverse when the membrane potential is made more negative than the potassium equilibrium potential, Engberg et al. (1979) suggested that the conductance mechanism linked to NMDA receptors shows voltage sensitivity; an analogous situation would be the action of muscarine on the M current present in sympathetic ganglion neurons (see Chapter 6). Subsequent studies on spinal neurons in culture revealed a different basis for the action of NMDA. Voltage-clamp recording was used by MacDonald et al. (1982), to show that L-aspartate produces a region of negative slope conductance in the membrane current–voltage relationship of mouse spinal neurons in culture. In physiological experiments with cultured neurons, L-aspartate acts relatively selectively at NMDA receptors. This behavior of NMDA and L-aspartate reflects voltage sensitivity of the conductance mechanism linked to NMDA receptors and suggests that instead of reducing an outward current, NMDA directly activates an inward current. The negative slope conductance (i.e., voltage sensitivity) of these agonists underlies the *apparent* membrane resistance increase that accompanies depolarizations evoked by the voltage-dependent excitatory amino acids.

Using voltage clamp, Mayer and Westbrook (1984) obtained current–voltage plots of amino acid responses over a wide range of membrane potential, from -100 to $+70$ mV, and showed that NMDA has a "J-shaped" relationship with a reversal potential close to 0 mV (Fig. 1A). Using the driving force for ionic current, we found that the conductance linked to NMDA receptors increases exponentially with an e-fold increase per 25 mV depolarization over the voltage range -80 to -10 mV. These results substantially confirmed earlier suggestions that NMDA receptors were linked to a voltage-sensitive conductance but revealed little about the mechanism gating the NMDA-activated conductance. MacDonald et al. (1982) suggested that in spinal neurons NMDA modulates a voltage-sensitive sodium conductance. A similar hypothesis was put forward by Flatman et al. (1983), who observed loss of voltage sensitivity and a shift in the reversal potential for the response evoked by NMDA in neocortical pyramidal cells in brain slices bathed in sodium-deficient solutions. Based on the results of current-clamp experiments on CA_1 pyramidal neurons in brain slices prepared from the hippocampus, Dingledine (1983) proposed that NMDA modulates a voltage-sensitive calcium conductance.

Neurotransmitter-mediated modulation of ionic currents gated by voltage-dependent mechanisms has precedent, and by analogy a similar action of NMDA seemed plausible. However, it now appears that the genesis of the voltage-dependency of the response to NMDA has a different mechanism. Responses to NMDA in both spinal cord and hippocampal neurons are antagonized by low concentrations of divalent cations, some of which (Ni^{2+}, Co^{2+}, Mn^{2+}) are potent calcium-channel blockers (Ault et al., 1980; Dingledine, 1983). Paradoxically Mg^{2+} is an effective NMDA antagonist at micromolar concentrations, yet the extracellular fluid *in vivo* and in experimental recording solutions usually contains 1–1.5 mM Mg^{2+}. Furthermore this blocking action of Mg^{2+} on NMDA responses shows voltage dependence; it is prominent at the resting potential yet virtually absent when the membrane potential is made positive to 0 mV (Mayer and Westbrook, 1985; Nowak et al., 1984). Thus when Mg^{2+} is omitted from recording solutions, NMDA responses lose their voltage sensitivity, and current–voltage plots of NMDA responses do not show a region of negative slope conductance (Fig. 1B).

Voltage jump experiments show that the blocking action of Mg^{2+} reaches equilibrium within 5–10 msec after a step change in membrane potential. Thus the voltage-dependent action of Mg^{2+} has rapid kinetics that are only marginally slower than responses due to calcium currents that are activated by a voltage-dependent gating mechanism.

The voltage-dependent blocking action of Mg^{2+} is reminiscent of charged channel blockers acting at a variety of other sites, and this led us to suggest that the voltage sensitivity of NMDA responses is due to channel block by Mg^{2+} rather than modulation of voltage-sensitive Na^+ or Ca^{2+} currents (Mayer and Westbrook, 1985; Mayer et al., 1984). Using the patch-clamp technique, Nowak et al. (1984) have been able to directly show the blocking action of

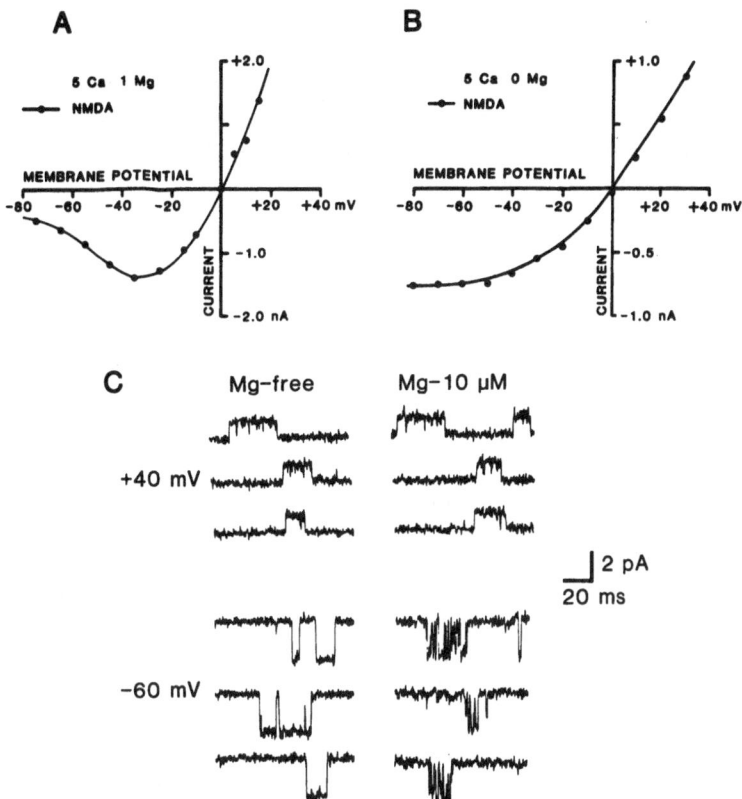

Figure 1. The voltage sensitivity of NMDA (and L-glutamate) is due to to voltage-dependent channel block by Mg^{2+}. (A,B) Current–voltage relationships of NMDA-evoked currents of cultured mouse spinal cord neurons. The neurons were voltage-clamped with two microelectrodes and responses to brief pressure applications of NMDA (1 mM) were examined at holding potentials from -80 mV to $+30$ mV, either in the presence of 1 mM Mg^{2+} (A) or in "Mg^{2+}-free" (less than 10 μM by atomic absorption spectroscopy) solutions (B). Microelectrodes were filled with 1 M CsCl, and the bath contained HEPES-buffered saline with 5 mM Ca^{2+}. Note that the negative slope conductance at potentials negative to -35 mV present in 1 mM Mg^{2+} is not present in Mg^{2+}-free solutions (B), demonstrating that the Mg^{2+} antagonism of NMDA is voltage-dependent. (C) Glutamate (1–10 μM)-evoked single-channel currents obtained from outside-out patches of cultured mouse striatal neurons demonstrate that Mg^{2+} acts directly on the channel to block inward current flow. Note at a holding potential of $+40$ mV, 10 μM Mg^{2+} had little effect, while at -60 mV the addition of 10 μM Mg^{2+} results in "bursts" with no change in the peak amplitude, characteristic of "fast" open channel block. The internal solution contained Cs^+ and 2 mM Mg^{2+}. The external solution contained HEPES-buffered saline with 1 mM Ca^{2+}. (A,B, from Mayer and Westbrook, 1985; C, From Nowak et al., 1984, with permission.)

Mg^{2+} on single channels linked to NMDA receptors. Thus, when outside-out patches are bathed in Mg^{2+}-free solutions and the membrane potential is held at $+40$ mV or -60 mV, NMDA channels activated by 1–10 μM L-glutamate show transitions between two states, open and shut, with a mean open time of approximately 5 msec (27°C). Addition of 10 μM Mg^{2+} to the extracellular solution does not alter the mean open time at $+40$ mV, but when the membrane potential is hyperpolarized to -60 mV the channels show complex bursting behaviour due to rapid blocking and unblocking of open channels (Fig. 1C). At physiological concentrations of Mg^{2+} (~ 1 mM), the frequency of blocking is so rapid that the recording system is unable to resolve the open-blocked-open transitions, and the elementary conductance appears to decrease (not shown). These results provide a satisfying explanation for the unusual behavior of the response evoked by NMDA, but rigorous quantitative analysis will be required to determine if this is the sole basis for the action of NMDA. It seems unlikely that these results are limited to neurons in dissociated culture, for Crunelli and Mayer (1984), using a brain slice preparation, have shown that the *apparent* increase in membrane resistance evoked by NDMA in hippocampal CA_1 pyramidal neurons and granule cells only occurs in the presence of Mg^{2+}.

The reversal potential of agonists acting at NMDA receptors is similar to that of kainate and quisqualate and close to 0 mV, suggesting a mixed ionic mechanism with an increase in permeability to both Na^+ and K^+. Voltage- and patch-clamp experiments have shown that Cs^+ ions can substitute for K^+, and thus in an analogous situation to acetylcholine-activated channels at the neuromuscular junction, it is probable that the ion channels linked to both NMDA and non-NMDA receptors show little discrimination between monovalent cations (Mayer and Westbrook, 1984; Nowak et al., 1984). Therefore, one would expect a hyperpolarizing shift in the reversal potential for amino acid responses on lowering the extracellular Na^+ concentration. In spinal cord neurons in culture, the response to kainic acid behaves as predicted, the reversal potential shifting by approximately -16 mV on lowering $[Na]_o$ to 10 mM (Mayer and Westbrook, 1985). However the response to NMDA does not behave in such a simple fashion. MacDonald (1984) has shown near complete block of the response of spinal cord neurons to L-aspartate in sodium-free solution, while Flatman et al. (1983) describe loss of voltage sensitivity of the response of neocortical pyramidal cells to NMDA, coupled with a hyperpolarizing shift for the reversal potential for the residual response. Using voltage clamp, we find a much smaller hyperpolarizing shift for the NMDA reversal potential in 10 mM $[Na]_o$ compared to that recorded for kainate on the same neurons. In addition, responses to NMDA in 10 mM $[Na]_o$ show enhanced desensitization compared to responses in normal extracellular sodium. We suggest that an increase in cytoplasmic calcium activity as a result of impaired Na^+/Ca^{2+} exchange in low sodium solutions could be responsible for this enhanced desensitization (Mayer and Westbrook, 1985).

2.2. Glutamate and Aspartate

The agonists used experimentally to selectively activate each of the amino acid receptors on vertebrate neurons are synthetic or of plant origin and are not present in the nervous system. Two acidic amino acids, L-glutamate and L-aspartate, are present in high concentration, but it is unlikely that this simply reflects a neurotransmitter role, since there is substantial evidence that L-glutamate and L-aspartate have metabolic functions and act as major intracellular anions. However, L-glutamate and L-aspartate are potent excitants, and there is evidence that these amino acids are present in vesicles in nerve terminals and secreted in a calcium-dependent manner (see Chapter 4). Thus, there is considerable interest in their mechanisms of action.

Experimentally it is difficult to mimic the highly localized action of synaptically released transmitter substances, and application of glutamate and aspartate to neurons in vivo by microiontophoresis, or in vitro by local pressure ejection or bath application, almost certainly activates receptors located in both subsynaptic and extrasynaptic regions. Moreover, the action of experimentally applied amino acids may reflect activation of more than one receptor species, unless the agonist acts specifically at only one receptor type.

Current–voltage plots of L-glutamate responses recorded under voltage clamp in mouse spinal neurons in culture are nonlinear, i.e., voltage dependent: from -80 to -30 mV the slope of the current-voltage plot is shallow and may approach zero in some neurons; at membrane potentials positive to -30 mV the slope increases steeply to large positive values (Fig. 2). This behavior can be explained by simultaneous activation of NMDA receptors (producing a response with a negative slope conductance from -30 to -80 mV) and either kainate or quisqualate receptors (producing a response with a positive slope conductance). Binding studies (Olverman et al., 1984) suggest that the affinity of L-glutamate for NMDA receptors is greater than that of NMDA itself and other amino acids, such as L-aspartate and L-homocysteate, which also activate NMDA receptors. Thus, although L-glutamate is a potent agonist at non-NMDA receptors, Nowak et al. (1984) were able to use L-glutamate as a ligand to study the blocking kinetics of Mg^{2+} on ion channels linked to NMDA receptors.

Block of NMDA receptors with the antagonist 2-APV, or omission of Mg^{2+} from the extracellular fluid (thus removing the voltage sensitivity of the NMDA receptor response) converts the response evoked by L-glutamate to one similar to that evoked by the conventional agonists, kainate and quisqualate (Fig. 2). A consequence of the near zero slope conductance for the action of L-glutamate in medium containing physiological concentrations of Mg^{2+} will be an apparent lack of resistance change during L-glutamate responses. However, if 2-APV is used to block NMDA receptors, then L-glutamate responses are accompanied by a membrane conductance increase (Westbrook and Mayer, 1984) similar to that evoked by kainate and quisqualate (Fig. 2B). If high concentrations of Mg^{2+} (10 mM) are used to block the ion channels linked to NMDA receptors, then L-glutamate responses are again accompanied by a membrane conductance increase (MacDonald and Wojtowicz, 1982). This paradoxical result is predicted by a depolarizing shift of the titration curve for voltage-dependent block of ion

A

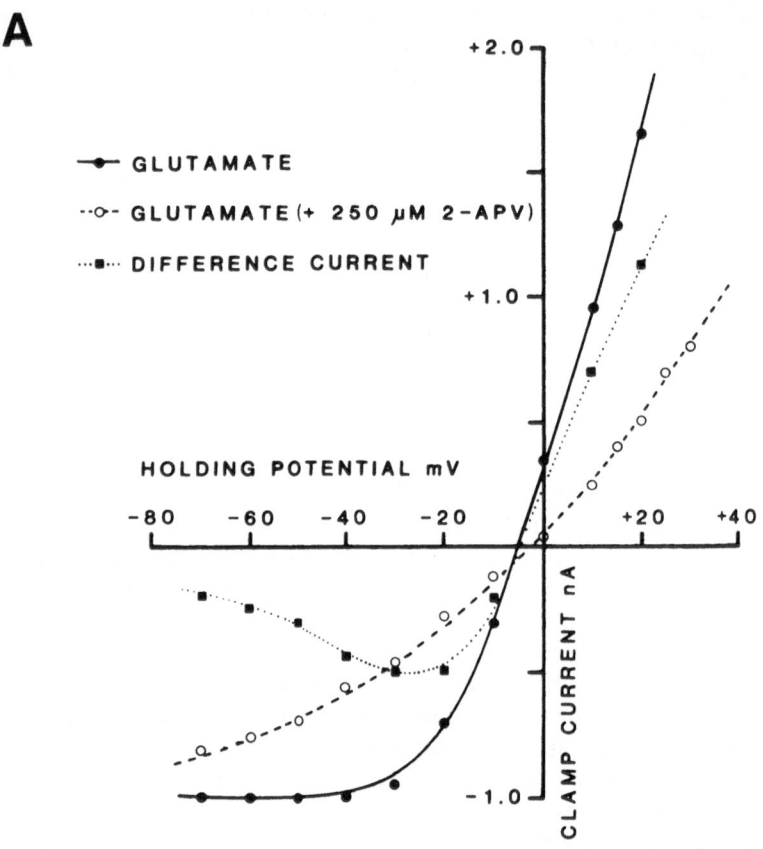

B1

GLUTAMATE

B2

GLUTAMATE + 250 µM 2-APV

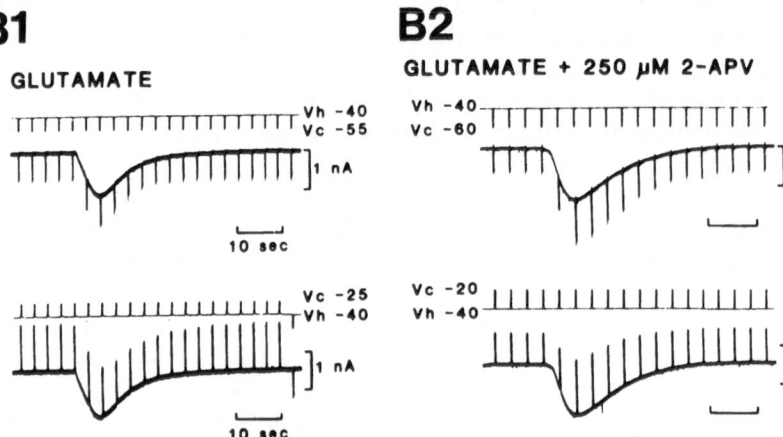

channels with increasing concentration of blocker (Woodhull, 1973) such that with 10 mM Mg^{2+} the probability of NMDA channels remaining blocked is close to one at membrane potentials negative to approximately 0 mV.

Since *in vivo* it has been difficult to detect a membrane resistance change during depolarizing responses to iontophoretically applied L-glutamate, it is probable that with this technique L-glutamate activates both NMDA and either kainate or quisqualate receptors. L-Glutamate can also evoke biphasic changes in membrane resistance both *in vivo* and *in vitro*. Two mechanisms probably contribute to this effect: firstly, the highly nonlinear membrane potential slope conductance relationship for L-glutamate has the consequence that when the membrane potential is depolarized beyond the value at which the slope conductance increases to large positive values (approximately − 30 mV in Fig. 2A), then L-glutamate responses will be accompanied by appreciable conductance increases; this transition zone from a region of low to high slope conductance occurs quite abruptly. Secondly, it is likely that calcium ions pass through the ion channels activated by L-glutamate (Buhrle and Sonnhof, 1983), along with sodium and potassium ions (Hablitz & Langmoen, 1982). Thus, during prolonged application of L-glutamate, there is ample opportunity for the activation of calcium-dependent potassium channels. The degree to which this response occurs will depend on the density of calcium-dependent potassium channels in individual neurons, the calcium flux generated by L-glutamate, and the activity of intracellular calcium-regulating mechanisms, all of which may vary from cell to cell. The end result will be to counterbalance the depolarizing inward current evoked by L-glutamate and to increase membrane conductance.

In spinal neurons in culture, L-aspartate behaves in a similar fashion to NMDA and acts fairly selectively at this one receptor. Measurement of the

---

Figure 2. L-Glutamate activates a voltage-sensitive and a voltage-insensitive conductance. (A) Current-voltage relationship of L-glutamate-evoked current obtained under voltage clamp from a cultured mouse spinal cord neuron. Responses were generated as described in Fig. 1A. The solid line indicates the current–voltage relationship of L-glutamate responses in media containing 5 mM Ca^{2+} and 1 mM Mg^{2+}. Note that at membrane potentials negative to − 30 mV the slope conductance of the L-glutamate-evoked responses is close to zero. However, when 250 μM 2-APV (a selective NMDA antagonist) was added to the bath, responses of the same neuron (dashed line) became nearly linear, suggesting that the voltage-sensitive component of the L-glutamate response is due to activation of NMDA receptors. The component of the response that was blocked by 2-APV (difference current, dotted line) strongly resembles the current–voltage relationship of NMDA (see Fig. 1A). (B1,B2) Membrane conductance changes accompanying inward current responses evoked by L-glutamate in the absence (B1) and presence of the NMDA antagonist, 2-APV (B2). In each case the membrane was clamped at − 40 mV (V_h) and hyperpolarizing 200-msec voltage jumps were used to measure membrane conductance. The upper trace is the membrane potential under voltage clamp; the lower trace is membrane current with a peak L-glutamate response of 1.15 nA in (B1) and 1.3 nA in (B2). Note that there is little change in conductance (G_m) during the glutamate response in (B1); control G_m was 43.3 nS; at peak of the L-glutamate response, G_m was 46.7 nS. However, in (B2), the same amplitude L-glutamate response results in a conductance increase from 27.5 nS to 55 nS. (From Westbrook and Mayer, 1984 with permission.)

voltage sensitivity of amino acid responses under voltage clamp provides a measure of the selectivity of amino acid action at NMDA versus non-NMDA receptors. Using this approach, we find L-aspartate to be slightly less specific than NMDA but considerably more selective than L-glutamate. The relative voltage sensitivity of responses evoked by acidic amino acids can be compared using a ratio of the chord conductance at +20 mV and −70 mV ("outward rectification ratio"), (Fig. 3). This demonstrates the three categories of voltage sensitivities observed: voltage-insensitive (kainate and quisqualate); highly voltage-sensitive (L-aspartate and NMDA); and an intermediate voltage sensitivity for the mixed agonists (L-glutamate and D-homocysteate). The specificity of action of L-glutamate is dose-dependent,

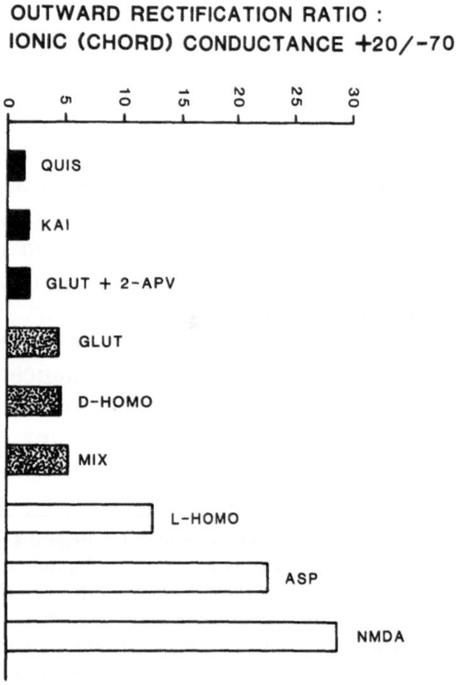

OUTWARD RECTIFICATION RATIO :
IONIC (CHORD) CONDUCTANCE +20/−70

Figure 3. Excitatory amino acids can be divided into three categories on the basis of their voltage sensitivity. Current–voltage relationship for amino acid-evoked currents were obtained under voltage clamp using methods described in Fig. 1A. Chord conductances (G_m) were computed using the directly measured reversal potential (V_{rev}) at potentials between −70 mV and +20 mV with the following equation, $G_m = I_m (V_m - V_{rev})$. In order to compare agonists an "outward rectification ratio" was calculated by dividing the chord conductance at +20 mV by the chord conductance at −70 mV. The voltage-insensitive agonists, kainate, and quisqualate, had the lowest rectification ratios while the strongly voltage-sensitive agonist, NMDA, had the highest rectification ratio. Aspartate and L-homocysteate also behaved as strongly voltage-sensitive agonists, whereas L-glutamate and D-homocysteate had intermediate voltage-sensitivities and rectification ratios. A mixture of kainate and NMDA ("mix") also produced an intermediate voltage sensitivity, consistent with the results of Fig. 2 demonstrating the L-glutamate acts as a mixed agonist. (From Mayer and Westbrook, 1984, with permission.)

the proportion of the response due to activation of NMDA receptors declining with increasing dose of L-glutamate (Mayer and Westbrook, 1984). It is probable that a similar, though weaker, mixed agonist effect occurs with L-aspartate and that at high doses this agonist will have a significant action at non-NMDA receptors.

3. EXCITATORY SYNAPTIC TRANSMISSION

3.1. The 1a EPSP

The excitatory synapse made by 1a primary afferent axons with motoneurons has been the subject of intense analysis following measurement of the 1a excitatory postsynaptic potential (1a EPSP) reversal potential by Coombs et al. (1955). Subsequently, a number of groups were unable to demonstrate reversal, and for several years doubt existed as to whether this synapse operated via chemical or electrical transmission (see review by Redman, 1979, and Engberg and Marshall, 1979). Recently, Redman and his colleagues have obtained a wealth of morphological and electrophysiological information clearly demonstrating the quantal nature of transmission at 1a synapses. It is quite plausible that an amino acid is the excitatory transmitter producing the 1a EPSP, but pharmacological experiments with selective antagonists are required to test this.

Finkel and Redman (1983) have recently been able to record the 1a excitatory postsynaptic current (EPSC) using a one-electrode, high-frequency, discontinuous voltage-clamp amplifier. The peak current of the 1a EPSC has a linear current–voltage relationship over the range -50 to $+20$ mV and a reversal potential close to $+5$ mV. The time constant of decay (T_d) of the 1a EPSC appears to decrease with hyperpolarization. The decay time constant of the EPSC provides an estimate of the mean open time of the transmitter-activated channel if the transmitter concentration at the receptor decreases rapidly compared to the channel lifetime (Magleby and Stevens, 1972). The brief decay time constant of the 1a EPSC (typically 0.4 msec at 37°C), and its linear voltage dependence suggest that the mean channel lifetime and voltage dependence of the transmitter-activated conductance mechanism are different than NMDA-activated channels. Thus NMDA receptors would appear not to be activated during transmission at 1a synapses. Although it has not been possible to resolve the single channel currents activated by non-NMDA receptor agonists with present day patch-clamp recording systems, estimates of the channel properties by noise analysis have indicated that the kainate and possibly quisqualate channels have lower unitary conductances and briefer open times than do NMDA channels (Nowak and Ascher, 1984). Whether one of these channels or some other mediates the 1a EPSC remains to be determined.

3.2. Excitatory Transmission in the Hippocampus

The one-electrode voltage-clamp technique has also been used to examine the properties of the excitatory synaptic response produced by granule cell mossy fiber axons synapsing on CA_3 pyramidal neurons. Brown and Johnston (1983) recorded a linear current–voltage relationship for the peak current of the mossy fiber EPSC, with a reversal potential close to 0 mV. The time constant of decay of the mossy fiber EPSC is voltage-dependent, but with an opposite polarity to that of the 1a EPSC, i.e., decreasing with depolarization. The mossy fiber EPSC also appears to have a longer time course (T_d, 3–4 msec) than the 1a EPSC (T_d, 0.2–0.6 ms).

The pharmacology of excitatory synaptic transmission in the hippocampus has been relatively well studied, reflecting the accessibility of defined synaptic pathways offered by use of the brain slice technique. γ-D-glutamylglycine, an antagonist which blocks the excitatory action of NMDA, kainate, and quisqualate, reduces the size of EPSPs evoked by stimulation of mossy fibers in CA_3 pyramidal neurons (Sawada et al., 1983). In addition excitatory synaptic transmission between perforant path fibers and granule cells (Crunelli et al., 1983) and Schaffer collaterals and CA_1 pyramidal neurons (Collingridge et al., 1983) is blocked by γ-D-glutamylglycine, but not the selective NMDA receptor antagonist 2-APV. Thus in the hippocampus, the linear current-voltage relationship of the mossy fiber CA_3 EPSC, and the sensitivity of this and other excitatory synaptic responses to kainate and quisqualate but not NMDA receptor antagonists, suggests that a synaptically released excitatory amino acid acts on either kainate or quisqualate receptors to produce the EPSP. Since L-glutamate and L-aspartate appear to be mixed agonists capable of acting at both NMDA and non-NMDA receptors, it has not been possible to determine which, if either, of these endogenous amino acids is the synaptic transmitter.

3.3. Excitatory Transmission in Spinal Cord Cultures

The excitatory synaptic connections between mouse spinal cord neurons (SC–SC) in culture has been well characterized both electrophysiologically and morphologically (Nelson et al., 1983; Neale et al., 1983a). SC–SC EPSPs that may be representative of a subset of interneuronal synapses present *in vivo* have a reversal potential near 0 mV (Macdonald et al., 1983). These synaptic responses are antagonized by the nonselective amino acid antagonist, cis-2,3-piperidine dicarboxylic acid (PDA), but not by the NMDA antagonist, 2-APV (Pun and Nelson, personal communication). Preliminary studies of the SC–SC EPSC using a two-electrode voltage clamp have revealed a linear current-voltage relationship of the peak current, and no detectable voltage dependence of the decay time constant. The time constant of decay of the SC–SC EPSC was about 0.5 msec at 25°C (Nelson et al., 1983b). Taken together, these findings suggest that an excitatory amino acid receptor, other than NMDA, may be the postsynaptic receptor.

4. SUMMARY AND COMMENTARY

The use of isolated preparations, especially dissociated cultures of CNS neurons, is beginning to reveal the mechanisms involved in the excitatory action of amino acids on mammalian neurons. However a number of questions are unresolved. Detailed voltage- and patch-clamp studies are required to determine the properties and ionic selectivity of the channels linked to kainate and quisqualate receptors. Quantitative simulation of the interaction between the negative slope conductance produced by the action of Mg^{2+} on NMDA channels and the negative slope conductance due to persistent inward Na^+ or Ca^{2+} conductances gated by Hodgkin-Huxley mechanisms could be of use in modeling the complex physiological response of excitable cells to NMDA. The role of calcium-activated potassium conductance in the bursting response to NDMA (see Gorman et al., 1981) and the source of the rise in intracellular calcium activity triggered by NMDA need to be resolved. The search for more potent and specific antagonists acting at amino acid receptors is a prerequisite for further evaluation of the role of amino acids in synaptic transmission. Here, too, biophysical measurements of the voltage-sensitivity and decay time constant of the EPSC, compared to the fundamental properties of the response of amino acid receptors to various agonists, may help to identify the natural transmitter. With the plethora of agonists and antagonists and biophysical techniques currently available for the study of amino acid action, it can only be a matter of time before it can be said with complete confidence that at an identified synapse in the mammalian CNS, an amino acid is the excitatory transmitter.

ACKNOWLEDGMENTS. We thank Maxine Schaefer for help in the preparation of this manuscript.

REFERENCES

Ault, B., Evans, R. H., Francis, A. S., Oakes, D. J., and Watkins, J. C., 1980, Selective depression of excitatory amino acid induced depolarizations by magnesium ions in isolated spinal cord preparations, *J. Physiol. (Lond.)* **307:**413–428.

Brown, T. H., and Johnston, D., 1983, Voltage-clamp analysis of mossy fiber synaptic input to hippocampal neurones, *J. Neurophysiol.* **50:**487–507.

Buhrle, Ch. Ph., and Sonnhof, U., 1983, The ionic mechanism of the excitatory action of glutamate upon the membrane of motoneurones of the frog, *Pflügers Arch.* **396:**154–162.

Collingridge, G. L., Kehl, S. J., and McLennan, H., 1983, Excitatory amino acids in synaptic transmission in the Schaffer collateral-commissural pathway of the rat hippocampus, *J. Physiol. (Lond.).* **334:**33–46.

Coombs, J. S., Eccles, J. C., and Fatt, P., 1955, Excitatory synaptic action on motoneurones, *J. Physiol. (Lond.)* **130:**374–395.

Crunelli, V., Forda, S., and Kelly, J. S., 1983, Blockade of amino acid-induced depolarizations and inhibition of excitatory post-synaptic potentials in rat dentate gyrus, *J. Physiol. (Lond.)* **341:**627–640.

Crunelli, V., and Mayer, M. L., 1984, Mg^{2+} dependence of membrane resistance increases evoked by NMDA in hippocampal neurones, *Brain Res.* **311**:392–396.

Curtis, D. R., Phillis, J. W., and Watkins, J. C., 1960, The chemical excitation of spinal neurones by certain acidic amino acids, *J. Physiol. (Lond.)* **150**:656–682.

Curtis, D. R., and Watkins, J. C., 1960, The excitation and depression of spinal neurones by structurally related amino acids, *J. Neurochem.* **6**:117–141.

Dingledine, R., 1983, N-Methyl aspartate activates voltage-dependent calcium conductance in rat hippocampal pyramidal cells, *J. Physiol. (Lond.)* **343**:385–405.

Engberg, I., Flatman, J. A., and Lambert, J. D. C., 1978, The action of N-methyl-D-aspartic and kainic acids on motoneurones with emphasis on conductance changes, *Br. J. Pharmacol.* **64**:384–385P.

Enberg, I., Flatman, J. A., and Lambert, J. D. C., 1979, The actions of excitatory amino acids on motoneurons in the feline spinal cord, *J. Physiol (Lond.)* **288**:227–261.

Engberg, I., and Marshall, K. C., 1979, Reversal potential for Ia excitatory post-synaptic potentials in spinal motoneurones of cats, *Neuroscience* **4**:1383–1591.

Finkel, A. S., and Redman, S. J., 1983, The synaptic current evoked in cat spinal motoneurones by impulses in single group Ia axons, *J. Physiol. (Lond.)* **342**:615–632.

Flatman, J. A., Schwindt, P. C., Crill, W. E., and Stafstrom, C. E., 1983, Multiple actions of N-methyl-D-aspartate on cat neocortical neurones *in vitro*, *Brain Res.* **266**:166–173.

Gorman, A. L. F., Hermann, A., and Thomas, M. V., 1981, Intracellular calcium and the control of neuronal pacemaker activity, *Fed. Proc.* **40**:2233–2239.

Hablitz, J. J., and Langmoen, I. A., 1982, Excitation of hippocampal pyramidal cells by glutamate in the guinea pig and rat, *J. Physiol. (Lond.)* **325**:317–331.

Hayashi T., 1954, Effects of sodium glutamate on the nervous system, *Keio J. Med.* **3**:183–192.

Hodgkin, A. L. and Huxley, A. F., 1952, A quantitative description of membrane current and its application to conduction and excitation in nerve, *J. Physiol. (Lond.)* **117**:500–544.

MacDonald, J. F., 1984, Substitution of extracellular sodium ions blocks the voltage-dependent decrease of input conductance evoked by L-aspartate, *Can. J. Physiol. Pharmacol.* **62**:109–115.

MacDonald, J. F., and Wojtowicz, J. M., 1982, The effects of glutamate and its analogues upon the membrane conductance of central murine neruones in culture, *Can. J. Physiol. Pharmacol.* **60**:282–296.

MacDonald, J. F., Porietis, A. V., and Wojtowicz, J. M., 1982, L-Aspartic acid induces a region of negative slope conductance in the current voltage relationship of cultured spinal cord neurones, *Brain Res.* **237**:248–253.

Macdonald, R. L., Pun, R. Y. K., Neale, E. A., and Nelson, P. G., 1983, Synaptic interactions between mammalian central neurons in cell culture. I. Reversal potentials for excitatory postsynaptic potentials, *J. Neurophysiol.* **49**:1428–1441.

Magleby, K. L., and Stevens C. F., 1972, The effect of voltage on the time course of end-plate currents, *J. Physiol. (Lond.)* **223**:151–171.

Mayer, M. L., and Westbrook, G. L., 1984, Mixed-agonist action of excitatory amino acids on mouse spinal cord neurones under voltage clamp, *J. Physiol. (Lond.)*, **354**:29–53.

Mayer, M. L, and Westbrook, G. L., 1985, The action of N-methyl-D-aspartic acid on mouse spinal neurones in culture, *J. Physiol. (Lond.)* **361**:65–90.

Mayer, M. L., Westbrook, G. L., and Guthrie, P. B., 1984, Voltage-dependent block by Mg^{2+} of NMDA responses in spinal cord neurones, *Nature*, **309**:261–263.

Neale, E. A., Nelson, P. G., Macdonald, R. L., Christian, C. N., and Bowers, L. M., 1983, Synaptic interactions between mammalian central neurons in cell culture. III. Morphophysiological correlates of quantal synaptic transmission, *J. Neurophysiol.* **49**:1459–1468.

Nelson, P. G., Marshall, K. C., Pun, R. Y. K., Christian, C. N., Sheriff, W. H., Jr., Macdonald, R. L., and Neale, E. A., 1983a, Synaptic interactions between mammalian central neurons in cell culture. II. Quantal analysis of EPSPs, *J. Neurophysiol.* **49**:1442–1458.

Nelson, P. G., Pun, R. Y. K., and Westbrook, G. L., 1983b, Monosynaptic excitatory postsynaptic potentials and responses to putative amino acid neurotransmitters in spinal cord cultures: A voltage clamp study, *Soc. Neurosci. Abst.* **9**:1144.

Nowak, L. M. and Ascher, P., 1984, N-methyl-D-aspartic, kainic and quisqualic acids evoked currents in mammalian central neurones, *Soc. Neurosci. Abst.* **10**:23.

Nowak, L., Bregestovski, P., Ascher, P., Herbet, A., and Prochiantz, A. 1984, Magnesium gates glutamate-activated channels in mouse central neurones, *Nature* **307**:462–465.

Olverman, H. J., Jones, W. S., and Watkins, J. C., 1984, L-Glutamate has higher affinity than other amino acids for [³H]-D-AP5 binding sites in rat brain membranes, *Nature* **307**:460–462.

Redman, S. J., 1979, Junctional mechanisms at group 1a synapses, *Prog. Neurobiol.* **12**:33–83.

Sawada, S., Takada, S., and Yamamoto, C., 1983. Selective activation of synapses near the tip of drug-ejecting microelectrode, and effects of antagonists of excitatory amino acids in the hippocampus, *Brain Res.* **267**:156–160.

Watkins, J. C., 1981, Pharmacology of excitatory amino acid receptors in: *Glutamate: Transmitter in the Central Nervous System* (P. J. Roberts, J. Storm-Mathisen, and G. A. R. Johnston, eds.) Wiley, New York, pp. 1–29.

Westbrook, G. L., and Mayer, M. L., 1984, Glutamate currents in mammalian spinal neurones: Resolution of a paradox, *Brain Res.* **301**:375–379.

Woodhull, A. M., 1973, Ionic blockage of sodium channels in nerve, *J. Gen. Physiol.* **61**:687–708.

Zieglgänsberger, W., and Puil, E. A., 1972, Tetrodotoxin interference of CNS excitation by glutamic acid, *Nature New Biol.* **234**:205–205.

PART II
ACETYLCHOLINE

6

Acetylcholine

JOHN S. KELLY and MICHAEL A. ROGAWSKI

1. INTRODUCTION

1.1. Overview

Although acetylcholine (ACh) was first isolated from the brain more than 50 years ago by Chang and Gaddum (see Dale, 1938) and the experiments of Curtis and Eccles (1958) identified the Renshaw cell as cholinoceptive more than 25 years ago, since that time no other synapse in the central nervous system (CNS) has been conclusively shown to be cholinergic. Indeed, the often repeated finding that the action of iontophoretic ACh on central neurons is slow in onset and highly variable in its action has led a number of workers to suggest that ACh does not function as a conventional synaptic transmitter in the brain and instead plays what has come to be known as a neuromodulatory role; i.e., it operates on single neurons by increasing or decreasing the potency of the more conventional synaptic inputs (see Bloom, 1980).

In keeping with Dale's original classification of the excitatory action of choline esters at peripheral synapses, the actions of ACh on central neurons have also been classified as nicotinic or muscarinic. Typically the action of ACh at nicotinic receptors is said to be quick in onset, short-lasting, and blocked by nicotine or d-tubocurarine. In contrast, the excitatory action at muscarinic receptors is slow in onset, prolonged, and blocked by atropine (see review by Krnjević, 1974). Unfortunately, this straightforward approach to the classification of ACh receptive neurons in the CNS is complicated by the presence of neurons that fit neither category and others that have been shown, using conventional antagonists, to possess both types of receptors. However, it should be remembered that the use of the original classification was absolutely decisive when Curtis and Eccles (1958) first showed the recurrent branches of the axons of motoneurons within the spinal cord to excite Renshaw cells by a nicotinic action that was identical to the action of ACh at the neuromuscular junction.

As at the neuromuscular junction, ACh synthesis in the brain is catalyzed by choline acetyltransferase (CAT) and is regulated by the availability of choline and acetyl CoA. Choline seems to be supplied by "de novo" synthesis and is taken up from the extracellular space by a high-affinity uptake system.

Although ligand binding studies have shown brain tissue to contain both muscarinic and nicotinic receptors, the concentration of muscarinic receptors is 100 times greater than that of nicotinic. The highest concentration of muscarinic receptors is found in the striatum and neocortex. Although there appears to be both high- and low-affinity sites, it is the low-affinity sites that are involved in the binding of muscarinic agonists and the biochemical response coupled to guanylate cyclase and phosphatidylinositol turnover. Once released from nerve terminals, ACh is hydrolyzed by acetylocholinesterase (AChE) and the choline is taken up into adjacent nerve terminals for resynthesis of ACh. Since ACh cannot be selectively stained, cholinergic pathways have been mapped predominantly by histochemical and immunohistochemical methods that stain either AChE or CAT.

As in the peripheral nervous system, ACh in the brain is contained predominantly in nerve terminals. High concentrations of ACh in any part of the brain or spinal cord imply a dense cholinergic innervation. However, study of its distribution in the CNS is hampered by lack of an easy physicochemical assay. Although, in general, bioassays are laborious, they are at present among the most sensitive (1 ng/ml) and perhaps the most specific methods available for determining the concentrations of ACh in small regions of the CNS. Equally sensitive physicochemical assays utilize enzymic, radiochemical, fluorimetric, and gas chromatographic techniques (including gas chromatography coupled to a mass spectrometer, which increases specificity). However, none of these techniques is entirely satisfactory and as a result attention has focused on the ACh synthetic enzyme choline acetyltransferase (CAT).

The highest levels of CAT activity are in the caudate nucleus, the retina, and the ventral spinal cord. In contrast, the dorsal roots contain only traces of the enzyme, as does the cerebellum. Histochemical methods using CAT specific antibodies allow CAT-containing neurons to be localized by both light and electron microscopy (see below).

Since it is possible that only terminals of cholinergic neurons possess an uptake system with a high affinity for choline, localization of uptake sites has also been used to map cholinergic pathways and quantify the activity of cholinergic neurons. High-affinity uptake is greatest in synaptosomes taken from regions of the brain where the concentrations of ACh and CAT are highest. Moreover, after specific lesions of cholinergic pathways, such as from the septal area to the hippocampus or from the medial habenular nucleus to the interpeduncular nucleus, a decrease in the uptake of [^{3}H]choline into synaptosomes accompanies the loss of ACh and CAT activity. Neuronal activity in cholinergic pathways may be reflected by the rate at which homogenates from the region take up choline by the high-affinity uptake process. Thus, availability of choline at nerve terminals may be a controlling factor in the synthesis of transmitter acetylcholine.

1.2. Acetylcholine Release

Acetylcholine is released from several regions of the brain, and in particular can be recovered from the surface of the cerebral hemispheres using a cortical cup. Release is increased by arousal and cortical activation, but diminished during sleep and in deep anaesthesia. Suspensions of ACh-containing synaptosomes release the transmitter when they are stimulated by electrical pulses or excess K^+.

1.3. Inactivation of Acetylcholine

The histochemical demonstration of the distribution of the esterase enzyme in the brain is a useful method of mapping cholinergic pathways. AChE has to be distinguished from nonspecific cholinesterases, and this can be carried out using specific inhibitors and substrates. Because AChE is distributed throughout the neuron, it is impossible to determine from any given section whether stained axons are efferent or afferent to a given brain area. However, after an acute lesion, AChE accumulates on the cell body side of the cut axon and disappears from the terminal side.

Unfortunately, AChE is not exclusively located in the cell bodies, axons, and synaptic terminals of cholinergic neurons, but is also present in the cell membranes of neurons that receive a cholinergic input. Indeed, AChE is not confined to the immediate postsynaptic membrane but spreads over both the body and dendrites of the postsynaptic cell. AChE staining of cell bodies cannot, therefore, be used as the sole criterion for labeling a neuron as cholinergic. For example, the cell bodies of the noradrenergic neurons of the locus coeruleus stain intensely for AChE, as do the noradrenergic neurons of peripheral sympathetic ganglia, yet they are almost certainly not cholinergic neurons.

1.4. Cholinergic Receptors

The specific binding of cholinergic ligands to cell membranes has been used to map and characterize ACh receptors in the brain. Unfortunately, it was not at first realized that the physiological actions of ACh in the brain are most commonly mediated by muscarinic receptors, and the binding of the nicotinic antagonists d-tubocurarine, hexamethonium, α-bungarotoxin, and of various cobra neurotoxins to brain homogenates was examined in great detail. Later, however, equilibrium dialysis was used to show the presence of binding sites for muscarinic drugs and now much easier assays are available, which allow the concentration of ACh binding sites to be determined in discrete areas of the brain. These methods depend on the availability of either a slowly reversible muscarinic antagonist, such as 3-quinuclidinylbenzilate (QNB) labeled with tritium to a high specific activity, or of a radioactively labeled, irreversibly binding antagonist such as the alkylating nitrogen mustard homolog of propyl-benzilycholine ([^{3}H]PrBCM). As might be expected, if the binding of [^{3}H]-QNB and [^{3}H]-PrBCM reflect a specific interaction with muscarinic receptors, the relative potency of muscarinic antagonists such as scopolamine, isopropamide, and atropine in preventing radioligand binding parallels their pharmacological activity. By contrast, nicotinic antagonists such as d-tubocurarine, pempidine, hexamethonium, and cobra venom have no effect. Subcellular fractionation shows [^{3}H]-QNB binding to be associated with synaptic membranes. After lesions that interrupt the septal-hippocampal cholinergic pathway, [^{3}H]-QNB binding in the hippocampus is unaltered, even when hippocampal CAT is reduced by 80%. This suggests that QNB binding sites are located postsynaptically and are not present on the presynaptic membrane of the cholinergic terminals.

The regional distribution of specific [^{3}H]-QNB binding in the rat and monkey brain parallels that of CAT and AChE and is therefore highest in the corpus striatum and lowest in the cerebellar cortex (Kuhar and Yamamura, 1976; Wamsley et al., 1981; Kobayashi et al., 1978). In other regions, however, this correlation is less good because there is a mixed population of nicotinic and muscarinic receptors on central neurons.

1.5. Central Cholinergic Pathways

Shute and Lewis (1967) were the first to produce a map of cholinergic fibers in the rat brain by combining a histochemical method for determining the AChE distribution with surgical lesions. However as noted above, not all neurons that stain for AChE are cholinergic, and it is now recognized that other approaches must be used to definitively map cholinergic pathways. The main cholinergic pathways shown in Fig. 1, therefore, have been established by mapping changes in AChE and CAT in discrete areas of the brain following destruction of specific subcortical nuclei and the use of new immunohistochemical techniques for the visualization of CAT (Fibiger, 1982).

Based upon CAT immunocytochemistry, cholinergic neurons have been localized to various specific areas of the brain and spinal cord. These neurons

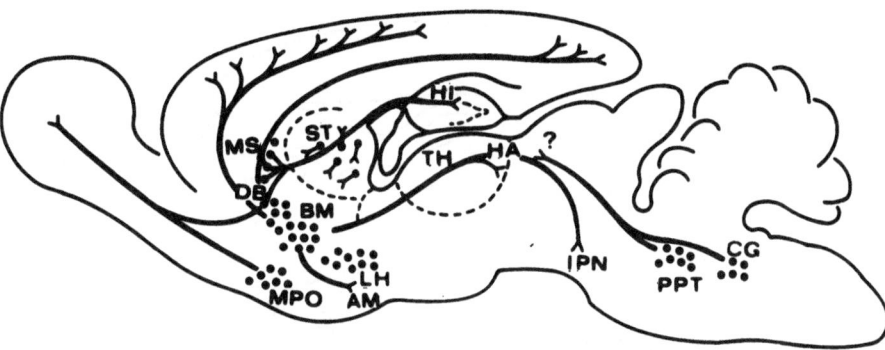

Figure 1. Schematic drawing of the main cholinergic pathways in the rat brain. Abbreviations: AM, amygdala; BM, nucleus basalis magnocellularis; CG, central grey; DB, nuclei of the diagonal band; HA, habenula; HI, hippocampus; IPN, interpeduncular nucleus; LH, lateral hypothalamus; MPO, magnocellular preoptic nucleus; MS, nucleus of the medial septum; PPT, peduncolo-pontine tegmental nucleus; ST, striatum; TH, thalamus. (From Pepeu, 1983, with permission.)

can be conveniently catagorized into three main groups: (1) basal forebrain and pontomesencephalic neurons that have ascending projections to cortex and thalamus, respectively; (2) intrinsic neurons of the striatum; and (3) motoneurons of the brainstem and spinal cord (Kimura et al., 1980; Armstrong et al., 1983; Mesulam et al., 1983). Interestingly, although all morphological types of cortex (i.e., paleo-, archi- and neocortex) receive cholinergic projections, no cholinergic cell bodies have been demonstrated in cortical areas. A similar situation holds for the dienchephalon: CAT staining fibers are found in many nuclei but there are no immunoreactive cell bodies.

1.5.1. Cholinergic Projection Neurons of the Basal Forebrain and Upper Brainstem

Mesulam et al. (1983) have proposed a simple scheme for labeling the forebrain and upper brainstem cholinergic nuclei based on their observations in the macaque monkey and the rat. The subsets of cholinergic neurons within the relevant nuclei are designated Ch1 through Ch6 (Fig. 2). Ch1 and Ch2 are contained within the medial septal nucleus and ventral limb nucleus of the diagonal band and collectively provide the cholinergic projections to the hippocampus. Ch3 lies within the horizontal limb nucleus of the diagonal band and is the major source of the projection to the olfactory bulb. Ch4 would compare most closely with the nucleus basalis of Meynert in primates (Pearson et al., 1983) and in addition would include cholinergic neurons within the nuclei of the ansa lenticularis, ansa peduncularis, the medullary laminae of the globus pallidus, and the substantis innominata; it provides the principal cholinergic innervation of the amygdala and neocortical areas. Ch4 is the most extensive cholinergic cell group and contains the largest

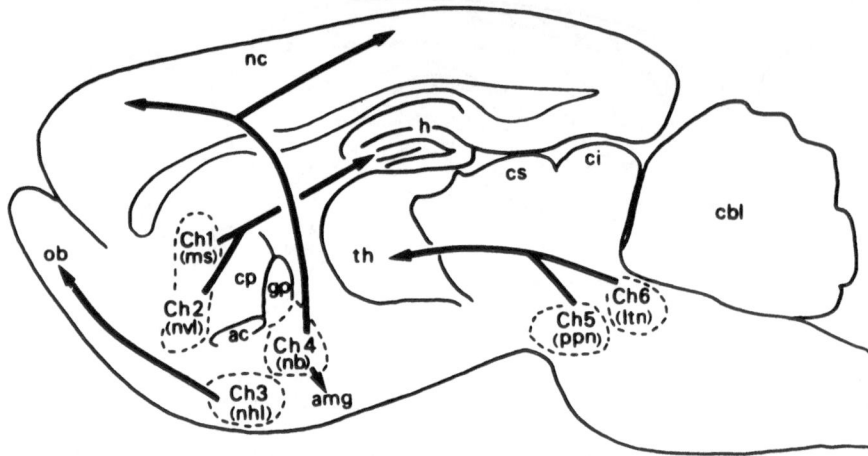

Figure 2. Schematic representation of the organization of the central cholinergic pathways. The traditional nuclear groups that most closely correspond to the Ch subdivisions are indicated in parentheses (see Table 1 for index to abbreviations). (From Mesulam et al., 1983, with permission.)

Table 1. Nomenclature for Cholinergic Projection Neurons of the Basal Forebrain and Upper Brainstem in the Rat[a]

Cholinergic cell groups	Major destination of cholinergic innervation	Traditional nomenclature for the nuclei that are the source of the cholinergic innervation
Ch1	Hippocampus (h)	Medial septal nucleus (ms)
Ch2	Hippocampus	Vertical limb nucleus of the diagonal band (nvl)
Ch3	Olfactory bulb (ob)	Lateral part of the horizontal limb nucleus of the diagonal band (nhl)
Ch4	Neocortex (nc) and amygdala (amg)	Nucleus basalis of Meynert (nb), globus pallidus (gp), substantia innominata, nucleus of the ansa lenticularis, neurons lateral to the vertical limb nucleus, and those on the medial parts of the horizontal limb nucleus of the diagonal band
Ch5	Thalamus (th)	Nucleus pedunculopontinus (ppn), neurons within the cuneiform nucleus and in the parabrachial area
Ch6	Thalamus	Laterodorsal tegmental nucleus (ltn)

[a]Based on the scheme of Mesulam et al. (1983). Abbreviations used in Fig. 2 are given in parentheses. Additional abbreviations in Fig. 2: ac, nucleus acumbens; cp, caudate putamen; cs, superior colliculus; ci, inferior colliculus; cbl, cerebellum.

neurons. Thus, the Ch1 to Ch4 neurons project topographically to the entire neocortical mantel as well as to limbic and olfactory structures. The neurons of Ch5 and Ch6 are located in the pontomesencephalic reticular formation and collectively provide the major cholinergic innervation of the thalamus (Table 1). These neurons are also a minor source of cholinergic innervation of neocortex and hippocampus. Although the widespread cholinergic pathway from Ch5 and Ch6 to the thalamus could be looked on as the origin of the classical reticular activating system, there is now a substantial amount of work that suggests that there must be a noncholinergic segment between the thalamus and the cortex that brings about arousal.

1.5.2. Intrinsic Cholinergic Neurons of the Neostriatum

The neostriatum (caudate nucleus and putamen) contains the highest concentration of CAT, AChE, and ACh in the brain, and all three markers appear to be contained solely within intrinsic neurons.

1.5.3. Motoneurons of the Brainstem and Spinal Cord

As might be predicted from our knowledge of the cholinergic nature of the neuromuscular junction, motoneurons are readily stained for both CAT and AChE. This holds true for motoneurons in the brainstem as well as in the ventral horn of the spinal cord (Kimura et al., 1981).

1.6. Functional Correlates of Identifiable Cholinergic Pathways

On the basis of AChE histochemistry combined with brain lesions, Shute and Lewis (1967) originally conceived of two major ascending cholinergic pathways, the first from the mesencephalic reticular formation (nucleus cuneiformis), and the second from the ventral tegmental area and substantia nigra, which were known as the dorsal and ventral tegmental pathways, respectively. As noted above, contemporary neuroanatomical studies with CAT immunohistochemistry have focused attention on the ascending projections from the basal forebrain and pontomesencephalic region (Ch1-Ch6). From the point of view of functional studies, two pathways are of particular importance. The first is from the magnocellular forebrain nuclei (MFN; Ch4), which provides a topographically organized cholinergic projection to the entire neocortical mantle.

Unilateral destruction of the MFN in the rat is associated with a decrease in the output of ACh from the ipsilateral frontal-parietal cortex, whereas stimulation of these nuclei results in an increase in ACh release (Fig. 3). In lesioned rats, the electrocorticogram shows a reduction in the electrical activity of the cortex overlying the lesioned nuclei, and this is associated with

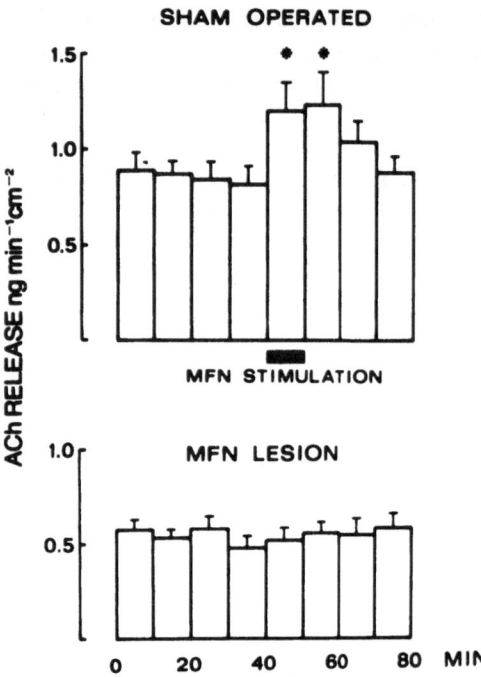

Figure 3. ACh release from the cerebral cortex of unanaesthetized rats. ACh diffuses from the cortex into a Perspex cylinder implanted epidurally into the skull 2 days before the experiment and filled with Ringer solution containing an inhibitor of AChE. ACh was quantified by bioassay every 10 min. The upper graph shows the increase in ACh output that occurs during and immediately after electrical stimulation of the peripallidal region of the magnocellular forebrain nuclei (*, P<0.01, n = 5). In the lower graph spontaneous ACh release from the ipsilateral cortex of rats (n = 5) with unilateral lesions of the magnocellular forebrain nuclei is shown. The ACh output is significantly (P<0.01) lower than the spontaneous unstimulated release in the sham-operated rats as shown above. (From Pepeu, 1983, with permission.)

a reduction in exploratory activity. The reduction in exploratory activity appears to be accompanied by a reduction in the acquisition of active and passive avoidance conditioned responses. Thus the pathways from the MFN to the cortex are thought to enhance the cortical activity associated with acquisition of new information. In man, an important feature of senile dementia of the Alzheimer type appears to be destruction of the nucleus basalis of Meynert and presumably as a consequence there is a marked decrease in cortical ACh levels and CAT activity (Coyle et al., 1983). Therefore it has been suggested that this pathway may be essential for cognitive function.

The second major pathway of functional interest originates from the large AChE staining neurons of the nucleus tractus diagonalis of Broca and the medial septum and runs from the septum through the fimbria to the hippocampus. Electrolytic lessions of the septum, or transections of the fimbria, have been shown to extensively deplete ACh, AChE, and CAT from the hippocampus.

The septohippocampal pathway appears to be essential for the hippocampal theta rhythm, which is known to be blocked by muscarinic antagonists. Although the function of this pathway has been a matter of controversy it appears to be necessary for the exploration of novel environments and the acquisition of avoidance behavior.

Although little is known about the function of the intrinsic cholinergic neurons of the striatum, it is suspected that these neurons are involved in the control of movement. Thus, in Parkinson's disease, it is believed that there is a functional hyperactivity of striatal cholinergic neurons due to a loss of dopaminergic control, whereas in Huntington's chorea there is a decrease in striatal CAT activity, indicating a loss of cholinergic neurons. The existence of cholinergic defects in these human neurological disorders has led to the suggestion that striatal cholinergic neurons play a pivotal role in movement control.

As evidence for the participation of dopamine in the regulation of striatal cholinergic neurons, biochemical studies have shown that dopamine receptor blocking agents enhance ACh release and turnover with a consequent decrease in ACh levels. Opposite changes occur after the administration of dopamine agonists. However, as yet, anatomical evidence of a direct synaptic interaction between dopaminergic afferents to the striatum and intrinsic cholinergic neurons is lacking.

2. EXTRACELLULAR STUDIES IN THE CENTRAL NERVOUS SYSTEM

2.1. Nicotinic Excitation

The earliest described cholinergic synaptic interaction in the CNS was that between spinal motoneurons and Renshaw cells, a type of interneuron that mediates feedback inhibition via recurrent collaterals of motoneurons in the spinal cord. Acetylcholine readily excites Renshaw cells and this action is mediated by receptors of the nicotinic type. Moreover, the initial excitation of Renshaw cells produced by antidromic stimulation of ventral roots (which sets up impulses in the axon collaterals of motoneurons that synapse on Renshaw cells) is due to activation of nicotinic receptors. Although more than three decades have elapsed since the original pioneering work on Renshaw cells was begun by Eccles and his collaborators, there is no other clear example of a central synaptic interaction mediated by nicotinic cholinergic receptors.

Renshaw cells are particularly sensitive to ACh and can be excited by the iontophoretic application of as little as 10^{-14} mole. Firing begins within 30 msec and rarely lasts more than 1 sec after the end of the ACh application (Curtis and Eccles, 1958; Biscoe and Krnjević, 1963; Curtis and Ryall 1966a). Afterdischarges are only a feature of ACh applications accompanied by an anticholinesterase or when a nonhydrolyzable cholinomimetic such as carbachol, succinylcholine, or nicotine is used.

The excitation evoked by antidromic stimulation of the recurrent branches of the motoneuron is brief in latency and gives rise to a high-frequency burst that is readily blocked by the nictonic antagonists hexamethonium and dihydro-β-erythroidine (DHβE). Unfortunately, the neuromuscular blocking agent d-tubocurarine applied by microiontophoresis excites most central neurons and cannot be shown to block the response of the Renshaw cells to ACh. Thus, the pharmacological specificity of the receptors is more characteristic of the nicotinic receptors of autonomic ganglia than those of skeletal muscle. The cholinergic nature of synaptic transmission at the Renshaw cells is supported by experiments that show evoked excitation to be blocked by the application of hemicholinium, a drug that competes with the uptake of choline into nerve terminals and in this way blocks the synthesis of ACh.

In all probability, ACh acts at central nicotinic receptors by increasing membrane permeability to cations much as is the case for nicotinic receptors of the neuromuscular junction (see Section 4.1). However, intracellular recording from Renshaw cells is difficult and there are no reliable measurements of the effects of ACh or synaptic transmission on membrane potential or conductance.

Although elsewhere in the CNS the response of a number of cells to ACh has been shown to be either reproduced by nicotine or blocked by d-tubocurarine-like drugs, the response itself is rarely comparable in speed of onset or offset with that of ACh on Renshaw cells. Such nicotinic effects have been observed in the medulla, lateral geniculate nucleus, cerebellum, and septal nucleus. As yet, however, there is no conclusive evidence that any of these neurons receive a cholinergic pathway that can be blocked by nicotinic antagonists.

2.2. Muscarinic Excitation

Muscarinic excitation is seen throughout the CNS. For example, the effect is particularly clear when ACh is applied to neurons within the deep layers of the cerebral cortex (Krnjević and Phillis, 1963a,b; Spehlmann, 1963; Crawford and Curtis, 1966; Salmoiraghi and Stefanis, 1967; Crawford, 1970; Stone, 1972). Characteristically, the increase in firing has a relatively slow onset and may be preceded by an initial depression. The excitation continues for some minutes after the application of ACh is terminated. The slowness of the onset of firing and the prolonged afterdischarge is in striking contrast to the abrupt onset and offset in firing evoked by glutamate. Moreover, the response to iontophoretic ACh is less predictable than that to glutamate in that it varies in intensity from preparation to preparation and from application to application in the same preparation. Presumably the variability could be related to its peculiar vulnerability to deep anaesthesia, metabolic inhibitors, and hypoxia (Krnjević, 1974). The excitation evoked by ACh in cortex is readily mimicked by the muscarinic agonists acetyl-β-methylcholine, propronylcholine, carbamylcholine (carbachol), and muscarine. Oxytremorine and pilocarpine have particularly slow and prolonged effects. In contrast, nicotine, butyrylcholine, tetramethylamonium, and other nicotinic agents are very much less effective. The action of ACh is blocked by atropine or scopolamine given systemically or by local application but is insensitive to the nicotinic antagonists tubocurarine, DHβE, and other toxiferines (Krnjević, 1974). Thus, a wide variety of consistent pharmacological evidence confirms the muscarinic character of the response.

2.3. Muscarinic Inhibition

A depressant action of ACh on single neurons in the cerebral cortex was first reported by Randić et al. (1964) and its occurrence has been confirmed by several groups of workers (Legge et al., 1966; Crawford and Curtis, 1966; Phillis and York, 1967a,b, 1968; Jordan and Phillis, 1972; Stone, 1972; Ben-Ari et al., 1976a,b; Dingledine and Kelly, 1977). The pharmacological properties of the response appear to be predominantly muscarinic: i.e., it is blocked by atropine and more readily evoked by muscarinic than nicotonic agonists. (Phillis and York [1968], however, were also able to elicit the inhibition with nicotine and found that it could be blocked by d-tubocurarine and strychnine [cf. Stone, 1972].) Similar inhibitory effects of ACh are seen in the olfactory bulb (Bloom et al., 1964), the caudate nucleus (Bloom et al., 1965; McLennan and York, 1966), the thalamus (Phillis, 1971; Tebēcis, 1972), the midbrain (Davis and Vaughan, 1969; Straschill and Perwein, 1971), the medulla (Salmoiraghi and Steiner, 1963; Bradley et al., 1966; Tebēcis, 1972), the cerebellar cortex (Crawford and Ryall, 1966a,b; McCance and Phillis, 1964), and the spinal cord (Curtis, 1966; Weight and Salmoiraghi, 1966). Since in most regions of the mammalian brain only a small percentage of the neurons detected with multibarrelled iontophoretic micropipettes are inhibited by ACh (whereas frequently many nearby cells are excited by smaller doses of ACh), and moreover since both the inhibitory and excitatory actions of ACh are antagonized by the same pharmacological agents, it has been suggested that the inhibitory action of ACh is mediated indirectly, i.e., through the excitation of neighboring cholinoceptive interneurons whose inhibitory transmitter is a substance other than ACh (Duggan and Hall, 1975; Randić et al., 1964). However, a number of authors (Randić et al., 1964; McLennan, 1970; Phillis and York, 1967a,b, 1968; Jordan and Phillis, 1972) have questioned this interpretation since in the most superficial layers of the cerebral cortex a strong inhibitory action of ACh predominates.

More recently, in the dorsolateral nucleus reticularis of the thalamus (nucR), Ben-Ari et al. (1976a,b) and Dingledine and Kelly (1977) have also shown short iontophoretic pulses of ACh to inhibit the spontaneous discharge of virtually every cell found to lie within the nucleus. Histological analysis showed that microelectrode tracks in which only ACh-inhibited cells were encountered lay solely within the nucR, while tracks containing ACh-excited cells lay deep to the ACh-inhibited cells in the ventrobasal complex of the thalamus, a region long known to contain ACh-excited cells (Andersen and Curtis, 1964a,b). In contrast to the rather long latency of onset (4-8 sec) for the ACh-evoked excitation of cells in the ventrobasal thalamus, the onset of the ACh-evoked inhibition of the spontaneously active cells in nucR was rapid. Indeed, on many occasions the onset was as fast as that for the onset, on the same cell, of equally potent doses of GABA and glutamate. The ACh-evoked inhibitions proved extremely sensitive to iontophoretic applications of atropine and relatively resistant to DHβE, thus revealing their muscarinic character. In the cortex, Jordan and Phillis (1972) also found the ACh-evoked inhibitions to be more readily blocked by atropine than by DHβE.

2.4. Synaptic Actions of Ascending Cholinergic Projections and the Possible Role of Acetylcholine-Mediated Disinhibition

High-frequency stimulation of the mesencephalic reticular formation (MRF) facilitates transmission through the major thalamic relay nuclei, including the lateral geniculate (Singer, 1973), medial geniculate (Symmes and Anderson, 1967), ventroposteriolateral nucleus (Steriade, 1970), and the ventrolateral nucleus (Purpura et al., 1966). In the case of the ventrolateral and lateral geniculate nuclei, intracellular recording has shown facilitation to result from an attenuation of recurrent inhibitory potentials (Purpura et al., 1966; Singer, 1973), and thus MRF-evoked facilitation has been attributed to disinhibition.

The observation that the MRF evokes such disinhibitory potentials in the thalamo-cortical relay cells raises the possibility that the MRF stimulation inhibits the neurons of the nucR, and there is indeed some evidence that stimulating the MRF leads to a decrease in unit activity in the rostral pole of nucR (Schlag and Waszak, 1971; Waszak, 1974; Yingling and Skinner, 1975). Anatomically, a direct pathway from the MRF to nucR has been identified (Schiebel and Scheibel, 1967; Edwards and de Olmos, 1976), and it may well be cholinergic (Shute and Lewis, 1967; however, see Section 1.5).

Poststimulus interval histograms (PSIH) show most neurons in the dorsolateral nucR and adjacent ventrobasilar complex to respond to repetitive stimulation of the MRF with alternating periods of inhibition and excitation. Dingledine and Kelly (1977) found there to be a highly significant correlation between the direction of the initial response of a cell to MRF stimulation and its response to ACh. However, the MRF evoked responses were not antagonized by massive iontophoretic or intravenous doses of atropine. It is worth noting that with the exception of the nicotinic synapse on the Renshaw cell (Curtis and Ryall, 1966a,b), it has proved very difficult to block other putative cholinergic synapses in the CNS with cholinergic antagonists, even in the habenulo-interpenduncular (Lake, 1973; Brown et al., 1983) and septohippocampal (Salmoiraghi and Stefanis, 1967) pathways, which are now known to have all the biochemical properties expected of cholinergic tracts (Lewis et al., 1967; Katasaka et al., 1973; Kuhar et al., 1975; Lebranth et al., 1975; Storm-Mathisen, 1975).

The rapid onset of the ACh-evoked inhibition of cells of the nucR is quite unlike the slow onset of the muscarinic inhibition of peripheral sympathetic ganglion cells (Section 4.2.6). However, this difference could be due to the special characteristics of nucR cells, which have a particularly high rate of spontaneous firing, possibly as a result of an abnormally high Na^+ permeability. In this situation, even small reductions in Na^+ permeability could cause the immediate onset of inhibition. Indeed, Krnjević (1974) has suggested that the often seen initial depressant action of ACh on ACh-excited cells is a characteristic feature of cells with a high spontaneous firing rate.

The finding that the spontaneous irregular firing of nucR neurons is intermittently interrupted by high-frequency bursts with long intervening silent periods also raises the possibility that synaptically released ACh may play a role in the physiological function of the nucR. For instance, it is now firmly established that during "slow wave sleep" (i.e., periods of electrocortical synchronization), the firing pattern of nucR cells is composed almost entirely of burst activity separated by long silent periods, and conversely during periods of wakefulness the same cells discharge continuously in a more regular and evenly spaced manner (Mukhametov et al., 1970; Lamarre et al., 1971). Indeed, the firing patterns seen during sleep (Lamarre et al., 1971) are indistinguishable from histograms of the firing that remains during the inhibitory action of iontophoretic ACh. This comparison suggests the existence of an inhibitory cholinergic input to the nucR that is active during slow-wave sleep. Shute and Lewis (1967) have shown the nucR to contain moderate levels of AChE and the CAT activity of this region is high (Brownstein et al., 1975). However, as mentioned earlier, MRF-evoked inhibition is atropine-insensitive and high-frequency stimulation of the MRF in unanaesthetized animals produces electrocortical desynchronization and behavioral arousal, precisely the opposite characteristics of slow-wave sleep.

2.5. Multiple Responses of Individual Neurons and Complexities to the Receptor Classification Scheme

A complicating factor in analyzing the cellular actions of acetylcholine in the CNS is that there are comparatively few cells that show only one type of response to ACh. Indeed, the depressant effect described above is perhaps the one most often seen alone. Although an almost pure muscarinic excitation is said to occur in the forebrain (Krnjević and Phillis, 1963a,b; Crawford and Curtis, 1966; Stone, 1972; Legge et al., 1966; Biscoe and Straughan, 1966; McLennan and York, 1966), it is often associated with an initial depressant effect that may be (although this is only one possibility) analogous to the inhibitory action described above. Furthermore, cortical neurons in the more superficial cortical layers (Stone, 1972) or in the medial wall of the hemisphere (Krnjević, 1969) or the parietal cortex (Legge et al., 1966) may exhibit nicotinic or intermediate characteristics.

The cells of the supraoptic nucleus of the hypothalamus appear to have nicotinic excitatory and muscarinic inhibitory receptors (Barker et al., 1971). In general, however, with the exception of some other diencephalon cells

(Phillis et al., 1967; Tebēcis, 1972) and some cells in the rat medulla (Bradley and Dray, 1972), most neurons give responses to ACh that cannot be simply classified as predominantly muscarinic or nicotinic but usually have inter-mediate characteristics. For example, ACh receptors can be blocked by both atropine and nicotinic antagonists in the ventral basal thalamus (Anderson and Curtis, 1964b), the lateral geniculate (Phillis et al., 1967; Rogawski and Aghajanian, 1982), the medial geniculate (Tebēcis, 1972), in the medulla and pons (Bradley et al., 1966), the cerebellum (Crawford et al., 1966; McCance, 1972), and hippocampus (Segal, 1978).

In addition to nicotinic receptors as discussed above, Renshaw cells in the spinal cord seem to have muscarinic receptors that mediate slow exci-tation. Moreover, recent studies have indicated that the nicotinic responses have complex pharmacological properties. In the cat, for instance, King and Ryall (1981) have shown both DHβE and atropine to block ACh-evoked excitation of Renshaw cells leaving excitation by DL-homocysteic acid un-affected. Although atropine was less effective than DHβE, the antagonism of the nicotinic agonists by the muscarinic antagonist appeared to be com-petitive, as judged by the parallel shift of dose response curves. In contrast, DHβE failed to block a component of the excitation evoked by the muscarinic agonist acetyl-β-methylcholine which was effectively blocked by atropine.

Thus, *muscarinic* receptors on Renshaw cells can be activated by ago-nists such as ACh, acetyl-β-methylcholine, muscarine and carbachol, but not by nicotine, and these receptors can be blocked by atropinelike sub-stances but not by DHβE, which is a selective antagonist of nicotinic recep-tors. The *nicotinic* receptors can be activated either by nicotinic agonists such as ACh, nicotine, and carbachol and also to a certain degree by agents that act at peripheral muscarinic receptors, such as acetyl-β-methylcholine and muscarine. This type of receptor is blocked by DHβE and only to a lesser extent by atropinelike substances. The new results of King and Ryall (1981) in the cat confirm similar observations of Headley et al. (1975) in the rat.

3. IONIC EVENTS UNDERLYING MUSCARINIC EXCITATION OF CENTRAL NEURONS

3.1. Intracellular Studies *In Vivo* and in the Hippocampal Slice

Krnjević et al. (1971) were the first to use intracellular electrodes and extracellular iontophoresis to demonstrate *in vivo* that the slow ACh-evoked excitation of cortical neurons was the result of a slow depolarization. How-ever, they point out that the depolarization itself did not seem sufficient to produce the strong discharge of spikes that is observed. It was therefore suggested that ACh might act in a modulatory fashion to potentiate other excitatory synaptic inputs or that it may produce an increased tendency to repetitive firing. The specific cellular bases for these phenomena have been the subject of intense investigation in more accessible *in vitro* preparations, and much is now known about the possible mechanisms that could underly these novel transmitter actions.

On the basis of the *in vivo* experiments, it was also possible to show the depolarization evoked by ACh to be accompanied by an increase in membrane resistance (Fig. 4). This was believed to be the result of a decrease in K^+ conductance as the reversal potential for ACh (E_{ACh}) was consistently more negative than the resting potentials and moreover, was in close agreement with the reversal level for K^+ determined by the inversion of the hyperpolarizing afterpotential of the action potential (AHP). As shown in Fig. 5, a possible decrease in Cl^- conductance was excluded by showing the ACh reversal level to be insensitive to intracellular injections of Cl^- ions that were of sufficient magnitude to cause the reversal of inhibitory post-synaptic potentials (IPSP) evoked in the same cells by cortical stimulation. (See Chapter 2 for discussion of the ionic basis of the IPSP.)

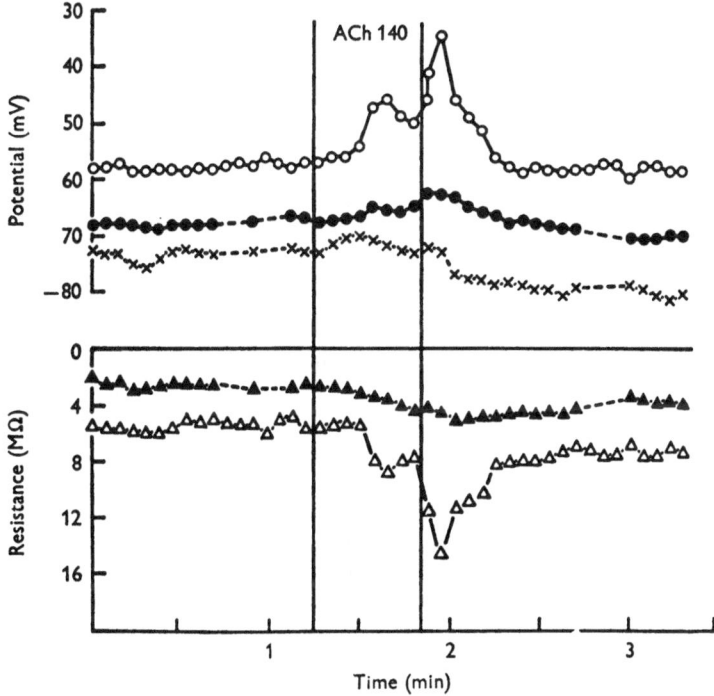

Figure 4. Effect of ACh on the membrane potential, membrane resistance, and IPSP of a cortical (precrutiate) neuron showing the correlation between depolarization and increase in membrane resistance. ACh (140 nA) was applied by iontophoresis during the period marked by vertical lines. The graphs plot membrane potential at rest (open circles) and during IPSP (filled circles), IPSP reversal level (crosses) and membrane resistance at rest (open triangles) and during IPSP (filled triangles). Each point calculated from regression lines drawn through series of eight voltage-current points. Note increasing resistance downward. (From Krnjević et al., 1971, with permission.)

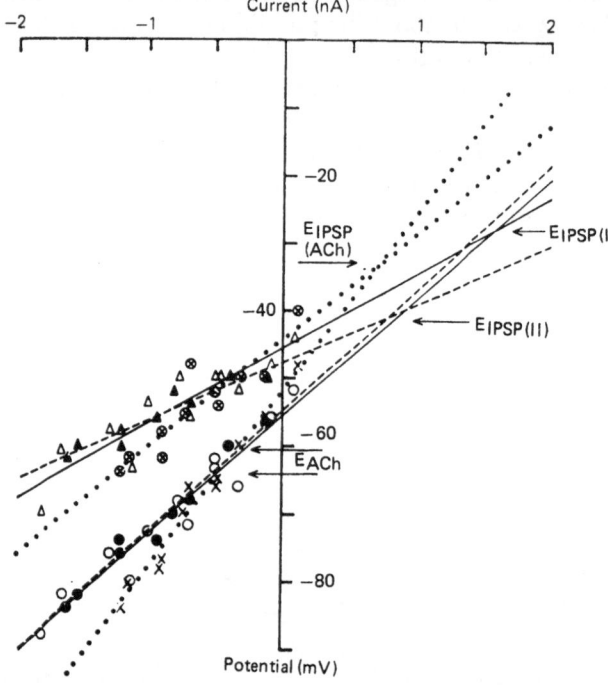

Figure 5. Voltage-current lines from a cortical neuron showing (in another format from that of Fig. 4) the effect of ACh on membrane resistance at rest and during the IPSP from a cortical neuron in which the IPSP was first reversed by the injection of KCl from the intracellular electrode. Vertical axis indicates maximum voltage deflection evoked by 20 msec pulses of current. Open and filled circles are initial and final "resting" control points; open and filled triangles are corresponding values near the peak of the IPSP; crosses and crossed circles are "resting" and IPSP points recorded during application of ACh (100 nA). Continuous lines show initial controls at rest and during the IPSP; dotted lines, during ACh and during the IPSP; dashes show final controls at rest and during the IPSP. Arrows indicate reversal levels for IPSP and for ACh. (From Krnjević et al., 1971, with permission.)

The *in vitro* slice preparation provides an opportunity to analyze the membrane actions of ACh in more detail. The major focus of attention has been on the hippocampal slice because of technical advantages of the preparation, including good viability *ex vivo* and its laminar organization that allows specific cell populations to be impaled under visual control and various afferent and efferent pathways to be electrically stimulated. In initial experiments on identified CA_1 and CA_3 pyramidal cells of the guinea pig hippocampal slice, ACh applied by microiontophoresis was shown to invariably cause membrane depolarization associated with an increase in membrane resistance (Dodd et al., 1981). The depolarization was typically 2–25 mV and was accompanied by an average increase in resistance of 39%. The action of ACh was mimicked by the muscarinic agonist acetyl-β-methacholine and the response of both agonists were readily blocked by 1 μM atropine added to the bath.

In the rat hippocampal slice, the action of equipotent applications of ACh and glutamate were compared, and the onset, peak, and recovery of the ACh-evoked depolarization was shown to be delayed. For example, the onset of the ACh response averaged 13 sec, whereas the onset of that evoked by glutamate occurred within less than 1 sec. As shown in Fig. 6, the delayed onset of the ACh-evoked depolarization was often associated with a transient period of decreased excitability. Thus, during the peak of the depolarization, there is typically a decline in the amplitude of the action potentials and an increase in firing threshold, presumably due to Na^+ inactivation. In addition, there is some widening of the action potential at this time.

As shown in Figs. 7 and 8, the relationship between depolarization and increase in membrane resistance is not a simple one, in that the onset of the increase in resistance is delayed with respect to the onset of the depolari-

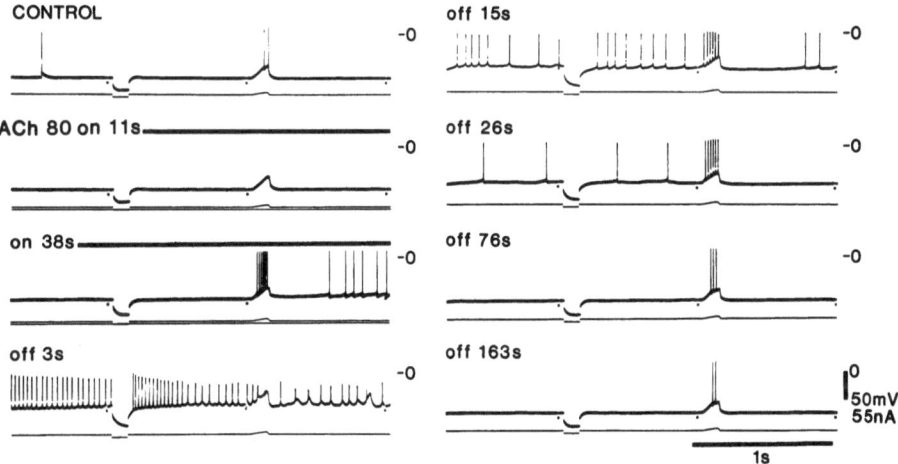

Figure 6. Response of a hippocampal neuron in the *in vitro* slice preparation to an iontophoretic application of acetylcholine (ACh). Intermittent records show the voltage response of the cell to hyperpolarizing rectangular pulses and depolarizing ramps of current passed through the intracellular microelectrode immediately before and at various intervals during and after the application of ACh. The total duration of the ACh application was 100 sec and the entire response is shown graphically in Fig. 7. Decreases and increases in excitability are indicated by an initial decrease and a later increase in the number of action potentials evoked by the depolarizing ramp of current and the appearance of spikes between the ramps. During the application of ACh, the response evoked by the rectangular hyperpolarizing pulse grew larger and less square and reached a maximum amplitude 3 sec after the iontophoretic application of ACh was terminated. Near the peak of the ACh-evoked depolarization, the action potentials were increased in width and decreased in amplitude, and became more difficult to evoke by the passage of current through the electrode. Although recovery of the action potential was rapid, the recovery of the resting level excitability and membrane resistance did not occur for 163 sec. (From Dodd et al., 1981, with permission.)

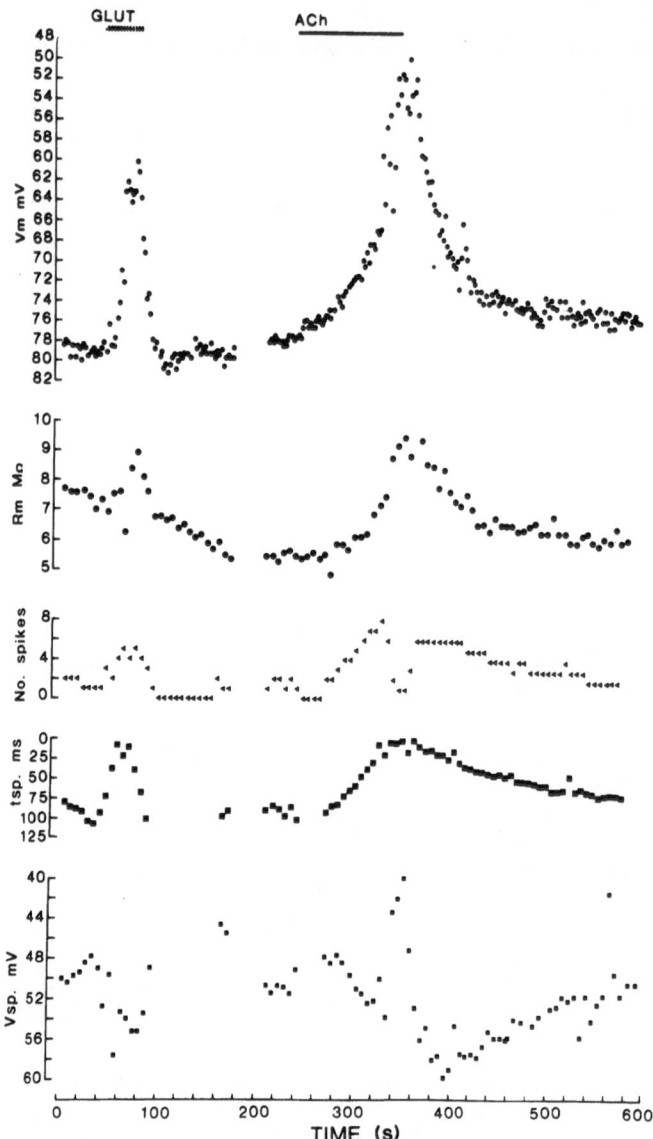

Figure 7. Graphical representation of the time course of the responses evoked by glutamate (GLUT; 20 nA) and acetylcholine (ACh; 80 nA) from the cell whose oscilloscope records are shown in Fig. 6. The depolarization evoked by ACh is one of the fastest seen. However, the response to glutamate is very much faster. The ACh-evoked depolarization is associated with a slowly developing increase in membrane resistance and excitability. The membrane resistance was determined from the amplitude of the hyperpolarizing pulse evoked by the passage of a constant amplitude rectangular pulse of current through the microelectrode. The excitability was determined by counting the number of spikes evoked by the passage of a depolarizing ramp of current through the electrode and from the latency (tsp) of the first spike on the ramp. The threshold voltage (Vsp) at which the first spike was evoked by the ramp was also determined. Near the peak of the ACh-evoked depolarization, the excitability of the cell suddenly declined, presumably due to an increase in sodium inactivation. The reduction in firing on the ramp was accompanied by an increase in threshold. (From Dodd et al., 1981, with permission.)

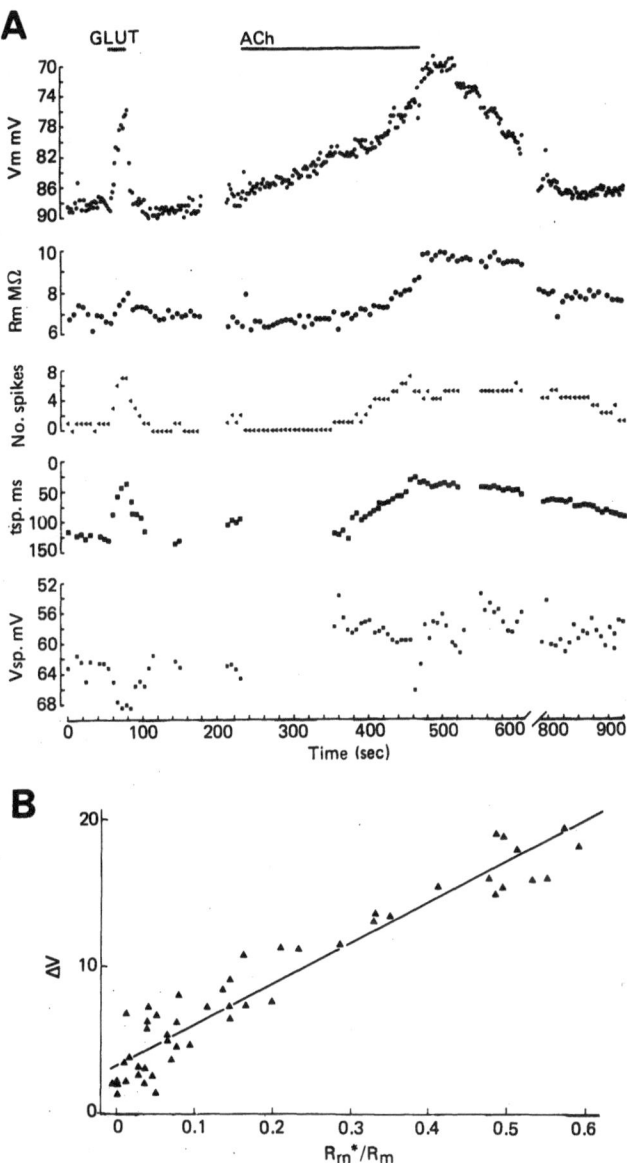

Figure 8. (A) Records prepared in the same way as shown in Fig. 7 from another CA$_1$ neuron comparing the time course of the response to glutamate (320 nA) with that of one of the slowest responses to ACh ever recorded. Again the ACh-evoked depolarization (80 nA) is associated with a slowly developing increase in membrane resistance and excitability. (B) Regression analysis shows the linearity of the relationship of the depolarization evoked by ACh (ΔV) to the corresponding increase in membrane resistance (R^*_m) expressed as a function of the membrane resistance measured before and after the response to ACh (R_m). The linearity of the lines suggests that the reversal for ACh remained constant throughout the entire application of ACh. The correlation coefficient was 0.96 and the difference between the reversal potential and the membrane potential was 37 mV. (From Dodd et al., 1981, with permission.)

zation. However, the peaks of both coincide. Indeed, regression analysis showed there to be a linear relationship between the amplitude of the depolarization and the increased membrane resistance expressed as a fraction of the resting input resistance of the cell. Figure 8A indicates how the depolarization evoked by ACh, ΔV, and the instantaneous input resistance of the cell during the application of ACh, R^*_m, expressed as a proportion of the resting input resistance R_m, was linear as predicted by the equation

$$\Delta V = (E_{ACh} - V_m) (R^*_m / R_m - 1)$$

where V_m is the mean resting membrane potential before and after the application of ACh, and E_{ACh} is the reversal potential of the ACh-evoked response. Furthermore, the slope of the regression line could be used to calculate the average E_{ACh}. This was -105 mV and agrees well with the value obtained *in vivo* by Krnjević et al. (1971).

3.2. Acetylcholine and Anomalous Rectification

As noted above, Dodd et al. (1981) adopted the view that their data showed the depolarization of hippocampal neurons by ACh to be accompanied by an increase in membrane resistance, since it was obtained from cells in which a passive depolarization of the cell membrane or a depolarization evoked by glutamate of the same magnitude did not cause substantial increases in membrane resistance measured by relatively short duration hyperpolarizing current pulses. However, in a number of other laboratories, slightly larger amplitude depolarizations of the same neurons have been shown almost invariably to be accompanied by an *apparent* increase in membrane resistance that is believed to result from activation of voltage-dependent inward currents (carried by sodium and/or calcium) that tend to depolarize the cell. This apparent increase in resistance, known as "anomalous (inward) rectification," occurs within a membrane potential range extending from about -70 mV to the firing threshold (Hotson et al., 1979). (Membrane resistance in these studies was measured with small hyperpolarizing current pulses from various holding potentials.)

Further studies of the phenomenon of anomalous rectification have provided insight into several possible ways in which ACh might depolarize neurons and modify their excitability. Thus, ACh has been demonstrated to promote anomalous rectification in CA_1 neurons of the guinea pig hippocampal slice (Benardo and Prince, 1981, 1982a,b). However, before describing this work in detail, it is worth pointing out that these experiments were conducted by applying concentrated solutions of ACh to the surface of the brain slice, either as droplets or as additions to the bathing medium, rather than by iontophoresis as used by Dodd et al.

Under normal circumstances, depolarization of hippocampal pyramidal neurons activates conductances for Ca^{2+} and Na^+, as well as for K^+; however, the increases in Na^+ and Ca^{2+} conductance seem to be responsible for the anomolous increase in input resistance accompanying depolarization. Thus a major component of anomalous rectification is reduced by the Na^+ channel blocker tetrodotoxin (TTX) or by a low-Na^+ solutions (see Benardo and Prince, 1982b). The addition of Mn^{2+} to the bathing solution blocks an additional component attributed to an increase in Ca^{2+} conductance.

Even in the control situation, the presence of TTX and Mn^{2+} or TTX alone causes a depolarizing shift in the membrane potential at which rectification first appears and the addition of ACh causes a further depolarizing shift in this level so that rectification only occurs at very much more depolarized potentials (Fig. 9). These experiments are compatible with the view that the rectification that remains in the presence of TTX and Mn^{2+} is due to a voltage-dependent K^+ current similar to that known as the M-current (I_M) in peripheral ganglia and that under these conditions ACh causes a marked reduction in this current (see Section 4.2.2). This idea was in part confirmed by experiments that show ACh to have no additional effect on membrane conductance in the presence of Ba^{2+}, which is believed to cause a maximal occlusion of I_M and other K^+ currents. In addition, however, Benardo and Prince (1982b) report that the depolarization evoked by ACh

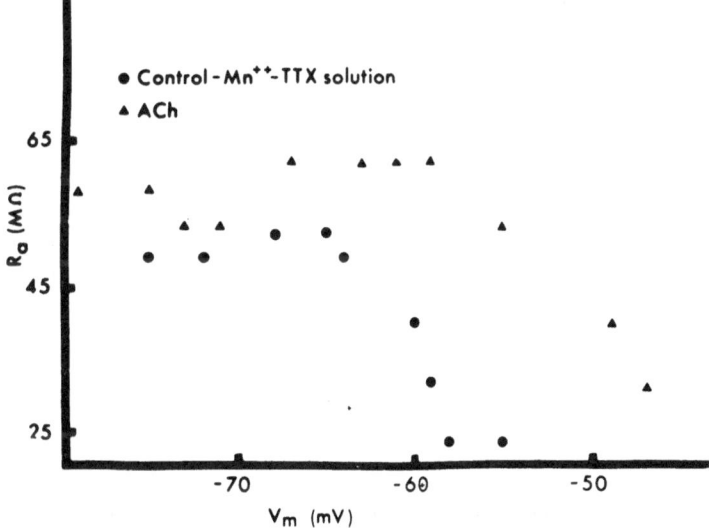

Figure 9. Plot of the apparent membrane resistance (R_a) in a guinea pig CA_1 hippocampal neuron measured by the injection of hyperpolarizing current pulses versus steady state membrane potential (V_M) to show how membrane rectification was modified by ACh. The entire experiment was conducted in the presence of TTX and Mn^{2+}. Outward rectification is evident in control conditions where R_a decreases about 50% as the cell was depolarized from -75 mV to -55 mV. After ACh, resting R_a increases, and rectification is still observed, but its activation is shifted to a more depolarized membrane potential. The voltage-dependent action of ACh is prominent for V_Ms less than -63 mV. Resting V_M, -61 mV. (From Benardo and Prince, 1982b, with permission.)

is partially attenuated by the presence of TTX and almost abolished by solutions containing Mn^{2+}. This fits with their suggestion that pyramidal cells have a persistent Ca^{2+}-dependent K^+ conductance that contributes to the normal resting potential. Thus, the attenuation of this current by ACh could account for the depolarization evoked by the application of ACh and muscarinic agents on cells held near or below their normal resting potential (Bernardo and Prince, 1982c) and outside the more depolarized potential range at which I_M appears to operate (see below).

Benardo and Prince (1982c) also showed the effects of ACh on membrane resistance and potential of guinea pig CA_1 neurons to be blocked by atropine (Fig. 10) and scopolamine, thus confirming the earlier observations in the rat (Dodd et al., 1981). In their study, only one cell out of seven tested was excited by nicotine, and this was not accompanied by a detectable change in membrane potential or resistance. As further evidence of the muscarinic nature of the response of CA_1 neurons, Benardo and Prince (1982c) showed the muscarinic agonist bethanechol to be more effective than ACh. Moreover,

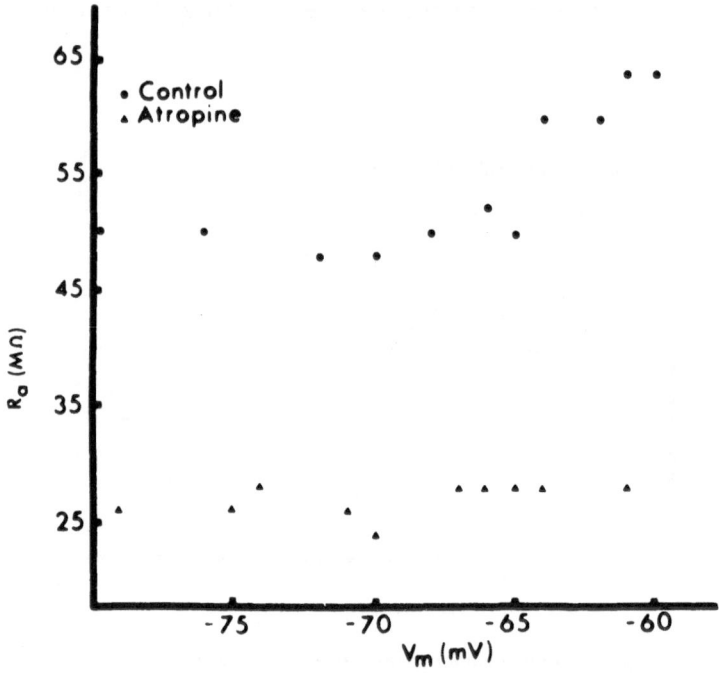

Figure 10. Atropine reduces anomolous inward rectification in hippocampal neurons. Experiments were similar to those shown in Fig. 9 except that control medium (lacking TXX and Mn^{2+}) was used so that anomolous rectification is observed (i.e., increase in apparent resistance, R_a, with depolarization of control cell). A second cell recorded in the presence of atropine (0.1 μM) demonstrates little rectification with depolarization. ACh or muscarinic agonists have the opposite effect to enhance the depolarization-induced increase in R_a (see text). Resting potential for both cells was -70 mV. (From Benardo and Prince, 1982c, with permission.)

this agonist had a longer-lasting effect than might have been predicted from its resistance to hydrolysis by acetylcholinesterase. This was interpreted as indicating that the effects of muscarinic agonists continue after they have been removed from the extracellular media. Indeed, Benardo and Prince (1982c) also indicate that the blocking action of atropine and scopolamine develop much more slowly than expected (since binding to the receptor is theoretically almost immediate), thus providing additional support for a complex intracellular mechanism.

Even in the absence of externally applied ACh, atropine causes a decrease in membrane rectification in the region of the resting potential (Fig. 10); the anticholinesterase eserine has the opposite effect. Thus, there appears to be a tonic release of ACh in the slice. Although it is speculated that the release occurs from septo-hippocampal axons which remain active in the slice even though they have been severed from their cell bodies, it is impossible to decide whether the process revealed by added atropine or enhanced by eserine results from events that occur prior to slicing or as a consequence of tissue release of ACh *in vitro* (Hadhazy and Szerb, 1977).

3.3. Studies on the M Current Under Voltage Clamp

Although conventional "current-clamp" intracellular recording can provide much information about the effects of neurotransmitters on passive membrane properties, the technique is of limited value when one or more voltage-dependent conductance mechanisms is involved. In this situation, voltage-clamp recording in conjunction with specific antagonists of interfering ionic currents is required. Halliwell and Adams (1982) have suggested that the "single electrode" voltage clamp technique, introduced by Wilson and Goldner in 1975, can be used to voltage-clamp hippocampal neurons in the slice preparation, provided the currents of interest have a relatively slow time course and are of low amplitude, and that one assumes that the hippocampal neurons are electrotonically compact.

Experiments with this method have revealed important similarities between the action of muscarinic agonists on CA_1 hippocampal neurons and neurons of the bullfrog sympathetic ganglion. As discussed in the previous section, recordings in the hippocampal slice using conventional techniques suggested that the action of ACh and muscarinic agonists is in part due to suppression of a persistent voltage-dependent K^+ current like the M current of sympathetic neurons. Using the voltage-clamp method, the existence of this current in hippocampal neurons has been confirmed, and, moreover, it has been shown to have a similar sensitivity to muscarinic receptor activation as in sympathetic neurons (Halliwell and Adams, 1982). However, these voltage-clamp recordings were carried out under conditions in which I_M could be observed in relative isolation (in the presence of TTX, at room temperature, and with voltage step protocols designed to maximize I_M in relation to other voltage-dependent currents). Therefore, effects on other ionic currents could easily be overlooked and the results do not give a complete picture of the complex actions of ACh on these neurons.

In Fig. 11, the two left-hand current records show that the conductance of the CA_1 cell increases dramatically when the holding potential of the cell is stepped from -62 to -42 mV. However, as demonstrated by the upper left trace, the current associated with the increased conductance at depolarized potentials turns off slowly during the hyperpolarizing step, causing a slow inward relaxation of the current trace (Fig. 11, top left). The central traces show that application of the cholinergic agonist carbachol causes the appearance of an apparent inward current due to the reduction of the steady (maintained) voltage-dependent outward current. In addition, the inward relaxation is almost completely eliminated. These observations agree with previous current-clamp studies described earlier, which show the depolarization of cortical neurons by cholinergic agents to be accompanied by a voltage-dependent increase in membrane resistance (Benardo and Prince, 1982b). Thus, the authors propose a unitary hypothesis that suggests that all

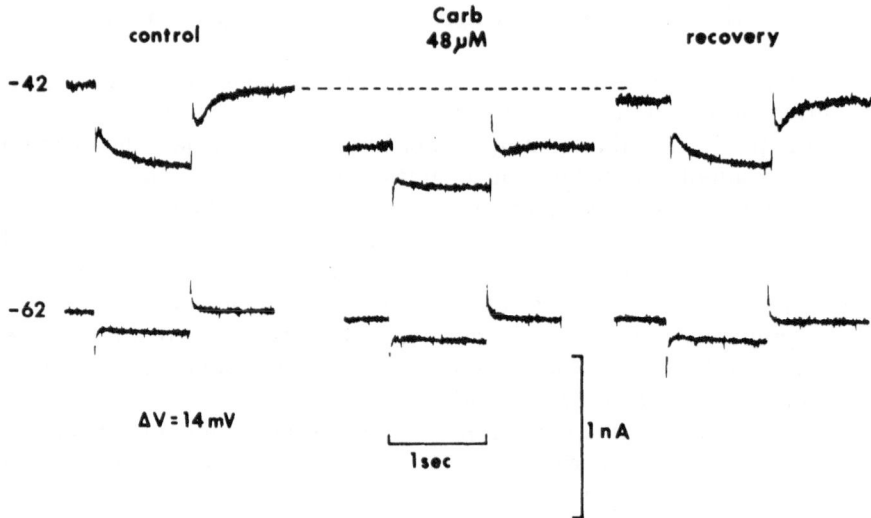

Figure 11. Single-electrode voltage-clamp recordings from a CA_1 hippocampal neuron showing the effect of carbachol on current relaxations at rest and at a depolarized holding potential. The traces show current steps initiated by a hyperpolarizing voltage-clamp step of 14 mV from a holding level of -42 mV (upper row) and from close to the resting potential of -62 mV (lower row), before, during, and 10 min after a brief (2 min) bath application of carbachol (48 μM). During administration of the drug, an inward current developed only at the more positive holding potential as indicated by the positioning of the traces. Note the approximately ohmic behavior of the cell at -62 mV, whereas a similar current response was only observed in the presence of carbachol at the depolarized level, i.e., when the time-dependent inward relaxation had been abolished. Tetrodotoxin (0.5 μM) was included in the bathing medium to abolish Na^+-dependent action potentials. The bath temperature was 23°C. (From Halliwell and Adams, 1982, with permission.)

phenomena associated with muscarinic excitation can be explained in terms of blocking I_M.

However, these results are complicated by the appearance of at least one other voltage and time-dependent current, the "anomalous rectifier." This current is activated by hyperpolarization of the membrane and probably accounts for the time-dependent sag in the hyperpolarizing electrotonic potential that is often seen in current clamp records (Fig. 6) (Dodd et al., 1981; Hotson et al., 1979; Schwartzkroin, 1975). As shown in Fig. 12, sufficient muscarine to completely abolish the phenomena thought to be related to I_M recorded at a holding potential of -40 mV (right panel) had no effect on the time-dependent component activated by hyperpolarization of the membrane observed at a holding potential of -70 mV (left panel). Clearly, the presence of this additional current at -70 mV, named I_Q by Halliwell and Adams (1982), complicates any attempt to interpret current clamp records in terms of the underlying ionic conductances.

With regard to pharmacology, Halliwell and Adams (1982) showed that I_M was sensitive to a variety of muscarinic agents including muscarine and bethanechol. Atropine always reversed these effects.

Other characteristics of I_M are as follows: An estimate of the reversal potential for I_M (E_M) obtained by extrapolating the instantaneous and steady state voltage current curves was -78 ± 4 mV, near E_K in these cells (Alger and Nicoll, 1981), thus suggesting that the current is carried predominantly by K^+ ions. The magnitude of I_M at -40 mV, was estimated to range from 30 to 350 pA. The effects of carbachol on I_M were unaffected by TTX. Similarly, cadmium, which blocks calcium conductance in these and other neu-

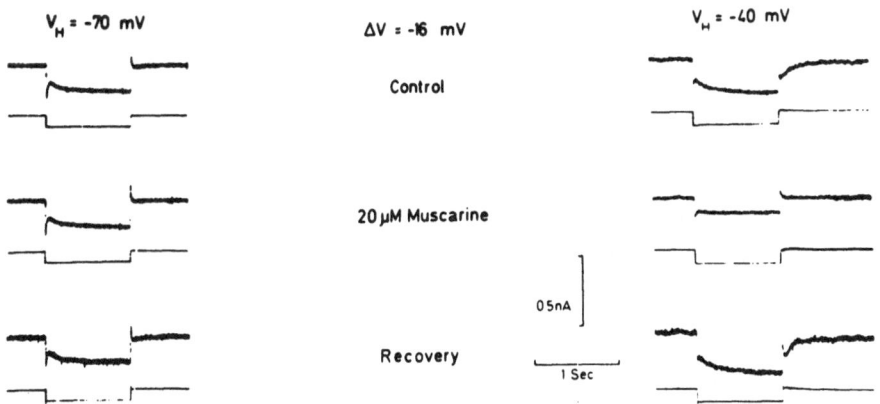

Figure 12. Single electrode voltage clamp records from a CA$_1$ hippocampal neuron showing the effect of holding potential on the response to muscarine. Traces show transmembrane currents (upper record of each pair) flowing in response to step hyperpolarizations (lower records) from a holding potential of -70 mV (left panel) and -40 mV (right panel). TTX (0.5 μM) was included in the bathing medium. Resting potential of the cell was -69 mV. The bath temperature was 23°C. (From Halliwell and Adams, 1982, with permission.)

rons (Adams, 1981; Kostyuk and Krishtal, 1977) was without effect. However I_M was readily blocked by Ba^{2+}, which is a selective blocker of this conductance in sympathetic neurons (Constanti et al., 1981). The effect of Ba^{2+} was unaltered by atropine, thus excluding any possible indirect effects resulting from the release of ACh. By progressively increasing the concentration of K^+ in the perfusing medium, Halliwell and Adams (1982) were able to show the dependence of E_M on the extracellular potassium concentration. As in rat sympathetic ganglia, the kinetics of I_M are strongly temperature dependent (Constanti and Brown, 1981) and at 37°C the current relaxations becomes so fast that they merge with the capacity transients of the voltage jumps. However, the effects of raising temperature on the input resistance of the cells are even more complicated and lead to an apparent increase in the whole cell time constant. Thus, the difference in temperature between the observations of Halliwell and Adams (1982) and those discussed earlier are yet a further complication when comparing the present data obtained under voltage clamp with that from experiments involving current clamp.

3.4. Muscarinic Inhibition of the Afterhyperpolarization

Hippocampal pyramidal neurons exhibit a slow afterhyperpolarization (AHP) following a short train of action potentials. This transient hyperpolarization is believed to result from activation of a Ca^{2+}-dependent K^+ conductance by the Ca^{2+} that enters during the spikes (see Meech, 1978). Benardo and Prince (1982a) were the first to observe that ACh caused an abolition of the AHP. Although the precise mechanism whereby this occurs in unknown, it may be different from the effect on I_M since the inhibition of the AHP is faster in onset and briefer in time course, i.e., within the time expected for ACh hydrolysis or passive diffusion. Moreover, nonmetabolized muscarinic agonists had an appreciably longer duration effect (Benardo and Prince, 1982c).

Although the Ca^{2+}-dependent K^+ conductance is strongly activated following a series of action potentials, Bernardo and Prince (1982a) suggest that it may be persistantly active at rest even in the absence of spikes. They speculate that ACh inhibits this resting K^+ conductance and that this contributes substantially to the ACh-induced membrane depolarization and increase in input resistance.

The effect of ACh on the AHP of CA_1 pyramidal neurons in the *in vitro* hippocampal slice has been confirmed by Cole and Nicoll (1983). These workers have also demonstrated that ACh blocks spike train accommodation (increases repetitive firing) to long depolarizing current pulses (Fig. 13) in a manner that is outwardly similar to the effect of norepinephrine on these cells (see Chapter 8). However, in the case of muscarinic receptor stimulation, the effect could be due to blockade of either the M current or the Ca^{2+}-dependent K^+ current or, more likely, both.

The pharmacological effects of ACh on the resting membrane properties,

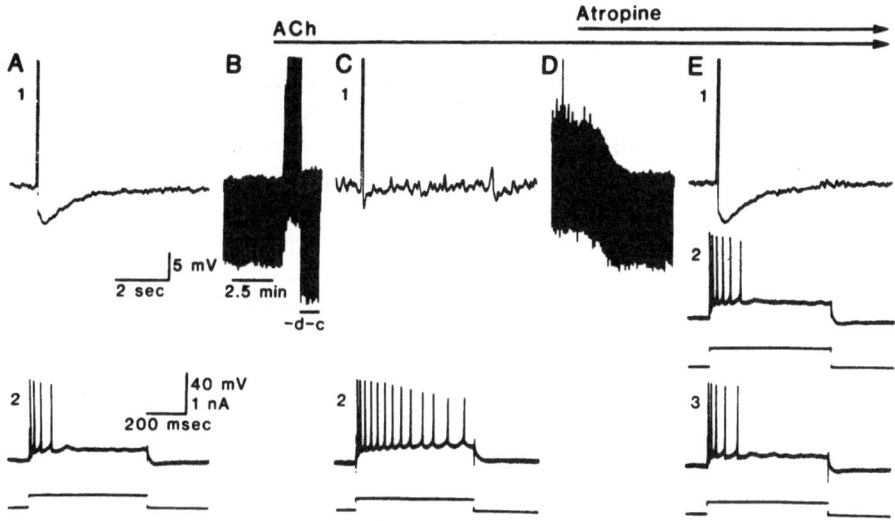

Figure 13. Intracellular (voltage) recordings from a CA_1 pyramidal cell showing the multiple effects of bath-applied ACh (200 μM) and their blockade by atropine (0.5 μM). (A) Control AHP after a 60-msec depolarizing pulse (trace 1) and response to a 600-msec pulse (trace 2). The current record is positioned below the voltage record. (B) ACh (200 μM) superfusion depolarized the membrane and increased the cell's input resistance. (C) Blockade of the AHP (trace 1) and accommodation (trace 2) in the presence of ACh. (D) Addition of atropine (0.5 μM) in the presence of ACh reversed the effects of ACh. (E) Atropine also reversed the effect of ACh on the AHP (trace 1) and on accommodation (traces 2 and 3). The current pulse in trace 3 was identical to those in trace 2 in (A) and (C). In trace 2 the current pulse was increased to match the depolarization evoked in the presence of ACh (trace 2 in [C]). Resting membrane potential, -57 mV. (From Cole and Nicoll, 1983, with permission. Copyright, 1983 by the AAAS.)

the AHP, and the excitability of CA_1 neurons were effectively reversed by atropine but not by the nicotinic antagonist dihydro-β-erythroidine. In addition, the pure muscarinic (or mixed nicotinic-muscarinic) agonists muscarine, pilocarpine, and carbachol mimicked the actions of ACh, whereas nicotine was without effect, thus providing strong evidence in favor of the muscarinic nature of all the responses to ACh. As expected, the cholinesterase inhibitor eserine prolonged the action of ACh.

Of particular interest in the studies of Cole and Nicoll is the observation that electrical stimulation of sites in the slice known to contain cholinergic fibers could produce a slow depolarization of CA_1 neurons that mimicked the pharmacological effects of exogenous ACh. These experiments are reviewed later in Section 3.7.

3.5. The Initial Inhibition Evoked by Acetylcholine

As mentioned earlier, Dodd et al. (1981) drew attention to a transient *decrease* in excitability of the hippocampal cell, which precedes the depolarization evoked by ACh (Fig. 6). This decrease in excitability was even more prominent in the experiments of Benardo and Prince (1981) where ACh was applied in the form of a droplet. This later phenomenon has been examined in detail by Haas (1982). In these experiments, the decrease in excitability was accompanied by hyperpolarization and an increase in membrane conductance. It was proposed that this effect is an indirect one and occurs because of the excitation of neighboring inhibitory interneurons. This concept is supported by the observations of both Benardo and Prince (1981) and Haas (1982) where the occurrence of spontaneous IPSPs increased during the application of ACh. In addition, the ACh-evoked hyperpolarization disappeared when the IPSP in the same cell was reversed by the injection of chloride ions from the KCl-filled pipette. Finally, the inhibition did not occur in the presence of synaptic blocks with TTX or Mn^{2+}. As additional supporting evidence, Benardo and Prince (1982a) recorded from interneurons and showed these cells to be excited by ACh. Thus it seems reasonable to suppose that the initial inhibition associated with a clear decrease in resistance is due to the excitation of inhibitory interneurons, although with more localized (iontophoretic) applications of ACh a different mechanism may be involved (Krnjević et al., 1971; Dodd et al., 1981).

3.6. Disinhibitory Effects of Acetylcholine

During their investigations of the action of carbachol and ACh on hippocampal neurons *in vivo* or in the slice *in vitro*, Herrling (1981) and Haas (1982) both noted a marked reduction in the IPSP evoked by either stimulation of the stratum radiatum or alveus. This occurred whether the agonists were applied by iontophoresis *in vivo* or added to the perfusion fluid of the slice, and was observed in spite of the depolarization and increase in resistance of the cell that would have been expected to cause an *increase* in the amplitude of the IPSP. In the slice, atropine reversed or blocked the inhibition of the IPSP produced by carbachol and by itself actually *increased* the amplitude of the IPSP. Haas argues from these findings that disinhibition is a regular feature of the excitatory action of ACh. Indeed, he suggests that the ability of TTX to attenuate the response to ACh is due to a blockade of this indirect effect. However, as discussed earlier, Bernardo and Prince (1982b) found that ACh could produce moderate depolarizations of hippocampal neurons even in the presence of TTX, so that disinhibition cannot account for the entire depolarizing effect.

Ben-Ari et al. (1981a,b) have confirmed these findings *in vivo* with intracellular recordings from CA_1 and CA_3 hippocampal neurons in rats anaesthetized with urethane. Iontophoretically applied ACh reduced the "potency" of inhibitory synaptic potentials evoked by fimbrial or entorhinal stimulation. This was observed as a depression of the conductance increase recorded near the peak of the IPSP. Such an effect cannot be attributed to a depression in K^+ conductance, which would, if anything, enhance the potential and conductance changes that accompany the IPSP (Kelly et al., 1969). Since ACh caused no reduction in the inhibitory action of iontophoretic GABA, Ben-Ari et al. suggest that ACh must act presynaptically.

Of course, one obvious possible explanation for this effect is that ACh has a specific inhibitory action on the firing of hippocampal inhibitory interneurons, as in the nucleus reticularis of the thalamus and perhaps in the neocortex (Krnjević, 1974; Ben-Ari et al., 1976a,b; Steriade, 1970). Alternatively, ACh may interfere with GABA release from inhibitory terminals. The sharp localization of this action of ACh to the pyramidal cell layer (Krnjević et al., 1981) (where the inhibitory nerve terminals appear to be concentrated) and the failure of Ben-Ari et al. to find interneurons that are inhibited by ACh has led them to favor the later hypothesis. In fact, Krnjević and his colleagues had previously suggested that the termination of the septo-hippocampal pathway on either side of the pyramidal layer (Storm-Mathisen, 1977; Lynch et al., 1978; Vijayan, 1979) may be especially well placed to interact with perisomatic inhibitory terminals (Krnjević and Ropert, 1981).

In addition to the effect of ACh on GABA release, there also appears to be some evidence for a regulatory effect of ACh on other noncholinergic terminals (Yamamoto and Kawai, 1976; Shepherd et al., 1978; Takagi and Yamamoto, 1978). For example, Hounsgaard (1978) has shown ACh to depress excitatory transmission in the hippocampal slice by what appears to be a presynaptic mechanism.

3.7. Cholinergic Synaptic Actions in the CNS

Only recently has it been possible to demonstrate with intracellular recording the similarity between electrical stimulation of a defined cholinergic pathway in the CNS and the pharmacological actions of ACh on target neurons of the pathway. This has been accomplished using the rat hippocampal slice preparation *in vitro*. Electrical stimulation of cholinergic fibers concentrated in the CA_2/CA_3 region of the slice (Kimura et al., 1980) has been demonstrated to mimic almost exactly the actions of ACh on hippocampal pyramidal cells in the CA_1 region (Cole and Nicoll, 1983). In Fig. 14, electrical stimulation not only caused a slow depolarization of CA_1 neurons (associated with an increase in input resistance), but also blocked the afterhyperpolarization (AHP) that follows a train of spikes, and reduced spike train accommodation during a prolonged depolarizing pulse. These effects were all effectively blocked by atropine and potentiated by eserine. However, a hyperpolarizing response 2–3 sec in duration that preceded the slow depolarization was not blocked by atropine, suggesting that it was mediated by noncholinergic fibers that had been inadvertently excited by the electrical stimulus.

These studies in the hippocampal slice provide important confirmatory evidence that the observed pharmacological actions of ACh and muscarinic agonists are of physiological relevance, and moreover, for the first time,

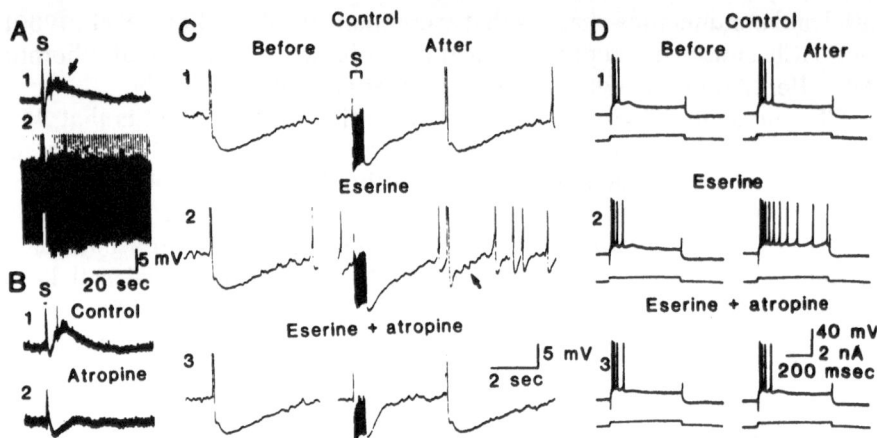

Figure 14. Stimulating the cholinergic pathway in the stratum oriens mimicks the action of exogenous ACh (see Fig. 13). (A) Immediately after a train of stimuli (S) the cell hyperpolarizes (condensed on this time scale) and then depolarizes (arrow in trace 1). In trace 2, the slow depolarization was manually voltage-clamped, which clearly shows the increase in resistance indicated by the size of the hyperpolarizing current pulses. Resting membrane potential, -53 mV. (B) In another cell, the slow depolarization (trace 1) was completely blocked by 1 μm atropine (trace 2). Resting membrane potential -59 mV. (C) AHPs before pathway stimulation and 4 sec after the stimulus. In control solution (trace 1) the AHP was slightly depressed after the stimulus; after the addition of 1 μM eserine (trace 2) the AMP was greatly reduced by the stimulus (arrow); and the AHP was restored to control amplitude by 1 μM atropine (trace 3). Resting membrane potential, -56 mV. (D) Identical experimental protocol as in (C) showing the accommodation during a 600-msec pulse before and after pathway stimulation. Resting membrane potential, -64 mV. (From Cole and Nicoll, 1983, with permission. Copyright 1983 by the AAAS.)

clearly demonstrates the nature of muscarinic synaptic actions in the CNS. The physiological response of CA$_1$ neurons to cholinergic stimulation is unlike the classical nicotinic EPSP involving a conductance increase with reversal potential near zero. Rather it consists of the blockade of at least two different potassium conductances that normally prevent the cell from firing repetitively. Thus, we have a situation in which the pyramidal cell may fire repetitively even though the synaptically evoked depolarization is minimal. Other transmitters can also facilitate repetitive firing by similar mechanisms, i.e., norepinephrine (see Chapter 8) and serotonin (see Chapter 7).

4. ACTIONS OF ACETYLCHOLINE IN THE PERIPHERY

4.1. Nicotinic Excitation at the Neuromuscular Junction

The most detailed biophysical understanding of the transmitter actions of acetylcholine, and indeed of any chemical transmitter, comes from work carried out over the past three decades on the skeletal neuromuscular junction. Although it is beyond the scope of this chapter to review the wealth of information that has been accumulated, recent advances provide insight into the direction of future research on ACh as a synaptic transmitter.

It is now generally believed that binding of ACh with nicotinic receptors in the postjunctional (end plate) membrane leads to a conformational change in the receptor, which then causes the formation of an ion channel in the receptor complex. This ion channel has poor selectivity for cations, admitting large positively-charged ions such as Ca^{2+}, NH_4^+, and even certain organic cations although it is impermeable to anions. Sodium and potassium are the major cations that flow through the channel in the open state, and this drives the membrane potential in the depolarized direction, near the compound reversal potential for the two ions (about -10 mV) (Takeuchi and Takeuchi, 1959).

The opening and closing of end-plate channels leads to fluctuations ("noise") in the membrane potential that can be seen superimposed on the steady depolarization (Katz and Miledi, 1972). Using statistical techniques, the mean size and duration of these voltage (or current, in voltage clamp experiments) fluctuations can be used to estimate the mean open time and conductance of the individual ion channels (Katz and Miledi, 1972; Anderson and Stevens, 1973). Since the half-life of the channels opened during an iontophoretic application of ACh appears to be similar to the decay rate of the end-plate potential evoked at the same junction (Magleby and Stevens, 1972; Anderson and Stevens, 1973), it has been suggested that the rate-limiting step in both cases is the same and may be either the relaxation (closing) rate of the open conformation of the ACh receptor complex or perhaps the rate at which ACh dissociates from the receptor.

More recent data has necessitated certain revisions of these earlier kinetic models. Thus, Adams (1975) and Dionne et al. (1978) have proposed that two ACh molecules must normally bind to the channel-receptor complex before it can open. This model can be formalized as follows:

$$R \rightleftharpoons AR \underset{\text{Very Fast}}{\overset{\text{Fast}}{\rightleftharpoons}} A_2R \underset{\text{Slow}}{\overset{\text{Fast}}{\rightleftharpoons}} A_2R^0$$

where R is the receptor channel complex, A is ACh and A_2R^0 is the open form of the receptor channel bound with 2 molecules of ACh.

Although patch clamp recordings of single ACh-activated channels have now confirmed the broad outlines of these models, important subtleties have emerged regarding the kinetics of channel gating and the conductance properties of the individual channels. On the basis of noise analysis experiments showing the spectral density function of agonist-induced current fluctuations to be fit well with a single Lorentzian function (and confirmatory voltage-jump-relaxation studies), it had been assumed that the distribution of open times for the ACh-activated channel would conform to a single exponential function (i.e., there is a single kinetically distinct open state). Suffice it to say that this model is now untenable as it is clear that the channel open time distribution is best fitted by the sum of two exponential functions (Colquhoun and Sakmann, 1981). The molecular basis for this phenomenon is unknown and a number of possible interpretations have been suggested, for example, that the short open times represent the combination of a single ACh molecule with the receptor and the longer open times a more stable state due to the binding of two ACh molecules. In addition, there are very brief (~50 μsec) closures known as "flickers" that often interrupt the channel openings; groups of openings separated by flickers are generally referred to as "bursts."

An additional complexity that has been uncovered through the use of single-channel recording is the apparent existence of multiple conductance states for the ACh-activated channel. For example, Hamill and Sakmann (1981) reported the existence of three, and possibly four, distinct long-lived conducting states in tissue-cultured rat muscle at low temperature. Other workers have confirmed the existence of various conducting states for the channel, although the details differ (see Sachs, 1983). It is now recognized that these various novel properties are not unique to the ACh-activated channel but may be a general feature of many receptor-channel systems.

4.2. Cholinergic Synaptic Actions in Autonomic Ganglia

In both the sympathetic and parasympathetic ganglia of the autonomic nervous system, acetylcholine mediates at least three distinct synaptic potentials and, in addition, may have a variety of other roles, including presynaptic inhibition and the regulation of the action potential afterhyperpolarization. The first type of synaptic potential, caused by activation of nicotinic receptors, is a rapid (< 15 msec) depolarization known as the "fast EPSP." This synaptic potential is observed in all ganglionic neurons. The other two cholinergic synaptic potentials result from muscarinic receptor activation. These are associated with a depolarization or hyperpolarization and are referred to as the "slow EPSP" and "slow IPSP," respectively. They are variable in their occurrence among different types of ganglion cells. In contrast to the rapid time course of the nicotinic EPSP, these muscarinic potentials may have a duration of seconds or even minutes (Nishi, 1974).

4.2.1. Nicotinic Excitation

The ionic basis of the nicotinic fast EPSP in autonomic ganglion neurons is similar to that of the end-plate potential at the neuromuscular junction. The kinetic properties of these potentials are also basically alike; however, there are certain important differences. Voltage-clamp recording and noise analysis have been used to characterize the fast EPSP of autonomic neurons in greater detail than any other synaptic potential in vertebrate neurons. Whereas conventional recordings of the EPSP provide only limited information regarding the kinetic properties of the underlying conductance mechanism because their form is governed predominately by the cell capacitance, analysis of the excitatory postsynaptic current (EPSC) obtained through voltage-clamp recordings allows an accurate characterization of the time course of the conductance change induced by the transmitter. Furthermore, as at the neuromuscular junction, noise analysis of current fluctuations under voltage clamp allow certain properties of the membrane channels to be estimated.

The characteristics of the EPSC and ACh-induced current fluctuations have been compared in a variety of sympathetic and parasympathetic ganglia (Connor and Parsons, 1983). The similarity between the EPSC decay constant and the estimated mean channel lifetime from fluctuation analysis has suggested that by and large the time course of the decay of the EPSC is primarily dependent on the kinetics of receptor-channel gating rather than the kinetics of transmitter release or ACh removal by diffusion or hydrolysis. The peak of the EPSC is reached within 3 msec. The decay occurs with a time constant of approximately 5 msec and is thus much longer than that of the end-plate current at the neuromuscular junction. The peak current is approximately 4 pA and the amplitude–voltage relationship is linear between -30 mV and -90 mV. The reversal potential, determined by extrapolation, is about -10 mV. In the presence of cholinesterase inhibitors, the EPSC decay is prolonged and no longer can be described by a single exponential function. The MEPCs and the estimates of the single-channel conductance are approximately 10–20 times smaller than those at the neuromuscular junction and values range between 5 and 15 pS. These observations support the suggestion that the density of nicotinic receptors on the postsynaptic cells may be much lower than at the neuromuscular junction and, in addition, the channels may be less powerful generators of current. However, the longer channel life time and associated increase in duration of the EPSC in sympathetic ganglia may in part offset the apparent reduction in the effectiveness of ACh.

In rat parasympathetic cells, the decay time course of the EPSC has been reported by Rang (1981) to consist of two exponential components whose time constants match the two time constants of ACh noise spectra in these cells. The time constant of the fast phase was 5–9 msec, while that of the slow phase was 27–45 msec. Clearly, the presence of more than one decay time raises the possibility that there might be more than one type of channel activated by nicotinic receptors with identical ion selectivity but mean lifetimes that differ fivefold.

4.2.2. Muscarinic Excitation

On the basis of two-electrode voltage clamp recordings from lumbar sympathetic ganglia of the bullfrog, Brown and Adams (1980) were the first to suggest that the prime target for muscarinic agents in sympathetic neurons might be the M current (I_M), a novel voltage-sensitive K^+ current. Unlike other K^+ currents in sympathetic neurons, the M current is blocked by

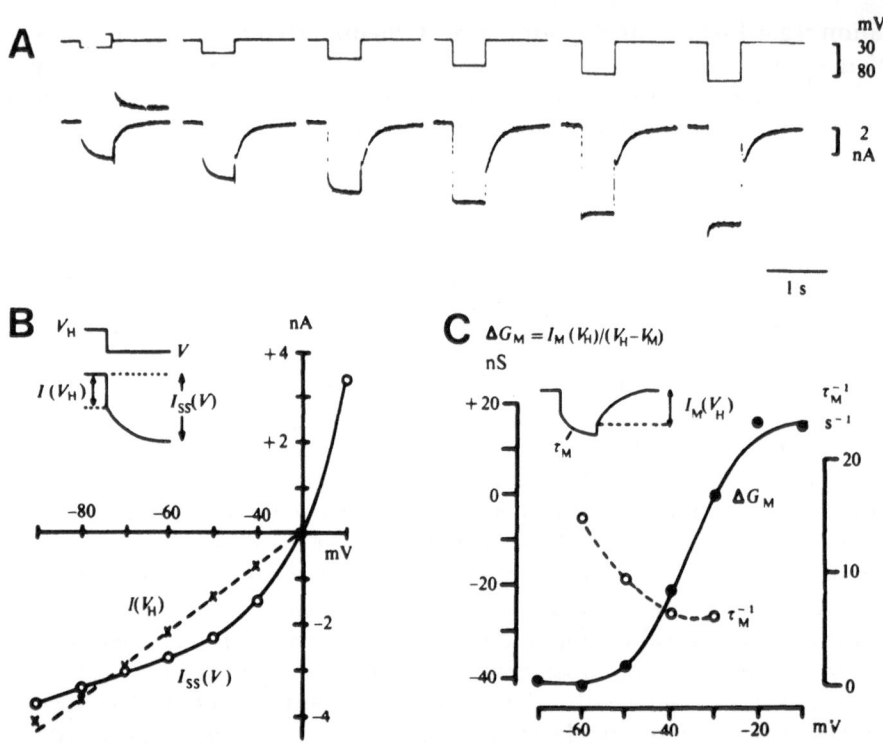

Figure 15. M currents in a voltage-clamped bullfrog sympathetic neuron. (A) The records show clamp currents (bottom trace; inward current is downwards) recorded during hyperpolarizing step comands from a holding potential (V_H) of -30 mV to command potentials (V) of -40 to -90 mV. The outward current in the first panel is the slow tail of repolarizing current after returning to V_H from a depolarizing step command to -20 mV; this current record is shifted upwards for clarity (the outward current during the command is offscale). (B) The instantaneous (x---x) and steady state (O---O) currents recorded in (A) are plotted against command potential (V). The instantaneous current is the amplitude of the fast transient $I(V_H)$ and the steady state current is the total current measured after the slow relaxation is complete, $I_{ss}(V)$ (see inset). The intersection gives the reversal potential (V_M) for the slow relaxation. The curves (C) show the change in conductance attributable to closing and opening of the M channels (ΔG_M) and the reciprocal of the time constant of the slow relaxation (τ_M^{-1}) plotted against command potential. ΔG_M was calculated from the amplitudes of the M current tails observed on repolarizing from V to V_H (-30 mV), divided by the driving force $V_M - V_M$. τ_M was calculated from semilogarithmic plots of the slow inward relaxations on hyperpolarizing from V_H to V. (From Brown and Adams, 1980, with permission.)

muscarinic agonists. The M current normally manifests itself as a substantial and steady outward current when a sympathetic neuron is held under voltage clamp at relatively depolarized potentials. The current is best illustrated (Fig. 15a) by applying hyperpolarizing command steps during which channels carrying the M current gradually close and give rise to slow inward current relaxation that follows the initial fast ohmic step. Channel closure during the relaxation is of course accompanied by a fall in membrane conductance, and this accounts for the smaller amplitude of the ohmic step at the end of the command than at the beginning. The repolarizing command then leads to a slow outward relaxation as the M channels re-open. (When the cell is held at potentials more negative than -70 mV the currents are complicated by the appearance of another K^+ current, the "transient outward current" that is analogous to the rapidly inactivating "A" current of molluscan neurons.) With increasing hyperpolarizing command steps of between -70 and -100 mV, the inward relaxation is first negated (Fig. 15A, 4th pulse of the series) and then reversed (5th and 6th pulse of the series). Since increases in the external K^+ from 2.5 to 8 and then 25 mM shift the reversal level in the depolarizing direction by 20–25 and 40–45 mV, respectively, it was concluded that the I_M is predominantly carried by K^+ ions (Brown and Adams, 1980; Adams et al., 1982a).

At -60 mV, near the resting potential, the channels carrying the M current are fully closed, and at membrane potentials more negative than -60 mV, hyperpolarizing command pulses yield only ohmic steps (Fig. 15C). Above -60 mV the conductance change attributable to the M channels opening increases sigmoidally until it reaches a maximum at about -20 mV.

As shown in Fig. 16, Brown and Adams (1980) illustrated the functional significance of the M current by comparing the actions of muscarine on ganglion cells recorded under current clamp and voltage clamp conditions.

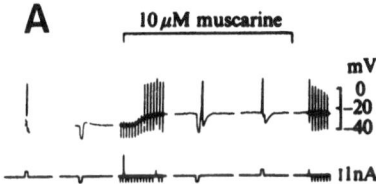

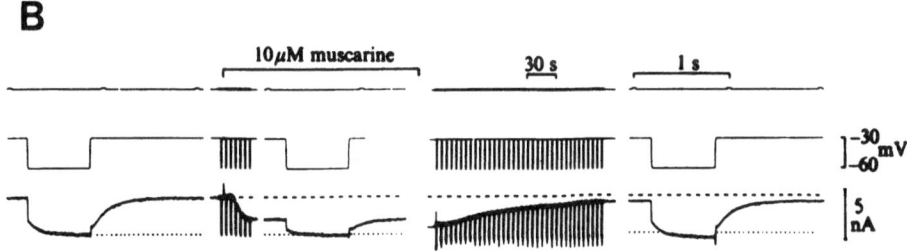

Figure 16. Effect of muscarine on a single neuron recorded under (A) current clamp and (B) voltage-clamp. The recorder was periodically accelerated to display the voltage and current transients. Muscarine was applied by rapid bath perfusion. In the voltage-clamp record, the membrane potential was held at -30 mV and stepped to -60 mV for 700 msec at 5-sec intervals. (From Brown and Adams, 1980, with permission.)

With conventional current clamp intracellular recording, muscarine produced a slow membrane depolarization associated with a conductance *decrease* (Fig. 16a). Under voltage clamp, muscarine caused a steady inward (depolarizing) current and there was a reduced current response to hyperpolarizing step commands (a reflection of the decreased membrane conductance). It was suggested that the steady state inward current and the reduced steady state conductance result solely from a reduction in the M current. In keeping with the characteristics of the M current shown in Fig. 15C, muscarine produced negligible inward current at -60 mV. Indeed, the net inward current was directly proportional to I_M measured with hyperpolarizing command steps throughout the voltage range. By studying the time course of the M current relaxations, Brown and Adams (1980) were able to show that muscarine simply depresses the amplitude of the M current without modifying the voltage sensitivity. In addition, they showed the action of muscarine to be concentration dependent and the concentration required for half channel closure to be 1.3 μM. This effect was fully antagonized by 1 μM atropine.

The uniqueness of I_M with respect to the delayed rectifier K^+ current was illustrated by showing that TEA, a specific blocker of the delayed rectifier, has little or no effect on I_M. Conversely, muscarine has no effect on the delayed rectifier. Although the precise role of I_M is unclear, it may serve to dampen cell firing near threshold for spike generation by reducing the rate of depolarization evoked by both steady and phasic inward currents. Thus, blockade of I_M during the slow EPSP would be expected to enhance the cell's responsiveness to other simultaneously occurring excitatory synaptic potentials, such as fast EPSPs (see below).

4.2.3. Features of the Muscarinic EPSP

On the basis of conventional current clamp recordings from bullfrog sympathetic neurons, it had been suggested that the slow EPSP was, in at least substantial part, due to the closure of K^+ channels (Weight and Votava, 1970; Kuba and Koketsu, 1976). With the discovery of the M current and its sensitivity to muscarinic agonists, Adams and Brown (1982) proposed that this current is selectively inhibited during the slow EPSP and that this entirely accounts for the synaptic potential. As evidence in favor of this concept, these workers demonstrated (1) that I_M relaxations recorded under voltage clamp were reduced during the slow EPSP, (2) that membrane conductance is diminished only at voltages where I_M is active, and (3) that the slow EPSP shows the same dependence on membrane potential as does I_M.

Although inhibition of the M current undoubtedly accounts for much of the depolarization and increase in excitability occurring during the slow EPSP, it is now clear that at least one other membrane conductance may at times be involved as well. Thus Kuffler and Sejnowski (1983) have found that the muscarinic EPSP increases in amplitude with hyperpolarization up to and beyond the equilibrium potential for K^+ (as judged by the reversal potential of the action potential AHP) in about half of the cells they recorded from in the paravertebral ganglia. This is an observation that had been previously reported by others (Kobayashi and Libet, 1968, 1974; Kuba and Koketsu, 1974, 1976). Moreover, using the single electrode voltage clamp technique, Kuffler and Sejnowski demonstrated that in some cells large synaptic potentials could be generated at membrane potentials more negative than -60 mV, where the M current was completely inactivated. Thus another conductance mechanism must be involved in the genesis of the slow EPSP in at least some cells. In other words, only in cells where the K^+ conductance is dominant does the slow EPSP null as the membrane is hyperpolarized toward the inactivation range for the M current and the equilibrium potential for K^+. In other cells a conductance increase predominates at hyperpolarized potentials; this may be contributed to by both Na^+ and Ca^{2+} (Kuba and Koketsu, 1976; Katayama and Nishi, 1977, 1982). In a more recent paper, Adams et al. (1983) appear to have conceded this point and agree that "in a fraction of cells" there is an additional and variable inward current accompanied by a conductance increase that persists during hyperpolarization.

The absence of a definite reversal potential in these cells is consistent with the observations of Brown et al. (1971) that in the presence of both increases and decreases of conductance the reversal level cannot lie between the equilibrium potentials of the two ionic species producing the response. In the present example, however, the voltage dependency of the conductance changes and their variability even at a fixed membrane potential complicate the arithmetical analysis still further.

4.2.4. Interactions between Nicotinic and Muscarinic EPSPs

Although all the evidence suggests that the slow muscarinic EPSP is activated by ACh released from the same nerves that produce the fast nicotinic EPSP, the muscarinic effects of ACh only become appreciable after repetitive stimulation. However, once activated they can last for as long as 1 min. As has been noted, during the muscarinic EPSP the neuron is more excitable. Therefore, each fast nicotinic EPSP, caused by ACh released by a single shock to the same nerve, is more certain to evoke a spike (Schulman and Weight, 1976). Thus high-frequency stimulation seems to be coupled to a mechanism for enhancing transmission through the ganglia. This concept is also supported by the finding that the muscarinic responses do not desensitize during prolonged applications of ACh and therefore tend to counteract the reduction of the nicotinic response that occurs with repetitive stimulation.

4.2.5. Similarities between Muscarinic and Peptidergic Synaptic Potentials

In addition to the three cholinergic synaptic potentials enumerated in the introduction to this section, there is a fourth synaptic response that can be evoked in some sympathetic neurons by sustained preganglionic stimulation—the late slow EPSP. It is believed that a peptide (teleost LHRH in the bullfrog), rather than acetylcholine, mediates this response (see Chapter 16). The ionic basis of the late slow EPSP appears to be identical with that of the slow muscarinic EPSP, although it is much more prolonged in duration, typically lasting several minutes.

As evidence that common conductance mechanisms mediate the muscarinic and peptidergic EPSPs, Kuffler and Sejnowski (1983) showed that they both had the same effects on membrane resistance and identical voltage sensitivities. Similar responses were also observed with exogenously applied agonists. In addition, they demonstrated that the peptidergic responses evoked either by nerve stimulation or the application of LHRH occluded the response to the muscarinic agonist bethanechol and vice versa (Fig. 17). The occlusion of one response by another supports the view that the postsynaptic muscarinic and peptidergic receptors act through a final common pathway. In fact, at least for the M current, a wide variety of agonists in addition to ACh and LHRH are capable of evoking a closure of the channel in bullfrog autonomic neurons. These include substance P, angiotensin, uridine nucleotides, and adenosine nucleotides, as well as the divalent cation Ba^{2+} (Brown et al., 1981; Adams et al., 1982b: Akasu et al., 1982).

4.2.6. The Slow Muscarinic IPSP

The muscarinic IPSP, as recorded in both sympathetic and parasympathetic ganglia in a large variety of species, is a hyperpolarizing synaptic potential with a time course measured in seconds or in minutes. Unlike the fast nicotinic EPSP, muscarinic IPSPs can be recorded in some, but not all, neurons in peripheral autonomic ganglia. In the bullfrog, mud puppy, rabbit, rat, and cat, the slow muscarinic IPSP is preceded by a fast nicotinic EPSP and is often followed by a late slow noncholinergic EPSP. The 9th and 10th paravertebral sympathetic ganglia of the bullfrog have been frequently used as a model system to study the slow IPSP as it is known that stimulation of spinal nerves 7 and 8 induces a slow IPSP in C cells within these ganglia (but not in other cell types). Although several hypotheses have been proposed for the genesis of the muscarinic IPSP, it is now generally accepted to be the result of a monosynaptic activation of a postsynaptic K^+ conductance.

Figure 17. Interaction between the responses to muscarinic agonists, LHRH, and the peptiderigic EPSP in two bullfrog sympathetic neurons. (A) Continuous (45 min) voltage-clamp recording during which a ganglion cell was held at its resting potential, -59 mV. Bethanechol and LHRH were applied for varying durations as indicated. (B) The neuron was voltage-clamped at its resting potential, -58 mV, and the cholinergic input stimulated ten times at 50 Hz. This was repeated at 2-min intervals. The fast nicotinic responses are cut off (small arrowheads). The size of the muscarinic current was reduced following a train of 100 stimuli at 20 Hz to the peptidergic nerves (7th and 8th trunks) (large arrowhead) and recovered with the decline of the peptidergic current. (From Kuffler and Sejnoski, 1983, with permission.)

A

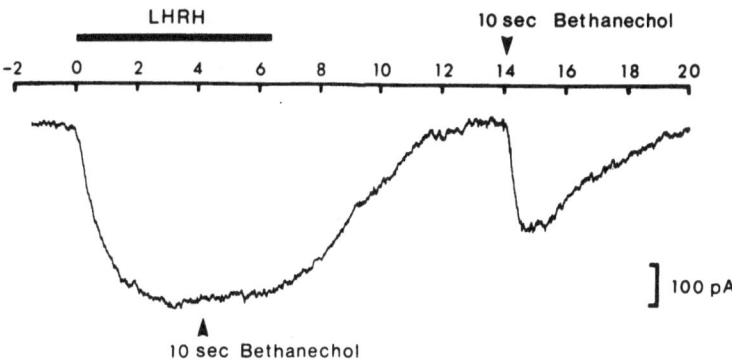

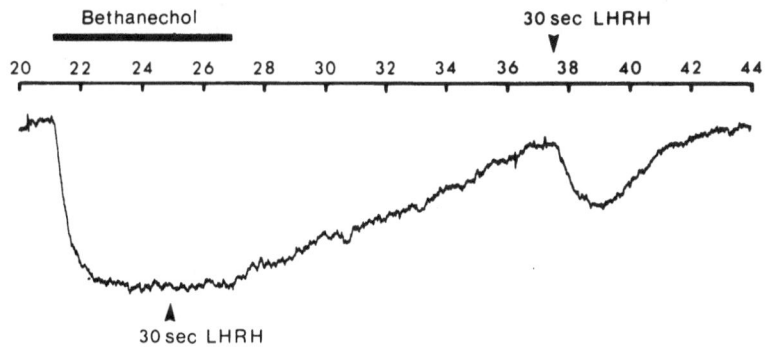

B

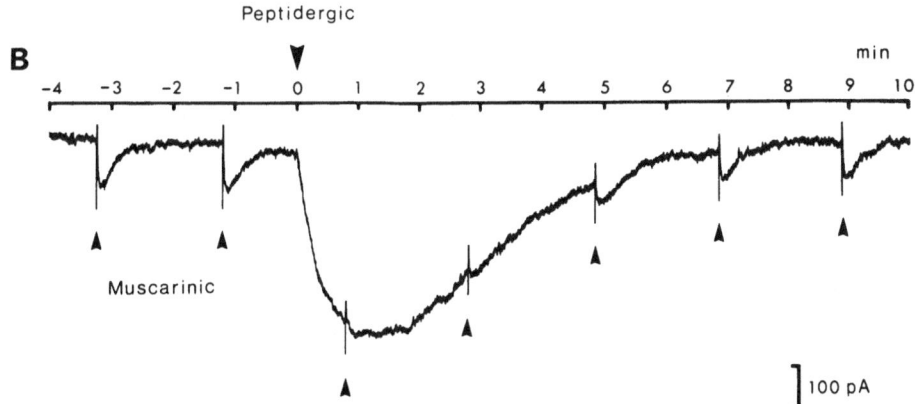

Evidence regarding the slow IPSP in the bullfrog that is consistent with this concept is summarized below.

On the basis of intracellular recordings, Dodd and Horn (1983) have shown the presynaptic threshold for eliciting the IPSP in C cells to be identical to that which produces the nicotinic EPSP. Sub-micromolar concentrations of atropine totally block the IPSP in a reversible manner (Tosaka et al., 1968; Horn and Dodd, 1981). The latency and time course of the IPSP are clearly mimicked by iontophoretically applied ACh (Fig. 18) and both exhibit the same voltage-dependent changes in kinetics. Thus the duration of the responses increased as the membrane was hyperpolarized from rest towards the reversal potential (Fig. 19). This change is closely connected with the rectifying properties of the C cells which leads to a sharp increase in resistance around -70 mV. Both events are produced by an increase in membrane conductance and they share a common reversal potential which varies as a Nernstian function of the extracellular K^+ concentration and is insensitive to changes in the Cl^- gradient. As is true of a variety of K^+-mediated events, low concentrations of Ba^{2+} totally, but reversibly, block the muscarinic conductance increase. Finally, the inhibitory effect of ACh on C cells is independent of Ca^{2+}-dependent transmitter release.

In addition to experimental studies designed to support the concept that

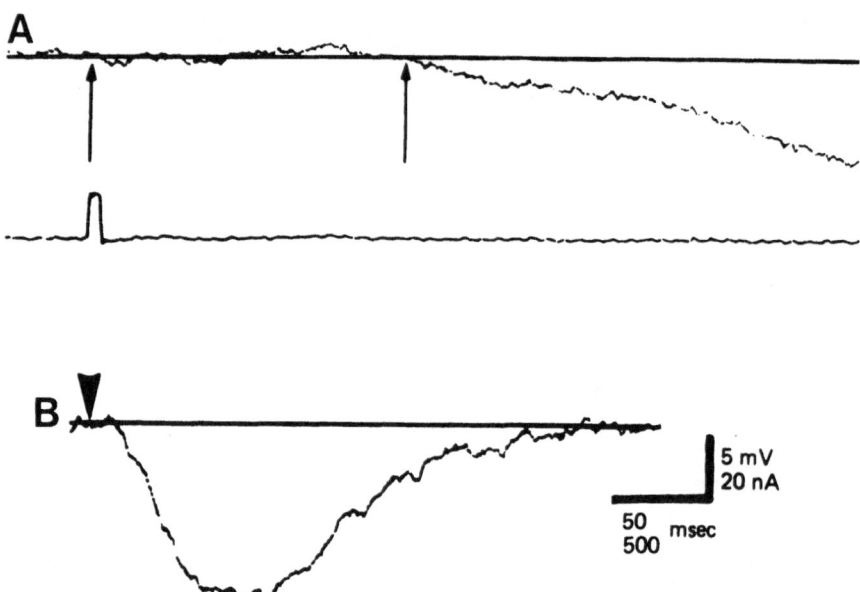

Figure 18. Time course of the inhibitory muscarinic response to a single ionophoretic pulse of ACh in a curarized bullfrog ganglion cell. (A) The latency of the response (between the arrows) was 160 msec. (B) On a slower time base the shape of the response resembles that of the IPSP evoked by a single nerve stimulus. T = 27°C. (From Dodd and Horn, 1983, with permission.)

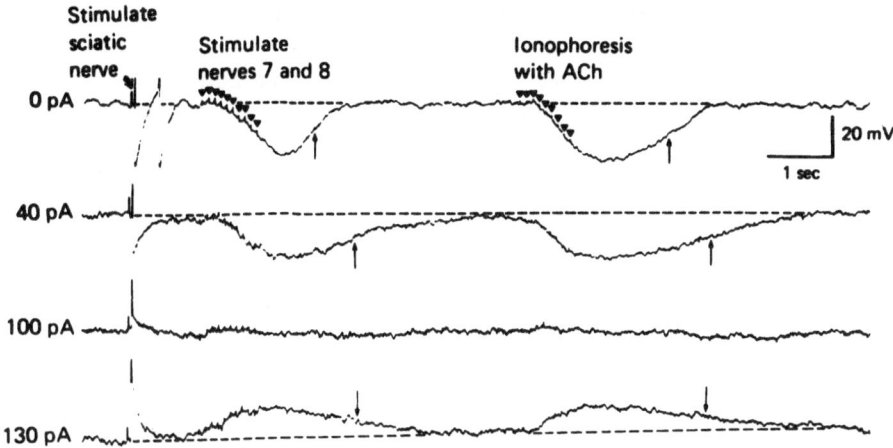

Figure 19. Reversal of the action potential afterpotential, the slow IPSP, and the muscarinic ACh response in a curarized bullfrog sympathetic ganglion neuron. The amount of polarizing current is at the left of each trace. The synaptic and ACh responses have the same reversal potential. Arrows denote the half decay points of the muscarinic responses. Note that as the cell was hyperpolarized from rest (about -50 mV), the decay times increased. T = 22°C. (From Dodd and Horn, 1983, with permission.)

ACh released from preganglionic neurons directly activates inhibitory muscarinic receptors on ganglionic neurons, various investigators have attempted to critically evaluate the original hypothesis of Eccles and Libet (1961) that a catecholamine-releasing inhibitory interneuron mediates the slow IPSP. These experiments have not supported the interneuron hypothesis. First, catecholamine antagonists that are known to be effective do not block the IPSP whether it is recorded extracellularly (Weight and Smith, 1980; Yavari and Weight, 1981) or intracellularly (Beddoe et al., 1971; Cole and Shinnick-Gallagher, 1980). Second, in order to mimic the IPSP, exogenous ACh must be applied close to the surface of the C cells, and this is inconsistent with the proposal that the hyperpolarization is mediated by neighboring catecholamine cells. Third, anatomical studies have demonstrated that the catecholamine-containing small intensely fluorescent (SIF) cells are sparsely distributed within the ganglion and lack processes. Finally, the pharmacological receptor for the catecholamine-induced hyperpolarization of ganglion neurons has now been clearly demonstrated to be of the α_2-type, and is not a dopamine receptor, although dopamine had been hypothesized to be the adrenergic transmitter of SIF cells (see Chapter 9).

More recently Cole and Shinnick-Gallagher (1984) have confirmed that in mammaliam sympathetic ganglia the slow IPSP is also due to the monosynaptic activation of muscarinic receptors and is probably mediated by an increase in potassium conductance. In addition, they suggest that the potassium conductance may be Ca^{2+}-activated, and that this Ca^{2+} sensitivity might explain the attenuation of the synaptic potential and the response to

ACh by the application of solutions containing zero Ca^{2+} and EGTA. These results may be compared with the observations based on patch clamp recording of Trautman and Marty (1984), in which carbamoylcholine was found to activate Ca^{2+}-dependent K^+ channels in rat lacrimal glands.

Within the next few years, the introduction of fluctuation (noise) analysis and single-channel recording to preparations of the central and peripheral nervous systems will allow the nature of the potassium channels opened by ACh to be defined more precisely. For example, Sakmann et al. (1983) used patch clamp recording to show that the muscarinic inhibitory action of ACh on pacemaker cells of the sinoatrial node in the rabbit heart is mediated by K^+ channels that could be differentiated on the basis of their gating and conductance properties from inward-rectifying resting K^+ channels (Fig. 20). This ACh-sensitive K^+ channel opens at low frequency even in the absence of ACh or muscarinic agonists; however, its probability of being in the open state increases dramatically with muscarinic stimulation. This is mainly due to shortening of the mean closed time; there is little effect on the mean open time, and the single channel conductance is unaffected by ACh (Soejima and Noma, 1984).

In further studies on rabbit atrial cells, Soejima and Noma (1984) demonstrated the power of the single-channel recording technique by showing that the frequency of ACh-sensitive K^+ channel opening increased only when

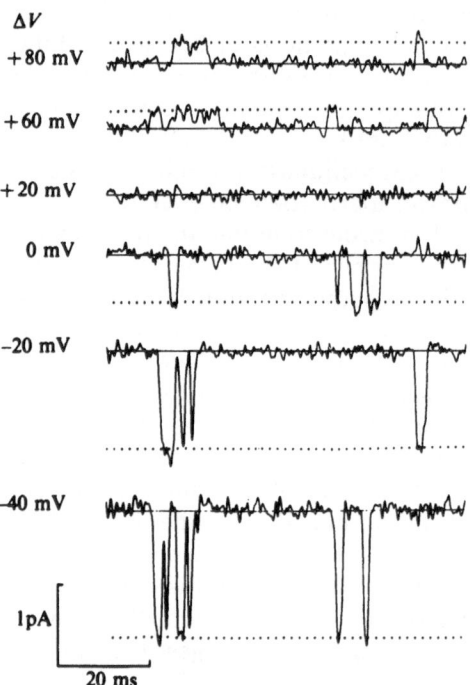

Figure 20. Patch clamp recording of ACh-activated single-channel currents of an atrioventricular nodal cell of the rabbit heart at various membrane potentials. The patch pipette contained 0.2 μM ACh in a high K^+ solution (20 mM). The numbers to the left of each trace indicate the shift in patch potential, ΔV, with respect to the cell's resting potential, V_r. Current steps reverse in polarity when the patch potential is made about 20 mV more positive than the resting potential. Inward current steps are downwards. The extrapolated reversal potential is about 20 mV more positive than V_r, or about -43 mV. This compares favorably with the calculated K^+ reversal potential of -45 mV with 20 mM extracellular K^+. The continuous lines indicate the fitted zero-current base-line; the dotted lines are the average single-channel amplitude at each potential. (From Sakmann et al., 1982, with permission.)

ACh was applied to the external surface of the patch of membrane within the patch pipette (by perfusion of the patch electrode); no effect was observed when the rest of the cell membrane was exposed to ACh. These observations were interpreted as suggesting that the muscarinic receptor is directly coupled to the ion channel and effectively excludes the possibility that the channel is activated by an intracellular second messenger that diffuses within the cell. These studies point out the qualitative similarity between muscarinic channels operating during inhibitory synaptic potentials and the nicotinic channels responsible for excitation at the neuromuscular junction. Thus, the inhibitory events mediated by ACh appear to involve conventional two-state (open-closed) ion channels coupled directly to the transmitter receptor. However, in the case of the channel mediating muscarinic inhibition, the ionic selectivity is more rigorously controlled to admit only K^+ and not other cations.

4.2.7. Presynaptic Inhibitory Actions in the Myenteric Plexus

There is a considerable amount of evidence that the activation of muscarinic receptors can lead to inhibition of ACh release from the myenteric plexus (Sawynok and Jhamandas, 1977; Fosbraey and Johnson, 1980; Kilbinger and Wessler, 1980; Szerb, 1980). In these experiments, muscarinic antagonists were shown to increase the overflow of ACh during electrical field stimulation of the plexus. More recently, on the basis of physiological recordings, Morita et al. (1982b) have shown the muscarinic agonist oxotremorine to inhibit transmitter release when applied in concentrations lower than those required to depolarize the neurons directly. In these experiments, release of ACh is assayed by monitoring the fast cholinergic EPSP; the amplitude of this potential is diminished by oxotremorine and this effect is blocked by muscarinic antagonists (Fig. 21A). In addition to mediating the autoinhibition of ACh release, presynaptic muscarinic receptors also seem to regulate the release of the noncholinergic transmitter that evokes the late slow EPSP (Johnson et al., 1981) (Fig. 21B). It is of interest that similar low concentrations of oxotremorine shorten the afterhyperpolarization (AHP) that follows bursts of action potentials in these neurons (Morita et al., 1982a). It is possible that this action and the reduction of transmitter release could have a common substrate, such as an enhancement of the ability of the neuron to sequester calcium ions. Thus, the presynaptic inhibition caused by oxotremorine may be mediated by a different mechanism from that which underlies the action of opiates (see Chapter 12).

The physiological significance of muscarinic autoinhibition of fast EPSPs is highlighted by experiments showing muscarinic antagonists to increase the amplitude of second and subsequent fast EPSPs evoked at a frequency of 1 Hz or greater. This implies that subsequent inhibition of transmitter release is brought about by the small amount of ACh released during the first fast EPSP. Moreover, muscarinic presynaptic inhibition is long-lasting,

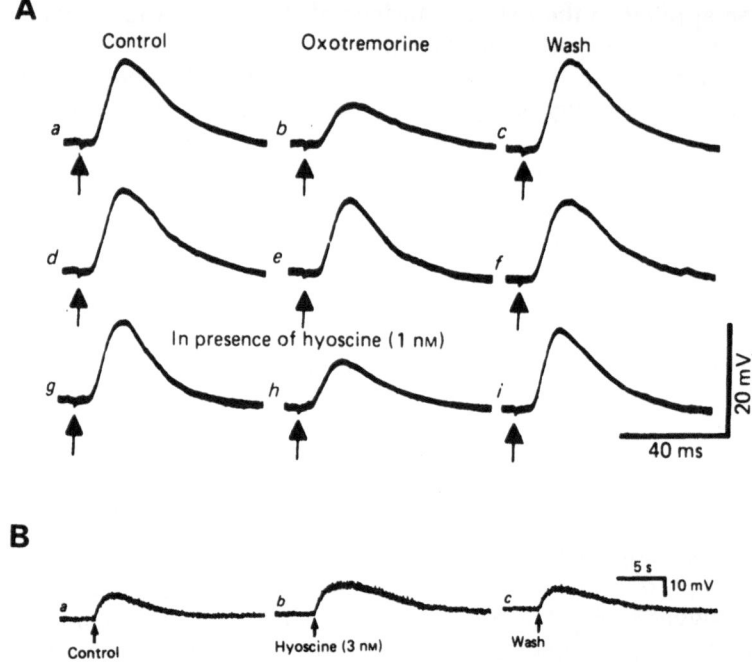

Figure 21. Muscarinic presynaptic inhibition of the nicotinic fast EPSP and the noncholinergic slow EPSP in guinea pig myenteric plexus neurons. (A) In these intracellular recordings, oxotremorine (30 nM) reduces the amplitude of the fast EPSP (panel b) and this effect is blocked in the presence of hyoscine (1 nM), a muscarinic antagonist (panel e). Hyoscine alone has no effect on the EPSP (panel d). After washout of hyoscine, oxotremorine regained its usual effect (panels g–i). (B) Late slow EPSPs evoked by repetitive nerve stimulation (5 Hz, 1 sec, arrow) showing the increase in amplitude and duration produced by hyoscine (3 nM). (From Morita et al., 1982b, with permission.)

comparable in duration to the postsynaptic muscarinic actions of ACh. It thus appears that ACh released under physiological conditions has significant presynaptic inhibitory effects, and it is apparent that muscarinic antagonists will have complex actions on interganglionic transmission.

5. INTRACELLULAR EVENTS RESULTING FROM MUSCARINIC RECEPTOR STIMULATION

Since the rates of ejection of glutamate and ACh from an iontophoretic pipette appear to be almost identical (Kelly, 1975) the greater latency and slower development of the muscarinic depolarizing ACh effect on central and peripheral neurons might be explained either by the location of the ACh receptors at greater distances from the microiontophoretic pipette (for example, on distant dendrites), or by some intrinsic property of the ACh receptor-ion channel complex that causes a delay between the arrival of the ligand and closure of the K^+ channel. However, in experiments with various *in vitro* preparations (Blackman et al., 1979; Bolton, 1972,1976; Ginsborg et al., 1974; Hill-Smith and Purves, 1978; Purves, 1974) where iontophoretic pipettes can be accurately placed at different distances from the cell membrane sites presumably bearing the receptors, the long latency and duration of the responses cannot be explained by a simple diffusion model (Dionne, 1976; Purves, 1977). Corrections for restricted diffusion of the neurotransmitter in the extracellular fluid, or a slow interaction between the neurotransmitter and the receptors were inadequate. Indeed, the slowness was best explained by postulating that a series of sequential chemical reactions (Niedergerke and Page, 1977) follows the formation of the neurotransmitter–receptor complex. Thus, the rate of depolarization evoked by ACh might be limited by the rate of formation of some intracellular product, and the long duration of the response by the time that would be required for its inactivation.

Certain limited biochemical and physiological evidence has suggested that intracellular cyclic guanosine-3',5'-monophosphate (cGMP) might mediate the muscarinic action of ACh. These data can be summarized as follows:

1. Activation of muscarinic receptors is associated with a rise in cGMP content in several tissues (George et al., 1970; Lee et al., 1972; Kebabian et al., 1975; Weight et al., 1974).
2. Extracellularly applied cGMP mimics the muscarinic effects of ACh on sympathetic ganglia neurons (McAfee and Greengard, 1972; but see below) and neocortical neurons (Stone et al., 1975; but see Phillis et al., 1974).
3. cGMP-dependent protein kinase has been described in a membrane preparation from ACh-sensitive mammalian smooth muscle (Casnellie and Greengard, 1974).

In recent years, a number of authors have pursued this hypothesis further with intracellular recordings in the brain and in sympathetic ganglia. For instance, Woody et al. (1978) found that the response of the cells in the cat somatosensory cortex to extracellular applications of ACh could be mimicked by intracellular iontophoretic injections of cyclic GMP. However, the magnitude and time course of the increase in resistance evoked by an intracellular pulse of cGMP was similar to that seen during extracellular iontophoresis of ACh and not faster, as would be suggested by the second messenger model.

On sympathetic ganglia, the excitatory muscarinic action of ACh cannot be mimicked by either extracellular (Dun et al., 1978; Hashiguchi et al., 1978) or intracellular (Gallagher and Shinnick-Gallagher, 1978) applications of cGMP. Similarly, in motoneurons, where the extracellular action of ACh also involves a depolarization and increase in membrane resistance (Zieglgänsberger and Bayerl, 1976; Zieglgänsberger and Reiter, 1974), intracellular injections of cGMP appear to have the opposite effect, i.e., there was a hyper-polarization associated with a fall in membrane resistance (Krnjević et al., 1976; Krnjević and VanMeter, 1976).

If these observations are confirmed, the general cGMP theory will have to be discarded or modified to include compartmentation; i.e., it might be postulated that the free cytoplasmic pool of cGMP does not have access to the cellular apparatus regulating ionic fluxes across the plasma membrane and that activation of muscarinic receptors generates a separate pool of cGMP that does have access to this apparatus.

Apart from the problem of characterizing the temporal sequence of events that link muscarinic activation to a change in membrane potential, the possibility should also be considered that the slow changes in membrane potential evoked by ACh may be an epiphenomenon of a more primary metabolic or trophic function at some muscarinic synapses (cf. Bloom, 1975). That is, one may conceive that a major role of some cholinergic synapses is to allow a presynaptic influence over the metabolic machinery of the postsynaptic cell. Many agents that depolarize nerve cells can cause an increase in tissue cGMP (Ferrendelli et al., 1970) so this effect need not be specific to ACh and may reflect a more general property of neurotransmission at certain sites.

In view of the difficulty of corroborating the hypothesis that muscarinic receptor activation is linked to changes in membrane channel activity via cyclic nucleotides, interest has now shifted to the observation that muscarinic receptor stimulation increases the rate at which membrane-bound phosphatidylinositol is broken down by hydrolysis (Michell, 1975). In fact, it has been demonstrated that muscarinic agonists stimulate the activity of a phospholipase C that degrades inositol phospholipids in brain slices (Jacobson et al., 1984; Fisher et al., 1983). However, the way in which these biochemical changes could result in specific effects on membrane ion channels remains unclear.

6. CONCLUSION

After more than 50 years of discovery, the pace of work on the transmitter physiology of acetylcholine continues to accelerate and the newest work encompasses a wealth of fresh and innovative ideas. It is now certain that for many central neurons, ACh has facilitatory actions that are different from those of ACh at the neuromuscular junction. These actions are mediated predominantly by muscarinic receptors, and the ultimate effect is facilitation of neuronal firing evoked by other depolarizing inputs. Although this facilitation occurs through several distinct mechanisms, the overall effect is a generalized increase in excitability, so that firing evoked by the action of synaptic inputs, the application of excitatory amino acids, or direct intracellular stimulation of single neurons, is enhanced. Some of the actions of

ACh are postsynaptic and range from a clearly identifiable reduction in a specific voltage-sensitive K^+ conductance associated with a current known as I_M and a reduction in the Ca^{2+}-dependent K^+ conductance underlying AHP and accommodation, to rather less well defined actions on other currents, which may or may not be associated with anomalous rectification or bursting. There are also a variety of essentially transynaptic mechanisms, of which the most obvious is a reduction in the effectiveness of inhibitory synaptic activity that occurs either by a depression of inhibitory interneuron discharge or by a suppression of the release of transmitter from inhibitory nerve terminals.

On the other neurons, however, the muscarinic action of ACh is reversed and can clearly be shown to cause both a direct and indirect inhibition of neural firing. Here again the mechanisms range from a clear-cut postsynaptic inhibition involving the opening of specific potassium channels to less well defined reductions in the release of either ACh from the same or neighboring nerve terminals, or the release of other transmitters. New work has also made it clear that some of the facilitatory actions of ACh are shared by a number of other transmitter substances and it is therefore necessary to put forward schemes that permit neural excitability to be controlled by the simultaneous release of a variety of such substances.

Although at first sight this degree of complexity may seem to rule out studies attempting to link the role of the now better defined ACh pathways to animal behavior, new understanding of the pharmacology of central cholinergic transmission coupled with the availability of specific agonists, antagonists, and other drugs acting on cholinergic systems, such as cholinesterase inhibitors, should make this all the more possible. Thus, drugs that have been known to act at peripheral muscarinic synapses and effector junctions for at least a half a century have taken on renewed usefulness as tools to understand central cholinergic function.

REFERENCES

Adams, P. R., 1975, An analysis of the dose-response curve at voltage-clamped frog endplates, *Pflügers Arch.* **360**:145–153.

Adams, P. R., 1981, The calcium current of a vertebrate neurone, in: *Advances in Physiological Science*, Vol. 4 (J. Salanki, ed.), Akademiai Kiado, Budapest, pp. 135–138.

Adams, P. R., and Brown, D. A., 1982, Synaptic inhibition of the M-current: Slow excitatory post-synaptic potential mechanism in bullfrog sympathetic neurones, *J. Physiol. (Lond.)* **332**:263–272.

Adams, P. R., Brown, D. A., and Constanti, A., 1982a, M-currents and other potassium currents in bullfrog sympathetic neurones *J. Physiol. (Lond.)* **330**:537–572.

Adams, P. R., Brown, D. A., and Constanti, A., 1982b, Pharmacological inhibition of the M-current, *J. Physiol. (Lond.)* **332**:223–262.

Adams, P. R., Brown, D. A., and Jones, S. W., 1983, Substance P inhibits the M-current in bullfrog sympathetic neurons, *Br. J. Pharmacol.* **79**:330–333.

Akasu, T., Hirai, K., and Koketsu, K., 1982, Modulatory actions of ATP on membrane potentials of bullfrog sympathetic ganglion cells, *Brain Res.* **258**:313–317.

Alger, B. E., and Nicoll, R. A., 1981, Epileptiform burst afterhyperpolarization: Calcium-dependent potassium potential in hippocampal CA1 pyramidal cells, *Science* **210**:1122–1124.

Andersen, P., and Curtis, D. R., 1964a, The excitation of thalamic neurones by acetylcholine, *Acta Physiol. Scand.* **61**:85–99.

Andersen, P., and Curtis, D. R., 1964b, The pharmacology of the synaptic and acetylcholine-induced excitation of ventrobasal thalamic neurons, *Acta Physiol. Scand.* **61**:100–120.

Anderson, C. R., and Stevens, C. F., 1973, Voltage clamp analysis of acetylcholine produced end-plate current fluctuations at frog neuromuscular junction, *J. Physiol. (Lond.)* **235**:655–691.

Armstrong, D. A., Saper, C. B., Levey, A. I., Wainer, B. H., and Terry, R. D., 1983, Distribution of cholinergic neurons in the rat brain demonstrated by the immunohistochemical localization of choline acetyltransferase, *J. Comp. Neurol.* **216**:53–68.

Barker, J. L., Crayton, J. W., and Nicoll, R. A., 1971, Noradrenaline and acetylcholine response of supraoptic neurosecretory cells, *J. Physiol. (Lond.)* **216**:19–32.

Beddoe, F., Nicholls, P. J., and Smith, H. J., 1971, Inhibition of the muscarinic receptor by dibenamine, *Biochem. Pharmacol.* **20**:3367–3376.

Benardo, L. S., and Prince, D. A., 1981, Acetylcholine-induced modulation of hippocampal pyramidal neurons, *Brain Res.* **211**:227–234.

Benardo, L. S., and Prince, D. A., 1982a, Cholinergic excitation of mammalian hippocampal pyramidal cells, *Brain Res.* **249**:315–331.

Benardo, L. S., and Prince, D. A., 1982b, Ionic mechanisms of cholinergic excitation in mammalian hippocampal pyramidal cells, *Brain Res.* **249**:333–334.

Benardo, L. S., and Prince, D. A., 1982c, Cholinergic pharmacology of mammalian hippocampal pyramidal cells, *Neuroscience* **7**:1703–1712.

Ben-Ari, Y., Dingledine, R., Kanazawa, I., and Kelly, J. S., 1967a, Inhibitory effects of acetylcholine on neurones in the feline nucleus reticularis thalami, *J. Physiol. (Lond.)* **261**:647–671.

Ben-Ari, Y., Kanazawa, I., and Kelly, J. S. 1976b, Exclusively inhibitory action of iontophoretic acetylcholine on single neurones of feline thalamus, *Nature (Lond.)* **259**:327–330.

Ben-Ari, Y., Krnjević, K., Reiffenstein, R. J., and Reinhardt, W., 1981a, Inhibitory conductance changes and action of γ-aminobutyrate in rat hippocampus, *Neuroscience* **6**:2445–2463.

Ben-Ari, Y., Krnjević, K., Reinhardt, W., and Ropert, N., 1981b, Intracellular observations on the disinhibitory action of acetylcholine in the hippocampus, *Neuroscience* **6**:2475–2484.

Biscoe, T. J., and Krnjević, K., 1963, Chloralose and the activity of Renshaw cells, *Exp. Neurol.* **8**:395–405.

Biscoe, T. J. and Straughan, D. W., 1966, Micro-electrophoretic studies of neurones in the rat hippocampus, *J. Physiol. (Lond.)* **183**:341–359.

Blackman, J. G., Ginsborg, B. L., and House, C. R., 1979, On the time course of the electrical response of salivary gland cells of *Nauphoeta cinerea* to iontophoretically applied dopamine, *J. Physiol. (Lond.)* **283**:81–92.

Bloom, F. E., 1975, The role of cyclic nucleotides in central synaptic function, *Rev. Physiol. Biochem. Pharmacol.* **74**:1–103.

Bloom, F. E., Costa, E., and Salmoiraghi, G. C., 1965, Anaesthesia and the responsiveness of individual neurons of the caudate nucleus of the cat to acetylcholine, norepinephrine and dopamine administered by microelectrophoresis, *J. Pharmacol. Exp. Ther.* **150**:244–252.

Bolton T. B., 1972, Rate of offset of action of slow-acting muscarinic antagonists is fast, *Nature (Lond.)* **270**:354–356.

Bolton, T. B., 1976, On the latency and form of the membrane responses of smooth muscle to the iontophoretic application of acetylcholine or carbachol, *Proc. R. Soc. Lond. B* **194**:99–119.

Borle, A. B., 1975, Modulation of mitochondrial control of cytoplasmic calcium activity, in: *Calcium Transport in Contraction and Secretion* (E. Carafoli, F. Clemented, W., Drabikowski, and A. Margietti, eds.) The North Holland Publishing Co., New York, pp. 77–80.

Bradley, P. B., and Dray, A., 1972, Short-latency excitation of brain stem neurones in rat by acetylcholine, *Br. J. Pharmacol.* **45**:372–374.

Bradley, P. B., Dhawan, B. N., and Wolstencroft, J. H., 1966, Pharmacological properties of cholinoceptive neurones in the medulla and pons of the cat, *J. Physiol. (Lond.)* **183**:658–673.

Brown, D. A,, and Adams, P. R., 1980, Muscarinic suppression of a novel voltage-sensitive K^+-current in a vertebrate neurone, *Nature (Lond.)* **283**:673–676.

Brown, D. A., Constanti, A., and Adams, P. R., 1981, Slow cholinergic and peptidergic transmission in sympathetic ganglia, *Fed. Proc.* **40**:265–2630.

Brown, D. A., Docherty, R. J., and Halliwell, J. V., 1983, Chemical transmission in the rat interpeduncular nucleus in vitro, *J. Physiol. (Lond.)* **341**:655–670.

Brown, J. E., Muller, K. J., and Murray, G., 1971, Reversal potential for an electrophysiological event generated by conductance changes: Mathematical analysis, *Science* **174**:318.

Brownstein, M., Kobayashi, R., Polkovits, M., and Saaverdra, J. M., 1975, Choline acetyltransferase levels in diencephalic nuclei of the rat, *J. Neurochem.* **24**:35–38.

Casnellie, J. E., and Greengard, P., 1974, Guanosine 3'5'-cyclic monophosphate-dependent phosphorylation of endogenous substrate proteins in membranes, *Proc Natl. Acad. Sci. USA* **71**:1891–1895.

Cole, A. E., and Nicoll, R. A., 1983, Acetylcholine mediates a slow synaptic potential in hippocampal pyramidal cells, *Science* **221**:1299–1301.

Cole, A. E., and Shinnick-Gallagher, P., 1980, Alpha-adrenoceptor and dopamine receptor antagonists do not block the slow inhibitory postsynaptic potential in sympathetic ganglia, *Brain Res.* **187**:226–230.

Cole, A. E., and Shinnick-Gallagher, P., 1984, Muscarinic inhibitory transmission in mammalian sympathetic ganglia mediated by increased potassium conductance, *Nature (Lond.)* **307**:270–271.

Colquhoun, D., and Sakmann, B., 1981, Fluctuations in the microsecond time range of the current through single acetylcholine receptor channels, *Nature (Lond.)* **294**:464–466.

Connor, E. A., and Parsons, R. L., 1983, Analysis of fast excitatory postsynaptic currents in bullfrog parasympathetic ganglion cells, *J. Neurosci.* **3**:2164–2171.

Constanti, A., Adams, P. R., and Brown, D. A., 1981, Why do barium ions imitate acetylcholine? *Brain Res.* **206**:244–250.

Coyle, J. T., Prince, D. L., and DeLong, M. R., 1983, Alzheimer's disease: A disorder of cortical cholinergic innervation, *Science* **219**:1184–1190.

Crawford, J. M., 1970, The sensitivity of cortical neurones to acidic amino acids and acetylcholine, *Brain Res.* **17**:287–296.

Crawford, J. M., and Curtis, D. R., 1966. Pharmacological studies on feline Betz cells, *J. Physiol. (Lond.)* **186**:121–138.

Crawford, J. M., Curtis, D. R., Voorhoeve, P. E., and Wilson, V. J., 1966, Acetylcholine sensitivity of cerebellar neurones in the cat, *J. Physiol. (Lond.)* **186**:139–165.

Curtis, D. R., and Eccles, R. M., 1958, The excitation of Renshaw cells by pharmacological agents applied electrophoretically, *J. Physiol (Lond.)* **141**:435–445.

Curtis, D. R., and Ryall, R. W., 1966b, The acetylcholine receptors of Renshaw cells, *Exp. Brain Res.* **2**:66–80.

Curtis, D. R., and Ryall, R. W., 1966b, The acetylcholine receptors of Renshaw cells, *Ex. Brain Res.* **2**:66–80.

Dale, H. H., 1938, Acetylcholine as a chemical transmitter of the effects of nerve impulses, *J. Mt. Sinai Hosp.* **4**:401–429.

Davis, R., and Vaughan, P. C., 1969, Pharmacological properties of feline red nucleus, *Int. J. Neuropharmacol.* **8**:475–488.

Dingledine, R., and Kelly, J. S., 1977, Brain stem stimulation and the acetylcholine-evoked inhibition of neurones in the feline nucleus reticularis thalami, *J. Physiol. (Lond.)* **271**:135–154.

Dionne, V. E., 1976, Characterization of drug iontophoresis with a fast micro assay technique, *Biophys. J.* **16**:705–717.

Dionne, V. E., Steinbach, J. H., and Stevens, C. F., 1978, An analysis of the dose response relationship at voltage-clamped frog neuromuscular junctions, *J. Physiol. (Lond.)* **281**:421–444.

Dodd, J., and Horn, J., 1983, Muscarinic inhibition of sympathetic C neurones in the bullfrog, *J. Physiol. (Lond.)* **334**:271–291.

Dodd, J., Dingledine, R., and Kelly, J. S., 1981, The excitatory action of acetylcholine on hippocampal neurones of the guinea pig and rat maintained in vitro, *Brain Res.* **207**:109–127.

Duggan, A. W., and Hall, J. G., 1975, Inhibition of thalamic neurones by acetylcholine, *Brain Res.* **100**:445–449.

Dun, N. J., Kaibara, K., and Karczmar, A. G. 1978, Muscarinic and cGMP induced membrane potential changes: Differences in electrogenic mechanisms, *Brain Res.* **150**:658–661.

Eccles, R. M., and Libet, B., 1961, Origin and blockade of the synaptic responses of curarized sympathetic ganglia, *J. Physiol. (Lond.)* **157**:484–503.

Edwards, S. B., and de Olmos, J. S., 1976, Autoradiographic studies of the projections of the midbrain reticular formation: Ascending projections of nucleus cuneiformis, *J. Comp. Neurol.* **165**:417–432.

Ferrendelli, J., Steiner, A., McDougal, D., and Kipnis, D., 1970, The effect of oxotremorine and atropine on cGMP and cAMP levels in mouse cerebral cortex and cerebellum, *Biochem. Biophys. Res. Commun.* **41**:1061–1067.

Fibiger, H. G., 1982, The organization and some projections of cholinergic neurons of the mammalian forebrain, *Brain Res.* **257**:327–388.

Fisher, S., K., Klinger, P. D., and Agranoff, B. W., 1983, Muscarinic agonist binding and phospholipid turnover in brain, *J. Biol. Chem.* **258**:7358–7363.

Fosbraey, P., and Johnson, E. S., 1980, Release-modulating acetylcholine receptors on cholinergic neurones of the guinea pig ileum, *Br. J. Pharmacol.* **68**:289–300.

Gallagher, J. P., and Shinnick-Gallagher, P., 1978, Electrophysiological effects of nucleotides injected intracellularly into rat sympathetic ganglion cells, in: *Iontophoresis and Transmitter Mechanisms in the Mammalian Central Nervous System* (R. W. Ryall, and J. S. Kelly, eds.), Elsevier/North-Holland Biomedical Press, Amsterdam, pp. 152–154.

George, W., J., Polson, J. B., O'Toole, A. G., and Goldberg, N. D., 1970, Elevation of guanosine $3',5'$-cyclic phosphate in rat heart after perfusion with acetylcholine, *Proc. Natl. Acad. Sci. U.S.A.* **66**:398–403.

Ginsborg, B. L., House, C. R., and Silinsky, E. M., 1974, Conductance changes associated with secretory potential in the cockroach salivary gland, *J. Physiol. (Lond.)* **263**:723–731.

Haas, H. L., 1982, Cholinergic disinhibition in hippocampal slices of the rat, *Brain Res.* **233**:200–204.

Hadhazy, P., and Szerb, J. C., 1977, The effect of cholinergic drugs on [³H]acetylcholine release from slices of rat hippocampus, striatum and cortex, *Brain Res.* **123**:311–322.

Halliwell, J. V., and Adams, P. R., 1982, Voltage clamp analysis of muscarinic excitation in hippocampal neurons, *Brain Res.* **250**:71–92.

Hamill, O. P., and Sakmann, B., 1981, Multiple conductance states of single acetylcholine receptor channels in embryonic muscle cells, *Nature* **294**:462–464.

Hashiguchi, T., Ushiyama, N. S., Kobayashi, H., and Libet, B., 1978, Does cyclic GMP mediate the slow excitatory synaptic potential in sympathetic ganglia? *Nature (Lond.)* **271**:267–268.

Headley, P. M., Lodge, D., and Biscoe, T. J., 1975, Acetylcholine receptors on Renshaw cells of the rat, *Eur. J. Pharmacol.* **30**:252–259.

Herrling, P. L., 1981, The effect of carbachol and acetylcholine on fornix evoked ipsps recorded from cat hippocampal pyramidal cells *in situ*, *J. Physiol. (Lond.)* **318**:26P.

Hill-Smith, I., and Purves, R. D., 1978, Synaptic delay in the heart: An iontophoretic study, *J. Physiol. (Lond.)* **279**:31–54.

Hotson, J. R., and Prince, D. A., 1980, A calcium-activated hyperpolarization follows repetitive firing in hippocampal neurons *J. Neurophysiol.* **43**:409–419.

Hotson, J. R., Prince, D. A., and Schwartzkroin, P. A., 1979, Anomalous inward rectification in hippocampal neurons, *J. Neurophysiol.* **42**:889–895.

Hounsgaard, J., 1978, Presynaptic inhibitory action of acetylcholine in area CA1 of the hippocampus, *Ex. Neurol.* **62**:787–797.

Jacobson, M. D., Wusteman, M., and Downes, C. P., 1985, Muscarinic receptors and hydrolysis of inositol phospholipids in rat cerebral cortex and parotid gland, *J. Neurochem.* **44**:465–472.

Johnson, S. M., Katayama, Y., Morita, K., and North, R. A., 1981, Mediators of slow synaptic potentials in the myenteric plexus of the guinea pig ileum, *J. Physiol. (Lond.)* **320**:175–186.

Jordan, L. M., and Phillis, J. W., 1972, Acetylcholine inhibition in the intact and chronically isolated cerebral cortex, *Br. J. Pharmacol. Chemother.* **45**:584–595.

Katasaka, K., Nakamura, Y., and Hassler, R., 1973, Habenulointerpenduncular tract: A possible cholinergic neuron in rat brain, *Brain Res.* **62**:264–267.

Katayama, Y. and Nishi, S. 1982, Voltage-clamp analysis of peptidergic slow depolarizations in bullfrog sympathetic ganglion cells, *J. Physiol. (Lond.)* **333**:305–315.

Katz, B., and Miledi, R., 1972, The statistical nature of the acetylcholine potential and its molecular components, *J. Physiol. (Lond.)* **224**:665–699.

Kebabian, J., Steiner, A., and Greengard, P., 1975, Muscarinic cholinergic regulation of cyclic guanosine 3'5'-monophosphate in autonomic ganglia: Possible role in synaptic transmission, *J. Pharmacol. Exp. Ther.* **193**:474–487.

Kelly, J. S., 1975, Microiontophoretic application of drugs onto single neurones, in: *Handbook of Psychopharmacology*, Vol. 2 (L. L. Iversen, S. D. Iversen, and S. Snyder, eds.), Plenum Press, New York, pp. 29–67.

Kelly, J. S., Krnjević, K., Morris, M. E., and Kim, G. K. W., 1969, Anionic permeability of cortical neurones, *Exp. Brain. Res.* **7**:11–31.

Kilbinger, H., and Wessler, I., 1980, Inhibition of acetylcholine of the stimulation evoked release of [³H]-acetylcholine from the guinea-pig myenteric plexus, *Neuroscience* **5**:1331–1340.

Kimura, H., McGeer, P. L., Peng, J. H., and McGeer, E. G., 1980, Choline acetyltransferase containing neurons in rodent brain demonstrated by immunohistochemistry. *Science* **208**:1057–1059.

King, K. T., and Ryall, R. W., 1981, A re-evaluation of acetylcholine receptors on feline Renshaw cells, *Br. J. Pharmacol.* **73**:455–460.

Kobayashi, H., and Libet, B., 1968, Generation of slow postsynaptic potential without increases in ionic conductance, *Proc. Natl. Acad. Sci. U.S.A.* **69**:1304–1311.

Kobayashi, R. M., Palkovits, M., Hruska, R. E., Rothschild, R., and Yamamura, H. I., 1978, Regional distribution of muscarinic cholinergic receptors in rat brain, *Brain Res.* **154**:13–23.

Kostyuk, P. G., and Krishtal, O. A., 1977, Separation of sodium and calcium currents in the somatic membrane of mollusc neurones, *J. Physiol. (Lond.)* **270**:569–580.

Krnjević, K., 1969, Central cholinergic pathways, *Fed. Proc.* **28**:113–120.

Krnjević, K., 1974, Chemical nature of synaptic transmission in vertebrates, *Physiol. Rev.* **54**:418–540.

Krnjević, K., and Lisiewicz, A., 1972, Injections of calcium ions into spinal motoneurons, *J. Physiol. (Lond.)* **225**:363–390.

Krnjević, K., and Phillis, J. W., 1963a, Acetylcholine sensitive cells in the central cortex, *J. Physiol. (Lond.)* **166**:296–327.

Krnjević, K., and Phillis, J. W., 1963b, Pharmacological properties of acetylcholine-sensitive cells in the cerebral cortex, *J. Physiol. (Lond.)* **166**:328–350.

Krnjević, K., and Ropert, N., 1981, Septo-hippocampal pathway modulates hippocampal activity by a cholinergic mechanism. *Can. J. Physiol. Pharmacol.* **59**:911–914.

Krnjević, K., and Van Meter, W. G., 1976, Cyclic nucleotides in spinal cells, *Can. J. Physiol. Pharmacol.* **54**:416–421.

Krnjević, K., Pumain, R., and Renaud, L., 1971, The mechanism of excitation by acetylcholine in the cerebral cortex, *J. Physiol. (Lond.)* **215**:247–268.

Krnjević, K., Puil, E., and Werman, R., 1976, Is cyclic guanosine monophosphate the internal 'second messenger' for cholinergic actions on central neurons? *Can. J. Physiol. Pharmacol.* **54**:172–176.

Krnjević, K., Reiffenstein, R. J., and Ropert, N., 1981, Disinhibitory action of acetylcholine in the rat's hippocampus: Extracellular observations, *Neuroscience* **6**:2465–2474.

Kuba, K., and Koketsu, K., 1974, Ionic mechanism of the slow excitatory postsynaptic potential in bullfrog sympathetic ganglion cells, *Brain Res.* **81**:338–342.

Kuba, K., and Koketsu, K., 1976, Analysis of the slow excitatory postsynaptic potential in bullfrog sympathetic ganglion cells, *Jpn. J. Physiol.* **26**:647–664.

Kuffler, S. W., and Sejnowski, T. J., 1983, Peptidergic and muscarinic excitation at amphibian sympathetic synapses, *J. Physiol. (Lond.)* **341**:257–278.

Kuhar, M. J., DeHaven, R. N., Yamamura, H. I., Rommelspacher, H., and Simon, J. R., 1975, Further evidence for cholinergic-habenulo-interpeduncular neurons: Pharmacologic and functional characteristics, *Brain Res.* **97**:265–275.

Kuhar, M. J., and Yamamura, H. I., 1976, Localization of cholinergic muscarinic receptors in rat brain by light microscopic radioautography, *Brain Res.* **110**:229–243.

Lake, N., 1973, Studies of the habenulo-interpeduncular pathway in cats, *Exp. Neurol.* **41**:113–132.

Lamarre. Y., Filion, M., and Cordeau, J. P., 1971, Neuronal discharges of the ventrolateral nucleus of the thalamus during sleep and wakefulness in the cat. I. Spontaneous activity, *Exp. Brain Res.* **12**:480–498.

Lebranth, C. S., Brownstein, M., Zabrosaky, L., Jaranyi, Z. S., and Palkovits, M., 1975, Morphological and biochemical changes in the rat interpeduncular nucleus following the transection of the habenulo-interpeduncular tract, *Brain Res.* **99**:124–128.

Lee, T.-P., Kuo, J. F., and Greengard, P., 1972, Role of muscarinic cholinergic receptors in regulation of guanosine 3':5'-cyclic monophosphate content in mammalian brain, heart muscle, and intestinal smooth muscle, *Proc. Natl. Acad. Sci. USA* **69**:3287–3291.

Legge, K. F., Randić, M., and Straughan, D. W., 1966, The pharmacology of neurones in the pyriform cortex, *Br. J. Pharmacol.* **26**:87–107.

Lehman, J., and Langer, S. Z., 1982, Muscarinic receptors on dopamine terminals in the cat caudate nucleus: Neuromodulation of [^{3}H]dopamine release in vitro by endogenous acetylcholine, *Brain Res.* **248**:61–69.

Lewis, P. R., Shute, C. C. D., and Silver, A., 1967, Confirmation from choline acetylase of a massive cholinergic innervation to the rat hippocampus, *J. Physiol. (Lond.)* **191**:215–224.

Lynch, G., Rose, G., and Gall, C., 1978, Anatomical and functional aspects of the septo-hippocampal projections, in: *Functions of the Septo-Hippocampal System*, CIBA Foundation Symposium 58 (new series) (K. Elliot and J. Whelan, eds.) Elsevier, Amsterdam, pp. 5–20.

McAfee, D. A., and Greengard, P., 1972, Adenosine 3',5'-monophosphate: Electrophysiological evidence for a role in synaptic transmission, *Science* **78**:310–312.

McCance, I., 1972, The role of acetylcholine in the intracerebellar nuclei of the cat, *Brain Res.* **48**:265–279.

McCance, I., and Phillis, J. W., 1964, The action of acetylcholine on cells in cat cerebellar cortex, *Experientia* **20**:217–218.

McLennan, H., 1970, Inhibition of long duration in the cerebral cortex, A quantitative difference between excitatory amino acids, *Exp. Brain Res.* **10**:417–426.

McLennan, H., and York, D. H., 1966, Cholinergic mechanisms in the caudate nucleus, *J. Physiol. (Lond.)* **187**:163–175.

Magleby, K. L., and Stevens, C. F., 1982, A quantitative description of end-plate currents, *J. Physiol. (Lond.)* **223**:173–197.

Meech, R. W., 1978, Calcium-dependent potassium activation in nervous tissues, *Ann. Rev. Biophys. Bioeng.* **7**:1–18.

Mesulam, M. M., Mufson, E. J., Wainer, B. H., and Levey, A. I., 1983, Central cholinergic pathways in the rat: An overview based on an alternative nomenclature (Ch1-Ch6), *Neuroscience* **10**:1185–1201.

Michell, R. H., 1975, Inositol phospholipids and cell surface receptor function, *Biochem. Biophys. Acta.* **415**:81–147.

Morita, K., North, R. A., and Tokimasa, T., 1982a, Muscarinic agonists inactivate potassium conductance of guinea-pig myenteric neurones, *J. Physiol. (Lond.)* **333**:125–139.

Morita, K., North, R. A., and Tokimasa, T., 1982b, Muscarinic presynaptic inhibition of synaptic transmission in myenteric plexus of guinea-pig ileum, *J. Physiol. (Lond.)* **333**:141–149.

Mukhametov, L. M., Rizzolatti, G., and Tradardi, V., 1970, Spontaneous activity of neurones of nucleus reticularis thalami in freely moving cats, *J. Physiol. (Lond.)* **210**:651–667.

Niedergerke, R., and Page, S., 1977, Analysis of catecholamine effects in single atrial trabeculae of the frog heart, *Proc. R. Soc. B.* **197**:333–362.

Nishi, S., 1974, Ganglionic transmission, in: *The Peripheral Nervous System* (J. I. Hubbard, ed.), Plenum Press, New York, pp. 225–255.

Nishi, S., and Koketsu, K., 1960, Electrical properties and activities of single sympathetic neurons in frogs, *J. Cell. Comp. Physiol.* **55**:15–30.

Pearson, R. C. A., Gatter, K. C., Brodal, P., and Powell, T. P. S., 1983, The projection of the basal nucleus of meynert upon the neocortex in the monkey, *Brain Res.* **259**:132–136.

Peng, H. B., Cheng, P.-C., and Luther, P. W., 1981, Formation of ACh receptor clusters induced by positively charged latex beads, *Nature* **292**:831–834.

Pepeu, G., 1983, Brain acetylcholine: An inventory of our knowledge on the 50th anniversary of its discovery, *Trends Pharmacol. Sci.* **4**:416–418.

Phillis, J. W., 1971, The pharmacology of thalamic and geniculate neurones, *Int. Rev. Neurobiol.* **14**:1–48.

Phillis, J. W., and York, D. H., 1967a, Cholinergic inhibition in the cerebral cortex, *Brain Res.* **5**:517–520.

Phillis, J. W., and York, D. H., 1967b, Strychnine block of neuronal and drug-induced inhibition in the cerebral cortex, *Nature* **216**:922–923.

Phillis, J. W., and York, D. H., 1968, Pharmacological studies on a cholinergic inhibition in the cerebral cortex, *Brain Res.* **10**:297–306.

Phillis, J. W., Tebēcis, A. K., and York, D. H., 1967, A study of cholinoceptive cells in the lateral geniculate nucleus, *J. Physiol. (Lond.)* **192**:695–713.

Phillis, J. W., Kosopolous, G. K., and Limacher, J. J., 1974, Depression of cortico-spinal cells by various purines and pyrimidines, *Can. J. Physiol. Pharmacol.* **52**:1226–1229.

Polak, R. L., 1970, An analysis of the stimulating action of atropine on release and synthesis of acetylcholine in cortical slices from rat brain, in: *Drugs and Cholinergic Mechanism in the CNS* (E. Heilbronn and A. Winter, eds.), Forsvarets Forskningsanstalt, Stockholm, pp. 323–338.

Pong, S. F., and Graham, L. T., 1972, N-Methyl bicuculline, a convulsant more potent than bicuculline, *Brain Res.* **42**:486–490.

Purpura, D. P., McMurtry, J. C., Maekawa, R., 1966, Synaptic events in ventrolateral neurons during suppression of recruitory responses by brain stem reticular stimulation, *Brain Res.* **1**:63.

Purves, R. D., 1974, Muscarinic excitation: A microelectric study on cultured muscle cells, *Brit. J. Pharmacol.* **52**:77–86.

Purves, R. D., 1977, The time course of cellular responses to iontophoretically applied drugs, *J. Theoret. Biol.* **65**:327–344.

Randić, M., Siminoff, R., and Straughan, D. W., 1964, Acetylcholine depression of cortical neurons, *Exp. Neurol.* **9**:236–242.

Rang, H. P., 1981, The characteristics of synaptic currents and responses to acetylcholine of rat submandibular ganglion cells, *J. Physiol.* **311**:23–55.

Rogawski, M. A., and Aghajanian, G. K., 1982, Activation of lateral geniculate neurons by locus coeruleus or dorsal noradrenergic bundle stimulation: Selective blockade by the alpha₁-adrenoceptor antagonist prazosin, *Brain Res.* **250**:31–39.

Sachs, F., 1983, Is the acetylcholine receptor a unit-conductance channel? in: *Single-Channel Recording* (B. Sakmann and E. Neher, eds.), Plenum Press, New York, pp. 365–376.

Sakmann, B., Noma, A., and Trautwein, W., 1983, Acetylcholine activation of single muscarinic K^+ channels in isolated pacemaker cells of the mammalian heart, *Nature* **303**:250–253.

Salmoiraghi, G. C., and Stefanis, C. N., 1967, A critique of iontophoretic studies of central nervous system neurons, *Int. Rev. Neurobiol.* **10**:1–30.

Salmoiraghi, G. C., and Steiner, F. A., 1963, Acetylcholine sensitivity of cat's medullary neurons, *J. Neurophysiol.* **26**:581–597.

Sawynok, J., and Jhamandas, K., 1977, Muscarinic feedback inhibition of acetylcholine release from the myenteric plexus in the guinea-pig ileum and its status after chronic exposure to morphine, *Can J. Physiol. Pharmacol.* **55**:909–916.

Schiebel, M. E., and Schiebel, A. B., 1967, Structural organization of nonspecific thalamic nuclei and their projection towards cortex, *Brain Res.* **6**:60–94.

Schlag, J., and Waszak, M., 1971, Electrophysiological properties of units of the thalami reticular complex, *Exp. Neurol.* **32**:79–97.

Schulman, J. A., and Weight, F. F., 1976, Synaptic transmission: Long lasting potentiation by a postsynaptic mechanism, *Science* **194**:1437–1439.

Schwartzkroin, P. A., 1975, Characteristics of CA1 neurons recorded intracellularly in the hippocampal slice, *Brain Res.* **85**:423–435.

Segal, M., 1978, The acetylcholine receptor in the rat hippocampus: Nicotinic, muscarinic or both? *Neuropharmacology* **17**:619–623.

Soejima, M., and Noma, A., 1984, Mode of regulation of the ACh-sensitive K-channel by the muscarinic receptor in rabbit atrial cells, *Pflügers Arch.* **400:**424–431.

Shepherd, J. T., Lorenz, R. R., Tyce, G. M., and Vanhoutte, P. M., 1978, Acetylcholine-inhibition of transmitter release from adrenergic nerve terminals mediated by muscarinic receptors, *Fed. Proc.* **37:**191–194.

Shute, C. C. D., and Lewis, P. R., 1967, The ascending cholinergic reticular system: Neocortical, olfactory, and subcortical projections, *Brain* **90:**497–520.

Singer, W., 1973, The effect of mesencephalic reticular stimulation on intracellular potentials of cat geniculate neurons, *Brain Res.* **61:**35–54.

Spehlmann, R., 1963, Acetylcholine and prostigmine electrophoresis at visual cortical neurons, *J. Neurophysiol.* **26:**127–139.

Steriade, M., 1970, Ascending control of thalamic and cortical responsiveness, *Int. J. Neurobiol.* **12:**87–144.

Stone, T. W., 1972, Cholinergic mechanisms in the rat somatosensory cerebral cortex, *J. Physiol. (Lond.)* **225:**485–499.

Storm-Mathisen, J., 1975, Choline acetyltransferase and acetylcholine in fascia dentata following lesion of the entorhinal afferents, *Brain Res.* **80:**181–197.

Storm-Mathisen, J., 1977, Localization of transmitter candidates in the brain: The hippocampal formation as a model, *Prog. Neurobiol.* **8:**119–181.

Straschill, M., and Perwein, J., 1971, Effect of iontophoretically applied biogenic amines and of cholinomimetic substances on neurons in the superior colliculus and mesencephalic reticular formation of the cat, *Arch. Cres. Physiol.* **324:**43–55.

Symmes, D., and Anderson, K. V., 1967, Reticular modulation of higher auditory centers in monkey, *Exp. Neurol.* **18:**161–176.

Szerb, J. C., 1980, Effects of low calcium and of oxotremorine on the kinetics of the evoked release of [³H]-acetylcholine from the guinea-pig myenteric plexus: Comparison with morphine, *Naunyn Schmiedebergs. Arch. Pharmacol.* **311:**119–127.

Takagi, M., and Yamamoto, C., 1978, Suppressing action of cholinergic agents on synaptic transmission in the corpus striatum of rats, *Exp. Neurol.* **62:**433–443.

Takeuchi, A., and Takeuchi, N., 1959, Active phase of frog's end-plate potential, *J. Neurophysiol.* **22:**395–411.

Tebēcis, A. K., 1972, Cholinergic and non-cholinergic transmission in the medial geniculate nucleus of the cat, *J. Physiol. (Lond.),* **226:**153–172.

Tosaka, T., Chichire, S., and Libet, B., 1968, Intracellular analysis of slow inhibitory and excitatory postsynaptic potentials in sympathetic ganglia of the frog, *J. Neurophysiol.* **31:**396–409.

Trautman, A., and Marty, A., 1984, Activation of Ca-dependent K channels by carbamoylcholine in rat lacrimal glands, *Proc. Natl. Acad. Sci. USA* **81:**611–615.

Vijayan, V. K., 1979, Distribution of cholinergic neurotransmitter enzymes in the hippocampus and the dentate gyrus of the adult and the developing mouse, *Neuroscience* **4:**137.

Wamsley, J. K., Lewis, M. S., Young, W. S., III, and Kuhar, M. J., 1981, Autoradiographic localization of muscarinic cholinergic receptors in rat brainstem, *J. Neurosci.* **1:**176–191.

Waszak, M., 1974, Firing pattern of neurones in the rostral and ventral part of nucleus reticularis thalami during EEG-spindles, *Exp. Neurol.* **43:**38–59.

Weight, F. F., and Padjen, A., 1973, Acetylcholine and slow synaptic inhibition in frog sympathetic ganglion cells, *Brain Res.* **55:**225–228.

Weight, F. F., and Smith, P. A., 1980, Small intensely fluorescent cells and the generation of slow postsynaptic inhibition in sympathetic ganglia, in: *Histochemistry and Cell Biology of Autonomic Neurons, SIF Cells, and Paraneurons,* (O. Eränkö, S. Soinila, and H. Päivärinta, eds.), Raven Press, New York, pp. 159–171.

Weight, F. F, and Votava, J., 1970, Slow synaptic excitation in sympathetic ganglion cells: Evidence for synaptic inactivation of potassium conductance, *Science* **170:**755–758.

Weight, F. F. and Salmoiraghi, G. C., 1966, Response of spinal cord interneurons to acetylcholine, norepinephrine and serotonin administered by microelectrophoresis, *J. Pharmacol. Exp. Ther.* **153:**420–427.

Weight, F. F., Petzold, G., and Greengard, P., 1974, Guanosine 3'5'-monophosphate in sympathetic ganglia; increase associated with synaptic transmission, *Science* **186**:942–944.

Wilson, W., and Goldner, M. A., 1975, Voltage-clamping with a single microelectrode, *J. Neurobiol.* **4**:411–422.

Wong, R. K. S., and Prince, D. A., 1981, Afterpotential generation in hippocampal pyramidal cells, *J. Neurophysiol.* **45**:86–97.

Woody, C. D., Swartz, B. E., and Gruen, E., 1978, Effects of acetylcholine and cyclic GMP on input resistance of cortical neurones in awake cats, *Brain Res.* **158**:373–395.

Yamamoto, C., and Kawai, N., 1967, Presynaptic action of acetylcholine in thin sections from the guinea pig dentate gyrus in vitro, *Exp. Neurol.* **19**:176–187.

Yavari, P., and Weight, F. F., 1981, Effect of phentolamine on synaptic transmission in bullfrog synpathetic ganglia, *Neurosci. Abst.* **7**:807.

Yingling, C. F., and Skinner, J. F., 1975, Regulation of unit activity in nucleus reticularis thalami by the mesencephalic reticular formation and the frontal granular cortex. *Electroenceph. Clin. Neurophysiol.* **39**:635–642.

Zieglgänsberger, W., and Reiter, C., 1974, A cholinergic mechanism in the spinal cord of cats, *Neuropharmacology* **13**:519–527.

Zieglgänsberger, W., and Bayerl, H., 1976, The mechanism of inhibition of neuronal activity by opiates in the spinal cord of cat, *Brain Res.* **115**:111–128.

PART III
BIOGENIC AMINES

Serotonin

C. P. VANDERMAELEN

1. HISTORICAL PERSPECTIVE AND OVERVIEW

Serotonin (5-hydroxytryptamine; 5-HT), along with dopamine and norepinephrine, is one of the biogenic amines. But unlike dopamine and norepinephrine, which are catecholamines, 5-HT is derived from an indole nucleus and is therefore classified as an *indoleamine*. Although the major focus of current research on serotonin concerns its role in the nervous system, historically the amine became known by viture of its presence in the blood and gut (see Cooper et al., 1978; Douglas, 1980).

Physiologists of the 19th century were aware of a substance in blood serum that caused constriction of blood vessels and increased vascular tone. In the late 1940s, scientists at the Cleveland Clinic in Ohio were successful in isolating this serum-borne substance, and named it "serotonin" (Rapport et al., 1948). They later deduced that the active component of their crystalline complex was the chemical 5-hydroxytryptamine (Rapport, 1949). About the same time, a group of Italian investigators was studying a substance found in high concentrations in enterochromaffin cells of the intestinal mucosa in the gut, which they called "enteramine," and which later was shown to be identical to serotonin (see Erspamer, 1954).

It is ironic that although serotonin was originally discovered in the blood and the gut, the reasons for its presence in enterochromaffin cells of the gut, and in platelets in the blood, are still unknown. On the other hand, research carried out since the early 1950s has shed considerable light on the role of serotonin as a neurotransmitter.

Because of the pioneering work done during the 1960s and early 1970s utilizing the techniques of extracellular recording and microiontophoresis (see review by Bloom et al., 1972), a general notion arose that serotonin functions mainly as an inhibitory neurotransmitter in the vertebrate nervous system. While this is probably true for many areas of the CNS, more recent research has revealed a wide variety of postsynaptic and presynaptic actions of serotonin in the peripheral, enteric (gut) and central nervous systems.

Table 1 provides a partial list of reported effects of 5-HT in the vertebrate nervous system. These include hyperpolarizations and depolarizations of neurons; modulation of membrane conductances to Na^+, K^+, and Ca^{2+}; depression of EPSP amplitude; inhibition of its own release from terminals; potentiation of norepinephrine and dopamine release; potentiation and inhibition of acetylcholine release; depression of postsynaptic nicotinic acetylcholine receptor sensitivity; and effects on adrenal functions, and vascular tone (see Table 1 for representative references or review articles). The purpose of Table 1 is to point out the diversity of effects attributed to serotonin and to provide the interested reader with a starting point for further study of any of these reported actions.

1.1. Distribution of Serotonergic Neurons

1.1.1. Central Nervous System

The presence of serotonin in the vertebrate CNS was first demonstrated with biochemical techniques by Twarog and Page in 1953. Then in the early 1960s, a group of Swedish scientists made what is undoubtedly the most important and influential discovery to date in the history of serotonin research. Using the technique of formaldehyde-induced fluorescence to visualize serotonin inside of cells, they found that virtually all of the serotonin-containing neurons in the CNS of the rat are located in discrete clusters within the midbrain, pons, and medulla (Dahlström and Fuxe, 1964). These groups of neurons, which were designated Groups B1-B9, corresponded in large part to the anatomically defined "raphe" nuclei. Figure 1 shows schematically the locations of these nine cell groups, and some of their projection pathways and target areas.

Over the years, improvements in techniques, including the introduction of tritiated-serotonin autoradiography (Aghajanian and Bloom, 1967), immunohistofluorescence (Steinbusch, 1981), and immunohistochemistry (Tramu et al., 1983) have helped to more clearly define the locations of serotonergic cell bodies, fibers, and terminals. These many studies have confirmed the original findings of Dahlström and Fuxe (1964) and extended them to show that serotonergic neurons are not confined to the raphe nuclei, nor to the confines of the originally described groups B1–B9 (see Steinbusch, 1981). In particular, some 5-HT neurons have been found in the interpeduncular nucleus at the level of the caudal portions of the substantia nigra, as well as within the borders of the locus coeruleus, and in the nearby nucleus subcoeruleus (Steinbusch, 1981). However, no serotonergic neurons have been found in the diencephalon or telencephalon, nor in the rodent spinal

Table 1. Some Reported Effects of Serotonin in the Vertebrate Nervous System

Preparation	Effects	Mechanism	References
CNS: Inhibitory actions			
Rat brain slice, serotonergic dorsal raphe neurons	Inhibition of firing; membrane hyperpolarization	Increase g_K	Aghajanian and Lakoski (1984)
Rat and guinea pig hippocampal slice, CA₁ pyramidal neurons	Membrane hyperpolarization	Increase g_K	Segal (1980), Jahnsen (1980)
Spinal motoneurons, anesthetized and unanesthetized cats	Membrane hyperpolarization	Not known, possibly "nonspecific action"	Phillis et al. (1968), Engberg et al. (1976)
Single unit recording and microintophoresis, numerous brain regions	Inhibits neuronal firing	Not known	Reviews by Aghajanian and VanderMaelen (1985), Bloom et al. (1972)
Guinea pig hippocampal slice, CA₁ pyramidal neurons	Reduced EPSP amplitudes	Possibly increased membrane conductance	Jahnsen (1980)
Guinea pig superior colliculus, isolated brain slice	Inhibition of electrically evoked excitatory responses	Not known	Kawai and Yamamoto (1969)
CNS: Excitatory and facilitatory actions			
Guinea pig hippocampal slice, CA₁ pyramidal neurons	Membrane depolarization	Possibly decreased membrane conductance	Jahnsen (1980)
Neostriatal neurons in anesthetized rat, dorsal raphe stimulation	EPSP	Not known	Park et al. (1982)
Facial motoneurons, anesthetized rat	Membrane depolarization	Decreased g_K	VanderMaelen and Aghajanian (1982b)
Spinal motoneurons, frog and rat, isolated spinal cord in vitro	Membrane depolarization	Not known	Neuman (1983)
Cultured mouse spinal cord neurons	Membrane depolarization	Increased or decreased conductance	Cottrell and Green (1982)

Table 1. Some Reported Effects of Serotonin in the Vertebrate Nervous System (continued)

Preparation	Effects	Mechanism	References
Lateral horn preganglionic sympathetic neurons, cat isolated spinal cord *in vitro*	Membrane depolarization	Increased input resistance	Yoshimura and Nishi (1982)
Single unit recording and microiontophoresis; numerous brain regions	Excitation or facilitation of neurons in various parts of the CNS	Decreased g_K or not known	Review, Aghajanian and VanderMaelen (1985)
CNS: Effects on transmitter release			
Rat hypothalamus, isolated brain slice	Inhibited the K$^+$-evoked release of serotonin from terminals	Not known	Ennis and Cox (1982)
Rat cerebral cortex, isolated brain slice	Inhibited the release of serotonin evoked by electrical stimulation, or changes in Ca^{2+}	Not known	Göthert and Weinheimer (1979)
Rat striatal slices *in vitro*	Inhibited the K$^+$-evoked release of dopamine from terminals	Not known	Ennis et al. (1981)
Homogenized fractionated retinal tissue	Caused a release of dopamine from fish and frog retina, but not rat	Not known	Kato et al. (1983)
Peripheral nervous system			
Isolated bullfrog dorsal root ganglion, A-type neurons	Membrane depolarization	Decreased input resistance	Holz et al. (1983)
Isolated bullfrog dorsal root ganglion, C-type neurons	Fast and transient depolarization Slow prolonged depolarization	Decreased input resistance Increased input resistance	Holz et al. (1983)

Preparation	Effect	Mechanism	Reference
Cultured chick dorsal root ganglion neurons	Decreased action potential duration	Decreased voltage dependent g_{Ca}	Dunlap and Fischbach (1978, 1981)
Anesthetized or decerebrate spinalized cat; recorded in sural nerve, stimulation and 5-HT application in spinal cord	Increased threshold for antidromic activation of C, Aδ, and Aβ fibers	Possibly increased membrane conductance and/or hyperpolarized nerve terminals	Carstens et al. (1981)
Rabbit sensory neurons in the isolated nodose ganglion of the vagus nerve	Membrane depolarization / Membrane hyperpolarization (a few neurons)	Possibly increased g_{Na} and g_K / Possibly increased g_K	Higashi (1977)
Isolated rabbit vagus nerve	Membrane depolarization	Possibly increased g_{Na}	Neto (1978)
Sympathetic neurons in isolated rabbit superior cervical ganglion	Membrane depolarization	Apparently increased g_{Na}, g_{Ca}, and g_K	Dun and Karczmar (1981), Wallis and Nash (1981), Wallis and North (1978)
Autonomic neurons of the isolated guinea pig celiac superior mesenteric plexus	Membrane depolarization	Increased input resistance	Kiraly et al. (1983)
Sympathetic neurons in isolated rabbit superior cervical ganglion	Reduced the amplitude of the fast EPSP	Apparently inhibited the release of ACh from terminals	Dun and Karczmar (1981)
Isolated rabbit heart	Increased heart rate	Stimulated release of norepinephrine from sympathetic nerve terminals	Fozard et al. (1979)
Isolated bullfrog lumbar sympathetic ganglion neurons	Increased EPSP amplitude and quantal content ["low" concentration of 5-HT (3 μM)] / Decreased EPSP amplitude and quantal content ["high" concentration of 5-HT (300 μM)]	Apparently increased the release of ACh from preganglionic sympathetic nerve terminals / Apparently inhibited the release of ACh from preganglionic sympathetic nerve terminals	Hirai and Koketsu (1980)

Table 1. Some Reported Effects of Serotonin in the Vertebrate Nervous System (continued)

Preparation	Effects	Mechanism	References
Peripheral nervous system (*cont.*)			
Isolated bullfrog lumbar sympathetic ganglion neurons	Reduced the amplitude of the ACh-induced postsynaptic current (5-HT, 300 μM)	Apparently depressed the sensitivity of postsynaptic nicotinic ACh receptors (curarelike)	Akasu et al. (1981)
Enteric nervous system			
AH-type neurons of isolated guinea pig myenteric plexus	Membrane depolarization and increased input resistance	Decreased calcium-activated g_K	Wood and Mayer (1979), Wood et al. (1979), Grafe et al. (1980)
S- and AH-type neurons of isolated guinea pig myenteric plexus	Membrane depolarization Membrane hyperpolarization	Decreased g_K Increased g_K	Johnson et al. (1980)
S-type neurons of isolated guinea pig myenteric plexus	Decreased the amplitude of the cholinergic fast EPSP	Decreased release of ACh from terminals	North et al. (1980)
Isolated guinea pig ileum in the presence of methysergide	Contraction	Caused release of ACh from terminals of postganglionic neurons of the intramural plexus	Fozard et al. (1979)
Striated muscle			
Isolated bullfrog sartorius muscle	Increased end plate potential (EPP) and quantal content (5-HT, 3 μM) Decreased EPP and quantal content (5-HT, 300 μM)	Apparently increased the release of ACh from nerve terminals Apparently decreased the release of ACh from nerve terminals	Hirai and Koketsu (1980)
Isolated bullfrog sartorius muscle	Reduced the amplitude of the ACh-induced postsynaptic current (5-HT, 300 μM)	Apparently depressed the sensitivity of postsynaptic nicotinic ACh receptors (curarelike)	Akasu et al. (1981)

	Smooth muscle and vasculature		
Isolated rat uterine muscle	Contraction	Not known	Gaddum (1953)
Isolated guinea pig ileum	Contraction	Direct effect	Gaddum and Picarelli (1957)
Isolated guinea pig stomach muscle	Inhibition of contraction	Apparently an indirect effect by exciting inhibitory ganglion cells	Bülbring and Gershon (1967)
Isolated vascular tissue; rat, guinea pig and dog	Contraction	Direct receptor-mediated effects	Apperley et al. (1980), Van Neuten et al. (1981), Peroutka et al. (1983), Leysen et al. (1982), Cohen et al. (1981)
	Blood, glands		
Platelets *in vitro*	Promotes platelet aggregation	Not known	Douglas (1980)
Adrenal medulla	Releases catecholamines from adrenal gland	Apparently increases Ca^{2+} influx, depolarizes cells	Douglas (1980)

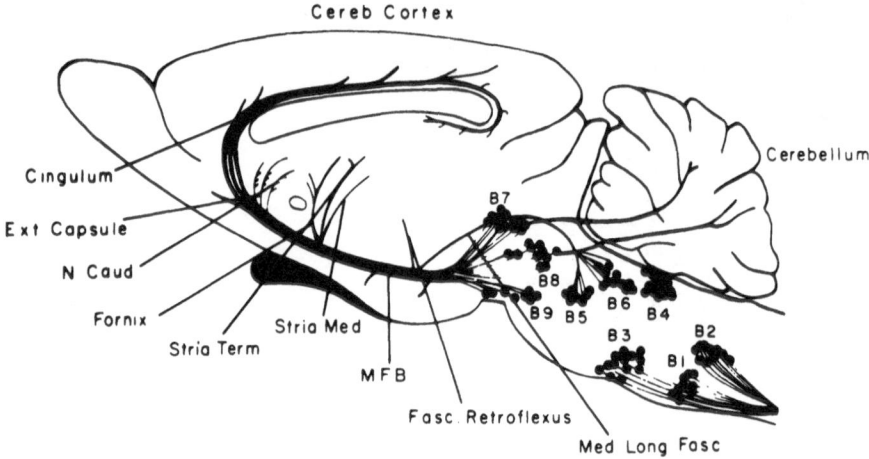

Figure 1. The major clusters of serotonergic neurons in the rat brain, designated areas B1–B9 by Dahlström and Fuxe (1964). (From Breese, 1975, with permission.)

cord, although a small number of serotonin-containing neurons have been reported to exist in the monkey spinal cord (LaMotte et al., 1982).

The serotonergic neurons of the midbrain, pons, and medulla send their axons rostral and caudal to innervate all levels of the CNS, from olfactory bulb and frontal cortex to sacral spinal cord. Very few major neuronal structures are spared at least some serotonergic innervation. Among the areas of the brain that receive little or no serotonergic innervation are certain thalamic nuclei such as the nucleus centro-medianus, nucleus reticularis, and nucleus ventralis; the lateral reticular nucleus in the medulla; the area postrema; and the subfornical organ (Steinbusch, 1981), although serotonergic fibers course very close to this latter structure (Tramu et al., 1983).

The most rostral serotonergic cell groups, B7 (dorsal raphe nucleus) and B8 (median raphe nucleus) are responsible for the serotonergic innervation of diencephalic and telencephalic structures. The dorsal raphe nucleus projects to the neocortex, the pyriform cortex, the olfactory bulb, the neostriatum, and the parafascicular nucleus of the thalamus (Andersen et al., 1983; Araneda et al., 1980; Jacobs et al., 1978; Van der Kooy and Hattori, 1980). The amygdala and hippocampus also receive inputs from the dorsal raphe nucleus, especially its dorsomedial portion, as well as from the caudal extension of the dorsal raphe nucleus (area B6). The dorsal raphe nucleus also projects to the substania nigra (Fibiger and Miller, 1977; Van der Kooy and Hattori, 1980), and caudal to the locus coeruleus (Segal, 1979). The median raphe nucleus (area B8) supplies the major serotonergic input to the hippocampus, the suprachiasmatic nucleus, the anterior hypothalamic area, and the medial preoptic area (Köhler and Steinbusch, 1982; Van de Kar and Lorens, 1979). The median raphe nucleus also projects to the cerebral cortex

(Van der Kooy and Hattori, 1980), the anterolateral hypothalamic area, the arcuate nucleus (Van de Kar and Lorens, 1979), and to its own close neighbor, the dorsal raphe nucleus (Mosko et al., 1977).

Serotonergic projections to the medulla and spinal cord originate from serotonergic cell groups B3 (raphe magnus), B2 (raphe obscurus), and B1 (raphe pallidus). The nucleus raphe magnus projects to the spinal cord via the dorsolateral funiculus and is believed to be involved in the descending control of pain transmission in the dorsal horn of the spinal cord (Basbaum, 1981). Areas B2 and B1 both project to the intermediolateral cell column and the ventral horn of the spinal cord. They are probably involved in the regulation of autonomic activity (Loewy and McKellar, 1981) and motoneuron excitability (White and Neuman, 1980).

An intriguing finding is that serotonergic fibers are present on the ependyma that line the ventricles of the brain, as well as in the pia over the spinal cord, and the arachnoid sheath around major cerebral blood vessels (Aghajanian and Gallager, 1975; Chan-Palay, 1976; Ternaux et al., 1977; Tramu et al., 1983). These fibers emanate from neurons located in numerous raphe nuclei, including raphe dorsalis, medianus, pallidus, pontis, and obscurus. Serotonergic nerve fibers are in direct contact with the cerebrospinal fluid (CSF) and the walls of blood vessels. Serotonin is definitely released into the CSF from some of these fibers (Ternaux et al., 1977). The functional significance of this is not yet known, but various hypothesized functions include effects on ependymal cells, modification of CSF formation and resorption by the choroid plexus, influences on hormone release, and involvement in body temperature regulation and the sleep-wake cycle (see Chan-Palay, 1976). In addition to serotonergic axons making contact with the CSF and with cerebral blood vessels, serotonergic neuronal cell bodies and dendrites sometimes make intimate contact with blood vessels and capillaries within the raphe nuclei (Felten and Crutcher, 1979; Scheibel et al., 1975). This apparent involvement of the serotonergic system in the regulation of cerebral blood flow is particularly interesting in light of the fact that certain serotonin receptor antagonists such as methysergide are used clinically for the prophylaxis of migraine ("vascular") headache.

Some neurons contain not only serotonin in their cell bodies and terminals but a neuropeptide as well. Serotonin-containing neurons have been found to contain substance P, enkephalin, thyrotropin-releasing hormone (TRH), and in some cases both substance P and TRH (Chan-Palay et al., 1978; Glazer et al., 1981; Johansson et al., 1981). Substance P, enkephalin, and serotonin have all been implicated in the transmission or modulation of pain impulses in the CNS (Basbaum, 1981). Substance P is thought to be an excitatory neurotransmitter for some pain-transmitting dorsal horn neurons, while both enkephalin and serotonin seem to suppress pain transmission in various parts of the spinal cord and brain. Just why substance P and enkephalin should exist in serotonergic neurons, and possibly be released with serotonin, remains a mystery.

1.1.2. *Peripheral Nervous System*

Serotonin is found in large amounts in the intestines. However, it is contained primarily in enterochromaffin cells in the intestinal mucosa, and not in serotonergic neurons.

The fact that there is so much serotonin present in the mucosa of the intestine actually hindered the discovery of serotonin as a neurotransmitter in the gut, and of serotonergic neurons in the submucosal layers of the intestine (see Gershon, 1982). The presence of 5-HT in submucosal layers was thought to reflect its high mucosal concentration, and not its presence in intrinsic neuronal elements. Serotonergic neurons and neuronal processes have now been shown by histofluorescence and immunocytochemical techniques to exist in the myenteric neuronal plexus (Auerbach's plexus) in the deeper layers of the intestine, between the circular and longitudinal layers of smooth muscle. In addition, certain neurons in the myenteric plexus that are believed to be involved in the regulation of peristaltic activity have been shown to be responsive to serotonin (Wood and Mayer, 1979). With so much serotonin present in the intestinal mucosa as a result of its secretion from enterochromaffin cells, one might think that this serotonin would affect, or even disrupt, the activity of serotonin-responsive neurons in the myenteric plexus. However, experiments performed using radioactively labeled serotonin have shown that a protective barrier of some sort exists to the transmural passage of serotonin from the mucosa to the deeper layers of the intestine containing the myenteric plexus (Gershon, 1982).

1.2. Serotonin Receptors

As can be seen in Table 1, serotonin has a multitude of reported actions, affecting vertebrate smooth muscle, neuronal cell bodies, dendrites, nerve fibers, terminals, blood platelets and glandular functions. Although the pharmacological principles are not as well defined as for other neurotransmitter systems, it has become clear that a number of pharmacologically distinct serotonin receptors exist in the periphery, and in the CNS. In the 1950s Gaddum and Picarelli (1957), defined two types of serotonin receptors in smooth muscle, the M and the D receptors. Responses mediated by the M receptor could be blocked by morphine, while those mediated by the D receptor could be blocked by dibenzyline (penoxybenzamine) and by LSD (d-lysergic acid diethylamide). Although today we recognize that the functional antagonism produced by morphine and phenoxybenzamine probably do not occur at the level of the serotonin receptor, while that by LSD does (Douglas, 1980), these early studies demonstrated the heterogeneity of serotonin receptors in the periphery.

More recently, receptor binding studies have defined two types of serotonin receptors within the CNS (Peroutka et al., 1981). The functional significance of these receptor subtypes, designated $5\text{-}HT_1$ and $5\text{-}HT_2$, is still not clear. Certain serotonin receptor-mediated behaviors in rats, such as the wet-dog shake (Yap and Taylor, 1983) and the head-twitch (Colpaert and Janssen, 1983) appear to be caused primarily by activation of 5-HT$_2$ receptors, since they can be blocked by selective 5-HT$_2$ antagonists such as ketanserin and pirenperone. Other serotonin receptor-mediated behaviors such as those making up the "serotonin-syndrome" (Jacobs, 1976) appear to be due primarily to activation of 5-HT$_1$ receptors (Lucki et al., 1984). Interestingly, some correspondence, or at least similarity, appears to exist between central 5-HT$_2$ receptors and certain peripheral serotonin receptors, since the 5-HT$_2$ antagonist ketanserin can effectively block the serotonin-induced contraction of various vascular smooth muscles (Van Neuten et al., 1981).

Different types of serotonin receptors within the CNS have also been distinguished based upon electrophysiological studies employing single-unit recordings in combination with systemic or microinotophoretic administration of drugs (see Aghajanian, 1981b; Aghajanian and VanderMaelen, 1985). Unfortunately, at this time a simple correspondence does not exist between serotonin receptor subtypes defined by electrophysiological studies and those defined by receptor binding or behavioral studies.

Electrophysiological studies indicate that there are at least three different types of serotonin receptors within the CNS: (1) a postsynaptic excitatory (or "facilitatory") receptor (S$_1$); (2) a postsynaptic inhibitory receptor (S$_3$); and (3) a serotonin "autoreceptor" on cell bodies and dendrites of serotonergic neurons (S$_2$) (Aghajanian, 1981b). Iontophorectic application of serotonin causes excitation of some neurons in the cerebral cortex (Roberts and Straughan, 1967), reticular formation (Haigler and Aghajanian, 1974b), neostriatum (Bevan et al., 1975), and spinal cord lateral horn (McCall, 1983). In other cases serotonin does not directly excite neurons (in anesthetized animals), but does facilitate the excitation of these cells by other excitatory agents (e.g., facial motoneurons, McCall and Aghajanian, 1979; spinal motoneurons, White and Neuman, 1980). The "classic" serotonin antagonist drugs such as metergoline, methysergide, cinanserin, and cyproheptadine, which are generally effective in blocking serotonin-induced responses in the periphery, are also effective in blocking the central postsynaptic excitatory and facilitatory serotonin receptors. In addition, LSD, which was originally defined as a serotonin antagonist in the periphery (Gaddum, 1953; Gaddum and Picarelli, 1957), is also an antagonist of excitatory serotonergic actions in the CNS (Boakes et al., 1969; Roberts and Straughan, 1967). However, LSD potentiates rather than antagonizes the effects of serotonin in the facial motor nucleus (McCall and Aghajanian, 1980a), suggesting that a further pharmacological subclassification of serotonin receptors may be necessary within the category of central postsynaptic excitatory and facilitatory serotonin receptors.

In contrast to the postsynaptic excitatory serotonin receptors, postsynaptic inhibitory serotonin receptors are not blocked by the classic serotonin antagonists metergoline, methysergide, cinanserin, and cyproheptadine (Haigler and Aghajanian, 1974b). These substances were ineffective when tested on neurons in the superior colliculus, ventral lateral geniculate, and amygdala. LSD, rather than acting as an antagonist, acts as a weak serotonin *agonist* on neurons receiving a postsynaptic inhibitory serotonergic input (Haigler and Aghajanian, 1974a).

Central serotonin-containing neurons are themselves inhibited by iontophoretically applied serotonin (Aghajanian et al., 1972), and the serotonin receptor that mediates this response has been termed the serotonin autoreceptor (Aghajanian and Wang, 1978). These receptors are located on the cell bodies and dendrites of serotonergic neurons and have been studied most extensively in the rat dorsal raphe nucleus. They appear to be pharmacologically distinct from the postsynaptic inhibitory serotonin receptors. This distinction is based on the finding that LSD is a much more potent serotonin agonist at the serotonin autoreceptor than at postsynaptic inhibitory serotonin receptors (Haigler and Aghajanian, 1974a). On the other hand, serotonin itself is about equally potent at both types of receptors. The term "serotonin autoreceptor" has also been used to describe a serotonin receptor that resides on serotonergic nerve terminals whose activation causes a reduction in serotonin release (Ennis and Cox, 1982; Göthert and Weinheimer, 1979). It is not yet known if these serotonin autoreceptors are pharmacologically identical to the autoreceptors on the serotonergic neuronal cell bodies and dendrites (Martin and Sanders-Bush, 1982). If they are, then the situation would be similar to what appears to be the case for somatodendritic and terminal autoreceptors on noradrenergic (see Chapter 8) and dopaminergic (see Chapter 9) neurons in the rat CNS.

2. CENTRAL SEROTONERGIC NEURONS

As described in Section I, serotonergic neurons innervate all levels of the brain and spinal cord (see Fig. 1). Numerous factors can potentially influence how much serotonin is released in the target areas. These include the brain levels of tryptophan that regulate how much serotonin is synthesized (Wurtman and Fernstrom, 1976), as well as the action of serotonergic autoreceptors (Ennis and Cox, 1982; Göthert and Weinheimer, 1979), noradrenergic α_2 receptors (Göthert et al., 1981), and dopamine receptors (Hery et al., 1980) that inhibit the release of serotonin. But the major determinant of how much serotonin is released from serotonergic terminals is the rate of action potential discharge of central 5-HT neurons.

Over the years, numerous electrophysiological studies have been performed recording from serotonergic neurons in anesthetized and unanesthetized rats and cats, including studies of unanesthetized freely moving cats (see reviews by Aghajanian, 1982; Aghajanian and VanderMaelen, 1985; Aghajanian and Wang, 1978; Trulson and Jacobs, 1981). These studies have indicated that although not all serotonergic neurons throughout the brainstem are alike in every way (Heym et al., 1982), a common characteristic of these neurons is their slow, regular, almost clocklike discharge pattern. For example, serotonergic neurons in the dorsal raphe nucleus (area B7), which have been studied most extensively because of their high density and accessibility, discharge at rates typically ranging from about 0.5–3.0 Hz (Aghajanian et al., 1972; Trulson and Jacobs, 1979). Presumed serotonergic neurons in the more caudal nucleus raphe pallidus (area B1) discharge somewhat faster, with an average discharge rate of 5.3 Hz (Trulson and Trulson, 1982). Yet, in all cases studied, central 5-HT neurons almost never discharge in bursts, but rather fire single action potentials separated by relatively uniform interspike intervals.

This slow and steady rate of discharge of central 5-HT neurons can be modified up and down as a function of the level of arousal of the animal (Trulson and Jacobs, 1981). If a cat is in a state of tonic arousal, the rate of discharge of serotonergic dorsal raphe neurons increases from about 3.0 Hz to about 4.0 Hz (Trulson and Jacobs, 1979). The rate momentarily shoots up to about 6.0 Hz during periods of auditory or visual stimulation. Conversely, dorsal raphe neurons slow during periods of drowsiness, and even more so during slow-wave sleep. A hallmark of serotonergic dorsal raphe neurons is their virtual complete cessation of activity during REM (rapid eye movement) sleep.

Most interesting is the finding that noradrenergic neurons in the locus coeruleus show a pattern of behavior over a wide range of behavioral states that is very similar to that of the serotonergic dorsal raphe neurons (Foote et al., 1983). Because norepinephrine-containing terminals make synaptic contacts with serotonergic dorsal raphe neurons (Baraban and Aghajanian, 1981), and iontophoretically applied norepinephrine excites these same neurons (Baraban and Aghajanian, 1980; VanderMaelen and Aghajanian, 1983a), it is tempting to speculate that central noradrenergic neurons help regulate the activity of central serotonergic neurons at a level of discharge appropriate to the behavioral state of the animal. For example, both noradrenergic and serotonergic neurons increase their discharge rates during periods of arousal and decrease their discharge rates during periods of slow-wave sleep and REM sleep (Foote et al., 1983; Trulson and Jacobs, 1981). The possible membrane mechanisms by which norepinephrine excites serotonergic dorsal raphe neurons are discussed in Chapter 8.

In contrast to norepinephrine, serotonin inhibits the firing of central serotonergic neurons, and it does so by activating serotonin autoreceptors on the cell bodies and dendrites of these neurons (see Aghajanian, 1982; Aghajanian and VanderMaelen, 1985; Aghajanian and Wang, 1978). This "autoinhibition" of serotonergic neuronal discharge by serotonin constitutes one of the mechanisms by which the activity of these neurons is regulated. Studies of serotonergic dorsal raphe neurons in rats suggest that autoinhibition of these cells might be due to release of serotonin from terminals of recurrent axon collaterals (Wang and Aghajanian, 1977a), or from dendrites of serotonergic neurons (Baraban and Aghajanian, 1981), or from axon varicosities within the dorsal raphe nucleus that do not make direct synaptic contacts with serotonergic neurons (Descarries et al., 1979). Of these three suggested mechanisms of autoinhibition, the release of serotonin from dendrites or axon varicosities seems most plausible, since electron-microscopic autoradiographic studies have failed to detect specialized synaptic contacts between 5-HT-concentrating axon terminals and the cell bodies or dendrites of dorsal raphe serotonergic neurons (Baraban and Aghajanian, 1981; Descarries et al., 1979).

The important question of just how serotonin inhibits the firing of central 5-HT neurons has been investigated with intracellular recording techniques. Aghajanian and VanderMaelen (1982b) found that systemic administration of LSD, which activates the serotonin autoreceptors on 5-HT neurons, caused a hyperpolarization of these cells that was accompanied by a decrease in neuronal input resistance. More recent studies by Aghajanian and Lakoski (1984) performed in rat brain slices have indicated that serotonin and LSD hyperpolarize serotonergic dorsal raphe neurons by increasing membrane conductance to K^+ (see Fig. 2).

As mentioned before, one of the defining characteristics of central serotonergic neurons is their slow and steady rate of discharge. This is seen in anesthetized and unanesthetized rats (Aghajanian and Wang, 1978), and in awake, freely moving cats (Trulson and Jacobs, 1981). Confirmation that the serotonergic neurons are in fact the neurons that exhibit this firing pattern, as well as the characteristic long duration (2–3 msec) extracellularly recorded action potentials, has been obtained (Aghajanian and Vander-Maelen, 1982a). Neurons in the rat dorsal raphe nucleus that displayed these characteristics were first recorded extracellularly and then impaled with an intracellular recording electrode that contained a red fluorescing dye (ethidium bromide). The dye was injected into the neuron and the tissue processed for formaldehyde-induced histofluorescence. When viewed in the fluorescent microscope, both the yellow fluorescence, indicative of the presence of serotonin, and the red fluorescence of the injected dye could be seen in these neurons.

The slow and steady discharge of serotonergic neurons would appear to be an intrinsic property of these cells, since it is still present in serotonergic dorsal raphe neurons in isolated midbrain slices from rats (Mosko and Jacobs, 1976; VanderMaelen and Aghajanian, 1983a) and mice (Trulson et al., 1982). Studies employing intracellular recording techniques both *in vivo* and in brain slices, have begun to shed some light on the membrane mechanisms responsible for the slow and steady discharge of serotonergic dorsal raphe neurons. These cells display a repeating cycle of membrane potential changes similar to "pacemaker potentials" seen in certain invertebrate neurons and vertebrate heart muscle cells. For this reason, the repeating changes in membrane potential of serotonergic dorsal raphe neurons have also been termed pacemaker potentials (Aghajanian and VanderMaelen, 1982b; Aghajanian, 1982).

The pacemaker potentials of rat serotonergic dorsal raphe neurons appear to be composed of at least five stages: (1) an action potential; (2) an

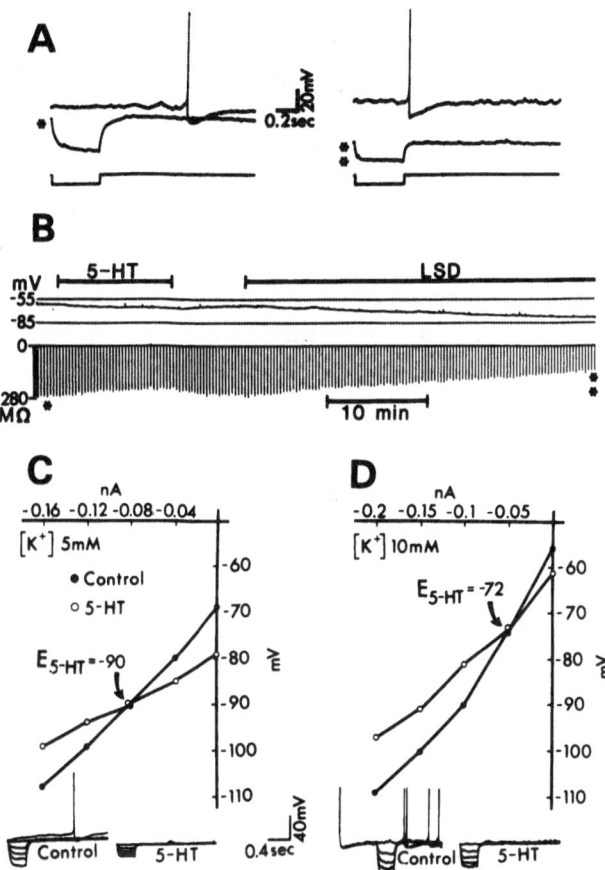

Figure 2. Intracellular recording from a dorsal raphe serotonergic neuron in the slice preparation showing the effect of 5-HT and LSD on membrane potential and input resistance. (A) Left panel: top trace shows a spike elicited by steady depolarization (0.04 nA) of this otherwise silent cell; middle trace shows voltage response to a 0.1-nA hyperpolarizing pulse; lower trace shows current monitor. Right panel: same except data was taken at a later time point from this same cell. (B) Top trace shows low-pass filtered record of membrane potential; note the reversible hyperpolarization (5 mV) in response to 5-HT (80 μM); also note the 18-mV hyperpolarization induced by LSD. Bottom trace shows isolated voltage deflections in response to repeated 0.1 nA hyperpolarizing pulses; asterisks correspond to time points at which the examples in (A) were taken. The voltage deflections were converted to resistance values by Ohm's law. (C, D) Current–voltage (IV) relationships before and during perfusion (15–20 min) of 5-HT (80 μM) in artificial CSF solutions containing either 5 or 10 mM KCl. In (C), in the presence of 5 mM KCl, the "control" and 5-HT IV curves intersect at −90 mV; insets beneath graph show superimposed voltage responses to incremental constant-current pulses from which the graphs were constructed. In (D), in the presence of 10 mM KCl, the intersection of control and 5-HT IV curves occurs at −72 mV; note in the inset that there is spontaneous activity that results from the depolarizing effect of the high potassium concentration. The points of intersection represent the reversal potentials, and the shift from −90 to −72 mV is almost exactly predicted by the Nernst equation for a K^+-mediated effect. (From Aghajanian and Lakoski, 1984, with permission.)

afterhyperpolarization (AHP) of 10–20 mV; (3) decay of the AHP during which the membrane gradually depolarizes; (4) a plateau phase during which the membrane potential appears to level off; and (5) a ramplike depolarization of 20–40 msec duration, which leads to the triggering of the next spike. Figure 3 illustrates these five stages. Pacemaker potentials composed of these five stages are seen in neurons recorded in anesthetized rats (Aghajanian and VanderMaelen, 1982a,b) and in isolated brain slices (Vander-Maelen and Aghajanian, 1983a). The plateau phase (stage 4) is not always present, especially in more rapidly firing neurons.

The characteristic slow and steady discharge of serotonergic dorsal raphe neurons is due to the presence of intrinsic pacemaker potentials and is not due to the rhythmic occurrence of excitatory postsynaptic potentials (EPSPs). This is demonstrated by the fact that no rhythmically occurring EPSPs or oscillations in membrane potential are seen in serotonergic neurons that are hyperpolarized to prevent action potential discharge, or in neurons that happen to be silent (VanderMaelen and Aghajanian, 1983a). This also means that unlike some types of pacemaker potentials, these pacemaker potentials are spike-dependent. Without an action potential, the rest of the events in the chain do not occur.

The underlying membrane conductances responsible for the pacemaker potentials in serotonergic dorsal raphe neurons are almost totally unknown.

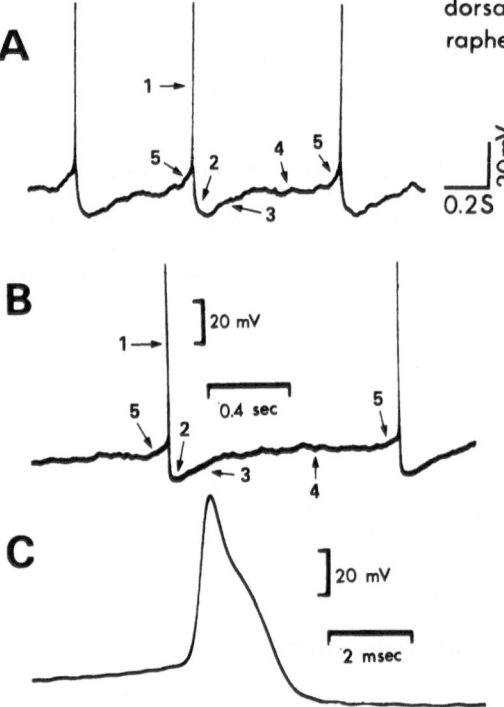

Figure 3. (A) *In vivo* intracellular recording from a rat serotonergic dorsal raphe neuron. Five stages of the pacemaker potentials can be discerned, consisting of (1) spike, (2) AHP, (3) decay of AHP, (4) plateau, (5) ramp depolarization. (Adapted from Aghajanian and Vander-Maelen, 1982a, with permission.) (B) *In vitro* intracellular recording from a rat serotonergic dorsal raphe neuron, with the five stages of the pacemaker potentials present. (C) Same cell as in (B) showing faster sweep speed of spike. Note slight shoulder on falling phase of spike. (Adapted from VanderMaelen and Aghajanian, 1983a, with permission.)

There is, however, some evidence indicating that at least a portion of the spike AHP is due to a calcium-activated g_K. Intracellular recording studies in brain slices indicate that the AHP is probably mediated by increased g_K and that it is reduced when Ca^{2+} is removed from the bathing medium or when calcium channels are blocked with Mn^{2+} (VanderMaelen and Aghajanian, 1983b). In addition, the action potential has a slight hump on its falling phase, suggestive of a calcium component (Fig. 3C). The AHP following a burst of spikes (artifically induced by injection of depolarizing current) is larger and more prolonged than that following a single spike, possibly due to greater calcium influx during the burst. Much additional research is needed to more fully elucidate the mechanisms responsible for the various components of the pacemaker potentials in central 5-HT neurons.

The fact that the slow and steady discharge of serotonergic dorsal raphe neurons is not produced by rhythmically occurring EPSPs does not mean that these neurons are totally independent of all extrinsic and synaptic input. On the contrary, conditions must be right for the expression of the pacemaker potentials. Various factors, including synaptic influences, probably determine if the pacemaker potentials will occur, and if so, how the different components will behave. A good example of such an important factor is the tonic noradrenergic synaptic input to serotonergic dorsal raphe neurons (Baraban and Aghajanian, 1980, 1981). Pharmacological manipulations that effectively remove the influence of norepinephrine from dorsal raphe neurons of anesthetized rats results in these neurons becoming silent. This may explain why in some brain slice preparations a relatively small number of serotonergic neurons are spontaneously active (Mosko and Jacobs, 1976; VanderMaelen and Aghajanian, 1983a), even though many of the silent cells are apparently perfectly healthy, and are responsive to norepinephrine, phenylephrine, glutamate, and intracellularly injected depolarizing current. But, noradrenergic stimulation is probably only one of a number of ways of providing the excitation necessary to bring the membrane potential to a level where action potentials will be triggered. Once this is done, however, the pacemaker potentials help ensure that only single spikes occur, and help regulate the interspike intervals.

3. POSTSYNAPTIC ACTIONS OF SEROTONIN IN THE CENTRAL NERVOUS SYSTEM

Ever since the discovery of serotonin in the vertebrate CNS (Twarog and Page, 1953), and especially since the mapping of serotonergic neurons in the rat brain (Dahlström and Fuxe, 1964), a major goal has been to understand the functional role of serotonin in the CNS. It is now apparent that among serotonin's functions in the CNS are included postsynaptic and presynaptic effects on neurons, and actions on cerebral vasculature (see Table 1).

Evidence that serotonin functions as a neurotransmitter or neuro-

modulator in the vertebrate CNS has come from biochemical, electrophysiological, and anatomical investigations, including electron-microscopic studies showing that serotonin is contained in nerve terminals that make
morphologically distinct synaptic contacts with target neurons (Aghajanian
and Bloom, 1967; Molliver et al., 1982). Scores of electrophysiological studies
have been carried out utilizing the techniques of extracellular single-unit
recording and microiontophoresis. These investigations have shown that
serotonin can have both inhibitory and excitatory (or "facilitatory") effects
on neuronal firing when applied by microiontophoresis to central neurons.

   Serotonin inhibits neuronal discharge in the hippocampus (Segal, 1975),
amygdala (Wang and Aghajanian, 1977b), neostriatum (Herz and Zieglgänsberger, 1968), dorsal lateral geniculate (Rogawski and Aghajanian, 1980),
hypothalamus (Moss et al., 1978), superior colliculus (Haigler and Aghajanian, 1974b), septum, thalamus, olfactory bulb, cuneate nucleus (see Bloom
et al., 1972), and the dorsal raphe nucleus (see Aghajanian and Vander-
Maelen, 1985; Aghajanian and Wang, 1978). Cerebellar Purkinje cells (Bloom
et al., 1972) and certain dorsal horn spinal neurons (see Basbaum, 1981) are
also inhibited by 5-HT. Cerebral cortical neurons can be either excited or
inhibited by serotonin (Szabadi et al., 1977), and evidence from intracellular
recordings indicates that some neostriatal neurons in the rat are excited by
serotonin as well (Park et al., 1982). Excitation or facilitation of neuronal
discharge by iontophoretically applied serotonin has been observed for cerebellar granule cells (Bloom et al., 1972), reticular formation neurons (Haigler
and Aghajanian, 1974b), and motor neurons in the facial nucleus (McCall
and Aghajanian, 1979, l980a) and spinal cord (White and Neuman, 1980).

   The membrane mechanisms responsible for these postsynaptic inhibitory, excitatory, and facilitatory actions of serotonin in the vertebrate CNS
are only just beginning to be discovered. A relatively small number of studies
have been carried out utilizing intracellular recording techniques to observe
membrane potential and resistance changes induced by the application of
serotonin onto central neurons. Interestingly, in those studies in which an
ionic mechanism for the action of serotonin has been deduced, they have
all involved changes in membrane conductance to K^+ (Aghajanian and
Lakoski, 1984; Segal, 1980; VanderMaelen and Aghajanian, 1982b). It will
be interesting to see if similar ionic mechanisms involving changes in g_K are
responsible for the actions of serotonin on other CNS neurons. What follows
is a description of intracellular recording studies on CNS neurons aimed at
understanding the postsynaptic actions of serotonin.

3.1. Hippocampal Pyramidal Neurons

   When applied iontophoretically in vivo, serotonin inhibits the firing of
hippocampal pyramidal neurons (Segal, 1975). The mechanisms by which
this occurs have been investigated in intracellular studies performed on
isolated brain slices in vitro. Segal (1980) used rat hippocampal slices, while

Jahnsen (1980) used slices from guinea pigs. Both of these studies showed that 5-HT causes a hyperpolarization of hippocampal CA_1 pyramidal neurons. This is accompanied by a decrease in neuronal input resistance (measured by injecting constant current hyperpolarizing pulses), indicative of increased membrane conductance to one or more ions.

Segal (1980) performed various manipulations of membrane potential and extracellular environment in his slice experiments, and concluded that the serotonin-induced hyperpolarization of hippocampal CA_1 neurons is due to an increase in g_K. Reasons for this conclusion included the findings that: (1) the reversal potential for the serotonin-induced response was in the neighborhood of the expected potassium equilibrium potential (E_K, -85 to -90 mV); (2) the response to serotonin changed predictably with changes in extracellular K^+ and with hyperpolarization of the membrane (see Fig. 4); (3) changes in extracellular Cl^- did not appreciably affect the response; and (4) the reversal potential for the 5-HT response was more negative than for the IPSP or for the response to iontophoretic GABA, two effects presum-

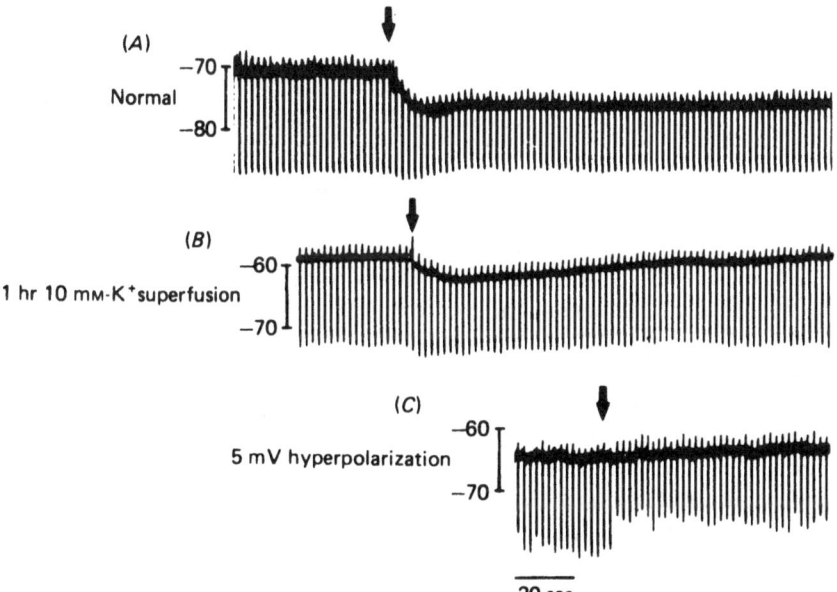

Figure 4. Response of a rat hippocampal CA_1 neuron *in vitro* to 5-HT applied by microdroplet (arrow). (A) 5-HT caused membrane hyperpolarization and decreased input resistance as indicated by the smaller deflections in membrane potential in response to constant-current hyperpolarizing pulses. (B) These responses are reduced, and the resting potential becomes depolarized when the extracellular K^+ concentration is raised to 10 mM. (C) Still in the same cell, hyperpolarizing the membrane by current injection brings it to the reversal potential for the 5-HT-induced response, while a resistance change is still evident. These results are indicative of a serotonin-induced hyperpolarization mediated by increased efflux of K^+. (From Segal, 1980, with permission.)

ably mediated by changes in g_{Cl}. In addition, the serotonin-induced hyperpolarization was still present when the bath contained no Ca^{2+} and elevated Mg^{2+} to depress synaptic transmission (Segal, 1980), or when other calcium channel blockers (Co^{2+}, Mn^{2+}; Jahnsen, 1980) were included. This implies that the effect is direct and postsynaptic, and not caused by serotonin exciting or inhibiting other neurons in the slice that then synaptically influence the CA_1 cells. This also implies that the serotonin response is not mediated by calcium influx, an important finding in light of other studies showing an involvement of Ca^{2+} in some 5-HT responses (e.g., myenteric plexus; Grafe et al., 1980). The particular population of K^+ channels involved is different from the voltage-dependent potassium channels responsible for repolarization of the action potential, since TEA (tetraethylammonium) caused broadening of action potentials but did not affect the response to 5-HT (Segal, 1980). As might be predicted from these findings, Segal and Gutnick (1980) found that serotonin also caused a transient rise in extracellular K^+ concentration in the slice, presumably because of K^+ efflux from neurons.

Thus, in a fashion similar to the action of 5-HT on serotonergic dorsal raphe neurons, 5-HT inhibits hippocampal CA_1 pyramidal neurons by increasing membrane conductance to K^+ and causing membrane hyperpolarization.

3.2. Neostriatal Neurons

Extracellular recording and microiontophoretic studies have usually shown that serotonin depresses the firing of neostriatal (caudate and putamen) neurons (Davies and Tongroach, 1978; Herz and Zeiglgänsberger, 1968). Likewise, electrical stimulation of the dorsal raphe nucleus, which projects to the neostriatum, causes a momentary inhibition of firing of neostriatal neurons (Miller et al., 1975; Olpe and Koella, 1977). On the other hand, some authors report mainly excitatory effects of iontophoretically applied 5-HT on neostriatal neurons (Bevan et al., 1975), and intracellular recording studies have revealed that the most immediate response in neostriatal neurons to electrical stimulation of the dorsal raphe nucleus is an EPSP (Park et al., 1982; VanderMaelen et al., 1979). The EPSP, which sometimes but not always triggers action potentials, is usually followed by an inhibitory postsynaptic potential (IPSP), which in turn is followed by a period of depolarization and action potential discharge. A study by Park et al. (1982) indicates that the initial EPSP, and it only, is mediated at least in large part by serotonin. Depleting serotonin stores with p-chlorophenylalanine (PCPA) pretreatment greatly reduced or abolished the initial EPSP normally elicited by dorsal raphe stimulation. This EPSP could be restored during the recording session by injecting 5-hydroxytryptophan, which acutely restores much of the lost serotonin in nerve terminals (see Fig. 5).

The ionic mechanisms responsible for this apparent serotonin-induced EPSP in rat neostriatal neurons are not known, but it is interesting to note

Figure 5. Intracellular recording from a rat neostriatal neuron showing growth of the EPSP evoked by electrical stimulation of the dorsal raphe nucleus following intravenous injection of 5-hydroxytryptophan (5-HTP), a precursor of 5-HT (traces A–D). 5-HT had been depleted by pretreatment with PCPA, and was restored

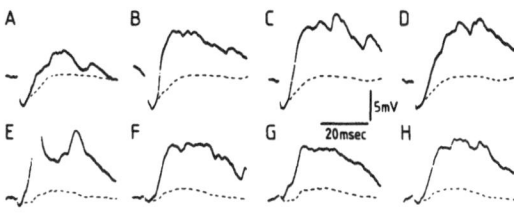

during the experiment by injection of 5-HTP (given 5 min before trace A). (E–H) The EPSP produced by substantia nigra stimulation recorded at corresponding times remained constant. The dotted lines are the field potentials in response to dorsal raphe and substantia nigra stimulation recorded with the electrode extracellular to the recorded neuron, and serve as control responses against which the EPSPs are measured. These results suggest that serotonin mediates the dorsal raphe-induced EPSP. (From Park et al., 1982, with permission.)

that the EPSP was elicited by a single brief (0.05 msec duration) stimulation pulse. In addition, the EPSP was similar in amplitude (2–20 mV) and duration (20–55 msec) to other EPSPs in rat neostriatal neurons elicited by stimulation of cerebral cortex, substantia nigra, or thalamus (VanderMaelen and Kitai, 1980). In other words, this putative serotonin-mediated EPSP was quite conventional in its appearance, and was not like the presumed serotonergic "slow EPSPs" seen in myenteric plexus neurons and celiac ganglion neurons following repetitive, but not single-shock, stimulation of afferent fibers (see Section 4).

3.3. Facial Motoneurons

Motor neurons in the rat facial nucleus are heavily innervated by serotonergic nerve terminals (Aghajanian and McCall, 1980). Extracellular recording, experiments have shown that iontophoretic application of serotonin onto quiescent facial motoneurons of anesthetized rats causes an apparent increase in excitability of these neurons, although usually the cells cannot be stimulated to fire action potentials by 5-HT alone without the simultaneous application of another excitatory stimulus (McCall and Aghajanian, 1979).

The membrane mechanisms responsible for this "facilitatory" action of serotonin on facial motoneurons were investigated with intracellular recording techniques by VanderMaelen and Aghajanian (1980, 1982b). They found that iontophoretically applied serotonin actually caused a depolarization of these neurons, but, for most neurons tested in their anesthetized rats, the membrane potential still remained below threshold for triggering action potentials. Thus, if one were recording extracellularly from these neurons, it would appear that serotonin by itself was having no direct effect. However, because the membrane potential was closer to spike threshold, these neurons could easily be excited by various forms of excitatory stimulation at levels that would normally be well below threshold for spike initiation. This is, in fact, exactly what had been found in the previous extracellular experiements where iontophoretically applied 5-HT did not directly excite facial motoneurons, but it greatly facilitated the excitatory actions of iontophoretically applied glutamate or of electrical stimulation of excitatory afferents (McCall and Aghajanian, 1979). In addition, the depolarization of facial motoneurons induced by serotonin was accompanied by an increase in neuronal input resistance. This increased input resistance would also be expected to contribute to the increase in neuronal excitability due to more effective electrotonic spread of excitatory membrane currents within the cell.

Thus, the facilitation of rat facial motoneuron excitation induced by serotonin, which was seen in extracellular recording experiments (McCall and Aghajanian, 1979), is due to a depolarization of the membrane and an increase in neuronal input resistance (VanderMaelen and Aghajanian, 1980, 1982b). Both of these factors contribute to the increase in excitability of these cells, which can be measured directly by intracellular injection of constant-current depolarizing pulses (see Fig. 6).

Some hint of the ionic mechanisms responsible for this action of serotonin was given by the fact that serotonin caused an increase rather than a decrease in measured neuronal input resistance. This suggests that 5-HT induces a decrease in membrane conductance to one or more ions. Intracellular experiments were performed *in vivo*, in which membrane potential and intracellular chloride concentrations were experimentally manipulated in conjunction with iontophoretic administration of various neurotransmitters (VanderMaelen and Aghajanian, 1982b). This investigation indicated that the serotonin-induced depolarization of rat facial motoneurons is caused by a decrease in the resting membrane conductance to potassium ions. Evidence supporting this conclusion included the findings that the serotonin response (1) was not affected by intracellular injection of Cl^- that reversed the responses to GABA and glycine, (2) was reduced or abolished by hyperpolarization of the membrane to the vicinity of E_K, and (3) was qualitatively different from depolarizations produced by excitatory amino acids.

Just how serotonin could be causing this decrease in resting g_K in rat facial motoneurons is not known. The response is similar in many respects to the serotonin-induced depolarization of guinea pig myenteric plexus neurons, which is thought to be due to a decrease in a calcium-activated g_K (see Section 4). It is also similar to the slow EPSP in bullfrog sympathetic neurons produced by muscarinic receptor activation, which causes a decrease in a voltage-dependent g_K (due to the "M current," see Chapter 6). The fact that a clear reversal of the serotonin response in rat facial motoneurons was not seen when the membrane was strongly hyperpolarized suggests that serotonin could be modulating a voltage-dependent conductance that is turned off at more hyperpolarized potentials.

Certain sensory neurons in Aplysia are depolarized by 5-HT, with an increase in input resistance and an increase in action potential duration.

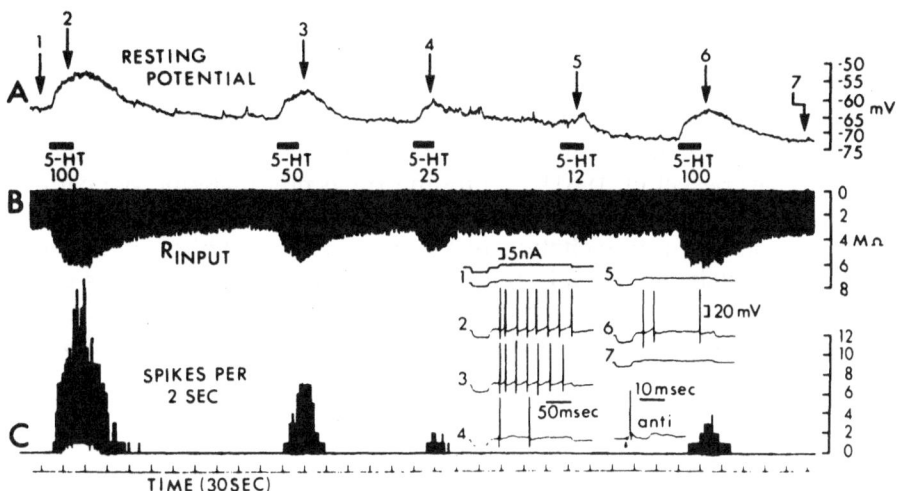

Figure 6. Responses of a facial motoneuron to varying amounts of ionophoretically applied serotonin, recorded intracellularly in an anesthetized rat. Panels A, B, and C are simultaneous chart recordings of resting membrane potential, neuronal input resistance, and number of spikes, respectively. Panel A shows resting potential, with electrotonic displacements of membrane potential and spike potentials electronically removed. B shows the amplitude of voltage displacements in response to 2.0-nA hyperpolarizing pulses with the scale on the right adjusted by Ohm's Law to give input resistance in MΩ. C shows the output of a spike counter that was reset every 2 sec. Most spikes that occurred were triggered by the intracellular depolarizing current pulse. The bars between panels A and B indicate the durations and ejection currents (in nA) of iontophoretically applied serotonin. Serotonin caused membrane depolarization, increased input resistance, and increased neuronal excitability. The inset shows individual oscilloscope traces taken at points indicated by the numbered arrows in A. The current monitor trace (above trace 1) indicates that a 30-msec 2.0-nA hyperpolarizing pulse used for input resistance measurement was followed, after a 20-msec delay, by a 140-msec 0.8-nA depolarizing pulse. This sequence occurred once every 2 sec. The depolarizing pulse had been adjusted to 62% of threshold to fire a single spike. The antidromic spike in response to stimulation of the facial nerve (small arrow) is shown below trace 7. Fifty millisecond time calibration applies to traces 1–7. The recording electrode contained 3 M KCl. (From VanderMaelen and Aghajanian, 1982b, with permission.)

Intracellular recording, voltage-clamp, and recent patch-clamp studies (see Siegelbaum et al., 1982) indicate that serotonin produces these effects by closing a subset of potassium channels. This effect seems to be mediated by stimulation of adenylate cyclase, and the increased levels of intracellular cyclic AMP produced as a consequence are believed to cause physphory-lation of a membrane protein that is somehow linked to the membrane channels. Whether a similar chain of events is responsible for the action of serotonin on rat facial motoneurons, or on neurons in other parts of the vertebrate nervous systems, is not yet known.

3.4. Spinal Cord

Serotonin can have both inhibitory and excitatory effects on spinal cord neurons. It inhibits the firing of dorsal horn neurons, including some spinothalamic tract neurons involved in the transmission of pain impulses to the brain (see Basbaum, 1981). Serotonin excites preganglionic sympathetic neurons in the lateral horn (McCall, 1983; Yoshimura and Nishi, 1982) and facilitates motoneuron excitation in the ventral horn (White and Neuman, 1980), very much as it does in the facial motor nucleus. In cultures of dissociated mouse spinal cord neurons, serotonin either has no effect or causes membrane depolarizations that can be associated with either increased or decreased neuronal input resistance (Cottrell and Green, 1982).

3.4.1. Preganglionic Sympathetic Neurons

Yoshimura and Nishi (1982) used intracellular recording techniques to study the effects of 5-HT, as well as other putative neurotransmitters, on presumed preganglionic sympathetic neurons in the lateral horn of cat spinal cord slices. They found that serotonin, in concentrations of 10–30 μM, produced a depolarization of the membrane and an increase in input resistance for most neurons tested (see Fig. 7). This was a direct postsynaptic effect since the response was not eliminated by adding tetrodotoxin (TTX) to the bath, or by switching to a low-Ca^{2+}, high-Mg^{2+} solution, treatments that would be expected to block synaptic transmission. These experiments also indicate that this serotonin response is not calcium-dependent, in contrast to a similar response in myenteric plexus neurons that may be due to blockade of a tonic calcium-activated g_K (Wood and Mayer, 1979; Grafe et al., 1980). This is particularly significant since it appears that the preganglionic sympathetic neurons in the cat possess a pronounced calcium-activated g_K that causes a large and very prolonged (up to 7 sec) hyperpolarization after each action potential.

5-HT (30 μM)

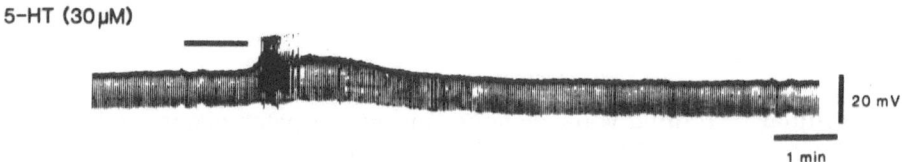

20 mV

1 min

Figure 7. Changes in membrane potential and input resistance induced by serotonin applied by superfusion to a preganglionic sympathetic neuron in the lateral horn of the spinal cord. Intracellular recordings were made from cat thoracic spinal cord slices maintained in vitro. The horizontal bar indicates time of drug application. Anelectrotonic potentials in record (downward deflections) were elicited by anodal current pulses (0.2 nA for 250 msec) applied through the recording electrode at 0.5 Hz and indicate changes in neuronal input resistance. Serotonin caused membrane depolarization and increased input resistance, with an elicitation of action potentials during the initial depolarization response (spikes were attenuated by the chart recorder). (From Yoshimura and Nishi, 1982, with permission.)

The ionic mechanism responsible for the serotonin-induced depolarization of cat lateral horn neurons is not yet known, but it could be the same as the one proposed for rat facial motoneurons (i.e. decreased persistent g_K). Also similar to rat facial motoneurons, most cat lateral horn cells respond to norepinephrine in a way identical to that of serotonin (see Chapter 8).

3.4.2. Spinal Motoneurons

In the ventral horn of the rat spinal cord, serotonin causes a facilitation of motoneuron excitation (White and Neuman, 1980), similar to that seen in the facial nucleus and possibly similar to the serotonin-induced excitation of lateral horn preganglionic sympathetic neurons. A study employing a modified sucrose-gap technique has shown that the serotonergic facilitation of spinal motoneuron excitation is also associated with a depolarization of the cell membrane (Neuman, 1983). Early intracellular studies *in vivo* found just the opposite. Cat spinal motoneurons became less excitable and were hyperpolarized by iontophoretically applied serotonin, norepinephrine, and histamine (Phillis et al., 1968). However, more recent intracellular studies indicate that this depressant effect of serotonin may have been "non-specific" (not receptor mediated) in that a number of other amines and drugs could also produce similar effects at appropriately high doses (Engberg et al., 1976). In addition, numerous studies employing single-unit, field potential, and reflex activity recording indicate that pharmacological or physiological manipulations that increase serotonin in the spinal cord also produce excitability of spinal motor neurons (see Aghajanian and VanderMaelen, 1985, for references).

Thus, it appears that one important function of serotonin in the mammalian CNS is to help regulate the excitability of motor neurons in the spinal cord and the facial nucleus, and quite possibly in other brain stem motor nuclei as well. Increasing the tonic serotonergic input to these motor neurons (e.g., as during the pharmacologically induced "serotonin syndrome") causes them to become partially depolarized and therefore more easily excited by various excitatory synaptic inputs. Conversely, decreasing the tonic serotonergic input to motor neurons (as probably occurs during REM sleep when central 5-HT neurons stop firing) would result in the membrane becoming more hyperpolarized and therefore less excitable. This would result in reduced muscle tone, such as occurs during REM sleep. One intracellular study has shown that systemic administration of two drugs which cause the serotonin syndrome, 5-methoxydimethyltryptamine (5-MeODMT) and p-chloroamphetamine, produce the same changes in rat facial motoneurons as seen with direct iontophoretic administration of 5-HT onto these neurons (VanderMaelen and Aghajanian, 1982a). This implies that the serotonin syndrome, at least in large part, is due to the drug-induced depolarization of motor neurons throughout the brain stem and spinal cord (i.e., actions on the "final common pathway") and is not due primarily to the numerous effects of these drugs on other neural systems.

4. POSTSYNAPTIC ACTIONS OF SEROTONIN IN THE PERIPHERAL NERVOUS SYSTEM

4.1. Myenteric Plexus Neurons

Serotonin has both presynaptic and postsynaptic effects in the myenteric plexus of the small intestine. With regard to presynaptic effects, serotonin inhibits the release of acetylcholine from terminals in the guinea pig ileum, causing a reduction in the cholinergic EPSP recorded in "S cells" or "Type 1" neurons (North et al., 1980). The mechanism for this presynaptic action is not known, but an interference with calcium influx at the terminal is one prominent possibility by analogy with studies showing that 5-HT reduces calcium influx in dorsal root ganglion neurons (see below).

As far as postsynaptic actions of 5-HT are concerned, serotonin can cause both depolarization and hyperpolarization of S cells and of AH (Type 2 or tonic type) neurons in the guinea pig myenteric plexus (Johnson et al., 1980). Both of these effects appear to be due to modulations in membrane conductances to K^+: hyperpolarizations are apparently caused by increased g_K, while the depolarizations are due to decreased g_K.

The depolarization of AH neurons by iontophoretically applied serotonin was virtually identical to the slow EPSP elicited in these cells by electrical stimulation of afferent fibers in the interganglionic connectives. Both responses were susceptible to the same pharmacological manipulations such as blockade by the serotonin antagonist methysergide and reduction after prolonged exposure to serotonin ("tachyphylaxis"; Wood and Mayer, 1979). For these reasons Wood and Mayer (1978, 1979) suggested that serotonin is the neurotransmitter that mediates the slow EPSP in guinea pig myenteric plexus neurons. However, this conclusion has been disputed by North and colleagues who have presented convincing evidence indicating that the transmitter is substance P and not serotonin (see Bornstein et al., 1984).

The serotonin- or fiber tract stimulation-induced depolarization of guinea pig AH myenteric plexus neurons was accompanied by an increase in input resistance, and an increase in neuronal excitability (Wood and Mayer, 1978, 1979). Figure 8 shows an example of this with iontophoretically applied serotonin. The underlying membrane mechanism responsible for the serotonin- and stimulation-induced depolarizations appear to be a reduction in a calcium-activated potassium conductance (Grafe et al., 1980; Wood et al., 1979). The depolarizing response reversed at membrane potentials close to E_K. In addition, blocking calcium influx into the cell by using a low-Ca^{2+}, high Mg^{2+} solution, or by adding Mn^{2+} to the bath had the effect of mimicking the action of serotonin or of interganglionic stimulation. In other words, serotonin acts like a calcium antagonist on these neurons. Whether serotonin actually blocks calcium influx into the cell (as with cultured dorsal root ganglion cells; see below) or interferes with calcium-activated g_K by

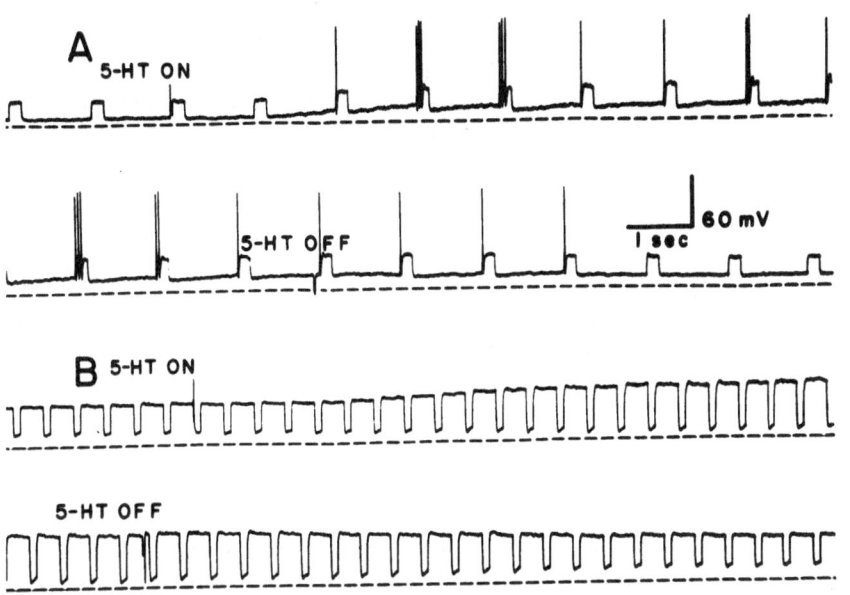

Figure 8. Membrane depolarization, increased input resistance, and increased excitability of a guinea pig myenteric plexus neuron recorded intracellularly *in vitro* in response to microiontophoretically applied serotonin. (A) A 200-msec subthreshold depolarizing pulse was injected every 1.2 sec. After 5-HT was turned on, the cell depolarized and became more excitable as indicated by the firing of action potentials during the depolarizing pulses. (B) Increased input resistance during the serotonin-induced depolarization is indicated by the larger amplitude voltage deflections in response to constant-current hyperpolarizing pulses. (From Wood and Mayer, 1979, with permission.)

another mechanism was not determined. However, it is interesting to note that serotonin not only causes quiescent neurons to depolarize but also results in a reduction in the afterhyperpolarization that follows a spike. This implies that serotonin blocks both a resting calcium-activated g_K as well as the calcium-activated g_K triggered by Ca^{2+} influx during the action potential.

4.2. Dorsal Root Ganglion Neurons

Serotonin has been reported to have two main effects on sensory neurons in dorsal root ganglia: (1) depolarization and (2) shortening the duration of the action potential.

The depolarizing effect of serotonin has been observed in bullfrog dorsal root ganglion (DRG) neurons recorded *in vitro* (Holz et al., 1983). Depending upon the cell type, different time courses of the response were obtained (see Table 1). Usually the depolarization was associated with a decrease in membrane resistance, although in C-type neurons serotonin sometimes produced a slow prolonged depolarization with *increased* input resistance, similar to responses seen in neurons of the myenteric plexus, the lateral horn of the spinal cord, and the facial motor nucleus. Due to the high serotonin concentrations required and the lack of serotonergic innervation of spinal sensory ganglia, the physiological relevance of these effects are uncertain. However, the responses could reflect similar membrane events at the inaccessible nerve terminals of sensory neurons and, as such, could provide insight into the mechanism of primary afferent depolarization and presynaptic inhibition in the bullfrog spinal cord.

The involvement of serotonin in presynaptic inhibition is intriguing in light of serotonin's possible role in the descending control of nociception at the spinal level (see Basbaum, 1981). A study of possible relevance here is that of Dunlap and Fischbach (1978) who found that serotonin, as well as norepinephrine and GABA, caused a shortening in the duration of the action potential recorded in chick DRG neurons grown in cell culture (see Fig. 9). In their study no changes in resting membrane potential or resistance were observed. The shortening of the action potential had the effect of greatly reducing the calcium component of the spike. If the same phenomenon occurs at nerve terminals of DRG neurons, it would be expected that less neurotransmitter would be released due to reduced calcium influx.

Dunlap and Fischbach (1981) performed additional studies using voltage clamp techniques to determine if the shortening of DRG action potentials produced by 5-HT, norepinephrine, and GABA was due primarily to a decrease in voltage-dependent g_{Ca}, or to an increase in voltage-dependent g_K. Their study indicates that the primary effect of these neurotransmitters is to reduce voltage-dependent g_{Ca}, probably by reducing single Ca^{2+} channel conductance or by reducing the number of available Ca^{2+} channels. The latter may be more likely in light of norepinephrine's ability to modify the number of available Ca^{2+} channels in heart cells, although in that case an increase rather than a decrease in Ca^{2+} channels is produced (Bean et al., 1983; see Chapter 8).

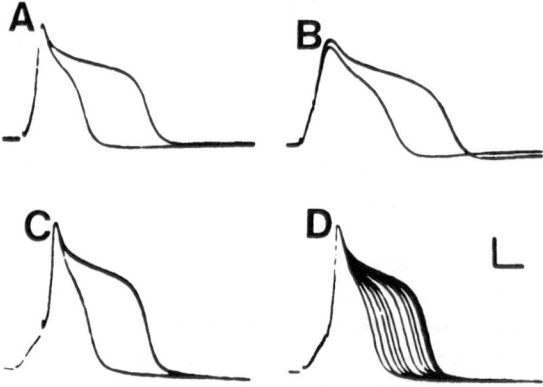

Figure 9. Serotonin (A), as well as GABA (B) and norepinephrine (C and D), cause a shortening in the duration of the soma action potential recorded in cultured chick dorsal root ganglion cells. Substances were applied by pressure ejection from micropipettes containing 10^{-5} M serotonin, 10^{-4} M GABA, and 10^{-4} M norepinephrine. Panels A, B, and C show spikes before (longer duration) and after drug application. Panel D shows return to control response, in 10-sec intervals, following norepinephrine application. Calibrations: vertical 20 mV; horizontal 2 msec. (From Dunlap and Fischbach, 1978, with permission.)

4.3. Autonomic Ganglia Neurons

Serotonin has been reported to have both presynaptic and postsynaptic effects in autonomic ganglia. Acting presynaptically, bath-applied 5-HT (1–100 μM) reduced the amplitude of the fast EPSP in rabbit superior cervical sympathetic ganglion neurons, apparently by inhibiting the release of acetylcholine from nerve terminals (Dun and Karczmar, 1981). Acting postsynaptically, serotonin usually has a depolarizing effect on autonomic ganglion neurons (Dun and Karczmar, 1981; Higashi, 1977; Kiraly et al., 1983; Wallis and Nash, 1981; Wallis and North, 1978), although under certain conditions hyperpolarizations are occasionally produced (Dun and Karczmar, 1981; Wallis and North, 1978).

Sensory neurons in the nodose ganglion of the rabbit vagus nerve are also responsive to serotonin. Higashi (1977) found that serotonin, when applied either by superfusion or iontophoresis, produced membrane depolarization in the vast majority of neurons studied. Effective concentrations for bath-applied 5-HT ranged from 10^{-7} M to greater than 10^{-4} M. As can be seen in Figure 10, the depolarizations were often large, being greater than 20 mV, and complex, consisting of a number of phases (e.g., Fig. 10a). In a small number of these cells, an initial hyperpolarizing response was seen (e.g., Fig. 10c). By manipulating the external concentrations of Na^+, K^+, and Cl^-, and by estimating the reversal potentials of the different responses, Higashi concluded that the depolarization was due to an increase in both g_{Na} and g_K, while the hyperpolarizations were caused by an increase in g_K.

Similarly, a study by Wallis and North (1978) indicates that 5-HT produces depolarization of rabbit superior cervical ganglion neurons by increasing both g_{Na} and g_K. A previous study suggested that an increase in g_{Ca} might also be involved (Wallis and Woodward, 1975). An important aspect of the results of the more recent study is that serotonin was only effective when administered by iontophoresis (see Fig. 11). Bath application of 5-HT produced weak or inconsistent effects, or no effect at all. This was apparently due to the rapid development of tachyphylaxis, which could also be seen with iontophoretic applications of serotonin if they were repeated too quickly (at about 0.1 Hz or more). Just why a rapid tachyphylaxis develops in some types of neurons and not others is not known, but this rather bothersome feature of the response of superior cervical ganglion neurons to serotonin can be turned into an experimental advantage. Wallis and North (1978) used the bath application of 5-HT (1–50 μM) to partially block the effects of iontophoretically applied 5-HT. This suggests that serotonin was acting at a specific serotonin receptor. Responses to iontophoretically applied 5-HT were also reduced by the bath application of the serotonin receptor antagonist cyproheptadine (50 μM).

The most convincing evidence for a role of serotonin in transmission in autonomic ganglia comes from work in the guinea pig celiac ganglia where serotonin apparently mediates a slow EPSP. Kiraly et al. (1983) found that

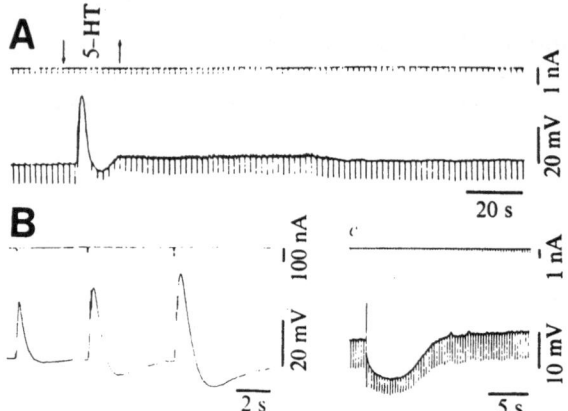

Figure 10. Serotonin-induced depolarizing and hyperpolarizing responses in afferent neurons of the rabbit nodose ganglion, recorded intracellularly *in vitro*. (A) Depolarization followed by hyperpolarization followed by a smaller depolarization, all associated with decreased input resistance, was seen in response to superfusion with 5-HT (5×10^{-5} M, between arrows). (B) Biphasic responses were seen with iontophoretic applications using 80-msec pulses and increasing ejecting currents (20, 35, and 85 nA, applied at blips in upper trace). (C) Initial hyperpolarization and decreased input resistance in response to iontophoretically applied serotonin (80 nA for 100 msec, at vertical artifact on voltage trace). Upper traces in (A) and (C) show intracellularly-injected constant current pulses. Action potentials that occurred on the rising phase of serotonin-induced depolarizations were attenuated by the recorder. (From Higashi, 1977, with permission.)

both electrical stimulation of the splanchnic nerve or iontophoresis of serotonin produced a depolarization of celiac ganglia neurons that was accompanied by an increase in input resistance (see Fig. 12). This increase in input resistance was not due to anomalous rectification since it was present when the membrane was "manually voltage-clamped" at the resting potential (Fig. 12B). Such a response could be caused by a decrease in the membrane

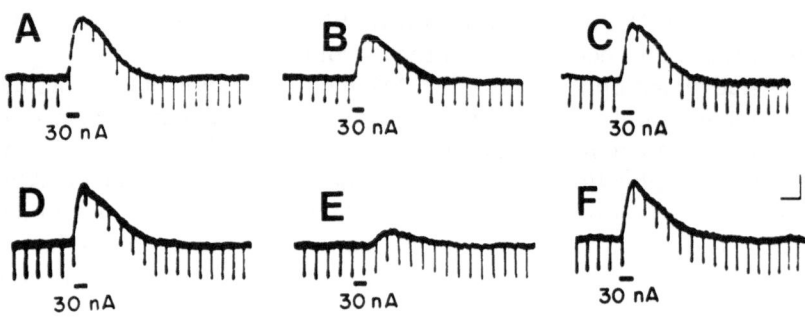

Figure 11. Depolarization and decreased input resistance in a rabbit superior cervical ganglion neuron recorded intracellularly *in vitro*, in response to iontophoretically-applied serotonin (30 nA for 1 sec). (A) Control response. (B) After 5-min perfusion of the ganglion with 1 μM 5-HT the response to iontophoretically applied 5-HT is reduced (tachyphylaxis). (C) Recovery of response after 18-min wash with normal Krebs solution. (D) Control response (later time, same neuron). (E) After 2.5-min perfusion with 50 μM 5-HT. (F) Recovery, after 3.5-min washing with normal Krebs solution. Repetitive constant-current hyperpolarizing pulses were 0.18 nA. Calibrations: vertical 5 mV, horizontal 2 sec. (From Wallis and North, 1978, with permission.)

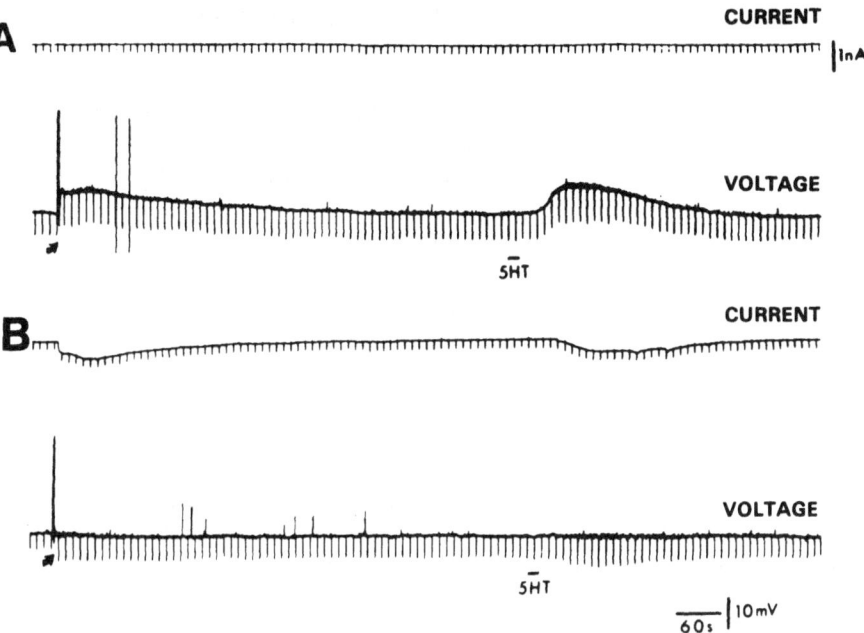

Figure 12. Slow EPSP and serotonin-induced depolarization in a guinea pig celiac ganglion neuron recorded intracellularly *in vitro*. An increase in input resistance accompanied each response. (A) Repetitive stimulation of the left splanchnic nerves (20 Hz, 2 sec; indicated by curved arrow) elicited a burst of spikes (dark vertical tracing) followed by an EPSP. The spikes are attenuated by the chart recorder. Atropine (2 μM) was continually present. Top tracings in (A) and (B) indicate current injected into cell; bottom traces indicate membrane potential. 5-HT (10 μM) was applied to the ganglion by superfusion for 15 sec each time as indicated by the short bars. (B) Slow EPSP and serotonin-induced depolarization were elicited in the same manner as in (A). However, the cell was "manually voltage-clamped" by passing hyperpolarizing current (note current trace) to keep the membrane potential at the resting level. Under these conditions the increases in neuronal input resistance, indicative of membrane resistance, were still seen. (From Kiraly et al., 1983, with permission.)

conductance to K^+. However, unlike the presumed serotonin-mediated slow EPSP in guinea pig myenteric plexus neurons (Wood et al., 1979; Grafe et al., 1980), the slow EPSP in celiac ganglia neurons does not appear to be due to a decrease in a calcium-activated g_K. This is because the depolarization induced by iontophoretically applied 5-HT was not reduced in a low-Ca^{2+} (0.2 mM) solution. It was, however, reduced by bath application of cyproheptadine (10–50 μM). suggesting that a specific serotonin receptor is involved. That the stimulation-evoked slow EPSP was really due to serotonin was further indicated by the fact that it was reduced by superfusing the ganglia with excess 5-HT (apparently because of tachyphylaxis) or with cyproheptadine, but not by the cholinergic blockers D-tubocurarine and atropine. Further research will help elucidate the exact mechanism by which serotonin depolarizes celiac ganglia neurons.

5. SUMMARY AND CONCLUSIONS

Serotonin (5-hydroxytryptamine; 5-HT) has multiple functions in the vertebrate nervous system. It affects sensory, motor, autonomic, and enteric (gut) neuronal activity, as well as influencing vascular and other smooth muscle responses. Besides being present in neuronal cell bodies, processes, and terminals, serotonin is also found in blood platelets, mast cells, and enterochromaffin cells of the intestine. Within the central nervous system, serotonin is thought to play a role in many normal and abnormal physiological and behavioral phenomena, including body temperature regulation, intestinal motility, reflex modulation, pain modulation, blood pressure regulation, locomotion, aggression, sexual behavior, learning, reinforcement, sleep, anxiety, and depression.

Very few areas of the CNS are spared at least some serotonergic innervation, with virtually all of the serotonin originating from neurons located in the midbrain, pons, and medulla, in areas coresponding closely to the anatomically defined raphe nuclei. Serotonin is contained in neuronal processes in at least some autonomic ganglia (Kiraly et al., 1983) and in neurons of the myenteric plexus in the gut.

Within the CNS, serotonin seems to function in both an inhibitory and excitatory (facilitatory) manner. In the few intracellular studies performed in which an ionic mechanism for the action of serotonin has been deduced, these have all involved a modulation of the membrane conductance to potassium. For example, the inhibitory effect of serotonin on hippocampal pyramidal cells and on serotonergic dorsal raphe neurons is apparently due to membrane hyperpolarization caused by an increase in g_K. The facilitatory action of serotonin on facial motoneurons seems to be caused by just the opposite effect, i.e., a depolarization of the membrane due to a decrease in g_K.

Generally, serotonin has inhibitory actions on CNS neurons involved in the tranmission of sensory information (e.g., dorsal horn spinothalamic tract neurons, lateral geniculate nucleus neurons), while facilitating the excitation of motor neurons in the brain stem and spinal cord. Thus, increasing serotonergic neurotransmission in the spinal cord can induce analgesia, while at the same time making motoneurons hyperexcitable. By appropriate increases and decreases in serotonergic neuronal activity, central serotonergic systems help to gate the influx of sensory information while modulating the tone of motor output systems.

Perhaps because of the largely modulatory role played by serotonin in the CNS, central 5-HT neurons discharge in a relatively slow and steady manner. However, this tonic activity is modulated by environmental influences and the behavioral state of the animal. Most of the complex neuronal interactions responsible for this modulation of 5-HT neuronal firing are unknown, but increases and decreases in the noradrenergic input to these neurons cause increases and decreases, respectively, in serotonergic dorsal raphe neuronal discharge. Intracellular recording experiments have revealed that the characteristic slow and steady discharge of serotonergic dorsal raphe neurons is due to the presence of pacemaker potentials in these cells, and is not due to some kind of rhythmically occurring synaptic input. The various membrane conductances responsible for the pacemaker potentials are mostly unknown. However, a calcium-activated g_K, triggered by Ca^{2+} entry during the action potential, is apparently responsible at least in large part for the prominent spike afterhyperpolarization. This afterhyperpolarization helps to regulate the interspike interval and also helps to ensure that these neurons virtually never spontaneously fire spikes in bursts.

In the periphery, serotonin has mostly excitatory postsynaptic actions on autonomic and enteric nervous system neurons, as well as producing contraction of smooth muscle in the uterus, ileum, and vasculature. The excitatory postsynaptic actions are generally mediated by decreases in membrane potassium conductance, although changes in sodium and calcium conductances are also involved in some cases.

Serotonin has presynaptic as well as postsynaptic actions. It can facilitate or inhibit the release of acetylcholine and can also inhibit the release of dopamine, norepinephrine, and serotonin, possibly by influencing calcium conductance at nerve terminals.

The multitude of effects produced by serotonin are mediated by various serotonin receptor types as delineated by biochemical, electrophysiological, and behavioral studies. As yet a consistent scheme applicable to these diverse approaches has not emerged. The $5\text{-}HT_2$ receptor defined by binding studies generally appears to correspond to the vascular 5-HT receptor and the receptor involved in certain serotonin-mediated behaviors such as the wet-dog shake and the head twitch. The $5\text{-}HT_1$ receptor defined by binding studies may be linked to an adenylate cyclase and appears to be primarily responsible for producing the behavioral serotonin syndrome in rats.

Continued multidisciplinary research will help clarify the pharmacology of serotonin receptors and will provide us with a deeper understanding of the physiological actions of serotonin in the nervous system.

ACKNOWLEDGMENTS. Sincere thanks are expressed to Dr. G.K. Aghajanian for helpful comments, Dr. A.L. VanderMaelen for encouragement and editorial assistance, and Ms. S. Genet and Ms. J. Higginbottom for expert secretarial assistance.

REFERENCES

Aghajanian, G. K., 1981b, The modulatory role of serotonin at multiple receptors in brain, in: *Serotonin Neurotransmission and Behavior* (B. L. Jacobs and A. Gelperin, eds.), Cambridge, Massachusetts, MIT Press, pp. 156–185.

Aghajanian G. K., 1982, Regulation of serotonergic neuronal activity: Autoreceptors and pacemaker potentials, in: *Serotonin in Biological Psychiatry* (B. T. Ho, J. C. Schoolar, and E. Usdin, eds.), Raven Press, New York, pp. 173–181.

Aghajanian, G. K., and Bloom, F. E., 1967, Localization of tritiated serotonin in rat brain by electron-microscopic autoradiography, *J. Pharmacol. Exp. Ther.* **156**(1):23–30.

Aghajanian, G. K., and Gallager, D. W., 1975, Raphe origin of serotonergic nerves terminating in the cerebral ventricles, *Brain Res* **88**:221–231.

Aghajanian, G. K., and Lakoski, J. M., 1984, Hyperpolarization of serotonergic neurons by serotonin and LSD: Studies in brain slices showing increased K^+ conductance, *Brain Res.* **305**:181–185.

Aghajanian, G. K., and McCall, R. B., 1980, Serotonergic synaptic input to facial motoneurons: Localization by electron-microscopic autoradiography, *Neuroscience* **5**:2155–2162.

Aghajanian, G. K., and VanderMaelen, C. P., 1982a, Intracellular identification of central noradrenergic and serotonergic neurons by a new double labeling procedure, *J. Neurosci.* **2**(12):1786–1792.

Aghajanian, G. K., and VanderMaelen, C. P., 1982b, Intracellular recordings from serotonergic dorsal raphe neurons: Pacemaker potentials and the effect of LSD, *Brain Res.* **238**:463–469.

Aghajanian, G. K., and VanderMaelen, C. P., 1985, Specific systems of the reticular core: Indoleamines—Serotonin, in: *Handbook of Physiology. The Nervous System. Intrinsic Regulatory Systems of the Brain* (F. E. Bloom, ed.), Am. Physiol. Soc., Bethesda, Maryland, in press.

Aghajanian, G. K., and Wang, R. Y., 1978, Physiology and pharmacology of central serotonergic neurons, in: *Psychopharmacology: A Generation of Progress* (M. A. Lipton, A. DiMascio, and K. F. Killam, eds.), Raven Press, New York, pp. 171–183.

Aghajanian, G. K., Haigler, H. J., and Bloom, F. E., 1972, Lysergic acid diethylamide and serotonin: Direct action on serotonin-containing neurons, *Life Sci.* **11**:615–622.

Akasu, T., Hirai, K., and Koketsu, K., 1981, 5-Hydroxytryptamine controls ACh-receptor sensitivity of bullfrog sympathetic ganglion cells, *Brain Res.* **211**:217–220.

Andersen, E., Rigor, B., and Dafny, N., 1983, Electrophysiological evidence of concurrent dorsal raphe input to caudate, septum, habenula, thalamus, hippocampus, cerebellum and olfactory bulb, *Int. J. Neurosci.* **18**:107–116.

Anderson, J., 1983, Serotonin receptor changes after chronic antidepressant treatments: Ligand binding, electrophysiological, and behavioral studies, *Life Sciences* **32**:1791–1801.

Apperley, E., Feniuk, W., Humphrey, P. P. A., and Levy, G. P., 1980, Evidence for two types of excitatory receptor for 5-hydroxytryptamine in dog isolated vasculature, *Br. J. Pharmacol.* **68**:215–224.

Araneda, S., Gamrani, H., Font, C., Calas, A., Pujol, J.-F., and Bobillier, P., 1980, Retrograde axonal transport following injection of [^{3}H]-serotonin into the olfactory bulb. II. Radioautographic study, *Brain Res.* **196**:417–427.

Baraban, J. M., and Aghajanian, G. K., 1980, Suppression of firing activity of 5-HT neurons in the dorsal raphe by alpha-adrenoceptor antagonists, *Neuropharmacology* **19**:355–363.

Baraban, J. M., and Aghajanian, G. K., 1981, Noradrenergic innervation of serotonergic neurons in the dorsal raphe: Demonstration by electron microscopic autoradiography, *Brain Res.* **204**:1–11.

Basbaum, A. I., 1981, Descending control of pain transmission: Possible serotonergic-enkephalinergic interactions, in: *Serotonin: Current Aspects of Neurochemistry and Function* (B. Haber, S. Gabay, M. R. Issidorides, and S. G. A. Alivisatos, eds.), Plenum Press, New York, pp. 177–189.

Bean, B. P., Nowycky, M. C., and Tsien, R. W., 1983, β-Adrenergic modulation of the number of functional calcium channels in frog heart cells, *Soc. Neurosci. Abst.* **9**:509.

Bevan, P., Bradshaw, C. M., and Szabadi, E., 1975, Effects of desipramine on neuronal responses to dopamine, noradrenaline, 5-hydroxytryptamine and acetylcholine in the caudate nucleus of the rat, *Br. J. Pharmacol.* **54**:285–293.

Bloom, F. E., Hoffer, B. J., Siggins, G. R., Barker, J. L., and Nicoll, R. A., 1972, Effects of serotonin on central neurons: Microiontophoretic administration, *Fed. Proc.* **31**(1):97–106.

Boakes, R. J., Bradley, P. B., Briggs, I., and Dray, A., 1969, Antagonism by LSD to effects of 5-HT on single neurones, *Brain Res.* **15**:529–531.

Bornstein, J. C., North, R. A., Costa, M., and Furness, J. B., 1984, Excitatory synaptic potentials due to activation of neurons with short projections in the myenteric plexus, *Neuroscience* **11**:723–731.

Breese, G. R., 1975, Chemical and immunochemical lesions by specific neurotoxic substances and antisera, in: *Biochemical Principles and Techniques in Neurophamacology*, Volume 1 (L. L. Iversen, S. D. Iversen, and S. H. Snyder, eds.), Plenum Press, New York, pp. 137–189.

Bülbring, E., and Gershon, M. D., 1967, 5-Hydroxytryptamine participation in the vagal inhibitory innervation of the stomach, *J. Physiol. (Lond.)* **192**:832–846.

Carstens, E., Klumpp, D., Randic, M., and Zimmerman, M., 1981, Effect of iontophoretically applied 5-hydroxytryptamine on the excitability of single primary afferent C- and A-fibers in the cat spinal cord, *Brain Res.* **220**:151–158.

Chan-Palay, V., 1976, Serotonin axons in the supra- and subependymal plexuses and in the leptomeninges: Their roles in local alterations of cerebrospinal fluid and vasomotor activity, *Brain Res.* **102**:103–130.

Chan-Palay, V., Jonsson, G., and Palay, S. L., 1978, Serotonin and substance P coexist in neurons of the rat's central nervous system, *Proc. Natl. Acad. Sci. USA* **75**:1582–1586.

Cohen, M. L., Fuller, R. W., and Wiley, K. S., 1981, Evidence of 5-HT$_2$ receptors mediating contraction in vascular smooth muscle, *J. Pharmacol. Exp. Ther.* **218**:421–425.

Colpaert, F. C., and Janssen, P. A. J., 1983, The head-twitch response to intraperitoneal injection of 5-hydroxytryptophan in the rat: Antagonist effects of purported 5-hydroxytryptamine antagonists and of pirenperone, an LSD antagonist, *Neuropharmacology* **22**:993–1000.

Cooper, J. R., Bloom, F. E., and Roth, R. H., 1978, *The Biochemical Basis of Neuropharmacology*, Oxford University Press, New York.

Cottrell, G. A., and Green, K. A., 1982, Responses of mouse spinal neurones in culture to locally applied serotonin, *J. Physiol. (Lond.)* **325**:25P–26P.

Dahlström, A., and Fuxe, K., 1964, Evidence for the existence of monoamine-containing neurons in the central nervous system. I. Demonstration of monoamines in cell bodies of brainstem neurons, *Acta Physiol. Scand.* **62** (Suppl. 232):1–55.

Davies, J., and Tongroach, P., 1978, Neuropharmacological studies on the nigro-striatal and raphe-striatal system in the rat, *Eur. J. Pharmacol.* **51**:91–100.

deMontigny, C., 1981, Enhancement of the 5-HT neurotransmission by antidepressant treatments, *J. Physiol. (Paris)* **77**:455–461.

deMontigny, C., and Aghajanian, G. K., 1978, Tricyclic antidepressants: long-term treatment increases responsivity of rat forebrain neurons to serotonin, *Science* **202**:1303–1306.

Descarries, L., Beaudet, A., Watkins, K. C., and Garcia, S., 1979, The serotonin neurons in nucleus raphe dorsalis of adult rat, *Anat. Rec.* **193**:520.

Douglas, W. W., 1980, Histamine and 5-hydroxytryptamine (serotonin) and their antagonists, in: *Goodman and Gilman's The Pharmacological Basis of Therapeutics*, Sixth Edition (A. G. Gilman, L. S. Goodman, and A. Gilman, eds.), MacMillan Publishing Company, New York, pp. 609–646.

Dun, N. J., and Karczmar, A. G., 1981, Evidence for a presynaptic inhibitory action of 5-hydroxytryptamine in a mammalian sympathetic ganglion, *J. Pharmacol. Exp. Ther.* **217**:714–718.

Dunlap, K., and Fischbach, G. D., 1978, Neurotransmitters decrease the calcium component of sensory neurone action potentials, *Nature* **276**:837–839.

Dunlap, K., and Fischbach, G. D., 1981, Neurotransmitters decrease the calcium conductance activated by depolarization of embryonic chick sensory neurones, *J. Physiol. (Lond.)* **317**:519–535.

Engberg, I., Flatman, J. A., and Kadzielawa, K., 1976, Lack of specificity of motoneurone responses to microiontophoretically applied phenolic amines, *Acta Physiol. Scand.* **96**:137–139.

Ennis, C., and Cox, B., 1982, The effect of tryptamine on serotonin release from hypothalamic slices is mediated by a cholinergic interneurone, *Psychopharmacology* **78**:85–88.

Ennis, C., Kemp, J. D., and Cox, B., 1981, Characterisation of inhibitory 5-hydroxytryptamine receptors that modulate dopamine release in the striatum. *J. Neurochem.* **36**(4):1515–1520.

Erspamer, V., 1954, Pharmacology of indolealkylamines, *Pharmacol. Rev.* **6**:425–487.

Felten, D. L., and Crutcher, K. A., 1979, Neuronal-vascular relationships in the raphe nuclei, locus coeruleus, and substantia nigra in primates, *Am. J. Anat.* **155**(4):467–481.

Fibiger, H. C., and Miller, J. J., 1977, An anatomical and electrophysiological investigation of the serotonergic projection from the dorsal raphe nucleus to the substantia nigra in the rat, *Neuroscience* **2**:975–987.

Foote, S. L., Bloom, F. E., and Aston-Jones, G., 1983, Nucleus locus coeruleus: New evidence of anatomical and physiological specificity, *Physiol. Rev.* **63**(3):844–914.

Fozard, J. R., Mobarok Ali, A. T. M., and Newgrosh, G., 1979, Blockade of serotonin receptors on autonomic neurones by (−)-cocaine and some related compounds, *Eur. J. Pharmacol.* **59**:195–210.

Gaddum, J. H., 1953, Antagonism between lysergic acid diethylamide and 5-hydroxytryptamine, *J. Physiol. (Lond.)* **121**:15P.

Gaddum, J. H., and Picarelli, Z. P., 1957, Two kinds of tryptamine receptor, *Br. J. Pharmacol.* **12**:323–328.

Gershon, M. D., 1982, Serotonergic neurotransmission in the gut, *Scand. J. Gastroenterol. (Norway)* **17**(71):26–41.

Glazer, E. J., Steinbusch, H. W. M., Verhofstad, A. A. J., and Basbaum, A. I., 1981, Serotonergic neurons in nucleus raphe dorsalis and paragigantocellularis of the cat contain enkephalin, *J. Physiol. (Paris)* **77**:241–245.

Göthert, M., and Weinheimer, G., 1979, Extracellular 5-hydroxytryptamine inhibits 5-hydroxytryptamine release from rat brain cortex slices, *Naunyn Schmiedebergs Arch. Pharmacol.* **310**:93–96.

Göthert, M., Huth, H., and Schlicker, E., 1981, Characterization of the receptor subtype involved in alpha-adrenoceptor-mediated modulation of serotonin release from rat brain cortex slices, *Naunyn Schmiedebergs Arch. Pharmacol.* **317**:199–203.

Grafe, P., Mayer, C. J., and Wood, J. D., 1980, Synaptic modulation of calcium-dependent potassium conductance in myenteric neurones in the guinea pig, *J. Physiol. (Lond.)* **305**:235–248.

Haigler, H. J., and Aghajanian, G. K., 1974a, Lysergic acid diethylamide and serotonin: a comparison of effects on serotonergic neurons and neurons receiving a serotonergic input, *J. Pharmacol. Exp. Ther.* **188**:688–699.

Haigler, H. J., and Aghajanian, G. K., 1974b, Peripheral serotonin antagonists: failure to antagonize serotonin in brain areas receiving a prominent serotonergic input, *J. Neural Transm.* **35**:257–273.

Hery, F., Soubrie, P., Bourgoin, S., Motastruc, J. L., Artaud, F., and Glowinski, J., 1980, Dopamine released from dendrites in the substantia nigra controls the nigral and striatal release of serotonin, *Brain Res.* **193**:143–151.

Herz, A., and Zieglgänsberger, W., 1968, The influence of microelectrophoretically applied biogenic amines, cholinomimetics and procain on synaptic excitation in the corpus striatum, *Int. J. Neuropharmacol.* **7**:211–230.

Heym, J., Steinfels, G. F., and Jacobs, B. L., 1982, Medullary serotonergic neurons are insensitive to 5-MEODMT and LSD, *Eur. J. Pharmacol.* **81**:677–680.

Higashi, H., 1977, 5-Hydroxytryptamine receptors on visceral primary afferent neurones in the nodose ganglion of the rabbit, *Nature* **267**:448–450.

Hirai, K., and Koketsu, K., 1980, Presynaptic regulation of the release of acetylcholine by 5-hydroxytryptamine, *Br. J. Pharmacol.* **70**:499–500.

Holz, G. A. IV, Shefner, S. A., and Anderson, E. G., 1983, Serotonin depolarizes A- and C-type primary afferents: an intracellular study in bullfrog dorsal root ganglion, *Soc. Neurosci. Abst.* **9**:254.

Jacobs, B. L., 1976, An animal model for studying central serotonergic synapses, *Life Sci.* **19**:777–785.

Jacobs, B. L., Foote, S. L., and Bloom, F. E., 1978, Differential projections of neurons within the dorsal raphe nucleus of the rat: A horseradish peroxidase (HRP) study, *Brain Res.* **147**:149–153.

Jahnsen, H., 1980, The action of 5-hydroxytryptamine on neuronal membranes and synaptic transmission in area CA1 of the hippocampus *in vitro*, *Brain Res.* **197**:83–94.

Johansson, O., Hökfelt, T., Pernow, B., Jeffcoat, S. L., White, N., Steinbusch, H. W. M., Verhofstad, A. A. J., Emson, P. C., and Spindel, E., 1981, Immunohistochemical support for three putative transmitters in one neuron: Coexistence of 5-hydroxytryptamine, substance P, and thyrotropin releasing hormone-like immunoreactivity in medullary neurons projecting to the spinal cord, *Neuroscience* **6**:1857–1881.

Johnson, S. M., Katayama, Y., and North, R. A., 1980, Multiple actions of 5-hydroxytryptamine on myenteric neurones of the guinea-pig ileum, *J. Physiol. (Lond.)* **304**:459–470.

Kato, S., Negishi, K., Teranishi, T., and Sugawara, K., 1983, 5-Hydroxytryptamine: Its facilitative action on [^{3}H]dopamine release from the retina, *Vision Res.* **23**(4):445–449.

Kawai, N., and Yamamoto, C., 1969, Effects of 5-hydroxytryptamine, LSD and related compounds on electrical activities evoked *in vitro* in thin sections from the superior colliculus, *Int. J. Neuropharmacol.* **8**:437–449.

Kiraly, M., Ma, R. C., and Dun, N. J., 1983, Serotonin mediates a slow excitatory potential in mammalian celiac ganglia, *Brain Res.* **275**:378–383.

Köhler, C., and Steinbusch, H., 1982, Identification of serotonin and non-serotonin-containing neurons of the mid-brain raphe projecting to the entorhinal area and the hippocampal formation. A combined immunohistochemical and fluorescent retrograde tracing study in the rat brain, *Neuroscience* **7**(4):951–975.

LaMotte, C. C., Johns, D. R., and DeLanerolle, N. C., 1982, Immunohistochemical evidence of indolamine neurons in monkey spinal cord, *J. Comp. Neurol.* **206**:359–370.

Leysen, J. E., Niemegeers, C. J. E., Van Nueten, J. M., and Laduron, P. M., 1982, [^{3}H]Ketanserin (R 41 468), a selective ^{3}H-ligand for serotonin$_2$ receptor binding sites, *Mol. Pharmacol.* **21**:301–314.

Loewy, A. D., and McKellar, S., 1981, Serotonergic projections from the ventral medulla to the intermediolateral cell column in the rat, *Brain Res.* **211**:146–152.

Lucki, I., Nobler, M. S., and Frazer, A., 1984, Differential actions of serotonin antagonists on two behavioral models of serotonin receptor activation in the rat, *J. Pharmacol. Exp. Ther.* **228**:133–139.

Martin, L. L., and Sanders-Bush, E., 1982, Comparison of the pharmacological characteristics of 5HT$_1$ and 5HT$_2$ binding sites with those of serotonin autoreceptors which modulate serotonin release, *Naunyn Schmiedebergs Arch. Pharmacol.* **321**:165–170.

McCall, R. B., 1983, Serotonergic excitation of sympathetic preganglionic neurons: A microintophoretic study, *Brain Res.* **289**:121–127.

McCall, R. B., and Aghajanian, G. K., 1979, Serotonergic facilitation of facial motoneuron excitation, *Brain Res.* **169**:11–27.

McCall, R. B., and Aghajanian, G. K., 1980a, Hallucinogens potentiate responses to serotonin and norepinephrine in the facial motor nucleus, *Life Sci.* **26**:1149–1156.

McCall, R. B., and Aghajanian, G. K., 1980b, Pharmacological characterization of serotonin receptors in the facial motor nucleus: A microiontophoretic study, *Eur. J. Pharmacol.* **65**:175–183.

Miller, J. J., Richardson, T. L., Fibiger, H. C., and McLennan, H., 1975, Anatomical and electrophysiological identification of a projection from the mesencephalic raphe to the caudate-putamen in the rat, *Brain Res.* **97**:133–138.

Molliver, M. E., Grzanna, R., Lidov, H. G. W., Morrison, J. H., and Olschowka, J. A., 1982, Monoamine systems in the cerebral cortex, in *Cytochemical Methods in Neuroanatomy*, Alan R. Liss, New York, pp. 255–277.

Mosko, S. S., and Jacobs, B. L., 1976, Recording of dorsal raphe unit activity *in vitro*, *Neurosci. Lett.* **2**:195–200.

Mosko, S. S., Haubrich, D., and Jacobs, B. L., 1977, Serotonergic afferents to the dorsal raphe nucleus: Evidence from HRP and synaptosomal uptake studies, *Brain Res.* **119**:269–290.

Moss, R. L., Kelly, M. J., and Dudley, C. A., 1978, Chemosensitivity of hypophysiotropic neurons to the microelectrophoresis of biogenic amines, Brain Res. **139**:141–152.

Neto, F. R., 1978, The depolarizing action of 5-HT on mammalian non-myelinated nerve fibres, Eur. J. Pharmacol. **49**:351–356.

Neuman, R. S., 1983, Serotonin induced depolarization of spinal motoneurones following blockade of synaptic transmission, Soc. Neurosci. Abst. **9**:1155.

North, R. A., Henderson, G., Katayama, Y., and Johnson, S. M., 1980, Electrophysological evidence for presynaptic inhibition of acetylcholine release by 5-hydroxytryptamine in the enteric nervous system, Neuroscience **5**:581–586.

Olpe, H.-R., and Koella, W. P., 1977, The response of striatal cells upon stimulation of the dorsal and median raphe nuclei, Brain Res. **122**:357–360.

Park, M. R., Gonzales-Vegas, J. A., and Kitai, S. T., 1982, Serotonergic excitation from dorsal raphe stimulation recorded intracellularly from rat caudate-putamen, Brain Res. **243**:49–58.

Peroutka, S. J., Lebovitz, R. M., and Snyder, S. H., 1981, Two distinct central serotonin receptors with different physiological functions, Science **212**:827–828.

Peroutka, S. J., Noguchi, M., Tolner, D. J., Allen, G. S., 1983, Serotonin-induced contraction of canine basilar artery: Mediation by 5-HT$_1$ receptors, Brain Res. **259**:327–330.

Phillis, J. W., Tebēcis, A. K., and York, D. H., 1968, Depression of spinal motoneurones by noradrenaline, 5-hydroxtryptamine and histamine, Eur. J. Pharmacol. **4**:471–475.

Rapport, M. M., 1949, Serum vasoconstrictor (serotonin). V. The presence of creatinine in the complex: a proposed study of the vasoconstrictor principle, J. Biol. Chem. **180**:961–969.

Rapport, M. M., Green, A. A., and Page, I. H., 1948, Serum vasoconstrictor (serotonin). IV. Isolation and characterization, J. Biol. Chem. **176**:1243–1251.

Roberts, M. H. T., and Straughan, D. W., 1967, Excitation and depression of cortical neurones by 5-hydroxytryptamine, J. Physiol. (Lond.) **193**:269–294.

Rogawski, M. A., and Aghajanian, G. K., 1980, Norepinephrine and serotonin: Opposite effects on the activity of lateral geniculate neurons evoked by optic pathway stimulation, Exp. Neurol. **69**:678–694.

Scheibel, M. E., Tomiyasu, U., and Scheibel, A. B., 1975, Do raphe nuclei of the reticular formation have a neurosecretory or vascular sensor function? Exp. Neurol. **47**:316–329.

Segal, M., 1975, Physiological and pharmacological evidence for a serotonergic projection to the hippocampus, Brain Res. **94**:115–131.

Segal, M., 1979, Serotonergic innervation of the locus coeruleus from the dorsal raphe and its action on responses to noxious stimuli, J. Physiol. (Lond.) **286**:401–415.

Segal, M., 1980, The action of serotonin in the rat hippocampal slice preparation, J. Physiol. (Lond.) **303**:423–439.

Segal, M., and Gutnick, M. J., 1980, Effects of serotonin on extracellular potassium concentration in the rat hippocampal slice, Brain Res. **195**:389–401.

Siegelbaum, S. A., Camardo, J. S., and Kandel, E. R., 1982, Serotonin and cyclic AMP close single K$^+$ channels in Aplysia sensory neurones, Nature **299**:413–417.

Steinbusch, H. W. M., 1981, Distribution of serotonin-immunoreactivity in the central nervous system of the rat—cell bodies and terminals, Neuroscience **6**(4):557–618.

Szabadi, E., Bradshaw, C. M., and Bevan, P., 1977, Excitatory and depressant neuronal responses to noradrenaline, 5-hydroxytryptamine and mescaline: The role of the baseline firing rate, Brain Res. **126**:580–583.

Ternaux, J. P., Hery, F., Hamon, M., Bourgoin, S., and Glowinski, J., 1977, 5-HT release from ependymal surface of the caudate nucleus in "encephale isole" cats, Brain Res. **132**:575–579.

Tramu, G., Pillez, A., and Leonardelli, J., 1983, Serotonin axons of the ependyma and circumventricular organs in the forebrain of the guinea pig, Cell Tissue Res. **228**:297–311.

Trulson, M. E., Howell, G. A., Brandstetter, J. W., Frederickson, M. H., and Frederickson, C. J., 1982, In vitro recording of raphe unit activity: Evidence for endogenous rhythms in presumed serotonergic neurons, Life Sci. **31**:785–790.

Trulson, M. E., and Jacobs, B. L., 1981, Activity of serotonin-containing neurons in freely moving cats, in: Serotonin Neurotransmission and Behavior (B. L. Jacobs and A. Gelperin, eds.), Cambridge, Massachusetts, MIT Press, pp. 339–365.

Trulson, M. E., and Jacobs, B. L., 1979, Raphe unit activity in freely moving cats: Correlation with level of behavioral arousal, *Brain Res.* **163**:135–150.

Trulson, M. E., and Trulson, V. M., 1982, Activity of nucleus raphe pallidus neurons across the sleep-waking cycle in freely moving cats. *Brain Res.* **237**:232–237.

Twarog, B. M., and Page, I. H., 1953, Serotonin content of some mammalian tissues and urine and a method for its determination, *J. Physiol. (Lond.)* **175**:157–161.

Van de Kar, L. D., and Lorens, S. A., 1979, Differential serotonergic innervation of individual hypothalamic nuclei and other forebrain regions by the dorsal and median midbrain raphe nuclei, *Brain Res.* **162**:45–54.

Van der Kooy, D., and Hattori, T., 1980, Bilaterally situated dorsal raphe cell bodies have only unilateral forebrain projections in rat, *Brain Res.* **192**:550–554.

VanderMaelen, C. P., and Aghajanian, G. K., 1980, Intracellular studies showing modulation of facial motoneurone excitability by serotonin, *Nature* **287**:346–347.

VanderMaelen, C. P., and Aghajanian, G. K., 1982a, Intracellular studies on the effects of systemic administration of serotonin agonists on rat facial motoneurons, *Eur. J. Pharmacol.* **78**:233–236.

VanderMaelen, C. P., and Aghajanian, G. K., 1982b, Serotonin-induced depolarization of rat facial motoneurons *in vivo*: Comparison with amino acid transmitters, *Brain Res.* **239**:139–152.

VanderMaelen, C. P., and Aghajanian, G. K., 1983a, Electrophysiological and pharmacological characterization of serotonergic dorsal raphe neurons recorded extracellularly and intracellularly in rat brain slices, *Brain Res.* **289**:109–119.

VanderMaelen, C. P., and Aghajanian, G. K., 1983b, Evidence for a calcium-activated potassium conductance in serotonergic dorsal raphe neurons, *Soc. Neurosci. Abst.* **9**:500.

VanderMaelen, C. P., Bonduki, A. C., and Kitai, S. T., 1979, Excitation of caudate-putamen neurons following stimulation of the dorsal raphe nucleus in the rat, *Brain Res.* **175**:356–361.

VanderMaelen, C. P., and Kitai, S. T., 1980, Intracellular analysis of synaptic potentials in rat neostriatum following stimulation of cerebral cortex, thalamus, and substantia nigra, *Brain Res. Bull.* **5**:725–733.

Van Neuten, J. M., Janssen, P. A. J., Van Beek, J., Xhonneux, R., Verbeuren, T. J., and Vanhoutte, P. M., 1981, Vascular effects of ketanserin (R 41 468), a novel antagonist of 5-HT$_2$ serotonergic receptors, *J. Pharmacol. Exp. Ther.* **218**(1):217–230.

Wallis, D., and Nash, H., 1981, Relative activities of substances related to 5-hydroxytryptamine as depolarizing agents of superior cervical ganglion cells, *Eur. J. Pharmacol.* **70**:381–392.

Wallis, D. I., and North, R A., 1978, The action of 5-hydroxytryptamine on single neurones of the rabbit superior cervical ganglion, *Neuropharmacol.* **17**:1023–1028.

Wallis, D. I., and Woodward, B., 1975, Membrane potential changes induced by 5-hydroxytryptamine in the rabbit superior cervical ganglion, *Br. J. Pharmacol.* **55**:199–212.

Wang, R. Y., and Aghajanian, G. K., 1977a, Antidromically identified serotonergic neurons in the rat midbrain raphe: Evidence for collateral inhibition, *Brain Res.* **132**:186–193.

Wang, R. Y., and Aghajanian, G. K., 1977b, Inhibition of neurons in the amygdala by dorsal raphe stimulation: Mediation through a direct serotonergic pathway, *Brain Res.* **120**:85–102.

White, S. R., and Neuman, R. S., 1980, Facilitation of spinal motoneurone excitability by 5-hydroxytryptamine and noradrenaline, *Brain Res.* **188**:119–127.

White, S. R., and Neuman, R. S., 1983, Pharmacological antagonism of facilitatory but not inhibitory effects of serotonin and norepinephrine on excitability of spinal motoneurons, *Neuropharmacology* **22**(4):489–494.

Wood, J. D., and Mayer, C. J., 1978, Slow synaptic excitation mediated by serotonin in Auerbach's plexus, *Nature* **276**:836–837.

Wood, J. D., and Mayer, C. J., 1979, Serotonergic activation of tonic-type enteric neurons in guinea pig small bowel, *J. Neurophysiol.* **42**(2):582–593.

Wood, J. D., Grafe, P., and Mayer, C. J., 1979, Slow synaptic modulation of excitability mediated by inactivation of calcium-dependent potassium conductance in myenteric neurons of guinea-pig small intestine, *Soc. Neurosci. Abst.* **5**:749.

Wooley, D. W., and Shaw, E., 1954, A biochemical and pharmacological suggestion about certain mental disorders, *Science* **119**:587–588.

Wurtman, R. J., and Fernstrom, J. D., 1976, Control of brain neurotransmitter synthesis by precursor availability and nutritional state, *Biochem. Pharmacol.* **25**:1691–1696.

Yap, C. Y., and Taylor, D. A., 1983, Involvement of 5-HT$_2$ receptors in the wet-dog shake behaviour induced by 5-hydroxytryptophan in the rat, *Neuropharmacology* **22**:801–804.

Yoshimura, M., and Nishi, S., 1982, Intracellular recordings from lateral horn cells of the spinal cord *in vitro*, *J. Autonom. Nerv. Syst.* **6**:5–11.

8

Norepinephrine

MICHAEL A. ROGAWSKI

1. INTRODUCTION

1.1. Historical Overview

The discovery of the biological importance of norepinephrine (NE) is inextricably tied to the development of the concept of chemical neurotransmission which took place in the 1920s and 1930s. The key figures in the genesis of this revolutionary idea were Loewi, who demonstrated that a substance similar to epinephrine was responsible for the acceleration of the heartbeat produced by sympathetic nerve stimulation, and Cannon, who established that an epinephrinelike substance is the chemical mediator liberated by sympathetic nerve impulses at neuroeffector junctions. Von Euler subsequently identified the substance in question as norepinephrine.

Using bioassay, Vogt and subsequently other investigators demonstrated that NE is widely and unevenly distributed throughout the mammalian CNS. Subsequently, an explosion in research on the role of brain NE as a transmitter was initiated by the comprehensive studies of a group of Swedish investigators in which the distribution of monoamine neurons was mapped using the histochemical fluorescence method of Falck and Hillarp (see Moore and Bloom, 1979, for references).

The biochemical features of noradrenergic neurotransmission in the peripheral and central nervous systems, that is, the synthesis, storage, release, reuptake, and metabolism of norepinephrine are now well understood (see Mayer, 1980). In this chapter, we briefly consider the anatomical distribution of norepinephrine-containing neurons and the pharmacological principles underlying the action of NE at adrenergic receptors ("adrenoceptors") as a prelude to discussing the physiological actions of the transmitter in the peripheral and central nervous systems.

1.2. Distribution of Norepinephrine Neurons

1.2.1. Peripheral Nervous System

Outside of the brain, NE neurons are confined to the sympathetic nervous system where their cell bodies are located in sympathetic ganglia. The ganglia are organized in three groups: the *vertebral sympathetic ganglia*, lying on either side of the vertebral column; the *prevertebral ganglia*, in the abdomen and pelvis; and a few *terminal ganglia*, lying near the organs innervated, particularly the bladder, colon and rectum. Norepinephrine-containing ("adrenergic") neurons in sympathetic ganglia are multipolar, with several short or long dendritic processes and one unmyelinated axon. These fibers provide autonomic control of the heart, blood vessels, glands, and viscera, via extensive plexuses located in these organs. The widely branching terminal axons of these neurons have multiple swellings ("terminal varicosities") packed with mitochondria and small (about 50 nm in diameter) "granular" or "dense core" vesicles. There are about 250 to 300 varicosities per millimeter in the terminal plexus, each containing 500 to 2000 vesicles. Histofluorescence studies indicate that the varicosities are the predominant site of NE storage. Typical synaptic specializations are not observed at peripheral neuroeffector junctions.

Because of its large size, the superior cervical ganglion has served as a model preparation for the study of the physiology and pharmacology of peripheral adrenergic neurons. Located in the carotid sinus, the superior cervical ganglion receives its input from the cervical sympathetic nerve, which is composed largely of axons originating from cholinergic neurons in the intermediolateral cell column of the thoracic spinal cord. In the rat, the ganglion itself consists of 35,000 to 50,000 postganglionic neurons and about 400 dopamine-containing "small intensely fluorescent" (SIF) cells. Output from the ganglion is carried in two major nerves: the external carotid nerve innervating blood vessels of the face and the internal carotid nerve, which enters the cranium where one branch innervates the pineal body and others distribute with the occulomotor nerves to innervate the iris, nictitating membrane, and eyelids (Burnstock and Costa, 1975; McAfee, 1982).

1.2.2. The Central Nervous System

The cell bodies of brain norepinephrine neurons are confined to the reticular formation of the pons and medulla. Based upon location and patterns of projection, there is a natural division of the cells into two major systems: the locus coeruleus cell group and the lateral tegmental cell system. The locus coeruleus [A6 of Dahlström and Fuxe (1964)], located near the wall of the fourth ventricle in the dorsal pontine tegmentum, is the largest NE nucleus in the mammalian brain and is densely packed with NE-containing perikarya (about 1600 on each side in the rat). These cells give rise to extensive projections that directly innervate large parts of the diencephalon and telencephalon, as well as the brainstem, cerebellum and spinal cord.

The remaining NE-containing perikarya are primarily located in scattered groups in the lateral tegmentum of the lower brainstem and in the dorsal medulla. Within the rostral pons there is the A7 or subcoeruleus group, extending from the parabrachial area to a region ventromedial to the motor nucleus of the trigeminal nerve. More caudally in the lateral pons, NE neurons are clustered in the A5 group near the facial nucleus and nerve and the superior olivary complex. The caudal extension of the lateral tegmental system in the medulla is the A1 cell group, located near the lateral reticular nucleus. In addition, NE-containing neurons are present in a column within the dorsomedial medulla (A2), primarily in and around the nucleus tractus solitarius and the area postrema. Lateral tegmental NE neurons have ascending and descending projections, principally to the hypothalamus, brainstem and spinal cord.

Brain NE neurons, whether of the locus coeruleus or lateral tegmental systems, characteristically give rise to axons that are highly collateralized so that a single cell may project to diverse regions of the neuraxis. However, recent studies have suggested that there is a regional topography to these projections. Moore and Bloom (1979) have concluded that each locus coeruleus neuron has an axon whose terminal area alone is at least 30 cm in length. Although there is variability to the degree of innervation among target areas, the axons typically form an extensive terminal plexus. Viewed using the fluorescence histochemical technique, terminal axons are typically fine, with regularly spaced, intensely fluorescent varicosities approximately 1–2 μm in diameter. Unlike peripheral NE boutons, CNS NE-containing terminals do not show small granular vesicles with routine fixation and staining. Rather, these terminals contain pleomorphic small vesicles (approximately 50 nM in diameter) and often large, dense-core vesicles. The degree to which NE terminals form ultrastructurally identifiable synaptic contacts is a matter of controversy (perhaps due to differences among various methods); however, recent work using dopamine-β-hydroxylase immunocytochemistry suggests that a high percentage of terminals may form conventional axodendritic membrane specializations (Molliver et al., 1982).

1.3. Adrenoceptors

Norepinephrine influences peripheral tissues via four pharmacologically distinct recognition sites, designated α_1, α_2, β_1, and β_2. The pharmacology of these adrenergic receptors is highly advanced. The impetus that has spurred this progress has come from the expected clinical importance of drugs that interact with the autonomic nervous system and the development of new drugs was made possible by the accessibility of peripheral test systems.

Recently, it has been found that the central synaptic actions of catecholamines may be mediated via receptors that correspond more or less closely with those present on peripheral sympathetic neurons or in peripheral sympathetic effector tissues. Therefore, a consideration of the principles of adrenergic pharmacology serves as a basis for the discussion of norepinephrine actions in autonomic ganglia and in the CNS.

Sir Henry Dale is credited with recognizing that the diverse effects of sympathetic neuron stimulation and sympathomimetic amines could be distinguished on the basis of the relative potencies of a series of agonists and through the use of selective antagonists (Dale, 1906; Barger and Dale, 1910). However, the concept of two distinct adrenergic receptor types, designated α and β, is the contribution of Ahlquist (1948). The α-type response, typified by smooth muscle constriction, shows a sensitivity to sympathomimetic amines characterized by the following order of potencies: epinephrine > NE > phenylephrine > α-methylnorepinephrine >> isoproterenol. This receptor is now designated as the α_1-adrenoceptor. The action of sympathomimetic amine agonists at α_1-adrenoceptors is blocked by antagonists such as the ergot preparations of Dale (1906), the haloalkylamine phenoxybenzamine, the 2-substituted imidazolines tolazoline and phentolamine, and the benzodioxans piperoxane and WB 4101.

In contrast to the usual smooth muscle-constricting effects of sympathetic stimulation, in the intestine sympathetic nerves mediate relaxation. This occurs through the inhibition of acetylcholine release from enteric cholinergic neurons (Paton and Vizzi, 1969; Kosterlitz, et al., 1970). Similarly, release of NE from noradrenergic neurons is regulated by adrenoceptors with similar pharmacological characteristics as those present on enteric cholinergic neurons (Langer, 1981). The pharmacological properties of these presynaptic actions is sufficiently different from the postjunctional response of smooth muscle to have necessitated the introduction of a new receptor subtype, designated α_2. Subsequently, α_2-adrenoceptors have been identified at sites other than on nerve terminals (such as on platelets, in some blood vessels, and on the somatodendritic region of certain CNS neurons) (Starke and Docherty, 1980).

On the basis of functional studies in intact tissues as well as with the use of radioligand binding to membrane preparations, it has been possible to identify relatively specific agonists and antagonists of α_1- and α_2-adrenoceptors. The following pharmacological principles are of significance (see Table 1). With regard to agonists, the imino-imidazolidine clonidine (as well as the clonidinelike guanidines guanabenz and guanfacin, and the arylimidazoline UK-14,304) are highly selective and potent α_2-agonists that have been particularly useful in physiological studies. It should be noted, however, that clonidine also binds to α_1 sites with high affinity, but acts as a partial agonist with low intrinsic potency (Ruffolo et al., 1980). The classical phenylethylamine agonists do not distinguish as well between α_1 and α_2 sites. Nevertheless, the rank order of potencies does differ, in particular, NE and phenylephrine are more potent than α-methylnorepinephrine at α_1-receptors, whereas the reverse is true at α_2 sites. Methoxamine is a selective, but weak, α_1-agonist.

Table 1. Relative Orders of Potency for Agonists and Antagonists at α_1- and α_2-Adrenoceptors[a]

α_1-Adrenoceptors

Agonists
  Epinephrine > norepinephrine > **phenylephrine**[b] > α-methylnorepinephrine >>
    isoproterenol
Antagonists
  Prazosin $\geqslant$ WB 4101 > phentolamine >> **corynanthine** > yohimbine > rauwolscine,
    piperoxane

α_2-Adrenoceptors

Agonists
  Guanabenz > **tramazoline** > **clonidine**[c] > **α-methylnorepinephrine** > norepinephrine,
    epinephrine > phenylephrine
Antagonists
  Phentolamine, **RX 781094 (idazoxan)** > **rauwolscine, yohimbine** > piperoxane

[a]Orders of potency may differ among experimental preparations.
[b]Compounds in bold type are selective for the specified receptor subtype.
[c]Clonidine is a partial agonist in some systems.

Recent advances have made it possible to easily distinguish α_1- and α_2-adrenoceptors on the basis of antagonist sensitivity. The older α antagonists, such as phentolamine, phenoxybenzamine, or piperoxane, show little selectivity between α_1 and α_2 sites. However, the newer drugs prazosin and corynanthine block mainly α_1-receptors, whereas yohimbine and its diastereoisomers rauwolscine (α-yohimbine) and β-yohimbine act preferentially at α_2 sites (Starke and Docherty, 1980). A particularly potent and selective α_2-antagonist is the imidazoline RX 781094 (idazoxan) with an almost 300-fold selectivity for α_2 versus α_1 sites (Doxey et al., 1983, 1984).

The second major category of adrenoceptor defined by Ahlquist is the β-adrenoceptor, which Lands and co-workers (1967) have subdivided into β_1 and β_2 subtypes. β_1-Adrenoceptors, defined by the sequence isoproterenol > NE > epinephrine >> salbutamol, cause stimulation of the heart, whereas β_2-receptors, defined by the sequence isoproterenol > epinephrine > salbutamol > NE, mediate relaxation of smooth muscle. A wide variety of β-antagonists are known including the nonselective compounds propranolol, pindolol, sotalol, and timolol, the selective β_1-blocking agents metoprolol and atenolol, and the selective β_2-antagonist butoxamine.

2. RESPONSES MEDIATED BY α_2-ADRENOCEPTORS

2.1. Sympathetic Ganglia

2.1.1. Presynaptic Actions

The major effect of catecholamines in sympathetic ganglia is to depress transmission by inhibiting acetylcholine release [although a direct action on ganglion cells occurs as well (see below)]. The initial observation that cate-cholamines inhibit ganglionic transmission was made by Marrazzi (1939) in crude but effective experiments where the compound action potential in the postganglionic nerve was recorded in response to repetitive stimulation of the preganglionic trunk. Intravenous injection of epinephrine reversibly de-pressed the postganglionic potential, but it was not until some four decades later that Christ and Nishi (1971) demonstrated this to be due primarily to an action on preganglionic nerve terminals. In these later experiments, neu-rons in the rabbit superior cervical ganglion (which had been removed from the animal and mounted in a chamber) were impaled with microelectrodes and the fast (nicotinic) EPSP was recorded in response to preganglionic nerve stimulation (see Chapter 6). Perfusion with epinephrine or NE depressed the amplitude of the EPSP with little or no effect on the electrical membrane properties of the postsynaptic cell. Moreover, there was no effect of epi-nephrine on the depolarizing response to iontophoretically applied acetyl-choline, indicating that the sensitivity of the postsynaptic membrane to the transmitter of the fast EPSP was not altered (see Fig. 1). Quantal analysis demonstrated that the number of quanta of transmitter released per stimulus ("quantal content," m) was decreased by epinephrine, but that the quantal size (q) was unchanged. These experiments were carried out in a low calcium, high magnesium perfusion solution to decrease the quantal content of each EPSP and produce a situation where some stimuli caused the release of no quanta ("failure"). Perfusion with epinephrine markedly increased the num-ber of failures; however, those EPSPs that occurred in the presence of epi-nephrine showed the same amplitude distribution as in the control situation, indicating that quantal size was unaffected (Fig. 2). In confirmatory exper-iments, it has been observed that epinephrine diminishes the stimulus-evoked release of [³H]acetylcholine from rat superior cervical ganglia preincubated with [³H]choline (see Brown and Caulfied, 1981).

Christ and Nishi found that the order of effectiveness of agonists con-formed to the series epinephrine > NE > isoproterenol. Moreover, α- but not β-agonists blocked the action of epinephrine, confirming that the re-

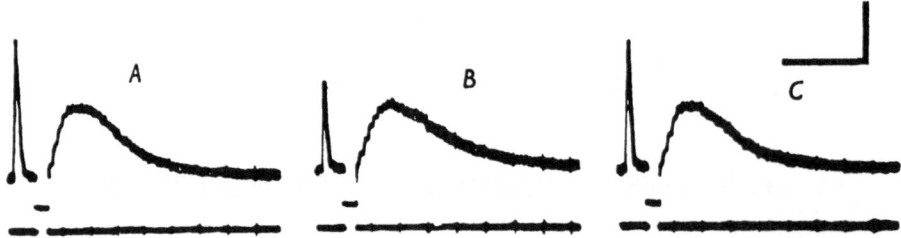

Figure 1. Intracellular recording from a neuron in the isolated rabbit superior cervical ganglion. EPSPs evoked in response to stimulation of the presynaptic nerve are shown to the left; the response to iontophoretically applied acetylcholine (80 nA) is shown on the right. (A) Control; (B) in the presence of epinephrine (10 μM); (C) recovery. Calibration: 20 mV, 300 msec. (From Christ and Nishi, 1971, with permission.)

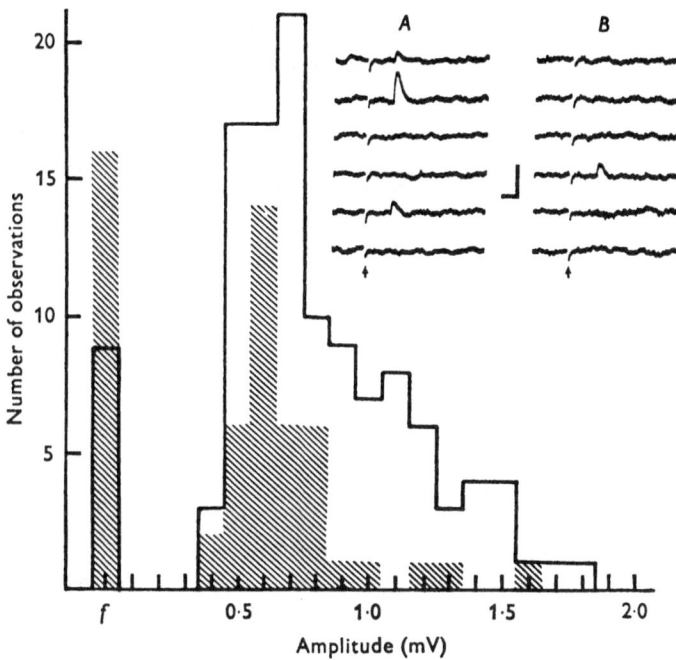

Figure 2. Histogram of EPSP amplitudes recorded in the rabbit superior cervical ganglion in response to preganglionic nerve stimulation. Epinephrine (10 μM, cross-hatched) increased the number of failures (f, plotted at 10 times the ordinate value) from 89 to 161 in 200 stimuli. Assuming a Poisson distribution, the average quantal content of the EPSP dropped from 0.81 to 0.22 quanta/stimulus. The first peak in the amplitude distribution indicates the size of single quanta, and its position (0.5–0.7 mV) is unchanged by epinephrine, demonstrating that quantal size is unaffected. Inset shows records of EPSPs before (A) and during (B) epinephrine perfusion. Indirect stimulation occurs at arrow. The ganglion is perfused in medium containing 0.5 mM $CaCl_2$ and 5.5 mM $MgCl_2$. Calibration: 2 mV, 10 msec. (From Christ and Nishi, 1971, with permission.)

sponse was mediated by an α-adrenoceptor. Recently, it has been demonstrated that the α-adrenoceptor is of the α_2-subtype, as clonidine is a powerful agonist and the response is blocked by yohimbine, but not prazosin (Brown and Caulfield, 1981).

2.1.2. Membrane Hyperpolarization

In some species, catecholamines have direct effects on the resting potential of sympathetic ganglion cells. Both hyperpolarization and depolarization can occur, although these effects are usually small in magnitude and the membrane mechanisms involved are at present obscure (Fig. 3A). The pharmacological properties of these effects were first characterized in the cat superior cervical ganglion by DeGroat and Volle (1966) who found that ganglionic hyperpolarization was mediated by α-adrenoceptors, whereas depolarization involved β-adrenoceptors. More recently, it has been clearly

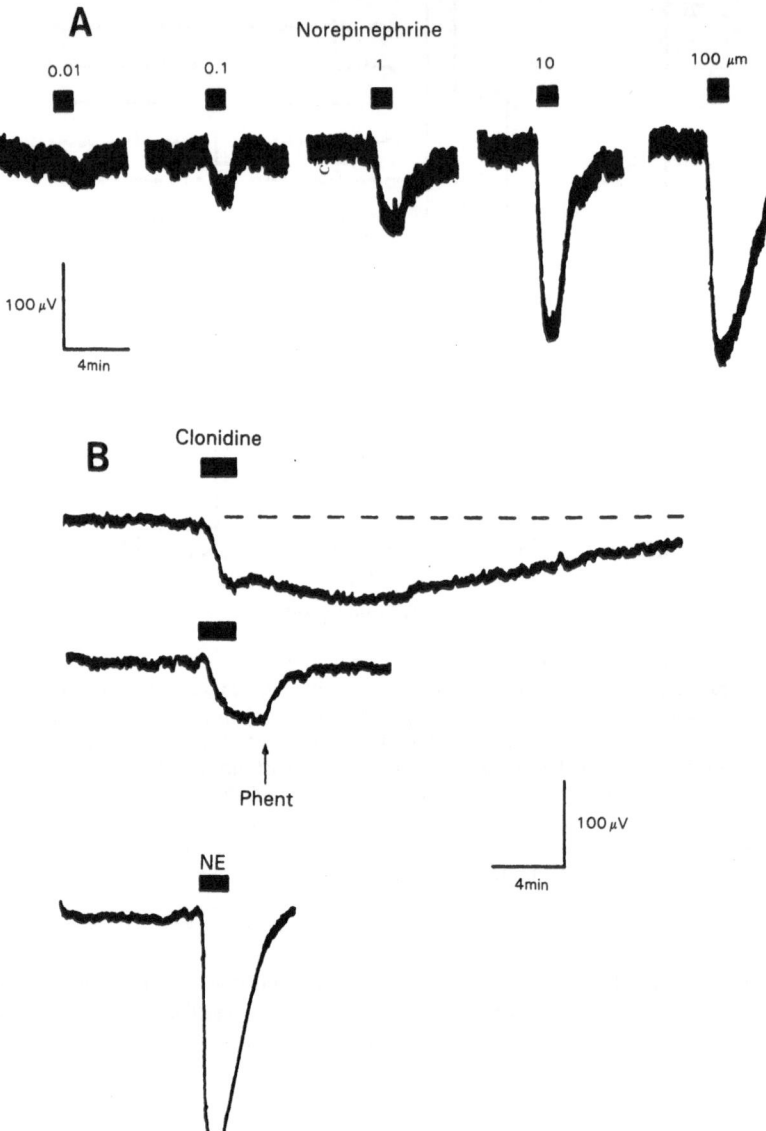

Figure 3. Hyperpolarization of isolated rat superior cervical ganglia recorded with the "air-gap" extracellular recording method. Bars indicate periods during which drug solutions were in contact with the preparation. (A) Dose response with increasing concentrations of NE in the perfusion. (B) Comparison of the maximum hyperpolarization produced by clonidine (1 μM) and NE (10 μM). Addition of phentolamine ("Phent"; 1 μM, at arrow) during the maintained hyperpolarization following the washout of clonidine produced a rapid restoration of the potential to baseline. (From Brown and Caulfield, 1979, with permission.)

demonstrated in both the rat (Brown and Caulfield, 1979, 1981), and the rabbit (Cole and Shinnick-Gallagher, 1981) that the hyperpolarizing response is due to adrenoceptors of the α_2-subtype. These experiments were carried out using the sucrose-gap or air-gap extracellular recording technique. The following rank order of agonists was obtained: epinephrine $\geq$ NE $>$ phenylephrine $>$ isoproterenol. Clonidine was active at low concentrations, but its effect was of lower maximal amplitude than that of the other agonists, indicating that it is a potent partial agonist (Fig. 3B). Yohimbine and phentolamine effectively block the hyperpolarizing effects of agonists, but prazosin or propranolol do not, confirming that the response is due to α_2- and not α_1- or β-adrenoceptors (Fig. 3B).

Although hyperpolarizing responses to α_2-agonists are readily demonstrated with extracellular recording, the effect is of small amplitude (< 0.4 to 0.7 mV). It has been difficult to consistently detect these hyperpolarizations when recording from single cells using intracellular techniques. However, when observed, the catecholamine-induced hyperpolarization is small (< 6 mV) and accompanied by no detectable change in input resistance as measured under current clamp (Horn and McAfee, 1980). Depolarizing responses of catecholamines in the rat appear to be due to activation of β_2-adrenoceptors (Brown and Dunn, 1983).

Like sympathetic neurons, parasympathetic cells in the cat urinary bladder exhibit a hyperpolarizing response to NE that is mediated by α_2-adrenoceptors. However, NE induced depolarizations of these neurons are due to activation of α_1-adrenoceptors (Nakamura et al., 1984).

2.1.3. Calcium Conductance Mechanisms

Recently, investigators have focused on the interaction between catecholamines and voltage-dependent calcium-current mechanisms in sympathetic ganglion neurons. Catecholamines, acting via α_2-adrenoceptors, are believed to suppress inward calcium current. These effects appear to be more robust and reproducible than the hyperpolarization, although both display similar pharmacological properties. The relationship between the hyperpolarization and the effect on calcium current is unclear.

Intracellular recordings from neurons of the rat superior cervical ganglion demonstrate a large (12 mV) and long-lasting (350 msec) hyperpolarizing afterpotential following each action potential. This afterpotential seems to be due to a calcium-dependent increase in potassium conductance (McAfee and Yarowsky, 1979). Catecholamines inhibit the hyperpolarizing afterpotential in a dose dependent manner with a rank order of potencies: epinephrine $>$ L-NE $>$ D-NE $>$ dopamine $>$ isoproterenol. Phentolamine (but not the β-blocker sotalol) antagonizes these effects, confirming that the response is α-adrenoceptor mediated.

Certain changes in the spike configuration brought about by NE suggest that the primary effect of α-adrenergic stimulation is on calcium-conductance mechanisms. In particular, the spike "shoulder," believed to reflect calcium entry, is blocked. In addition, the rate of rise and amplitude of regenerative calcium action potentials recorded in the presence of tetrodotoxin and tetraethylammonium (to block the sodium spike) are depressed by catecholamines (Horn and McAfee, 1979) (Fig. 4).

It has been possible to confirm these observations by recording the inward calcium current directly using the voltage-clamp technique (Galvan and Adams, 1982). In these experiments, opposing outward potassium currents were suppressed by bathing the cells in tetraethylammonium and using recording electrodes filled with cesium and tetraethylammonium. NE reduced the inward calcium current by up to 50% without any change in the voltage sensitivity or the time course of the residual calcium current (Fig. 5). In addition, NE substantially reduced the outward current that follows termination of the depolarizing command and corresponds with the spike afterhyperpolarization (calcium-dependent potassium conductance). The EC_{50} for these effects is about 2 μM, comparable to the EC_{50} for suppression of the hyperpolarizing afterpotential (1 μM, Horn and McAfee, 1980), the EC_{50} for hyperpolarization of ganglion cells (1.7 μM, Brown and Caulfield, 1981), and the K_i for inhibition of radioligand binding to rat superior cervical ganglion α_2-adrenoceptors (1.6 μM, Kafka and Thoa, 1979). Nevertheless, it has yet to be confirmed through the use of specific pharmacological agonists and antagonists that the effect on calcium current is mediated by α_2-adrenoceptors (see Williams and North, 1985).

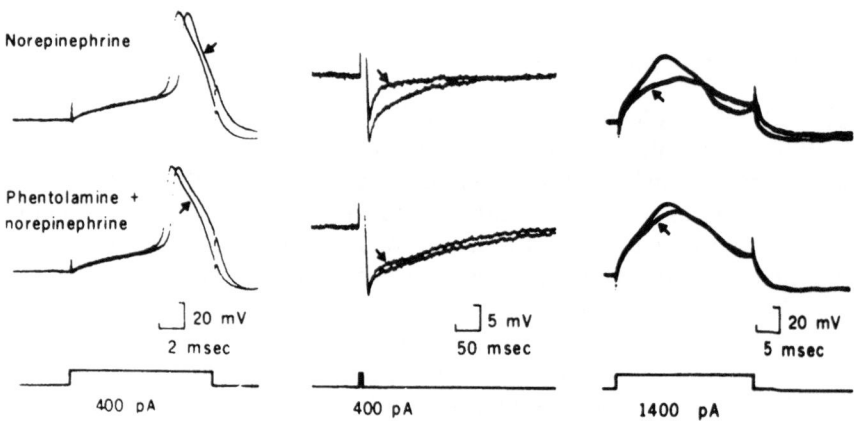

Figure 4. Intracellular records of calcium-dependent potentials in sympathetic neurons of the rat superior cervical ganglion. Each record is composed of superimposed oscilloscope traces of a control and experimental (arrow) response. These voltage responses were initiated by depolarizing currents passed through the microelectrode (rectangular pulses at bottom). Left-hand traces show the action potential "shoulder" at a rapid sweep speed. Traces in the middle show records obtained from the same cell at a slower sweep speed to best illustrate the hyperpolarizing afterpotential. Records of Ca^{2+} spikes are shown on the right from another cell bathed in tetrodotoxin (1 μM) and tetraethylammonium (5 mM). In the top horizontal row, the experimental traces (arrow) were recorded after exposure to 10 μM NE. In the bottom row, the experiment was repeated after incubation in 10 μM phentolamine. (From Horn and McAfee, 1979, with permission.)

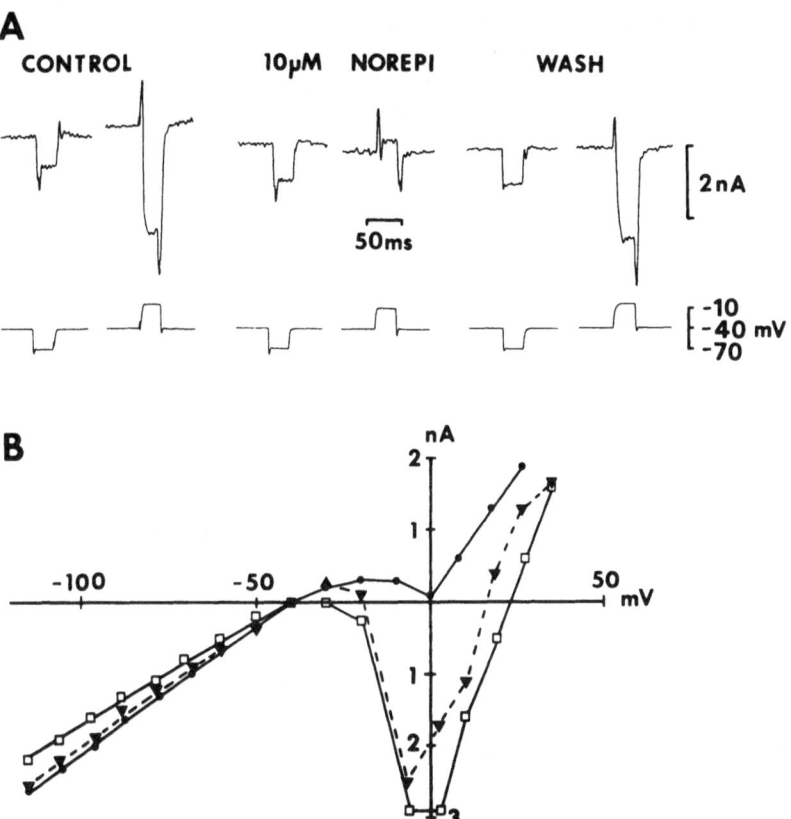

Figure 5. Voltage-clamp recordings from the rat superior cervical ganglion using the single-microelectrode technique. Microelectrodes were filled with 3 M CsCl and 1 M tetraethylammonium bromide to block potassium currents. The bathing medium also contained 20 mM tetraethylammonium. Sample records are shown in A and the peak current is plotted in B. (□), Control; (●), NE; (▼), recovery. (From Galvan and Adams, 1982, with permission.)

For comparison, it should be noted that catecholamines acting at β_1-receptors in cardiac muscle greatly *increase* the slow inward current carried by calcium (Reuter and Scholz, 1977). This effect is believed to be mediated by an increase in intracellular cyclic AMP that causes a cyclic AMP-dependent protein kinase to phosphorylate a membrane protein. Recent studies of single calcium channel currents recorded using the patch clamp technique indicate that β-receptor occupancy increases the probability that individual calcium channels are open (see Tsien et al., 1983; Reuter et al., 1983).

It has been suggested that the effect of NE on the calcium conductance of the ganglion cell soma may reflect similar consequences of α_2-adrenoceptor activation at nerve terminals, providing a mechanism to explain the presynaptic effect of catecholamines. Thus, presynaptic α_2-adrenoceptors would reduce neurotransmitter release by inhibiting calcium influx through voltage-sensitive calcium channels at the nerve terminal. Other than as a model for presynaptic nerve terminals, the functional role of α_2-adrenoceptors on the somal membrane of sympathetic ganglion cells is unclear, although it is possible that interference with calcium conductance might alter repetitive discharge characteristics through an effect on the calcium-dependent after-hyperpolarization.

2.2. Sensory Ganglia

Recordings from sensory neurons of dorsal root ganglia have demonstrated similar effects of NE on calcium currents as observed in sympathetic neurons (Dunlap and Fischbach, 1981; Canfield and Dunlap, 1984). These experiments used dissociated embryonic chick dorsal root ganglion neurons maintained in tissue culture. Sensory neurons have a large calcium conductance that is activated by depolarization and contributes a plateau phase to the action potential. NE (ED$_{50}$, 0.6 μM) produced a dose-dependent shortening of this plateau phase that seemed to be mediated by an α-adrenoceptor, as it was mimicked by phenylephrine, but not isoproterenol, and blocked by phentolamine and yohimbine, but not propranolol. However, the receptor was not a typical α_2-adrenoceptor in that clonidine and xylazine (a less selective α_2-agonist) were without effect. NE did not alter the resting membrane potential or conductance of the cells. Voltage-clamp studies proved that NE decreased inward calcium current independent of an effect on outward potassium current. This occurred without a change in the voltage dependence or kinetics of calcium current activation or the calcium reversal potential, indicating a depression of the maximum calcium conductance. As noted in the relevant chapters of this book, a number of other transmitter substances, including GABA, serotonin, and enkephalin have similar effects on the voltage-sensitive slow inward (calcium) current of sensory neurons. Because cultured embryonic tissue was used in these experiments, it is necessary to be cautious in extrapolating the results to the intact adult organism.

As in the case of sympathetic neurons, it has been suggested that the effects of NE on soma calcium conductance be taken as a model to understand the mechanism whereby NE suppresses release at nerve terminals. In the situation of primary sensory neurons such an interaction is hypothetical and direct physiological proof has been difficult to obtain. Descending noradrenergic neurons terminate in the marginal layer of the dorsal horn where they could interact with primary afferent fibers. In fact, the threshold for activation of single cutaneous afferent fibers is increased by adrenoceptor agonists (Jeftinija et al., 1983) and primary afferent terminals are hyperpolarized via α_2-adrenoceptors (Wohlberg et al., 1983), suggesting an additional presynaptic mechanism distinct from effects on calcium conductance. Nevertheless, it has not been possible to demonstrate that stimulation-induced descending inhibition of sensory evoked dorsal horn neuron responses is specifically mediated by noradrenergic fibers (Hodge et al., 1983). Moreover, it is now clear that NE, acting through α_2-adrenoceptors, can also directly inhibit the target neurons within the dorsal horn of nociceptive sensory afferents (see Section 2.6).

2.3. Myenteric Plexus

Sympathetic fibers to the intestine terminate primarily in the enteric plexuses where they arborize extensively around ganglion cells. Sympathetic stimulation relaxes nonsphincteric regions of the intestine, and α-adrenergic agonists including NE powerfully inhibit the contraction of longitudinal muscle produced by field stimulation. This reduction of the twitch response is due predominantly to inhibition of acetylcholine release from intrinsic enteric neurons rather than a direct effect on muscle, as α-agonists fail to affect the contractile response to exogenous acetylcholine. Detailed pharmacological studies indicated that twitch inhibition by α-adrenoceptor agonists is mediated by α_2-type receptors (Drew, 1978; Wilkberg, 1978). In radioligand binding studies with the α_2-agonist [^{3}H]clonidine, it has been demonstrated that α_2-receptors in the guinea pig small intestine are located exclusively on neurons of the myeteric plexus and not on the longitudinal muscle (Wikberg and Lefkowitz, 1982). Direct measurements of acetylcholine release from small intestine confirm that acetylcholine output is reduced by sympathetic nerve stimulation or α-agonists but increased by α-adrenoceptor blocking drugs (see Kilbinger, 1982).

Intracellular recordings by Hirst and McKirdy (1974) provide physiological evidence that sympathetic nerve stimulation can block acetylcholine release by a presynaptic mechanism. These workers recorded from myenteric neurons of the guinea pig small intestine. Cholinergic fast EPSPs were evoked by field stimulation or distention of the bowel with a balloon. Trains of stimuli applied to the periarteral sympathetic nerves produced no detectable change in the electrical properties of the myenteric neurons, but the occurrence of EPSPs was reduced or abolished in an all-or-none fashion. Other investigators have demonstrated that bath-applied NE or clonidine also reversibly suppresses cholinergic fast EPSPs and that this effect is prevented by the α-antagonists phenoxybenzamine or phentolamine (but not propranolol or prazosin)(Wood and Mayer, 1979; Morita and North, 1981; Nishi and North, 1973a,b) (Fig. 6). Moreover, the depolarizing response to exogenous acetylcholine applied to the cell soma is unaffected by NE. These observations confirm that the α_2-mediated inhibition of cholinergic transmission in the myenteric plexus is due to presynaptic mechanisms. Since NE inhibits the release of acetylcholine even when cholinergic axons are stimulated directly, the interaction between sympathetic and cholinergic neurons is presumably axon to axon. Recently, a morphological correlate for this has been provided by ultrastructural studies showing adrenergic-cholinergic axo-

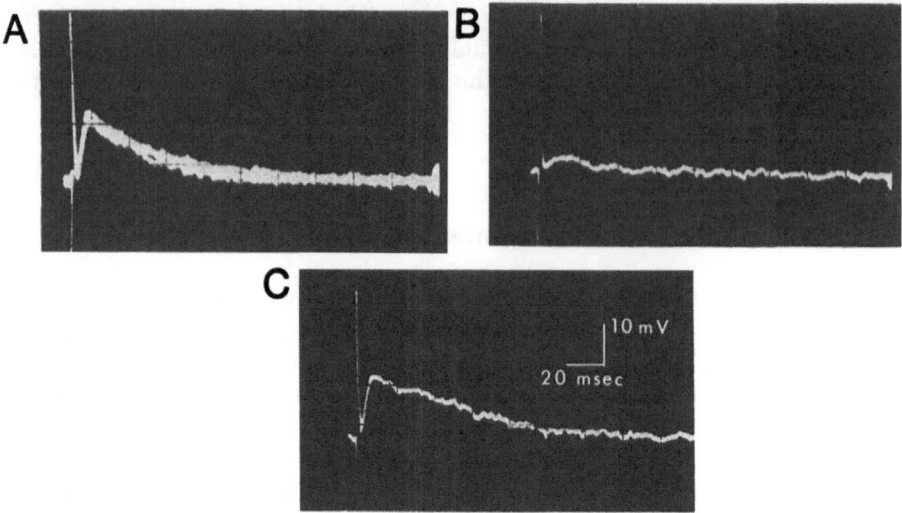

Figure 6. Intracellular recording from a neuron of the guinea pig myenteric plexus showing blockade of fast EPSPs by NE. (A) Superposition of three EPSPs evoked by fiber tract stimulation. (B) Reduction of EPSP amplitude in the presence of 2 μM NE. (C) Recovery. (From Wood and Mayer, 1979, with permission.)

axonic synapses in the myenteric plexus (see Gershon, 1981). Nevertheless, the precise mechanism whereby NE inhibits acetylcholine release remains to be determined.

A possible clue comes from studies of the direct effects of α_2-agonists on the membrane properties of myenteric neurons (Morita and North, 1981). In intracellular recordings, clonidine (100 pM to 30 nM) caused a concentration-dependent hyperpolarization of myenteric neurons of the guinea pig ileum that was accompanied by an increase in membrane conductance. These effects were shared by epinephrine and blocked by phentolamine and phenoxybenzamine, but not propranolol or prazosin. The clonidine induced hyperpolarization was increased by low-potassium (1–2 mM) solutions and reduced by high-potassium (10–20 mM) solutions, as expected if it was generated by an increase in potassium conductance. It can be postulated that if a similar hyperpolarization occurs at nerve terminals, this might prevent the invasion of action potentials so that synaptic release is reduced. As yet there is no evidence to suggest that α_2-agonists inhibit voltage-dependent calcium entry in myenteric neurons, as is the situation in sympathetic or sensory neurons, and, in fact, calcium-dependent afterhyperpolarizations seen in some cells are unaffected, indicating that this may not be the case.

In addition to effects on fast EPSPs, NE and clonidine block the slow EPSP that is elicited in myenteric neurons by repetitive fiber tract stimulation (Fig. 7). The slow EPSP may be mediated by serotonin, although this has been disputed (see Chapter 7 for discussion). Evidence in favor of a presynaptic locus for the action of NE include the observation that NE did not

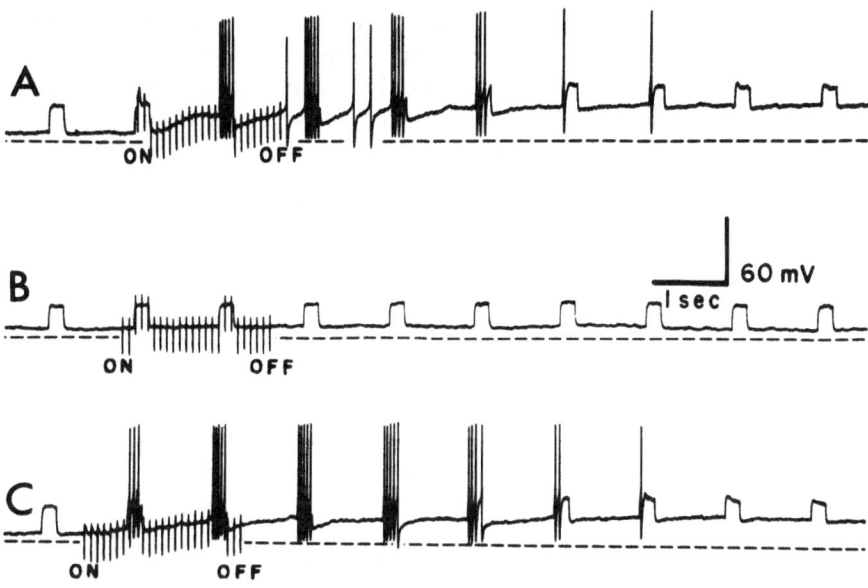

Figure 7. Intracellular recording from a guinea pig myenteric neuron showing blockade of slow EPSP by NE. Constant current depolarizing pulses were injected continuously to test the excitability of the neuron. (A) Control slow EPSP elicited by repetitive fiber tract stimulation during indicated period. (B) Complete blockade of response 3 min after perfusion with 2 μM NE. (C) Recovery after removal of NE from perfusion. (From Wood and Mayer, 1979, with permission.)

effect the response to exogenous serotonin and the interesting finding that NE did not influence the time course of the slow EPSP when it was applied *after* the cessation of fiber tract stimulation, presumably at a time following completion of the release of the excitatory transmitter. [Conflicting observations have been made with clonidine, however; see Morita and North (1981).] The blocking effect of NE on the slow EPSP is prevented by phentolamine, indicating that it is probably mediated by α-receptors as is the effect on the fast EPSP (Wood and Mayer, 1979).

2.4. Locus Coeruleus

Physiological analysis of central noradrenergic neurotransmission by single-cell recording techniques has, not surprisingly, lagged behind studies in peripheral systems. Nevertheless, in recent years, due in large measure to the availability of powerful pharmacological tools developed in peripheral systems, a coherent understanding of the functional role of adrenergic receptors in the CNS is beginning to emerge. The remainder of this chapter deals with the actions of NE in the brain and spinal cord.

The responsiveness of noradrenergic neurons in the locus coeruleus (LC) has been studied by extracellular unit recording *in vivo* and more recently by intracellular recording both *in vivo* and in tissue slices *in vitro*. In anesthetised rats, LC neurons fire spontaneously at a more or less regular rate of 0.5 to 5 Hz. Microiontophoretic application of NE readily suppresses this firing. This observation has led to the concept that LC neurons possess receptors for their own transmitter, i.e., "autoreceptors," that are presumably somatodendritic in location. Pharmacological analysis of these adrenoceptors using microiontophoresis has revealed the following rank order of potencies for agonists: clonidine $>>$ α-methylnorepinephrine $>$ epinephrine $=$ NE $>>$ phenylephrine, indicating that they are of the α_2 type (Cedarbaum and Aghajanian, 1977). Clonidine readily crosses the blood-brain barrier and its systemic administration powerfully suppresses LC neurons. As expected, the α_2-antagonists piperoxane and RX 781094 (idazoxan) block the response to NE or clonidine, whereas the β-antagonist sotalol does not (see Aghajanian and Rogawski, 1983; Freedman and Aghajanian, 1984). Noradrenergic neurons of the pontine lateral tegmental cell group (A5) and dorsal medulla (A2) appear to possess inhibitory α_2-receptors similar to those on LC neurons (Andrade and Aghajanian, 1982; Moore and Guyenet, 1983a,b).

Intracellular recordings from LC neurons *in vivo* indicate that systemically administered clonidine causes a marked hyperpolarization in association with an inhibition of firing (Fig. 8). This change in membrane potential is accompanied by a reduction in membrane input resistance. The hyperpolarization is not reversed when chloride-containing microelectrodes are used, suggesting that a change in chloride conductance is not primarily involved. It is likely therefore that activation of potassium conductance may underly the hyperpolarization and decrease in input resistance (Aghajanian and VanderMaelen, 1982).

Recordings from LC neurons in an *in vitro* slice preparation confirm these observations. Bath-applied NE or field stimulation of the slice produced a hyperpolarizing response that reversed at the potassium equilibrium potential (Fig. 9). The stimulation-induced hyperpolarization ("IPSP") was shown to be synaptically mediated as it was abolished in calcium-free and/or high-magnesium solutions. Pharmacological experiments demonstrated that the field stimulation-induced IPSP was indeed NE mediated. The IPSP could be blocked by the α-antagonists phentolamine or yohimbine (α_2 selective) (Fig. 10A) and the IPSP was potentiated by the NE reuptake blocker desmethylimipramine (Fig. 10B). The hyperpolarizing response produced in LC neurons *in vitro* by low concentrations of NE (1–30 μM) showed identical pharmacological properties except that it persisted in low-calcium/high-magnesium solutions, as expected if it were a direct postsynaptic effect (Egan et al., 1983). The hyperpolarization could be mimicked by the α_2-agonists clonidine and epinephrine, both of which were more potent than NE, but not by isoproterenol or phenylephrine (Williams et al., 1985). Desmethylimipramine decreased the effective concentration of NE 10- to 30-fold, suggesting that a significant amount of the amine is taken up by cells in the slice. [At somewhat higher concentrations NE can inhibit calcium spikes in LC neu-

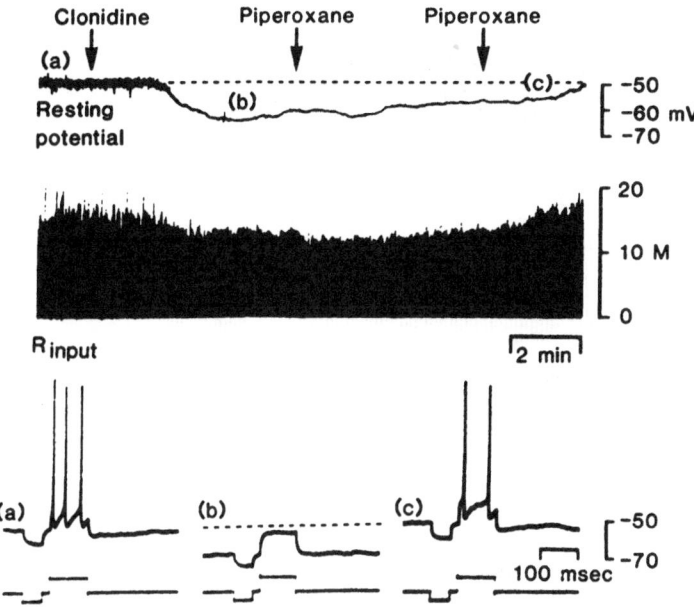

Figure 8. Intracellular recording from a locus coeruleus neuron *in vivo* showing hyperpolarizing effect of clonidine (200 μg/kg, i.p.) and reversal by piperoxane (2 μ/kg, i.p. $\times$ 2). Upper trace shows filtered record of membrane potential; the middle trace indicates input resistance (MΩ), determined from the voltage deflections of hyperpolarizing constant-current pulses; the lower traces are sample oscilloscope sweeps at points a, b, and c showing responses to hyperpolarizing (0.5 nA) and depolarizing (1 nA) pulses. (From Aghajanian and VanderMaelen, 1982, with permission.)

rons; however this effect does not appear to be adrenoceptor mediated (Williams and North, 1985)].

Studies with several α_2-antagonists indicated that these drugs block the hyperpolarizing response to NE or clonidine in a competitive manner with a rank order of potencies: RX 781094 (idazoxan) > yohimbine > phentolamine > piperoxane; neither propranolol nor prazosin affected the response to NE.

Locus coeruleus neurons in explant cultures from newborn mice are also hyperpolarized by NE via α_2-adrenoceptors. However, early in the development of these neurons (less than 26 days in culture) depolorizations mediated by α_1-adrenoceptors are also observed (Finlayson and Marshall, 1984).

Single-electrode voltage-clamp recordings from LC neurons in the *in vitro* slice have confirmed that α_2-agonists hyperpolarize these neurons by increasing membrane potassium conductance (Williams et al., 1984). In these experiments, NE or clonidine induced a membrane current whose amplitude varied linearly with membrane potential within the range -50 to -120 mV; the current was outward at depolarized potentials but reversed in polarity at the potassium equilibrium potential, -100 to -110 mV. Thus the specific

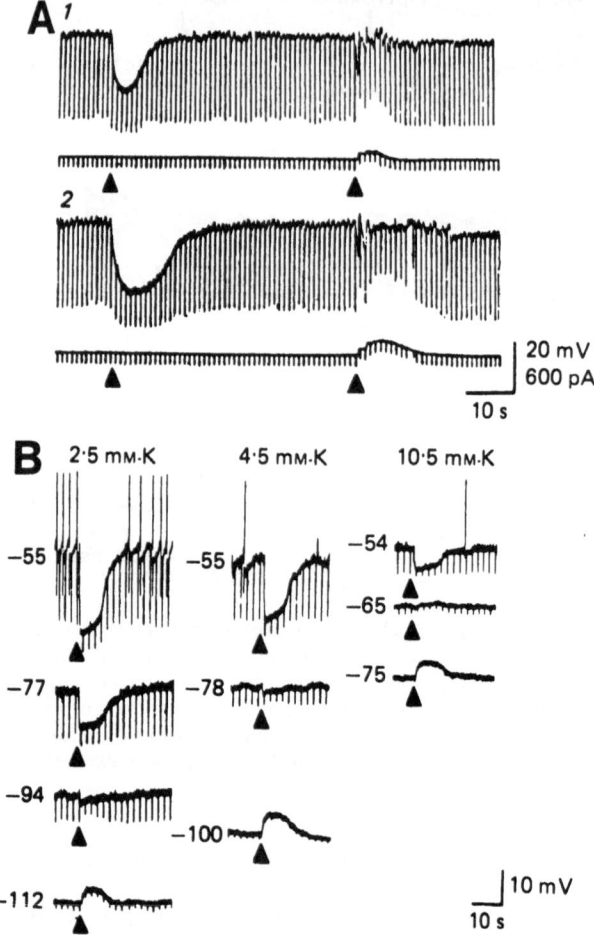

Figure 9. Intracellular recording from locus coeruleus neurons in slices of rat pons *in vitro*. NE was applied (arrowheads) by pressure application from a micropipette placed in the bathing solution above the slice. (A,1) Manual clamp of NE-induced hyperpolarization. The full amplitude of NE-induced response is seen on the first application. During the second application, the membrane potential was held constant. Top traces are membrane potential and bottom traces are membrane current. Note the increase in membrane conductance during NE as measured by constant current hyperpolarizing pulses. (A,2) Same as A,1 but with twice the dose of NE. (B) Determination of the NE reversal potential in solutions of varying potassium concentration. The reversal potential varies linearly with the log of the extracellular potassium concentration as predicted by the Nernst equation. (From Egan et al., 1983, with permission.)

potassium channels coupled to α_2-adrenoceptors in LC neurons seem to be relatively insensitive to membrane potential.

In addition to mediating the effects of extrinsic catecholaminergic influences on LC neurons, it has been suggested that somatodendritic α_2-adrenoceptors also participate in direct NE-mediated inhibition within the LC. In support of this concept are the observations that orthodoromic stimulation of LC afferents or antidromic activation of LC axons in the dorsal noradre-

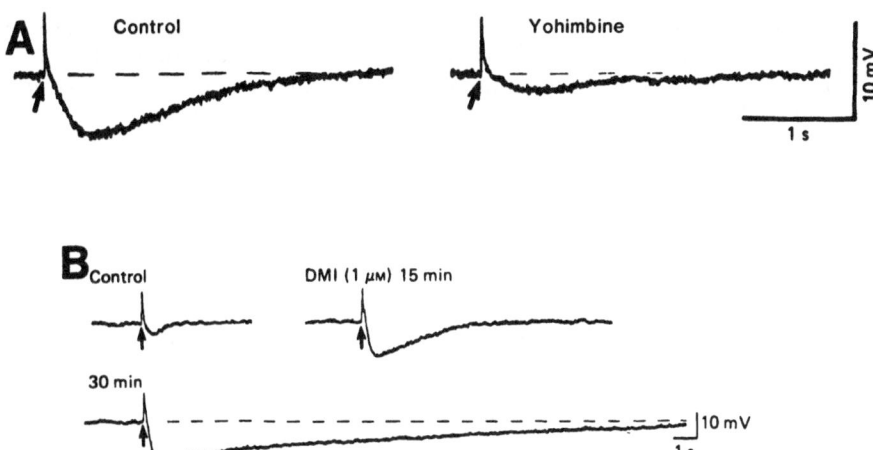

Figure 10. Intracellular recording from a locus coeruleus neuron *in vitro* showing the slow IPSP produced by field stimulation, its blockade by yohimbine, and its enhancement by desmethylimipramine. A (left): Typial EPSP–IPSP sequence recorded in locus coeruleus neurons following a single shock (20 V, 0.5 msec; arrow). A (right): Perfusion with yohimbine (100 mM) almost completely blocked the IPSP with minimal affect on the EPSP. B: Potentiation of the IPSP by desmethylimipramine (1 μM). (From Egan et al., 1983, with permission.)

nergic bundle produces a period of suppressed firing that can be blocked by the α-antagonist piperoxane (Aghajanian and Cederbaum, 1977; Cedarbaum and Aghajanian, 1978).

More recently, intracellular recordings *in vivo* (Aghajanian et al., 1983) and in brainstem slices *in vitro* have shown that LC neurons exhibit a prolonged afterhyperpolarization following single or multiple spikes, which could correspond with the period of postactivation inhibition recorded extracellularly. This appears to be predominantly the result of activation of a calcium-dependent potassium conductance rather than an effect mediated via α_2-adrenoceptors (Andrade and Aghajanian, 1984a). In contrast to the earlier view, these more recent studies have indicated that postactivation inhibition is largely an intrinsic property of LC neurons, and it is not due to local inhibitory interactions between cells within the nucleus (Andrade and Aghajanian, 1984b).

α_2-Adrenoceptors may also be of importance in regulating the release of NE at the nerve terminals of LC axons. In biochemical studies it has been observed that release of NE from brain slices or synaptosomes is depressed by α_2-receptors with similar pharmacological characteristics to the somatodendritic adrenoceptors of LC neurons (see Reichenbacher et al., 1982; Wemer et al., 1982; Frankhuyzen and Mulder, 1982). By analogy with the situation at the soma, it is possible, but not yet proven, that α_2-adrenoceptor-mediated inhibition of NE release from noradrenergic nerve terminals could occur as a result of a hyperpolarization induced by increased potassium conductance. Consistent with this hypothesis is the observation that noradrenergic axon terminals in the frontal cortex become less excitable following

α_2-receptor stimulation by clonidine (Nakamura et al., 1981). Local infusion of clonidine raises the threshold current necessary to antidromically activate coeruleo-cortical axons. The α-antagonist phentolamine blocks this effect (and actually produces an increase in terminal excitability), indicating that it is specifically mediated by α_2-adrenoceptors. Hyperpolarization accompanied by shunting of the membrane resistance is one mechanism whereby axon excitability could be decreased, and this would be in accord with the known effects of clonidine at the soma of LC neurons.

2.5. Preganglionic Sympathetic Neurons

Although most electrophysiological studies of CNS α_2-adrenoceptors have focused on the locus coeruleus, recent work suggests that inhibitory α_2-adrenoceptors are also present on preganglionic sympathetic neurons of the spinal intermediolateral cell column and on interneurons of the dorsal horn. The identification of α_2-receptors on cholinergic preganglionic sympathetic neurons and spinal interneurons is of special significance since they cannot be considered autoreceptors but, rather, presumably mediate responses from descending catecholaminergic projections originating in the brain stem.

In the case of preganglionic sympathetic neurons, postsynaptic α_2-adrenoceptors could play a role in cardiovascular regulation. Characterization of these receptors was accomplished by extracellular recordings from antidromically identified preganglionic neurons in the thoracic sympathetic column of the pigeon. In these studies, microiontophoretically applied α-agonists depressed the spontaneous firing of preganglionic neurons with a rank order of potencies identical to that found in the LC: clonidine $> \alpha$-methynorepinephrine $>$ epinephrine $>$ NE $>$ phenylephrine. Moreover, the inhibitory effects of clonidine and NE were antagonized by the α_2-selective antagonist yohimbine as well as the nonselective α-antagonists piperoxane and phentolamine, but not the α_1-antagonist prazosin or the β-agonist sotalol (Guyenet and Cabot, 1981).

Intracellular recordings from identified preganglionic sympathetic neurons in the intermediolateral cell column of cat spinal cord slices have failed to confirm the response seen in the pigeon (Yoshimura and Nishi, 1982). The primary effect of *bath-applied* NE is depolarization accompanied by an increase in cell input resistance, although some unidentified lateral horn neurons are hyperpolarized by NE. The different mode of administration of NE may explain the discrepancy.

2.6. Substantia Gelatinosa

As noted previously, the spinal cord dorsal horn, in particular the substantia gelatinosa, receives a prominent supraspinal noradrenergic innervation. This lamina is also known to contain a high density of α_2-binding sites as determined by autoradiography (Young and Kuhar, 1980). Descending noradrenergic neurons seem to suppress spinal nociceptive transmission, however the precise site in the dorsal horn where this occurs is unknown. There is some evidence that NE may act presynaptically on sensory afferents (see Section 2.2). On the other hand, physiological studies have clearly demonstrated that NE, acting via α_2-adrenoceptors, can directly inhibit dorsal horn interneurons by a postsynaptic mechanism.

Extracellular recordings in vivo have shown that iontophoretically applied NE reduces the spontaneous firing of dorsal horn neurons and suppresses their responsiveness to noxious stimuli (Belcher et al., 1978; Headly et al., 1978).

More recently, NE, acting specifically at α_2-adrenoceptors, has been found to selectively inhibit nociceptive responses of identified dorsal horn neurons with long ascending projections; activation of these neurons by innocuous stimuli or the excitatory amino acid DL-homocysteate was unaffected (Fleetwood-Walker et al., 1985).

Intracellular recordings in rat spinal cord slices in vitro indicated that NE causes a dose-dependent hyperpolarization of substantia gelatinosa interneurons in association with a fall in input resistance (North and Yoshimura, 1984). This effect was reversibly blocked by phentolamine and yohimbine, but not prazosin or propranolol. Clonidine mimicked the effect of NE, but its action was more prolonged, whereas isoproterenol was inactive. These results clearly establish that NE hyperpolarizes substantia gelatinosa neurons through α_2-adrenoceptors. The NE hyperpolarization is due to a direct postsynaptic action as it persists in low-calcium/high-magnesium solution or in medium containing cobalt and high magnesium. At various external potassium concentrations, the reversal potential of the response was near the potassium equilibrium potential as predicted by the Nernst equation, demonstrating that the hyperpolarization is associated with an increase in potassium conductance. Therefore, α_2-mediated activation of potassium conductance occurs on certain postsynaptic target neurons as well as on the noradrenergic cells themselves. From a functional point of view, hyperpolarizing α_2-adrenoceptors on dorsal horn interneurons are likely to be a major target of descending catecholaminergic fibers. However, it is yet to be established that the specific modulation of nociceptive transmission occurs at this site.

3. RESPONSES MEDIATED BY α_1-ADRENOCEPTORS

3.1. Facial and Spinal Motoneurons

Discussion of central α_1-adrenoceptor-mediated responses begins with a consideration of motoneurons in the brain and spinal cord. (The properties of motoneurons and their responsiveness to serotonin is discussed in detail in Chapter 7.) Noradrenergic nerve terminals are scattered throughout the spinal cord ventral horn and brainstem somatic motor nuclei. Spinal noradrenergic projections appear to be derived exclusively from pontine NE neurons, predominantly the locus coeruleus as well as the A7 and A5 cell groups, whereas brainstem primary motor nuclei receive their innervation entirely from the NE-containing cells of the lateral tegmental system (Westlund et al., 1983; Levitt and Moore, 1979).

Early intracellular recordings in the cat indicated that iontophoretically applied NE had a hyperpolarizing action on spinal α motoneurons that was accompanied by a decrease in membrane conductance (Engberg and Marshall, 1971). Later, however, it was concluded that this response was probably not mediated by specific adrenoceptors, since a wide variety of other substances including local anesthetics, hydrogen ions, and adrenoceptor antagonists could evoke similar effects (Engberg et al., 1976).

In contrast to these initial studies, Barasi and Roberts (1977) reported that NE *increased* the amplitude of field potentials originating from antidromically activated motoneurons. This observation set the stage for the current view of the facilitatory action of NE on motoneurons which is believed to be mediated by α_1-adrenoceptors. In anesthetized rats, brainstem and spinal motoneurons are quiescent, presumably in part due to suppression of excitatory synaptic activation. Although iontophoretic NE fails to excite motoneurons in the facial nucleus of anesthetized rats, McCall and Aghajanian (1979) noted that it did produce a long lasting facilitation of synaptically-activated or glutamate-induced excitation. NE and serotonin (see Chapter 7) produce similar effects on neuronal excitability in the facial nucleus, but these responses are mediated by pharmacologically distinct receptors, i.e., the effects of NE, but not serotonin, are blocked by the α-antagonist piperoxane. Similar effects of NE on spinal motoneurons were obtained by White and Neuman (1980). Moreover, electrical stimulation in the vicinity of the LC has been observed to facilitate the spinal monosynaptic reflex and this effect is blocked by α-adrenoceptor antagonists (Strahlendorf et al., 1980).

Intracellular recordings from spinal motoneurons in the cat have demonstrated that stimulation of the LC with trains of pulses produces a slowly rising, low amplitude depolarization (EPSP). In addition, there is an enhancement of the responsiveness of motoneurons to afferent (dorsal root) stimulation that is blocked by phenoxybenzamine, indicating that the effect is mediated by α-adrenoceptors (Fung and Barnes, 1981).

The membrane mechanisms underlying the facilitatory action of NE on motoneurons were further examined by intracellular recordings in the facial nucleus *in vivo* (VanderMaelen and Aghajanian, 1980). Extracellular iontophoresis of NE produced a long-lasting depolarization of a few millivolts associated with a decrease in membrane conductance. It thus seemed possible to account for the failure of NE to excite quiescent facial motoneurons, since the degree of depolarization produced by NE was not sufficient to bring cells to threshold. Nevertheless, NE did markedly enhance neuronal excitability, as indicated by a reduction in the threshold for the triggering of action potentials by intracellularly injected current. The membrane effects produced by NE could account for this enhancement of excitability as depolarization would tend to bring the cell closer to threshold for action potential generation while decreased membrane conductance should theoretically enhance the voltage excursion produced by excitatory synaptic currents and decrease the membrane length constant, thus enhancing spatial summation. (However, other specific membrane mechanisms may also play a role; see Section 3.4).

Due to the limited viability of motoneurons in slice preparations, it has not yet been possible to use *in vitro* systems to further characterize the α_1-mediated action of NE on these cells. However, as noted in Section 2.6, spinal dorsal horn neurons can maintain viability *ex vivo* and it has been found that a small proportion of these depolarize in response to NE (North and Yoshimura, 1984). This effect is delayed in onset and prolonged in duration, reminiscent of the effect of NE on motoneurons. Moreover, the response is clearly mediated by α_1-adrenoceptors, as it is blocked by prazosin, but not yohimbine, and isoproterenol does not mimic the depolarization.

Similar responses to NE have been observed in dissociated spinal cord neurons grown together in tissue culture with explants of the LC. In a subpopulation of spinal neurons (most frequently those that appeared to be innervated by catecholamine-containing fibers), NE caused a slow depolarization and increase in input resistance that was blocked by the α-adrenoceptor antagonists phenoxybenzamine, phentolamine or piperoxane (Pun et al., 1985). Of particular interest is the observation that electrical stimulation of the explant caused a pharmacologically similar slow depolarizing response usually only in those cells that were depolarized by NE, thus providing clear evidence that synaptically released NE (acting on α-adrenoceptors) can induce the same specific effects on membrane properties as exogenous NE.

3.2. Lateral Geniculate Nucleus

The dorsal lateral geniculate nucleus (LGNd), the primary thalamic relay center for vision in the rat, receives a dense noradrenergic innervation derived exclusively from the locus coeruleus. Unlike facial motoneurons whose NE innervation originates from the scattered cells of the nearby lateral tegmental cell groups, the relatively long and discrete LC pathway is amenable to electrical stimulation studies. This has been exploited to gain an understanding of central noradrenergic pathways acting on target cells through α_1-adrenoceptors.

In 1974, Nakai and Takaori discovered that conditioning stimulation of the LC could facilitate the responsiveness of LGNd relay neurons to afferent stimulation. Subsequently it was observed that local (iontophoretic) application of NE enhances the spontaneous or evoked firing of LGNd neurons. Detailed pharmacological studies demonstrated that the response to NE is mediated by α_1-adrenoceptors (Rogawski and Aghajanian, 1980a) (Fig. 11). The actions of NE on LGNd relay neurons and motoneurons are similar in many respects. In particular, if ongoing excitatory stimulation of relay neurons is suppressed by acute transection of the afferent optic pathways, NE is unable to excite neuronal firing (although it still enhances excitation due

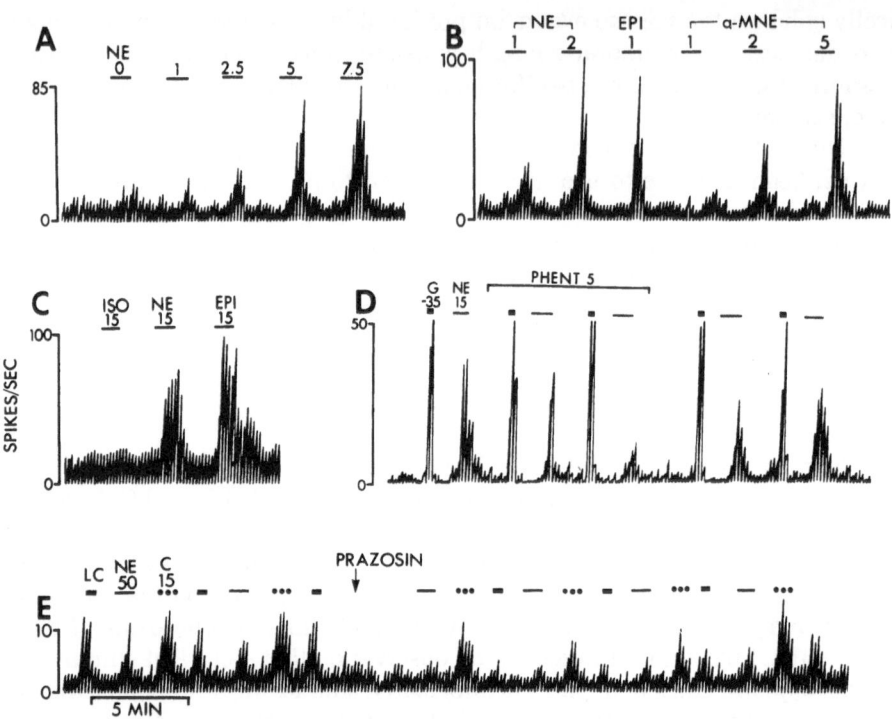

Figure 11. Extracellular recordings from rat dorsal lateral geniculate neurons *in vivo*. (A) Rate-meter record showing activation by various iontophoretic doses of NE. (B) Comparison of NE, epinephrine (EPI), and α-methylnorepinephrine (α-MNE). (C) Comparison of isoproterenol (ISO), NE, and epinephrine at equal ejection currents. (D) Selective blockade of NE, but not glutamate (G), excitations by phentolamine. (E) Selective blockade of NE and LC stimulation (trains at 10 Hz), but not carbachol, by prazosin (125 µg/kg, i.v.). Drugs were applied by iontophoresis (with currents as indicated) except for prazosin, which was administered intravenously. (From Rogawski and Aghajanian, 1980a, 1982, and unpublished, with permission.)

to glutamate). Electrical stimulation of the LC facilitates the firing of LGNd relay neurons via α_1-adrenoceptors, but this effect is also lost when ongoing excitation of relay neurons is reduced (Rogawski and Aghajanian, 1980b).

Trains of stimuli to the LC are required to produce a detectable effect on the excitability of target neurons in the LGNd but the response, once generated, is long-lasting. These characteristics are comparable to those of slow synaptic potentials in peripheral systems. Although it seems likely that the membrane mechanisms underlying the α_1-mediated actions of NE on LGNd relay neurons and motoneurons are similar, proof of this awaits intracellular recording in the LGNd.

3.3. Neocortex

Since the development of the iontophoretic technique over 20 years ago, the response of cerebral cortical neurons *in vivo* to NE has been intensively studied—perhaps more so than any other brain region—yet, until recently, the results have been unsatisfying due to inconsistencies in the experimental data brought about by complexities that will be considered in the following section.

The earliest studies of Krnjević and Phillis (1963) found NE to be purely depressant on spontaneously active cortical neurons of barbiturate anesthetized cats. It was later observed that although this depressant response almost universally occurred under barbiturate anesthesia, excitation was frequent in unanesthetized (*encephale isolé*) preparations or when other general anesthetic agents were used (Johnson et al., 1969). A spirited controversy raged for a number of years in which it was claimed that the excitatory effects of NE were pH artifacts or due to hypoxia induced by constriction of small cerebral blood vessels. It was also noted that factors such as baseline firing rate or iontophoretic dose could influence the direction of the response to NE (see Szabadi, 1979).

Recent studies applying an elegant technique in which a single microelectrode is used to simultaneously monitor the extracellular NE concentration and record spike activity have gone a long way toward resolving this controversy (Armstrong-James and Fox, 1983). The *in situ* assay of NE is based upon a fast electrochemical (polarographic) method using a carbon fiber microelectrode that can be electronically switched to monitor NE concentration or record extracellular potentials. NE is iontophoresed from an adjacent barrel of a multibarrel array in the conventional manner except that the ejecting current is continuously adjusted to maintain a constant concentration of NE at the electrode tip. Experiments carried out in the primary somatosensory cortex of lightly anesthetized rats demonstrated that the spontaneous activity of superficial cells (0 to 800 μm in depth) were uniformly suppressed by NE at concentrations of 5–6 $\times$ 10^{-8} M. This corresponded to ejection currents in the range of 0–4 nA, far lower than had been used in previous studies. Deep cortical neurons (800–1400 μm), on the other hand, could often be excited by very low NE concentrations ($< 10^{-8}$ M), but the firing of these same neurons was suppressed when the concentration of NE rose to levels 10 to 100 times greater (Fig. 12). Thus, some deep cortical neurons can respond to NE with either excitation or inhibition; however, the inhibitory response occurs at much higher doses than are required to inhibit superficial neurons. Since the response of neocortical neurons to NE is critically dependent upon dose and is not uniform in all cortical layers, it is clear why inconsistencies had arisen in earlier uncontrolled studies.

Detailed studies characterizing the pharmacological properties of NE-induced excitation and inhibition have also helped to resolve the controversy regarding the true physiological effects of NE in neocortex, although the evidence here is incomplete and is flawed by conflicting observations. Experiments of Szabadi and his co-workers (see Szabadi, 1979) have demonstrated that the α-adrenergic agonists phenylephrine and methoxamine produce exclusively excitatory effects on cortical neurons, whereas the β_2-agonist salbutamol only causes depressant responses. The nonselective β-agonist isoproterenol is also predominantly depressant, although at higher doses

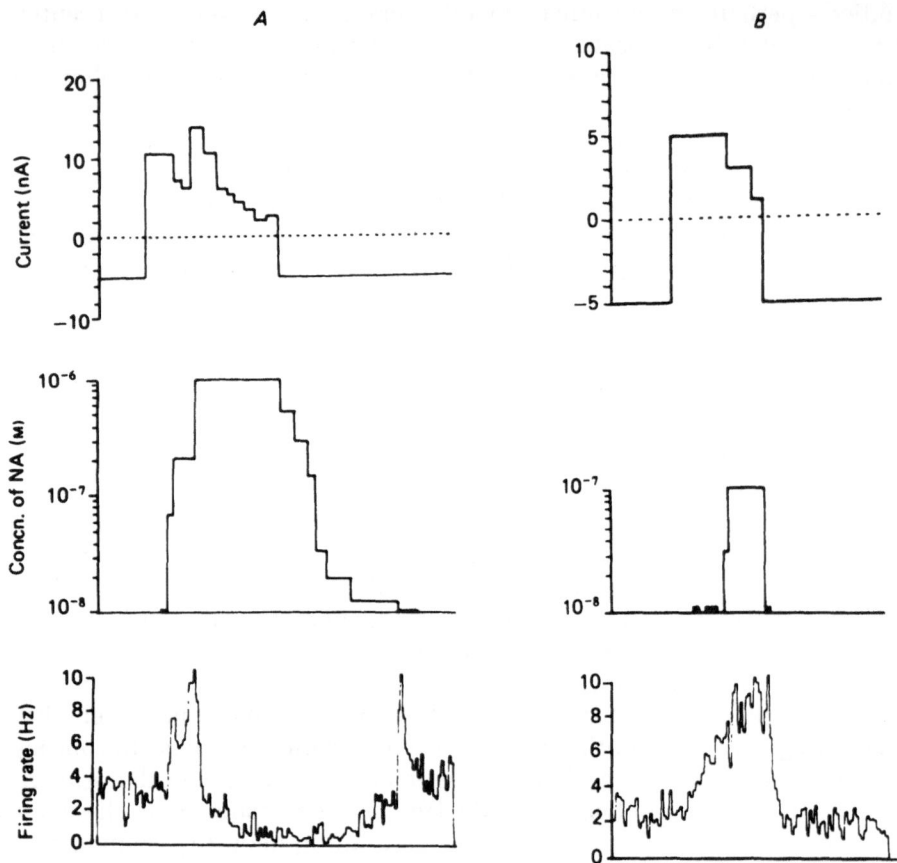

Figure 12. Extracellular recording of the firing of a single neuron in the deep (1200 μm) zone of the somatosensory cortex whose receptive field was on the distal hind foot pad. Lower traces are rate-meter records; top traces show the iontophoretic current applied to the NE barrel; and the middle traces show the measured concentration of NE at the electrode tip as recorded by a carbon fiber. Panel A shows the predominantly depressant response to relatively high concentrations of NE with excitation apparent at the onset and offset of the NE ejection when the NE concentration is low. Panel B shows the excitatory response to low concentrations of NE. (From Armstrong-James and Fox, 1983, with permission.)

weak excitation could also be obtained. The α-antagonists phenoxybenzamine and phentolamine prevented the excitatory responses to all α-adrenoceptor agonists, whereas the depressant response could be antagonized by the β-adrenoceptor blocking drug sotalol. The β-blockers also seemed to inhibit the excitatory responses, but this may have resulted from the relatively high doses used.

Presumably as a result of dose-related nonspecific effects or bias with regard to selection of neurons (i.e., exclusively those in superficial layers, for example), some investigators have observed only depression of spontaneous activity for both α- and β-adrenergic agonists (Stone and Taylor, 1977; Waterhouse et al., 1981). Despite these conflicting findings, however, it is now clear that both excitatory and inhibitory effects of NE can occur in the cortex, even on the same neuron. The excitatory effect is mediated by α-adrenoceptors, whereas the depressant response seems to occur via receptors similar to β-adrenoceptors. Whether these various effects represent direct or indirect actions remains to be determined.

Although the way in which adrenergic agonists affect the spontaneous firing of cortical neurons has allowed a characterization of the receptor pharmacology of these neurons, it is apparent that determination of effects on spontaneous firing alone are insufficient to understand the role of NE in cortical information processing. A conceptualization of the functional role of NE has evolved from studies in somatosensory cortex of the interaction between iontophoretic NE and simultaneously applied transmitters (such as GABA or acetylcholine) or synaptically driven inhibition or excitation (Waterhouse et al., 1981; Waterhouse et al., 1982). NE or the β-agonist isoproterenol, even at doses below those that cause direct effects on spontaneous firing, can facilitate GABA-induced suppression of neurons in somatosensory cortex. This NE-induced enhancement of inhibition is blocked by β- but not α-antagonists. Similar effects of NE could be demonstrated for synaptic inhibition induced by somatosensory stimulation (Waterhouse et al., 1982). Conversely, NE has been found to facilitate iontophoretically applied acetylcholine, which excites cortical neurons. This effect is mimicked by the α-agonist phenylephrine, but not the β-agonist isoproterenol, and blocked by the α-antagonist phentolamine, but not the β-antagonist sotalol. Similar effects of NE on synaptic excitation have also been observed.

These studies have led to the suggestion that, despite direct effects of NE on neuronal firing, it is the interaction between NE and excitatory or inhibitory synaptic inputs to cortical neurons that is of crucial importance in understanding the role of the transmitter in cortical functioning. Although the precise nature of this interaction is as yet undefined, at least for the α-adrenoceptor-mediated facilitation of excitation, the mechanism is likely to be similar to that observed in facial motoneurons. On the other hand, the mechanism underlying the β-receptor-induced potentiation of inhibition is unclear.

NE has also been shown to modulate the responsiveness of visual cortical neurons to stimulation of their receptive fields with appropriate visual stimuli (Kasamatsu and Heggelund, 1982). This can take the form of either an increase or decrease in the absolute firing recorded in response to stimulation with a slit of light, but it is almost invariably noted that the background spontaneous firing of the cell is suppressed during iontophoresis of NE and that this reduction is greater than the reduction, if any, in the evoked signal (however, see Videen et al., 1984). Such an increase in evoked activity relative to background spontaneous discharge has been referred to as an enhancement of the "signal-to-noise ratio" and it seems to occur preferentially for more optimal stimuli of the cell's receptive field so that receptive field borders are sharpened (Madar and Segal, 1981). Although the mechanism whereby this occurs is unknown, similar effects of NE have been observed for the appropriate sensory stimulation in auditory cortex (Foote et al., 1975), somatosensory cortex (Waterhouse and Woodward, 1980), and cerebellum (Freedman et al., 1977; Moises et al., 1979).

3.4. Dorsal Raphe Nucleus

Physiological studies have demonstrated that the firing of serotonergic (5-HT) neurons in the dorsal raphe nucleus is regulated by adrenergic influences mediated via α_1-adrenoceptors. The anatomical substrate for this interaction is a dense noradrenergic innervation of the dorsal raphe and adjacent central grey whose origin is ill defined. Ultrastructural studies using specific labeling techniques have revealed synaptic contacts between noradrenergic nerve terminals and the dendrites of 5-HT neurons (Baraban and Aghajanian, 1981).

In anesthetized rats, the slow, regular spontaneous firing of 5-HT neurons is suppressed by α-adrenoceptor antagonists, suggesting that under these conditions an adrenergic excitatory input is required to maintain their firing. Iontophoresis of α-adrenoceptor agonists can reverse the effects of low doses of antagonists with a rank order of potency typical of α_1-adrenoceptors: NE > phenylephrine > α-methylnorepinephrine > isoproterenol. In the absence of α-antagonists, iontophoretic administration of NE also excites 5-HT neurons, but low iontophoretic currents must be used since at higher doses inhibition is the predominant effect (Baraban and Aghajanian, 1980).

In the in vitro slice preparation where the adrenergic input has presumably been interrupted, many 5-HT neurons are quiescent but their normal spontaneous activity can be restored by bath application of the α-agonist phenylephrine or by iontophoresis of NE. These effects are prevented by bath-applied α-antagonists such as phentolamine, thymoxamine, or prazosin (VanderMaelen and Aghajanian, 1983). These observations are consistent with the existence of facilitatory α_1-adrenoceptors on dorsal raphe neurons. Intracellular recordings have provided insight into the membrane mechanisms whereby these receptors facilitate excitability. The regular firing of 5-HT neurons is due to a repeating cycle of membrane potential changes referred to as "pacemaker potentials" (see Chapter 7). Activation of these neurons by α_1-adrenoceptor agonists occurs by speeding of the pacemaker cycle. Conventional current-clamp as well as single microelectrode voltage-clamp intracellular recordings from raphe neurons in brainstem slices have indicated that this may occur by inhibition of a steady, resting potassium conductance so that the cells are depolarized. In addition, there is suppression of a voltage-activated, transient potassium conductance that gives rise to the "A-current" and is believed to regulate interspike interval (Aghajanian, 1985).

3.5. Hypothalamus

Hypothalamic neurons receive a dense noradrenergic innervation that is believed to play a role in regulating the hypothalamic control of neuroendocrine and autonomic function. In particular, the neurosecretory neurons of the supraoptic and paraventricular nuclei are especially heavily innervated by the A1 NE cell group of the ventrolateral medulla. Physiological studies *in vivo* have indicated that presumed vasopressin neurons (but not oxytocin neurons) are selectively activated by stimulation with trains of pulses to the A1 area. This response was absent in animals treated with the selective catecholamine neurotoxin 6-hydroxydopamine (Day and Renaud, 1984).

In hypothalamic explants *in vitro* similar excitatory effects of NE or the α-agonist methoxamine were obtained in extracellular recordings from supraoptic neurons. In contrast, the β-agonist isoproterenol was inactive. The effects of NE and methoxamine were blocked by prior application of low concentrations of the α-antagonists phenoxybenzamine or prazosin. The excitatory response to α-agonists was maintained when the explants were bathed in high magnesium medium that prevents synaptic transmission (Randle et al., 1984). These studies provide strong evidence that noradrenergic efferents from the A1 cell group directly facilitate the activity of magnocellular vasopressin neurons via α_1-adrenoceptors.

4. RESPONSES MEDIATED BY β-ADRENOCEPTORS

4.1. Cerebellum

Purkinje cells of the cerebellar cortex serve as a unique model system for the analysis of NE inhibitory actions in the CNS. In contrast to the situation in the neocortex and other postsynaptic target areas, the spontaneous firing of these neurons *in vivo* is invariably depressed by iontophoretically applied NE, although the dose required is high. This effect is mimicked by the β-agonist isoproterenol and reversibly blocked by the β-antagonist sotalol, providing support for the idea that it is mediated by β-adrenoceptors (Hoffer et al., 1971). Intracellular recording from Purkinje neurons *in vivo* has revealed that the inhibitory action of NE is associated with membrane hyperpolarization and an increase in input resistance (Siggins et al., 1971). The ionic basis underlying this effect is unknown.

The inhibition of spontaneous firing and membrane hyperpolarization produced by extracellular iontophoresis of NE is mimicked by electrical stimulation of the locus coeruleus, which provides a uniform noradrenergic innervation of the cerebellar cortex. The characteristics of the response of Purkinje neurons to LC stimulation define certain unique features of the noradrenergic inhibition mediated by the coeruleo-cerebellar pathway. Optimal depression of Purkinje cell discharge is produced by *trains* of stimuli at frequencies comparable to that of the firing of LC neurons (3 to 20 Hz) (Moises and Woodward, 1980; Hoffer et al., 1973) (Fig. 13). Following such a train, the spontaneous firing of Purkinje neurons is depressed for up to 1 min. Of significance is that a single shock to the LC usually produces little or no change in the probability of firing following the stimulus. However, in the infrequent situations where the effects of a single shock can be detected, the latency is about 150 msec. Thus, the coeruleo-cerebellar norad-

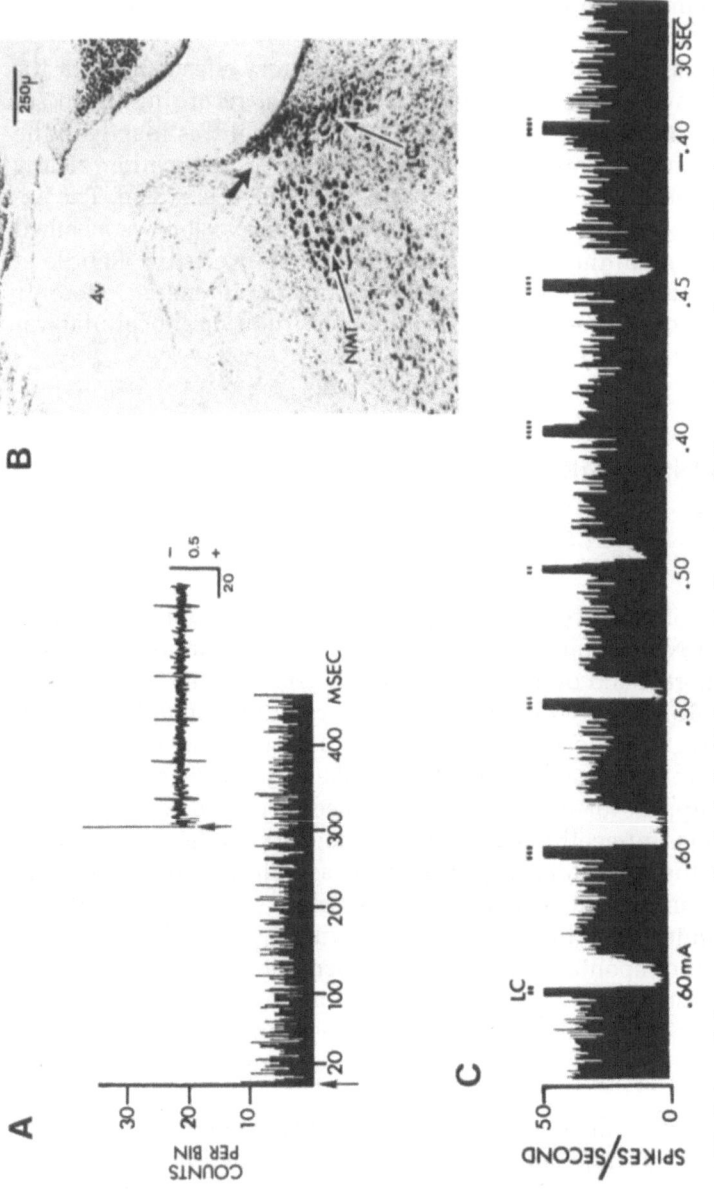

Figure 13. Extracellular response of a single Purkinje neuron in the rat cerebellar cortex to electrical stimulation of the ipsilateral locus coeruleus. (A) Stimulation with single shocks (0.5 mA) at 2 Hz produced no short latency response as shown by the poststimulus time histogram and oscilloscope (inset) records. Arrows denote stimulus artefacts. Spike record's vertical scale is in mV and the horizontal scale in msec. (B) Photomicrograph of Nissl-stained section showing the stimulation site in the locus coeruleus (thick arrow). (C) Continuous rate-meter record demonstrating inhibition produced by trains of stimuli at 10 Hz. Stimulation currents are given in mA below the record. Shock artefacts obscure spike counting during the stimulation. Abbreviations: LC, locus coeruleus, NTM, nucleus mesencephalic tract of V; 4V, fourth ventricle. (From Moises and Woodward, 1980, with permission.)

renergic pathway seems particularly well suited for the leisurely transmission of changes in the "state" of locus coeruleus activity as opposed to more conventional synaptic pathways that operate on the time scale of milliseconds.

Apart from a direct inhibitory action on the spontaneous firing of Purkinje cells, NE exerts a specific effect on GABA-mediated inhibition similar to that observed in the somatosensory cortex. Iontophoretic doses of NE subthreshold for producing direct suppression of spontaneous discharge augment the response to GABA or synaptic inhibition (Fig. 14). Pharmacological characterization of this effect indicates that it is mediated by β_1-adrenoceptors. Thus, the effect is mimicked by the β-agonist isoproterenol, but not the α-agonist phenylephrine, and is blocked by sotalol and practolol (β_1-selective) but not the α-antagonist phentolamine (Yeh and Woodward, 1983).

Extracellular recordings from single Purkinje neurons in the *in vitro* cerebellar slice have added unexpected complexity to the conception of NE's actions in the cerebellar cortex (Basile and Dunwiddie, 1984). Perfusion of these slices with low concentrations (0.5–10 μM) of NE elicited an *increase*

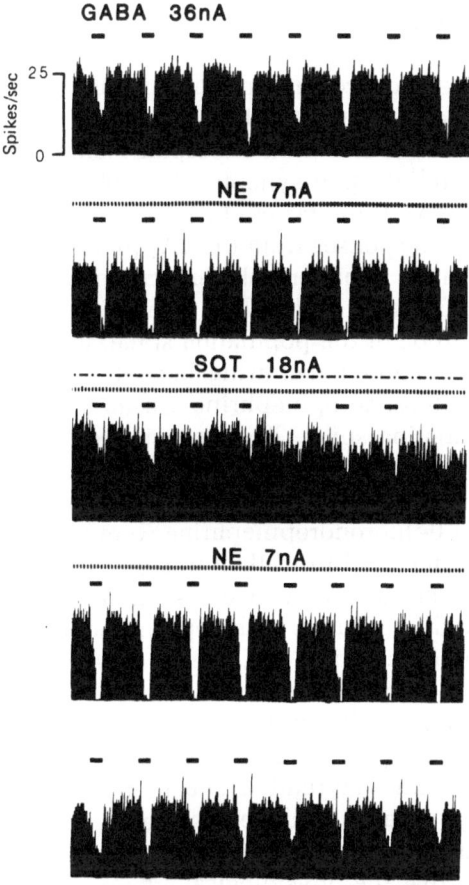

Figure 14. Extracellular recording from a Purkinje neuron in the rat cerebellar cortex showing augmentation of GABA inhibition by NE and blockade of the NE effect by sotalol (SOT). Drugs were applied by iontophoresis during the periods indicated by bars (GABA), dotted lines (NE), dashed line (sotalol), with the currents indicated. (From Waterhouse et al., 1982, with permission.)

in the spontaneous firing of Purkinje neurons, although at higher concentrations (> 25 μM) depression as observed *in vivo* was obtained. The excitatory effect of NE appeared to be due to an action on β-adrenoceptors as it was blocked by timolol, whereas the pharmacological specificity of the depressant responses was less clear (probably an α-receptor). The most plausible explanation for the divergent results obtained *in vivo* and *in vitro* is that dose and/or locus of drug application are critical to determining whether excitation or inhibition is observed. However, since pathway stimulation clearly mimics the inhibition obtained with iontophoresis *in vivo*, the physiological relevance of the *in vitro* observations are open to question.

4.2. Hippocampus

The accessibility of the hippocampal slice preparation for intracellular recording has allowed the cellular mechanisms underlying the action of NE to be examined in greater detail than in any other brain region. Prior to discussing intracellular recording, however, we will briefly consider two other approaches that have been used to study the role of NE in the hippocampus, first, extracellular unit recording, and, second, field potential analysis.

Iontophoretic application of NE *in vivo* depresses the spontaneous firing of virtually all hippocampal pyramidal cells (Segal and Bloom, 1974). Pharmacological studies have indicated that this is a β-adrenoceptor-mediated effect. Field potential analysis, which relies upon synaptically evoked activity, has provided a different perspective (Mueller et al., 1981, 1982). In the hippocampal slice, population spike responses from the CA_1 pyramidal cell layer can be driven by stimulation of Schaffer collateral-commisural afferents in the stratum radiatum. Superfusion of the slice with NE elicits weak and variable effects on the amplitude of the population spike, which represents the summed activity of CA_1 pyramidal cell firing. In contrast, the selective β-agonists isoproterenol or 2-fluoronorepinephrine caused a consistent increase in the size of the population spike. These effects were exquisitely sensitive to the potent β-agonist timolol and, at higher concentrations, also to propanolol and sotalol, but not phentolamine. Clonidine, at high doses, and the selective α-agonist 6-fluoronorepinephrine were found to depress the population spike amplitude, and this effect was blocked by phentolamine. Thus, it has been hypothesized that the inconsistent response to NE is due to stimulation of both α- and β-receptors with opposing actions. In support of this interpretation is the observation that after pretreatment with phentolamine or timolol, NE elicits a robust and consistent elevation or reduction, respectively, in the population spike, presumably due to stimulation of the unblocked receptor type. Drugs that release NE from presynaptic nerve terminals, such as d-amphetamine or tyramine (after pretreatment with a monoamine oxidase inhibitor), usually produced increases in the population spike amplitude that could be blocked by timolol but not phentolamine, thus supporting the concept that the physiological effects of endogenously released NE occur predominantly through an interaction with β-adrenoceptors. On the basis of studies using the population spike response the precise locus of NE action cannot be determined. Nevertheless, none of the adrenergic agonists affected the extracellular field EPSP, suggesting that they mainly act postsynaptically. This could be on pyramidal neurons themselves, on interneurons, or on the coupling between the two.

The field potential of granule cells in the dentate gyrus evoked by perforant path stimulation is also enhanced by NE (however, see Dahl et al., 1983). This has been demonstrated both *in vivo* with iontophoresis of NE (Neuman and Harley, 1983) and *in vitro* in the hippocampal slice (Lacaille and Harley, 1983; Stanton and Sarvey, 1985a). An interesting feature of the effect is that it often persists for 30 min or longer following a brief pulse of NE. As is the case in the CA_1 region, potentiation of the dentate gyrus population spike by NE is blocked by the β-antagonist timolol. Locus coeruleus stimulation also enhanced perforant path-evoked population spikes, and this effect was blocked by injection of the catecholamine neurotoxin 6-hydroxydopamine into the dorsal noradrenergic bundle (Assaf et al., 1979).

In addition to its *acute* effects on synaptically activated field responses, recent studies indicate that NE can modulate the *long term* effectiveness of certain synaptic pathways within the hippocampus. Brief, high frequency stimulation of the mossy fiber input to CA_3 pyramidal neurons can induce a long lasting (hours or more) increase in the field response to a test stimulus applied to the same pathway. This phenomenon is referred to as "long term potentiation" (LTP). In the hippocampal slice, superfusion with NE or isoproterenol during the high frequency stimulation markedly enhanced the magnitude, duration and probability of induction of LTP. These effects were reversibly blocked by the β-antagonists propranolol or timolol (Hopkins and Johnston, 1984).

LTP induced in granule cells of the hippocampal dentate gyrus by perforant path stimulation also appears to be modulated by NE. Thus, destruction of the NE innervation of the dentate with 6-hydroxydopamine reduces LTP *in vivo* (Bliss et al., 1983) or *in vitro* (Stanton and Sarvey, 1985b). Forskolin, a direct activator of adenylate cyclase, restored LTP in hippocampal slices from 6-hydroxydopamine-treated animals. In slices from normal animals, propranolol and the β_1-antagonist metoprolol also reduced LTP due to perforant path stimulation in granule cells. These various observations indicate that noradrenergic modulation of LTP in the hippocampus occurs via β-adrenoceptors, possibly through a cyclic AMP-dependent mechanism.

A third approach to investigating the action of NE in the hippocampus is intracellular recording. The predominant effect of NE on cat hippocampal neurons recorded *in vivo* is membrane hyperpolarization accompanied by an increase in input resistance (Herrling, 1981). Possibly as a result of the conductance change, evoked EPSPs are markedly increased in amplitude. Thus, despite membrane hyperpolarization and a decrease in the frequency of spontaneous action potentials, evoked spikes are more easily generated in the presence of NE because EPSPs are larger. It is apparent that these observations could be the intracellular correlates of the enhanced "signal-to-noise" ratio (i.e., evoked versus background spontaneous discharge) produced by NE in hippocampus (Segal and Bloom, 1976) and other systems.

Recordings in the hippocampal slice have provided additional information, although they have not always been consistent with observations *in vivo*. The discrepancy may result from metabolic changes occurring as a result of the artificial conditions *in vitro*, or the methods by which NE is applied, for example, a relatively high concentration drop touched to the surface of the slice or by bath perfusion. With this in mind, it can be stated that the predominant effect of low doses of NE on the resting properties of CA_1 pyramidal cells is a slow hyperpolarization accompanied by a decrease in the frequency of spontaneous action potential firing (Segal, 1981). However, the degree of hyperpolarization is smaller than that recorded *in vivo* and effects on cell input resistance have been inconsistent. Also in contrast to results obtained *in vivo*, in the slice, EPSPs evoked by stimulation of the Schaffer collateral-commisural system are depressed by NE. All of these effects are mimicked by isoproterenol and blocked by sotalol, indicating that they are due to activation of β-adrenoceptors. It has been hypothesized that the hyperpolarization of CA_1 cells by NE is due to stimulation of the Na^+-K^+ pump, but definitive proof is yet to be forthcoming.

In addition to the membrane hyperpolarization, it has been observed that NE also markedly attenuates the late afterhyperpolarization following action potentials in CA_1 pyramidal cells (Madison and Nicoll, 1982; Haas and Konnerth, 1983). The effect of NE on the spike afterhyperpolarization seems to be mediated by β-adrenoceptors as it is mimicked by isoproterenol (at 10-fold lower concentrations than NE), but not phenylephrine, and is blocked by propranolol, but not phentolamine. In addition, a similar effect is produced by extracellular application of 8-bromo-cyclic AMP, a nonhydrolyzable analog of cyclic AMP; by intracellular injection of cyclic AMP; or by forskolin, a stimulator of cyclic AMP synthesis. It has therefore been suggested that cyclic AMP could mediate the effects of NE as is the case for other β-adrenoceptor-coupled cellular processes (see Madison and Nicoll, 1982).

The late afterhyperpolarization is believed to reflect the turning on of a calcium-dependent potassium conductance by calcium ions that enter during the action potential. Madison and Nicoll (1982) observed little effect of NE on calcium action potentials and therefore concluded that the predominant effect of NE is to directly inhibit the potassium conductance. Recent voltage clamp studies have supported this view, and furthermore have suggested that a specific component of the calcium-activated potassium current is affected, i.e., the low amplitude, slowly inactivating I_{AHP} but not the more prominent, faster I_c (Adams and Lancaster, 1985).

Of particular significance to understanding the role of NE in the hippocampus is the observation that NE produces an increase in the number of spikes fired in response to depolarizing stimuli (Madison and Nicoll, 1982). Whereas under control conditions the spike frequency of CA_1 neurons rapidly diminishes with sustained depolarization ("accomodation"), in the presence of NE, prolonged trains of action potentials are fired (Fig. 15). This effect is believed to result from a depression of the late afterhyperpolarization. Potentiation of pyramidal cell responsiveness occurs even in the pres-

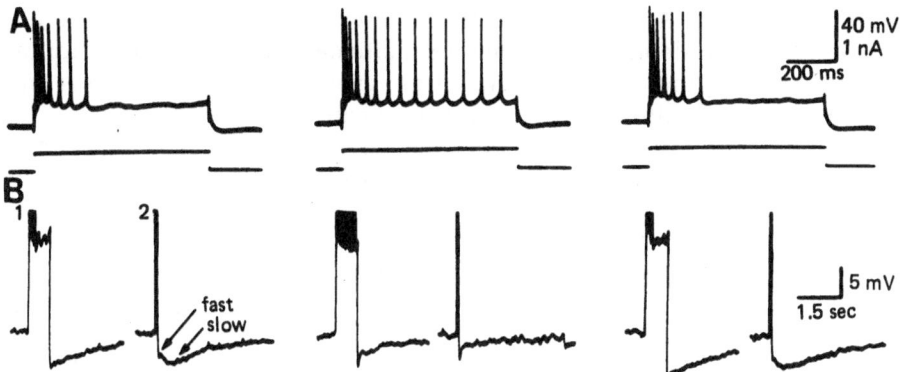

Figure 15. Intracellular recording from a CA_1 pyramidal cell in the rat hippocampal slice showing how NE blocks spike accomodation by supressing the spike afterhyperpolarization. (A) Response of the cell to depolarizing current pulses before (left), during (middle) and 30 min following (right) washout of 10 μM NE. There was no change in membrane potential during the application of NE. (B) High-gain records of the response shown in (A) (B_1) and the response to a short (100 msec) depolarizing current pulse (B_2). Note that NE blocks only the slow (Ca^{2+}-dependent), but not the fast (Ca^{2+}-independent), component of the afterhyperpolarization. (From Madison and Nicoll, 1982, with permission.)

ence of the weak membrane hyperpolarization that is sometimes produced by NE. This has suggested an alternative mechanism to explain the "signal-to-noise" enhancing effect of NE. Hyperpolarization would tend to decrease background firing induced by weak synaptic inputs. On the other hand, blockade of the spike afterhyperpolarization would selectively enhance repetitive spiking in response to strongly depolarizing synaptic inputs. In concert, these two effects—both mediated by β-adrenoceptors—would be expected to selectively favor transmission of activity elicited by strong stimuli and would allow a reconciliation of data obtained in various experimental paradigms.

5. RESPONSES MEDIATED BY INTERNEURONS

5.1. Olfactory Bulb

The suggestion has been made that the facilitatory action of NE in certain systems results from a suppression of tonically active inhibitory interneurons. Although this hypothesis is difficult to prove or disprove *in vivo*, the evidence reviewed in prior sections of this chapter suggests that in at least some situations the contrary is true, i.e., NE acts directly on principal neurons to enhance their responsiveness to synaptic excitation. Nevertheless, in some circumstances a synergistic effect may be produced by an additional suppression of inhibitory interneurons (see Kayama et al., 1982) or depression of recurrent inhibition could be the primary mechanism whereby NE exerts it facilitatory action. An example of this is provided by the olfactory bulb, where it has been demonstrated that NE facilitates the excitability of mitral cells by reducing the release of GABA from granule cells, interneurons that form recurrent inhibitory dendrodendritic synapses on the mitral cells. The experimental support of this concept comes from intracellular recordings in the isolated turtle olfactory bulb (Jahr and Nicoll, 1982). IPSPs recorded in mitral cells, the principal output neurons of the olfactory bulb, were attenuated by NE (see Fig. 16, top). However, the resting membrane properties of these neurons (membrane potential and input resistance) were unaffected and, moreover, NE had no effect on exogenously applied GABA (Fig. 16, bottom). These observations lead to the conclusion that the NE-induced facilitation of mitral cells was not caused by an action on the mitral cells themselves but rather was due to a reduction in GABA release from granule cells.

Although the major effect of NE on mitral cells is believed to be mediated indirectly via granule cells, in some mitral cells it was noted that NE could actually raise the threshold for spike firing elicited by intracellular stimulation, presumably as a result of a direct effect on the mitral cell membrane. Moreover, recordings from rabbit olfactory bulb *in vivo* have demonstrated that NE produces a predominantly depressant effect on mitral cell *spontaneous* activity that obviously cannot be explained by depression of IPSPs but could be due to the effect on spike threshold (Bloom et al., 1964). As noted in prior sections of this chapter, NE can in certain situations suppress spontaneous firing yet enhance the evoked responsiveness of neurons. The observations in the olfactory bulb suggest a further mechanism whereby this could occur; i.e., NE could raise the threshold for firing spontaneous action potentials by a direct action yet facilitate evoked activity through an indirect effect on recurrent inhibition. Nevertheless, in the absence of studies using physiological olfactory stimuli, the true role of noradrenergic pathways in information processing in the olfactory bulb must remain speculative.

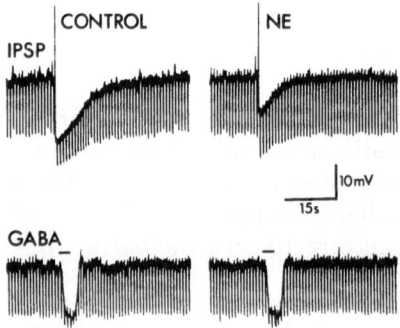

Figure 16. Intracellular recording from a mitral cell in the turtle olfactory bulb. (top) The recurrent IPSP occurring following a spontaneous action potential is diminished in the presence of NE (20 μM). (bottom) NE does not affect the response to iontophoretically applied GABA (80 nA) on the same cell. The resting potential was -54 mV throughout. (From Jahr and Nicoll, 1982, with permission.)

5.2. Lateral Geniculate Nucleus

Intrinsic interneurons within the dorsal lateral geniculate nucleus (LGNd) respond differently to NE than do principal (relay) neurons. In contrast to the excitatory effect of NE or LC stimulation on relay neurons (Section 3.2), these treatments *suppress* the spontaneous or light-evoked firing of intrinsic LGNd interneurons (Kayama et al., 1982). Because these interneurons are sparse (<7% of cells) and difficult to record from, their physiological role has been hard to ascertain. Nevertheless, it is believed that they exert an inhibitory influence on relay nuerons. It is unlikely that the activation of relay neurons by NE occurs via the suppression of these interneurons. However, there could be a synergistic effect produced by the combined action of NE on the two cell populations, resulting in an enhanced ability of the LC to influence signal transmission through the LGNd.

6. CONCLUSION

In recent years, the cellular mechanisms underlying the short-term transmitter actions of norepinephrine have been characterized in a number of peripheral and central systems. As for other transmitters, there are various pharmacological receptors through which NE acts, and in each case the receptor is coupled to one or more specific ionic mechanisms. α_2-Adrenoceptor-mediated actions can involve either an inhibition of calcium-conductance, leading to a reduction in transmitter release, or an activation of potassium conductance, resulting in an inhibition of target cell excitability. α_1-Adrenoceptors usually mediate a decreased-conductance depolarization of neurons, possibly by inhibition of resting potassium current, which leads to a facilitation of excitability. Equally critical in the facilitation of excitability by α_1-adrenoceptors may be suppression of the A current, a potassium current transiently activated by depolarization and implicated in the control of firing behavior (see Rogawski, 1985). β-Adrenoceptor-mediated actions are less well understood, although in the hippocampus the most prominent effect is inhibition of calcium-dependent potassium conductance, which results in enhanced excitability with little change in resting membrane properties. In this latter situation, there is good evidence that cyclic AMP acts as an intracellular messenger.

This emerging understanding of the cellular bases of NE's transmitter actions can provide insight into the functional role of peripheral and central noradrenergic systems. In the periphery, NE neurons form the major final common pathway of the sympathetic nervous system and, as such, take part in regulating the activity of glands and muscle. The predominant *neuronal* actions of NE within sympathetic and enteric ganglia are presynaptic inhibition of transmitter release via α_2-adrenoceptors.

Since the role of central NE systems are less easily described, a functional understanding of these neurons has been more difficult to achieve. Crucial here have been recordings from locus coeruleus NE neurons in awake, behaving rats and monkeys (Foote et al., 1980). The tonic rate at which these neurons fire closely reflects the animal's state of behavioral arousal. During periods of vigilance (high attentiveness to the external environment), spontaneous firing is maximum, whereas during inattentive waking and slow-wave sleep the neurons fire less frequently. The cells are silent in rapid-eye-movement sleep.

Superimposed upon this tonic activity are rapid phasic bursts of firing when the animal orients to a significant sensory stimuli (or to a spontaneous internal cue). The LC system transmits both the tonic and phasic behavioral state information to target areas throughout the neuraxis. In these postsynaptic target areas, the consequences of increased impulse flow along LC axons are diverse, but generally reflect facilitation or sharpening of transmission with respect to specific sensory modalities or other, as yet less well defined, synaptic inputs. Although the functional role of lateral tegmental noradrenergic systems is less well understood, these neurons have been implicated in cardiovascular regulation and the neuroendocrine control of pituitary hormone secretion by the hypothalamus (see Moore and Bloom, 1979).

This chapter has focused on the short-term consequences of NE release. However, it has been suggested that central noradrenergic neurons could exert a trophic influence on the developing nervous system or participate in long-term plastic changes occurring in mature animals (see Foote et al., 1983). An example of the latter is the role of NE in long term potentiation within the hippocampus. Characterizing the cellular bases underlying these potential actions are a challenge for the future.

REFERENCES

Adams, P. R., and Lancaster, B., 1985, Components of Ca-activated K current in rat hippocampal neurones *in vitro, J. Physiol. (Lond.)* **362**:23P.

Aghajanian, G. K., 1985, Modulation of a transient outward current in serotonergic neurones by α_1-adrenoceptors, *Nature* **315**:501–503.

Aghajanian, G. K., and Cedarbaum, J. M., 1977, Evidence for norepinephrine-mediated collateral inhibition of locus coeruleus neurons, *Brain Res.* **136**:570–577.

Aghajanian, G. K., and Rogawski, M. A., 1983, The physiological role of α-adrenoceptors in the CNS: New concepts from single-cell studies, *Trends Pharmacol. Sci.*, **4**:315–317.

Aghajanian, G. K., and VanderMaelen, C. P., 1982, α_2-Adrenoceptor-mediated hyperpolarization of locus coeruleus neurons: Intracellular studies *in vivo, Science* **215**:1394–1396.

Aghajanian, G. K., VanderMaelen, C. P., and Andrade, R., 1983, Intracellular studies on the role of calcium in regulating the activity and reactivity of locus coeruleus neurons in vivo, *Brain Res.* **273**:237–243.

Ahlquist, R. P., 1948, A study of adrenotropic receptors, *Am J. Physiol.* **153**:586–600.

Andrade, R., and Aghajanian, G. K., 1982, Single cell activity in the noradrenergic A-5 region: Responses to drugs and peripheral manipulations of blood pressure, *Brain Res.* **242**:123–135.

Andrade, R., and Aghajanian, G. K., 1984a, Locus coeruleus activity *in vitro:* Intrinsic regulation by a calcium-dependent potassium conductance but not α_2-adrenoceptors, *J. Neurosci.* **4**:161–170.

Andrade, R., and Aghajanian, G. K., 1984b, Intrinsic regulation of locus coeruleus neurons: Electrophysiological evidence indicating a predominant role for autoinhibition, *Brain Res.* **310**:401–406.

Armstrong-James, M., and Fox, K., 1983, Effects of ionophoresed noradrenaline on the spontaneous activity of neurones in rat primary somatosensory cortex, *J. Physiol. (Lond.)* **335**:427–447.

Assaf, S. Y., Mason, S. T., and Miller, J. J., 1979, Noradrenergic modulation of neuronal transmission between the entorhinal cortex and the dentate gyrus of the rat, *J. Physiol. (Lond.)* **292**:52P.

Baraban, J. M., and Aghajanian, G. K., 1980, Suppression of firing activity of 5-HT neurons in the dorsal raphe by alpha-adrenoceptor antagonists, *Neuropharmacology* **19**:355–363.

Baraban, J. M., and Aghajanian, G. K., 1981, Noradrenergic innervation of serotonergic neurons in the dorsal raphe: Demonstration by electron microscopic autoradiography, *Brain Res.* **204**:1–11.

Barasi, S., and Roberts, M. H. T., 1977, Responses of motoneurons to electrophoretically applied dopamine, *Br. J. Pharmacol.* **60**:29–34.

Barger, G., and Dale, H. H., 1910, Chemical structure and sympathomimetic action of amines, *J. Physiol. (Lond.)* **41**:19–59.

Basile, A. S., and Dunwiddie, T. V., 1984, Norepinephrine elicits both excitatory and inhibitory responses from Purkinje cells in the vitro rat cerebellar slice, *Brain Res.* **296**:15–25.

Belcher, G., Ryall, R. W., and Schaffner, R., 1978, The differential effects of 5-hydroxytryptamine, noradrenaline and raphe stimulation on nociceptive and non-nociceptive dorsal horn interneurones in the cat, *Brain Res.* **151**:307–321.

Bliss, T. V. P., Goddard, G. V., and Riives, 1983, Reduction of long-term potentiation in the dentate gyrus of the rat following selective depletion of monoamines, *J. Physiol. (Lond.)* **334**:475–491.

Bloom, F. E., Costa, E., and Salmoiraghi, G. C., 1964, Analysis of individual rabbit olfactory bulb neuron responses to the microiontopohresis of acetylcholine, norepinephrine and serotonin synergists and antagonists, *J. Pharmacol. Exp. Ther.* **146**:16–23.

Brown, D. A., and Caulfield, M. P., 1979, Hyperpolarizing 'α₂'-adrenoceptors in rat sympathetic ganglia, *Br. J. Pharmacol.* **65**:435–445.

Brown, D. A., and Caulfield, M. P., 1981, Adrenoceptors in ganglia, in: *Adrenoceptors and Catecholamine Action* (G. Kunos, ed.), John Wiley & Sons, New York, pp. 99–115.

Brown, D. A., and Dunn, P. M., 1983, Depolarization of rat isolated superior cervical ganglia mediated by β₂-adrenoceptors, *Br. J. Pharmacol.* **79**:429–439.

Burnstock, G., and Costa, M., 1975, *Adrenergic Neurons*, Chapman and Hall, London.

Canfield, D. R., and Dunlap, K., 1984, Pharmacological characterization of amine receptors on embryonic chick sensory neurons, *Br. J. Pharmac.* **82**:557–563.

Cedarbaum, J. M., and Aghajanian, G. K., 1977, Catecholamine receptors on locus coeruleus neurons: Pharmacological characterization, *Eur. J. Pharmacol.* **44**:375–385.

Cedarbaum, J. M., and Aghajanian, G. K., 1978, Activation of locus coeruleus neurons by peripheral stimuli: Modulation by a collateral inhibitory mechanism, *Life Sci.* **23**:1383–1392.

Christ, D. D., and Nishi, S., 1971, Site of adrenaline blockade in the superior cervical ganglion of the rabbit, *J. Physiol. (Lond.)* **213**:107–117.

Cole, A. E., and Shinnick-Gallagher, P., 1981, Comparison of the receptors mediating the catecholamine hyperpolarization and slow inhibitory postsynaptic potential in sympathetic ganglia, *J. Pharmacol. Exp. Ther.* **217**:440–444.

Dahl, D., Bailey, W. H., and Winson, J., 1983, Effect of norepinephrine depletion of hippocampus on neuronal transmission from perforant pathway through dentate gyrus, *J. Neurophysiol.* **49**:123–133.

Dahlström, A., and Fuxe, K., 1964, Evidence for the existence of monoamine-containing neurons in the central nervous system. I. Demonstration of monoamines in the cell bodies of brain stem neurons, *Acta Physiol. Scand.* **62** (Suppl. 232):1–55.

Dale, H. H., 1906, On some physiological actions of ergot, *J. Physiol. (Lond.)* **34**:163–206.

Day, T. A., and Renaud, L. P., 1984, Electrophysiological evidence that noradrenergic afferents selectively facilitate the activity of supraoptic vasopressin neurons, *Brain Res.* **303**:233–240.

De Groat, W. C., and Volle, R. L., 1966, The actions of the catecholamines on transmission in the superior cervical ganglion of the cat, *J. Pharmacol. Exp. Ther.* **154:**1–13.

Doxey, J. C., Roach, A. G., and Smith. C. F. C., 1983, Studies on RX 781094: A selective, potent and specific antagonist of α_2-adrenoceptors, *Br. J. Pharmacol.* **78:**489–505.

Doxey, J. C., Lane, A. C., Roach, A. G., and Virdee, N. K., 1984, Comparison of the α-adrenoceptor antagonist profiles of idazoxan (RX 781094), yohimbine, rauwolscine and corynanthine, *Naunyn-Schmiedeberg's Arch. Pharmacol.* **325:**136–144.

Drew, G. M., 1978, Pharamcological characterization of the presynaptic α-adrenoceptors regulating cholinergic activity in the guinea-pig ileum, *Br. J. Pharmacol.* **64:**293–300.

Dunlap, K., and Fischbach, G. D., 1981, Neurotransmitters decrease the calcium conductance activated by depolarization of embryonic chick sensory neurones, *J. Physiol. (Lond.)* **317:**519–535.

Egan, T. M., Henderson, G., North, R. A., and Williams, J. T., 1983, Noradrenaline-mediated synaptic inhibition in rat locus coeruleus neurones, *J. Physiol. (Lond.)* **345:**477–488.

Engberg, I., Flatman, J. A., and Kadzielawa, K., 1976, Lack of specificity of motoneurone responses to microiontophoretically applied phenolic amines, *Acta Physiol. Scand.* **96:**137–139.

Engberg, I., and Marshall, K. C., 1971, Mechanism of noradrenaline hyperpolarization in spinal cord motoneurons of the cat, *Acta Physiol. Scand.* **83:**142–144.

Finlayson, P. G. and Marshall, K. C., 1984, Hyperpolarizing and age-dependent depolarizing responses of cultured locus coeruleus neurons to noradrenaline, *Develop. Brain Res.* **15:**167–175.

Fleetwood-Walker, S. M., Mitchell, R., Hope, P. J., Molony, V., and Iggo, A., 1985, An α_2 receptor mediates the selective inhibition by noradrenaline of nociceptive responses of identified dorsal horn neurones, *Brain Res.* **334:**243–254.

Foote, S. L., Aston-Jones, G., and Bloom, F. E., 1980, Impulse activity of locus coeruleus neurons in awake rats and monkeys is a function of sensory stimulation and arousal, *Proc. Natl. Acad. Sci. U.S.A.* **77:**3033–3037.

Foote, S. L., Bloom, F. E., Aston-Jones, G., 1983, Nucleus locus ceruleus: New evidence of anatomical and physiological specificity, *Physiol. Rev.* **63:**844–914.

Foote, S. L., Freedman, R., and Oliver, A. P., 1975, Effects of putative neurotransmitters on neuronal activity in monkey auditory cortex, *Brian Res.* **86:**229–242.

Frankhuyzen, A. L., and Mulder, A. H., 1982, Pharmacological characterization of presynaptic α-adrenoceptors modulating [^{3}H]noradrenaline and [^{3}H]5-hydroxytryptamine release from slices of the hippocampus of the rat, *Eur. J. Pharmacol.* **81:**97–106.

Freedman, J. E. and Aghajanian, G. K., 1984, Idazoxan (RX 781094) selectively antagonizes α_2-adrenoceptors on rat central neurons, *Eur. J. Pharmac.* **105:**265–272.

Freedman, R., Hoffer, B. J., Woodward, D. J., and Puro, D., 1977, Interaction of norepinephrine with cerebellar activity evoked by mossy and climbing fibers, *Exp. Neurol.* **55:**269–288.

Fung, S. J., and Barnes, C. D., 1981, Evidence of facilitatory coerulospinal action in lumbar motoneurons of cats, *Brain Res.* **216:**299–311.

Galvan, M., and Adams, P. R., 1982, Control of calcium current in rat sympathetic neurons by norepinephrine, *Brain Res.* **244:**135–144.

Gershon, M. D., 1981, The enteric nervous system, *Ann. Rev. Neurosci.* **4:**227–272.

Guyenet, P. G., and Cabot, J. B., 1981, Inhibition of sympathetic preganglionic neurons by catecholamines and clonidine: Mediation by an α-adrenergic receptor, *J. Neurosci.* **1:**908–917.

Haas, H. L., and Konnerth, A., 1983, Histamine and noradrenaline decrease calcium-activated potassium conductance in hippocampal pyramidal cells, *Nature* **302:**432–434.

Headley, P. M., Duggan, A. W., and Griersmith, B. T., 1978, Selective reduction by noradrenaline and 5-hydroxytryptamine of nociceptive responses of cat dorsal horn neurons, *Brain Res.* **145:**185–189.

Herrling, P. L., 1981, The membrane potential of cat hippocampal neurons recorded in vivo displays four different reaction-mechanisms to iontophoretically applied transmitter agonists, *Brain Res.* **212:**331–343.

Hirst, G. D. S., and McKirdy, H. C., 1978, Presynaptic inhibition at mammalian peripheral synapse? *Nature* **250:**430–431.

Hodge, C. J., Jr., Apkarian, A. V., Stevens, R. T., Vogelsang, G. D., Brown, O., and Franck, J. I., 1983, Dorsolateral pontine inhibition of dorsal horn cell responses to cutaneous stimulation: Lack of dependence on catecholaminergic systems in cat, *J. Neurophysiol.* **50:**1220–1235.

Hoffer, B. J., Siggins, G. R., and Bloom, F. E., 1971, Studies on norepinephrine-containing afferents to Purkinje cells of rat cerebellum. II. Sensitivity of Purkinje cells to norepinephrine and related substances administered by microiontophoresis, *Brain Res.* **25:**522–534.

Hoffer, B. J., Siggins, G. R., Oliver, A. P., and Bloom, F. E., 1973, Activation of the pathway from locus coeruleus to rat cerebellar Purkinje neurons: Pharmacological evidence of noradrenergic central inhibition, *J. Pharmacol. Exp. Ther.* **184:**553–569.

Hopkins, W. F., and Johnston, D., 1984, Frequency-dependent noradrenergic modulation of long-term potentiation in the hippocampus, *Science* **226:**350–352.

Horn, J. P., and McAfee, D. A., 1979, Norepinephrine inhibits calcium-dependent potentials in rat sympathetic neurons, *Science* **204:**1233–1235.

Horn, J. P., and McAfee, D. A., 1980, Alpha-adrenergic inhibition of calcium-dependent potentials in rat sympathetic neurones, *J. Physiol. (Lond.)* **301:**191–204.

Jahr, C. E., and Nicoll, R. A., 1982, Noradrenergic modulation of dendrodendritic inhibition in the olfactory bulb, *Nature* **297:**227–229.

Jeftinija, S., Semba, K, and Randić, M., 1983, Norepinephrine reduces excitability of single cutaneous primary afferent C and A fibers in the cat spinal cord, in: *Advances in Pain Research and Therapy* (J. J. Bonica, ed.), vol. 5, Raven Press, New York, pp. 271–276.

Johnson, E. S., Roberts, M. H. T., and Straughan, D. W., 1969, The responses of cortical neurones to monoamines under differing anaesthetic conditions, *J. Physiol. (Lond.)* **203:**261–280.

Kafka, M. S., and Thoa, N. B., 1979, α-Adrenergic receptors in the rat superior cervical ganglion, *Biochem. Pharmacol.* **28:**2485–2489.

Kasamatsu, T., and Heggelund, P., 1982, Single cell responses in cat visual cortex to visual stimulation during iontophoresis of noradrenaline, *Exp. Brain Res.* **45:**317–327.

Kayama, Y., Negi, T., Sugitani, M., and Iwama, K., 1982, Effects of locus coeruleus stimulation on neuronal activities of dorsal lateral geniculate nucleus and perigeniculate reticular nucleus of the rat, *Neuroscience* **7:**655–666.

Kilbinger, H., 1982, The myenteric plexus-longitudinal muscle preparation, in: *Progress in Cholinergic Biology: Model Cholinergic Synapses* (I. Hanin and A. M. Goldberg, eds.), Raven Press, New York, pp. 137–167.

Kosterlitz, H. W., Lydon, R. J., and Watt, A. J., 1970, The effects of adrenaline, noradrenaline and isoprenaline on inhibitory α- and β-adrenoceptors in the longitudinal muscle of the guinea-pig ileum, *Br. J. Pharmacol.* **39:**398–413.

Krnjević, K., and Phillis, J. W., 1963, Actions of certain amines on cerebral cortical neurones, *Br. J. Pharmacol. Chemother.* **20:**471–489.

Lacaille, J. C., and Harley, C. W., 1983, In vitro superfusion of norepinephrine potentiates the perforant path evoked field potential in the dentate gyrus, *Soc. Neurosci. Abstr.* **9:**1001.

Lands, A. M., Arnold, A., McAuliff, J. P., Luduena, F. P., and Brown, T. G., Jr., 1967, Differentiation of receptor systems activated by sympathomimetic amines, *Nature* **214:**597–598.

Langer, S. Z., 1981, Presynaptic regulation of the release of catecholamines, *Pharmacol. Rev.* **32:**337–362.

Levitt, P., and Moore, R. Y., 1979, Origin and organization of brainstem catecholamine innervation in the rat, *J. Comp. Neurol.* **186:**505–528.

Madar, Y., and Segal, M., 1981, Differential effects of noradrenaline in the visual cortex, *Neurosci. Lett. (Suppl.)* **7:**S162.

Madison, D. V., and Nicoll, R. A., 1982, Noradrenaline blocks accomodation of pyramidal cell discharge in the hippocampus, *Nature* **299:**636–638.

Marrazzi, A. S., 1939, Electrical studies on the pharmacology of autonomic synapses. II. The action of a sympathomimetic drug (epinephrine) on sympathetic ganglia, *J. Pharmacol. Exp. Ther.* **65:**395–404.

Mayer, S. E., 1980., Neurohormonal transmission and the autonomic nervous system, in: *Goodman and Gilman's The Pharmacological Basis of Therapeutics*, 6th edition (A. G. Gilman, L. S. Goodman, and A. Gilman, eds.), Macmillan, New York, pp. 56–90.

McAfee, D. A., 1982, Superior cervical ganglion: Physiological considerations, in: *Progress in Cholinergic Biology: Model Cholinergic Synapses* (I. Hanin and A. M. Goldberg, eds.), Raven Press, New York, pp. 191–211.

McAfee, D. A., and Yarowsky, P. J., 1979, Calcium-dependent potentials in the mammalian sympathetic neurone, *J. Physiol. (Lond.),* **290:**507–523.

McCall, R. B., and Aghajanian, G. K., 1979, Serotonergic facilitation of facial motoneuron excitation, *Brain Res.* **169:**11–27.

Moises, H. C., and Woodward, D. J., 1980, Potentiation of GABA inhibitory action in cerebellum by locus coeruleus stimulation, *Brain Res.* **182:**327–344.

Moises, H. C., Woodward, D. J., Hoffer, B. J., and Freedman, R., 1979, Interactions of norepinephrine with Purkinje cell responses to putative amino acid neurotransmitters applied by microiontophoresis, *Exp. Neurol.* **64:**493–515.

Molliver, M. E., Grzanna, R., Lidov, H. G. W., Morrison, J. H., and Olschowka, J., 1982, Monoamine systems in the cerebral cortex, in: *Cytochemical Methods in Neuroanatomy* (S. L. Palay and V. Chan-Palay, eds.) Alan R. Liss, New York, pp. 255–277.

Moore, R. Y., and Bloom, F. E., 1979, Central catecholamine neuron systems: anatomy and physiology of the norepinephrine and epinephrine systems, *Ann. Rev. Neurosci.* **2:**113–168.

Moore, S. D., and Guyenet, P. G., 1983a, An electrophysiological study of the forebrain projection of nucleus commissuralis: Preliminary identification of presumed A2 catecholaminergic neurons, *Brain Res.* **263:**211–222.

Moore, S. D., and Guyenet, P. G., 1983b, Alpha-receptor mediated inhibition of A2 noradrenergic neurons, *Brain Res.* **276:**188–191.

Morita, K., and North, R. A., 1981, Clonidine activates membrane potassium conductance in myenteric neurones, *Br. J. Pharmacol.* **74:**419–428.

Mueller, A. L., Hoffer, B. J., and Dunwiddie, T. V., 1981, Noradrenergic responses in rat hippocampus: Evidence for mediation by α and β receptors in the in vitro slice, *Brain Res.* **214:**113–126.

Mueller, A. L., Kirk, K. L., Hoffer, B. J., and Dunwiddie, T. V., 1982, Noradrenergic responses in rat hippocampus: Electrophysiological actions of direct- and indirect-acting sympathomimetics in the *in vitro* slice, *J. Pharmacol. Exp. Ther.* **223:**599–605.

Nakai, Y., and Takaori, S., 1974, Influence of norepinephrine-containing neurons derived from the locus coeruleus on lateral geniculate neuronal activities of cats, *Brain Res.* **71:**47–60.

Nakamura, S., Tepper, J. M., Young, S. J., and Groves, P. M., 1981, Neurophysiological consequences of presynaptic receptor activation: changes in noradrenergic terminal excitability, *Brain Res.* **226:**155–170.

Nakamura, T., Yoshimura, M., Shinnick-Gallagher, J. P. and Akasu, T., 1984, α_2 and α_1-adrenoceptors mediate opposing actions on parasympathetic neurons, *Brain Res.* **323:**349–353.

Neuman, R. S., and Harley, C. W., 1983, Long-lasting potentiation of the dentate gyrus population spike by norepinephrine, *Brain Res.* **273:**162–165.

Nishi, S., and North, R. A., 1973a, Intracellular recording from the myenteric plexus of the guinea-pig ileum, *J. Physiol. (Lond.)* **231:**471–491.

Nishi, S., and North, R. A., 1973b, Presynaptic action of noradrenaline in the myenteric plexus, *J. Physiol. (Lond.)* **231:**29–39P.

North, R. A., and Yoshimura, M., 1984, The actions of noradrenaline on neurones of the rat substantia gelatinosa *in vitro, J. Physiol. (Lond.)* **349:**43–55.

Paton, W. D. M., and Vizi, E.S., 1969, The inhibitory action of noradrenaline and adrenaline on acetylcholine output by guinea-pig ileum longitudinal muscle strip, *Br. J. Pharmacol.* **35:**10–28.

Pun, R. Y. K., Marshall, K. C., Hendelman, W. J., Guthrie, P. B., and Nelson, P. G., 1985, Noradrenergic responses of spinal neurons in locus coeruleus-spinal cord co-cultures, *J. Neurosci.* **5:**181–191.

Randle, J. C. R., Bourque, C. W., and Renaud, L. P., 1983, α-Adrenergic activation of rat hypothalamic supraoptic neurons maintained in vitro, *Brain Res.* **307:**374–378.

Reichenbacher, D., Reimann, W., and Starke, K., 1982, α-Adrenoceptor-mediated inhibition of noradrenaline release in rabbit brain cortex slices. Receptor properties and role of the biophase concentration of noradrenaline, *Naunym Schmiedeberg's Arch. Pharmacol.* **319**:71–77.

Reuter, H., and Scholz, H., 1977, The regulation of the calcium conductance of cardiac muscle by adrenaline, *J. Physiol. (Lond.)* **264**:49–62.

Reuter, H., Cachelin, A. B., De Peyer, J. E., and Kokobun, S., 1983, Modulation of calcium channels in cultured cardiac cells by isoproterenol and 8-bromo-cAMP, *Cold Spring Harbor Symp. Quant. Biol.* **48**:193–200.

Rogawski, M. A., 1985, The A-current: How ubiquitous a feature of excitable cells is it? *Trends Neurosci.* **8**:214–219.

Rogawski, M. A., and Aghajanian, G. K. 1980a, Activation of lateral geniculate neurons by norepinephrine: Mediation by an α-adrenergic receptor, *Brain Res.* **182**:345–359.

Rogawski, M. A., and Aghajanian, G. K., 1980b, Modulation of lateral geniculate neurone excitability by noradrenaline microiontophoresis or locus coeruleus stimulation, *Nature* **287**:731–734.

Rogawski, M. A., and Aghajanian, G. K., 1982, Activation of lateral geniculate neurons by locus coeruleus or dorsal noradrenergic bundle stimulation: Selective blockade by the alpha$_1$-adrenoceptor antagonist prazosin, *Brain Res.* **250**:31–39.

Ruffolo, R. R., Jr., Waddell, J. E., and Yaden, E. L., 1980, Receptor interactions of imidazolines. IV. Structural requirements for *alpha* adrenergic receptor occupation and receptor activation by clonidine and a series of structural analogs in rat aorta, *J. Pharmacol. Exp. Ther.* **213**:267–272.

Sagen, J., and Proudfit, H. K., 1984, Effect of intrathecally administered noradrenergic antagonists on nociception in the rat, *Brain Res.* **310**:295–301.

Segal, M., 1981, The action of norepinephrine in the rat hippocampus: Intracellular studies in the slice preparation, *Brain Res.* **206**:107–128.

Segal, M., and Bloom, F. E., 1974, The action of norepinephrine in the rat hippocampus. I. Iontophoretic studies, *Brain Res.* **72**:79–97.

Segal, M., and Bloom, F. E., 1976, The action of norepinephrine in the rat hippocampus. IV. The effects of locus coeruleus stimulation on evoked hippocampal unit activity, *Brain Res.* **107**:513–525.

Siggins, G. R., Oliver, A. P., Hoffer, B. J., and Bloom, F. E., 1971, Cyclic adenosine monophosphate and norepinephrine: Effects of transmembrane properties on cerebellar Purkinje cells, *Science* **171**:192–194.

Stanton, P. K., and Sarvey, J. M., 1985a, Blockade of norepinephrine-induced long-lasting potentiation in hippocampal dentate gyrus by an inhibitor of protein synthesis, *Brain Res.* in press.

Stanton, P. K., and Sarvey, J. M., 1985b, Depletion of norepinephrine, but not serotonin, reduces long-term potentiation in the dentate of rat hippocampal slices, *J. Neurosci.* **5**:2169–2176.

Starke, K., and Docherty, J. R., 1980, Recent developments in α-adrenoceptor research, *J. Cardiovasc. Pharmacol.* **2**(Suppl. 3):5269–5286.

Stone, T. W., and Taylor, D. A., 1977, The nature of adrenoceptors in the guinea pig cerebral cortex: A microiontophoretic study, *Can. J. Physiol. Pharmacol.* **55**:1400–1404.

Strahlendorf, J. C., Strahlendorf, H. K., Kingsley, R. E., Gintautas, J., and Barnes, C. D., 1980. Facilitation of the lumbar monosynaptic reflexes by locus coeruleus stimulation, *Neuropharmacology* **19**:225–230.

Szabadi, E., 1979, Adrenoceptors on central neurones: Microelectrophoretic studies: *Neuropharmacology* **18**:831–843.

Tsein, R. W., Bean, B. P., Hess, P., and Nowycky, M., 1983, Calcium channels: Mechanisms of β-adrenergic modulation and ion permeation, *Cold Spring Harbor Symp. Quant. Biol.* **48**:201–212.

VanderMaelen, C. P., and Aghajanian, G. K., 1980, Intracellular studies showing modulation of facial motoneurone excitability by serotonin, *Nature* **287**:346–347.

VanderMaelen, C. P., and Aghajanian, G. K., 1983, Electrophysiological and pharmacological characterization of serotonergic dorsal raphe neurons recorded extracellularly and intracellularly in rat brain slices, *Brain Res.* **289**:109–119.

Videen, T. O., Daw, N. W., and Rader, R. K., 1984, The effect of norepinephrine on visual cortical neurons in kittens and adult cats, *J. Neurosci.* **4:**1607–1617.

Waterhouse, B. D., and Woodward, D. J., 1980, Interaction of norepinephrine with cerebro-cortical activity evoked by stimulation of somatosensory afferent pathways, *Exp. Neurol.* **67:**11–34.

Waterhouse, B. D., Moises, H. C., and Woodward, D. J., 1981, Alpha-receptor-mediated facilitation of somatosensory cortical neuronal responses to excitatory synaptic inputs and iontophoretically applied acetylcholine, *Neuropharmacology* **20:**907–920.

Waterhouse, B. D., Moises, H. C., Yeh, H. H., and Woodward, D. J., 1982, Norepinephrine enhancement of inhibitory synaptic mechanisms in cerebellum and cerebral cortex: Mediation by *beta* adrenergic receptors, *J. Pharmacol. Exp. Ther.* **221:**495–506.

Wemer, J., Frankhuyzen, A. L., and Mulder, A. H., 1982, Pharmacological characterization of presynaptic alpha-adrenoceptors in the nucleus solitarii and the cerebral cortex of the rat, *Neuropharmacology* **21:**499–506.

Westlund, K. N., Bowker, R. M., Ziegler, M. G., and Coulter, J. D., 1983, Noradrenergic projections to the spinal cord of the rat, *Brain Res.* **263:**15–31.

White, S. R., and Neuman, R. S., 1980, Facilitation of spinal motoneurone excitability by 5-hydroxytryptamine and noradrenaline, *Brain Res.* **188:**119–127.

Wikberg, J. E. S., and Lefkowitz, R. J., 1982, Alpha$_2$ adrenergic receptors are located prejunctionally in the Auerbach's plexus of the guinea pig small intestine: direct demonstration by radioligand binding, *Life Sci.* **31:**2899–2905.

Wilkberg, J., 1978, Differentiation between pre- and postjunctional α-receptors in guinea pig ileum and rabbit aorta, *Acta Physiol. Scand.* **103:**225–239.

Williams, J. T., and North, R. A., 1985, Catecholamine inhibition of calcium action potentials in rat locus coeruleus neurones, *Neuroscience* **14:**103–109.

Williams, J. T., Henderson, G., and North, R. A. 1985, Characterization of α_2-adrenoceptors which increase potassium conductance in rat locus coeruleus neurones, *Neuroscience* **14:**95–101.

Wood, J. D., and Mayer, C. J., 1979, Adrenergic inhibition of serotonin release from neurons in guinea pig Auerbach's plexus, *J. Neurophysiol.* **42:**594–603.

Wohlberg, C. J., Hackman, J. C., Ryan, G. P., and Davidoff, R. A., 1983, Hyperpolarization of primary afferent terminals mediated by α_2-adrenoceptors, *Soc. Neurosci. Abstr.* **9:**1001.

Yeh, H. H., and Woodward, D. J., 1983, Beta-1 adrenergic receptors mediate noradrenergic facilitation of Purkinje cell responses to gamma-aminobutyric acid in cerebellum of rat, *Neuropharmacology* **22:**629–639.

Yoshimura, M., and Nishi, S., 1982, Intracellular recordings from lateral horn cells of the spinal cord in vitro, *J. Autonom. Nerv. Syst.* **6:**5–11.

Young, W. S., and Kuhar, M. J., 1980, Noradrenergic α1 and α2 receptors: Light microscopic autoradiographic localization, *Proc. Natl. Acad. Sci. U.S.A.* **77:**1696–1700.

9

Dopamine

ANTHONY A. GRACE and BENJAMIN S. BUNNEY

1. INTRODUCTION

1.1. Historical Perspective

Appreciation of the role played by dopamine (DA) in brain function has undergone rapid change in recent years (Andén, 1979). Upon its discovery in brain in 1939, DA was proposed to act as an intermediate in the biosynthesis of norepinephrine and epinephrine. However, in 1958 DA was demonstrated to be present in brain in concentrations similar to that of norepinephrine, suggesting that DA not only serves as a precursor but might function as a neurotransmitter in its own right. When it was discovered that the striatum contained 70–80% of the brain's DA and that depletion of striatal DA was important in the pathogenesis of Parkinson's disease (Hornykiewicz, 1973), DA rapidly became the subject of intense interest among neuropharmacologists. The study of DA and other catecholamines was aided tremendously by the discovery that catecholamine systems could be visualized microscopically through the use of fluorescence histochemical techniques. This permitted the precise anatomical localization of dopaminergic neurons and fibers and, when combined with biochemical data, unequivocally demonstrated the existence of a dopamine-containing neuronal population distinct from other catecholamine systems. The development of the histochemical fluorescence technique was also crucial to the neurophysiological analysis of brain DA systems, which relies upon knowledge of the anatomical location of these neurons and their projection areas.

1.2. Distribution of Dopamine Neurons and Fibers

Although the neuroanatomical location of catecholamine systems may be visualized specifically using formaldehyde or glyoxylic acid-induced fluorescence histochemistry, distinguishing *which* catecholamine is located in a particular region is more difficult. One recent anatomical solution to this problem has been the use of immunocytochemical techniques to localize enzymes specific for the synthesis of each neurotransmitter. The catecholamine specific enzyme *tyrosine hydroxylase*, which acts on tyrosine to produce the immediate precursor of DA, L-dihydroxyphenylalanine (L-DOPA), is a marker for catecholamine neurons, but cannot be used to distinguish between DA and other catecholamine neurons. L-DOPA is converted to DA by the enzyme DOPA decarboxylase (aromatic amino acid decarboxylase). This enzyme is widely distributed among various neuronal systems and is also unsuitable for use as a specific marker. In contrast to the other catecholamine biosynthetic enzymes, norepinephrine and epinephrine neurons alone contain the enzyme dopamine-β-hydroxylase, which converts DA to norepinephrine; thus, this enzyme is a marker for differentiating dopaminergic from other catecholamine-containing neuronal systems [see Cooper et al. (1982) for discussion].

The anatomy of DA systems appears to differ in at least one important respect from that of the other monoamines. Whereas noradrenergic and serotonergic systems project diffusely to a large number of areas, the DA systems innervate specific brain structures and are often oriented in distinct topographical projections within these structures. Categorized on the basis of their site of origin and termination, they can be divided into eight different systems (Moore and Bloom, 1978). (1) The nigrostriatal DA system has cell bodies in the substantia nigra zona compacta and innervates the striatum (caudate-putamen nucleus). This system, which forms the major component of the A9 cell group (Dahlström and Fuxe, 1964), is probably the best studied DA system to date due to its involvement in Parkinson's disease. (2) Mesocortical and mesolimbic DA systems have their somata primarily located in the ventromedial tegmental region of the mesencephalon (designated A10 by Dalström and Fuxe, 1964) and project either to cortical areas, including the prefrontal, cingulate, and entorhinal cortices, or to limbic structures such as the amygdaloid system and nucleus accumbens. It has been hypothesized that a dysfunction in one or more of these systems may be involved in the pathogenesis of schizophrenia. (3) The cell bodies of the tuberohypophyseal DA system are located in the arcuate nucleus of the hypothalamus and project to the median eminence and pituitary. These neurons are involved in regulating the release of pituitary hormones, the best studied of which is prolactin. (4) DA is also present within the inner nuclear layer of the retina in neurons known as interplexiform cells, which constitute 5–10% of the cells in the region (Gallego, 1971). These neurons send processes into the inner and outer plexiform layers of the retina. Four other CNS DA systems have been described although little is known about their functional role: (5) the incertohypothalamic DA system, (6) the periventricular DA neurons (7) the periglomerular DA cells located in the olfactory bulb, and (8) the diencephalospinal DA projection neurons.

Some dopamine neurons are located outside of the central nervous system. For example, DA can be found in glomus cells of the carotid body, as well as in small intensely fluorescent (SIF) cells of sympathetic ganglia. A subpopulation of dorsal root ganglion cells that contains DA has also been identified (Price and Mudge, 1983).

1.3. Dopamine Receptors

As is the case for other transmitters, there are more than a single class of receptor for DA. These receptor subtypes have been differentiated using a variety of techniques, such as ligand binding, linkage to adenylate cyclase, effects on neuronal firing or passive membrane properties, and gross behavioral effects. Although these various means of describing receptor subtypes have not been in total agreement with regard to subclassification schemes and nomenclature, one useful classification system based on behavioral, anatomical, and electrophysiological evidence subdivides DA receptors into two categories: "postsynaptic receptors" and "presynaptic receptors" ("autoreceptors"). Postsynaptic DA receptors are located on neurons innervated by DA cells, and can be preferentially blocked by the antipsychotic drug sulpiride. In contrast, autoreceptors are located on the DA neurons themselves, either on the DA cell body or on presynaptic terminals. Autoreceptors show a different pharmacological profile from postsynaptic DA receptors in that they are preferentially blocked by drugs such as metoclopramide (Alander et al., 1980).

1.3.1. Dopamine Postsynaptic Receptors

The ability of DA to stimulate cyclic AMP synthesis was first demonstrated in bovine superior cervical ganglia and later in brain (Kebabian and Calne, 1978). This neurochemical observation forms an important part of the current subclassification of DA receptors where a distinction is made between those DA receptors whose occupancy is linked to stimulation of adenylate cyclase (leading to increased cyclic AMP production) and those that either decrease or have no effect on cyclic AMP production. The receptor mediating stimulation of adenylate cyclase, designated D1, has been localized to both the striatum and the substantia nigra. Within the striatum D1 receptors appear to be located on cell bodies, as kainic acid lesions of the striatum result in their loss. Although there are D1 receptors in the substantia nigra, lesions of nigral DA neurons do not reduce the number of these receptors. However, these nigral D1 receptors are eliminated by lesions of the striatonigral feedback loop, indicating that D1 receptors in the substantia nigra are located not on DA cells, but on the terminals of striatonigral afferents.

DA receptors not linked to adenylate cyclase have been termed D2 receptors, and can be differentiated from D1 receptors on the basis of their preferential binding of butyrophenone DA antagonists and agonists such as apomorphine. Furthermore, the neuroleptics sulpiride and molindone preferentially block D2 receptors, while having little or no effect on D1 receptors (Kebabian and Calne, 1979). D2 receptors are present within the substantia nigra and striatum. Nigral D2 receptors are greatly reduced following lesions of DA neurons, suggesting that they reside on DA cell bodies. Within the striatum, these receptors are located both on cell bodies (since they are reduced by intrastriatal kainic acid) and on corticostriatal terminals (since decortication reduces the number of striatal D2 binding sites). Furthermore, this subclass of striatal DA receptors becomes supersensitive after DA lesions. D2 receptors have been associated with behavioral responses to DA agonists and antagonists and it is believed that dopaminergic drugs act at these sites to ameliorate the symptoms of Parkinson's disease. Seeman (1980) has proposed, based on differential binding of DA agonists and antagonists, the existence, of two additional DA receptor subtypes designated D3 and D4, but the physiological relevance of these sites is unclear.

Although in vitro binding techniques have proven useful in describing binding characteristics of receptors, they are limited in their ability to localize the receptors to specific brain regions. A recent advance has been the ability to visualize DA binding sites autoradiographically. Radioactively labeled ligands, such as the D2 antagonist [³H]spiroperidol, when injected intravenously specifically accumulate at DA binding sites thus allowing the in situ localization of the receptors (Kuhar et al., 1978). A shortcoming of the in vivo labeling techniques is the inability to control conditions during binding, making delineation of receptor subtype difficult. One solution to this problem was the adoption of in vitro autoradiographic binding methods in which brain slices are incubated with the appropriate ligands, and the resultant sections subjected to autoradiography (Fig. 1; Palacios et al., 1981). A variant of these labeling techniques that can be applied to human subjects uses positron emission tomography (PET) (Wagner et al., 1983). Intravenous injection of the positron-emitting ligand 3-N-[¹¹C]methylspiperone into baboons and humans both in the presence and absence of excess unlabeled blockers allowed the visualization of specific DA binding sites in the awake experimental subject. This technique may prove itself of great value in assessing the functional state of DA receptors in a number of clinical syndromes.

1.3.2. Dopamine Autoreceptors

In addition to DA receptors that exist on cells located in the postsynaptic target areas of DA neurons, there is biochemical and physiological evidence

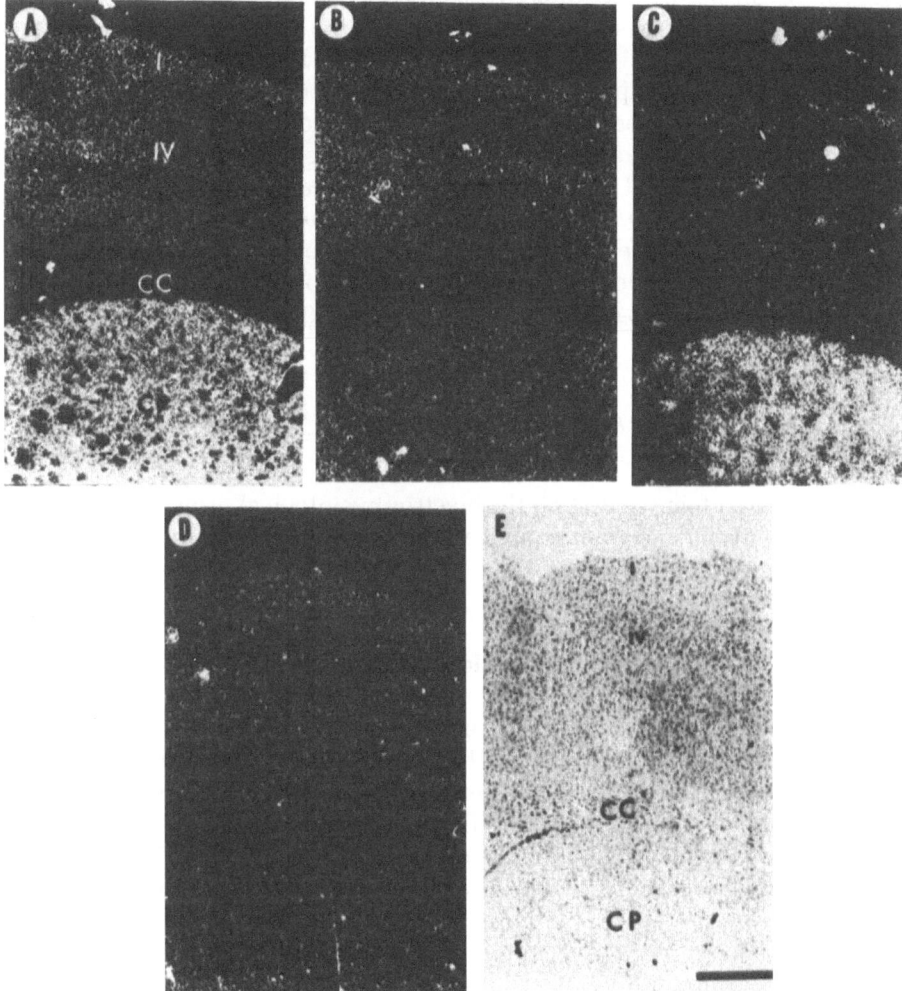

Figure 1. Autoradiography of [³H]spiroperidol binding sites in rat cortex and striatum. (A),(B),(C), and (D) are dark-field illumination micrographs and show autoradiographic grain distributions over tissue sections consecutive to the one shown in (E), a bright-field micrograph, where the autoradiographic grains cannot be seen. (A) Total binding, i.e. all [³H]spiroperidol (0.4 nM) binding sites. (B) What remains after 10⁻⁶ M ADTN; that which is displaced represents dopaminergic receptor binding. The binding in laminae I and IV is unaffected while the binding in the caudate (CP) is markedly decreased. (C) Cinanserin (3 × 10⁻⁷ M) displaceable binding; that which is displaced represents serotonin receptor binding. Note the blockade of binding in lamina IV of the cortex and the lack of effect in striatum. (D) Haloperidol (10⁻⁷ M) displaceable binding; some binding remains in lamina I. Bar = 500 μm. The corpus callosum (CC) shows low total binding levels and no detected displaceable binding. (From Palacios et al., 1981, with permission.)

for DA receptors on DA neurons themselves. These "autoreceptors" (Carlsson, 1975) can be divided into two classes: (1) those located on the axon terminals of DA neurons which participate in the local control of DA synthesis and release, and (2) those located on the DA cell somatodendritic region which may be important in controlling DA cell firing rate (Aghajanian and Bunney, 1977). These somatodendritic autoreceptors have been shown to be much more sensitive to the effects of DA agonists than their postsynaptic counterparts (Skirboll et al., 1979). Autoreceptors are not, however, present on all central DA cells. DA neurons that project to the prefrontal and cingulate cortices, as well as those making up the tuberohypophyseal DA system, are devoid of both somatodendritic and terminal autoreceptors (Bannon et al., 1982; Chiodo et al., 1984; Moore and Demarest, 1982).

2. CENTRAL DOPAMINE NEURON ELECTROPHYSIOLOGY

This section focuses first on the electrophysiological properties of brain dopamine neurons and then considers the action of dopamine in postsynaptic target areas.

2.1. Electrophysiological Identification

Midbrain DA neurons in the A9 and A10 areas were the first DA neurons to be identified electrophysiologically (Bunney et al., 1973). This identification was accomplished through the use of four approaches, which established that the characteristic extracellular electrical activity of a set of neurons in these areas belonged to cells that contained DA (Fig. 2). The experimental observations were: (1) anatomical localization of the characteristic extracellular spike waveform to an area known to contain DA neurons, (2) absence of such spikes following treatment with the specific catecholamine neurotoxin 6-hydroxydopamine, (3) changes in the firing rate of these neurons induced by drugs believed to be specific dopamine agonists and antagonists, and finally (4) an increase in the fluorescence intensity of neurons surrounding the tip of the recording electrode induced by extracellular iontophoresis of the DA precursor L-DOPA (L-dihydroxyphenyl-alanine). Although these techniques were by their nature indirect, in combination they provided strong evidence that the characteristic extracellular units recorded in the A9 and A10 areas belonged to DA neurons. More recently, DA neurons have been unequivocally identified using intracellular recording combined with the injection of various compounds that increase intracellular DA levels and allow the specific cell recorded from to be identified with fluorescence histochemistry using the glyoxylic acid technique (Grace and Bunney, 1980, 1983a). The following compounds were used: (1) L-DOPA, to increase DA levels by precursor loading; (2) tetrahydrobiopterin,

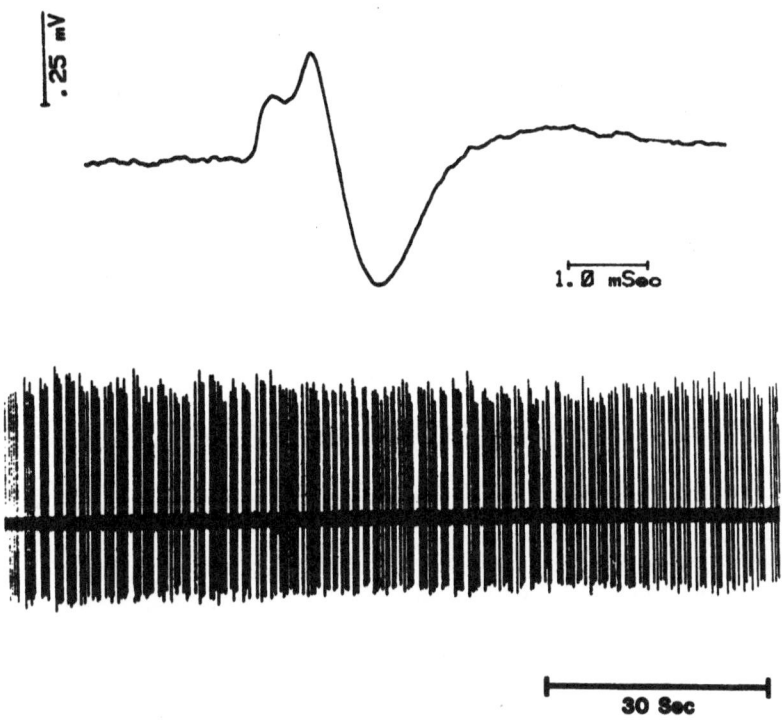

Figure 2. (Top) Representative oscilloscope tracing of a DA neuron action potential recorded extracellularly. The action potentials are long in duration and typically have a notch in the positive phase of the action potential (positive is up in all extracellular recordings shown). (Bottom) Extracellular recording of a train of DA neuron action potentials firing spontaneously, observed at a slower time base than above. The pattern is characteristically irregular, and often shows bursting, i.e., a train of 3–6 spikes of decreasing amplitude.

an analog of the cofactor of tyrosine hydroxylase (the rate-limiting enzyme of DA synthesis) to increase DA synthesis; and (3) colchicine, to allow accumulation of DA in the soma. In each case, the fluorescence intensity of the injected DA cell was enhanced relative to its neighbors. However, no fluorescence was observed following injection of these compounds into nondopaminergic neurons (Fig. 3).

Nigrostriatal and mesocortical/mesolimbic DA neurons were also identified by antidromic activation from their terminal fields (Guyenet and Aghajanian, 1978; Thierry et al., 1978; Grace and Bunney, 1980, 1983a). Cells in both areas demonstrated the characteristic features of antidromically activated DA neurons: (1) slow conduction velocity of the axon (approximately 0.5 m/sec) and (2) activation of only an initial segment (IS) spike under most circumstances. If a full IS-SD (initial segment and somatodendritic) spike was activated, it rapidly deteriorated to an IS spike with stimulation rates above 10 Hz. Both the IS and the IS-SD spikes were found to collide with spontaneously occurring or directly elicited action potentials (Fig. 4).

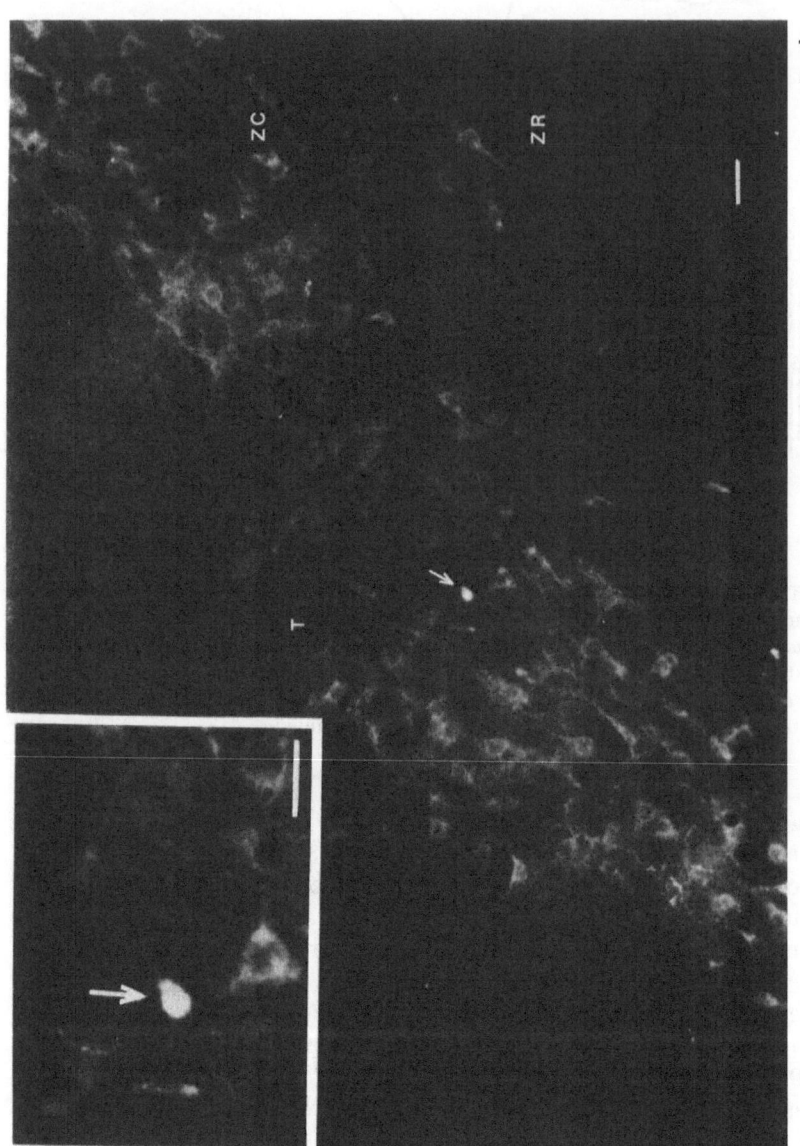

Figure 3. A DA cell injected intracellularly with L-DOPA (arrow) is seen fluorescing at a much greater intensity than the neighboring noninjected DA cells after processing for catecholamine histofluorescence. Inset shows higher magnification of same cell. An electrode track (T) leads to the injected neuron. ZC = zona compacta; ZR = zona reticulata. Scale bar = 50 μm (inset: bar = 25 μm).

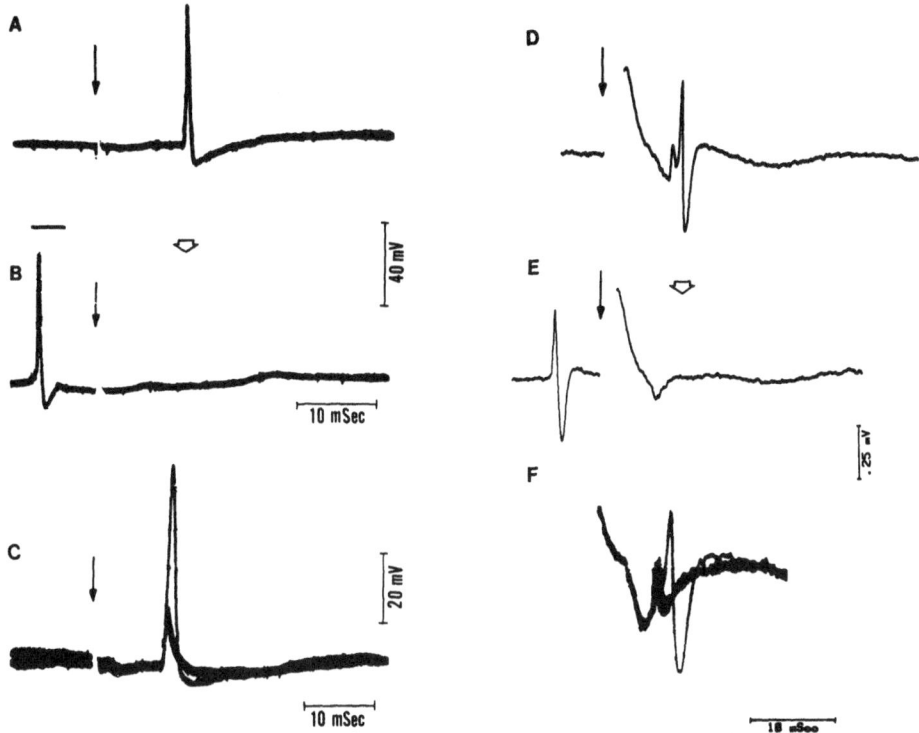

Figure 4. Antidromic activation and collision of dopaminergic neuron action potentials during intracellular (A,B,C) and extracellular (D,E,F) recording. (A) Stimulation of the caudate (arrow) during intracellular recording resulted in an action potential which demonstrated constant latency (not shown). (B) Intracellular current injection (0.15 nA at bar) resulted in an action potential which collided with the antidromically elicited action potential (open arrow marks spike failure). (C) High frequencies of antidromic stimulation (e.g., 20 Hz) reduced the action potential to the axon hillock spike after an initial full amplitude spike was activated by the first stimulus in the train. (D) During extracellular recording, caudate stimulation (arrow) resulted in an antidromic action potential in DA neurons at a constant latency. (E) Collision of the antidromically elicited action potential (open arrow) with a spontaneously occurring extracellular action potential. (F) High-frequency stimulation reduced the extracellular action potential to the axon hillock spike (time calibration slightly longer than in D and E for clarity). (From Grace and Bunney, 1983a, with permission.)

2.2. Morphology

Most morphological studies of neurochemically identified DA neurons have been carried out in the A9 region using either catecholamine histofluorescence (Lindvall and Björklund, 1978) or intracellular injections of the fluorescent dye Lucifer yellow (Grace and Bunney, 1983b) (Fig. 5). DA cells lie in a thin band in the most dorsal region of the substantia nigra, the zona compacta. The more ventral substantia nigra is called the zona reticulata; it contains a number of non-DA containing interneurons and projection cells. Zona compacta DA cells are reported to have small (12–30 μm diameter),

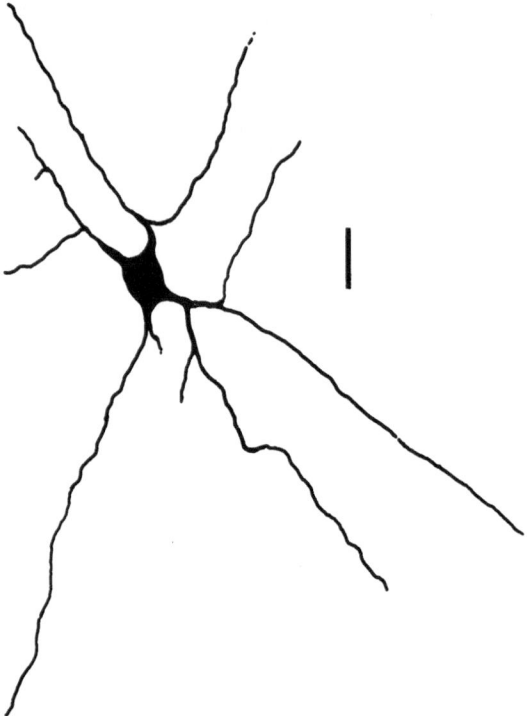

Figure 5. Tracing of a serially recon-
structed DA neuron following intracellular injection of the dye Lucifer
yellow. Dendrites emerge from the
neuron's poles and bifurcate approximately 15–30 μm from the soma. Four
major dendrites were seen to course
100–200 μm laterally and ventrally into
the zona reticulata, with the axon typically arising from one of these processes (not shown). Scale bar = 25
μm.

pyramidal or polygonally shaped somata with 3–6 large (4–8 μm diameter)
dendrites extending from their poles. These dendrites extend over 30 μm
before bifurcating, then continue to course laterally and ventrally through
the zona reticulata for distances of over 300 μm. The dendrites join together
in bundles with closely apposed membranes that may represent the morphological correlate of the electrical or chemical (DA-mediated) coupling
between DA neurons (see below). The thin (0.5 μm diameter), unmyelinated
axon arises from one of these major dendrites at a distance of approximately
30 μm from the soma before travelling medially to join the medial forebrain
bundle where it ascends to rostral structures. Nigral neurons displaying a
similar morphology have also been observed in studies using the Golgi staining technique (Juraska et al., 1977).

2.3. Electrophysiological Characteristics

The membrane electrophysiology of DA neurons has been studied in
the rat using *in vivo* intracellular recording techniques (Grace and Bunney,
1983a,b,c). DA neurons have a comparatively large input resistance (31 MΩ)
and long time constant (15 msec). The intracellularly recorded action potential duration is quite long (2–5 msec) and corresponds closely to that
observed extracellularly (Bunney et al., 1973).

The DA cell action potential has a prominent notch in its rising phase, corresponding to the initial segment (IS) spike. If, as suggested on the basis of morphological studies, the IS spike is indeed generated at a dendritic segment distal to the soma, one would expect a low safety factor for somatodendritic invasion. This would result in the IS spike having low reliability for triggering a full action potential. Such low reliability was, indeed, observed during antidromic activation. It can be overcome and a full IS-SD spike obtained by injecting depolarizing current into the soma. Further depolarization, however, leads to a progressive decrease in amplitude and increase in duration of the SD spike until it completely inactivates.

The relative ease with which DA neurons undergo depolarization inactivation appears to be a fundamental characteristic of these cells. Thus, DA cell inactivation is obtained by injection of the potent excitatory amino acid analog kainic acid into the caudate nucleus, or by local application of the excitatory amino acid glutamate or the excitatory peptide cholecystokinin by means of iontophoresis. A state of tonic depolarization inactivation can be induced by chronic administration of the DA receptor blocking agent haloperidol, which excites DA neurons (see below) (Bunney and Grace, 1978).

2.4. Endogenous Pacemaker Activity

The slow, irregular spontaneous firing pattern of DA neurons seems to result from a spontaneously occurring slow depolarization of about 15 mV which brings the membrane potential from its resting level (typically 58–62 mV) to spike threshold (40–42 mV) over a period of about 70 msec (Fig. 6). This depolarization triggers the IS spike and supplies the depolarized condition necessary for the IS spike to trigger the SD spike with high reliability despite the low safety factor. The SD spike, which is at least partially calcium mediated, is followed by a hyperpolarizing afterpotential. Evidence suggests that this hyperpolarization is caused by calcium entry during spike generation resulting in a potassium efflux (calcium-activated potassium conductance or $I_{K(Ca)}$ [Meech, 1978]). The hyperpolarization then decays into the next slow depolarization and spike. DA cells can be made to fire in a pacemaker pattern by interfering with the $I_{K(Ca)}$. Thus, intracellular injection of the calcium chelator EGTA into DA neurons in vivo (Fig. 7b; Grace and Bunney, 1983d, 1984b) or removal of calcium from the bathing medium in in vitro nigral slice preparations (Sanghera et al., 1983) causes DA cells to fire in a very regular, nonbursting pattern.

2.5. Firing Pattern

Dopamine neurons typically fire in one of two patterns: (1) slow (3–6 Hz) irregularly spaced single action potentials generated by the pacemaker activity described above or (2) bursts of spikes separated by longer silent intervals. Burst firing consists of groups of 3–10 action potentials with a

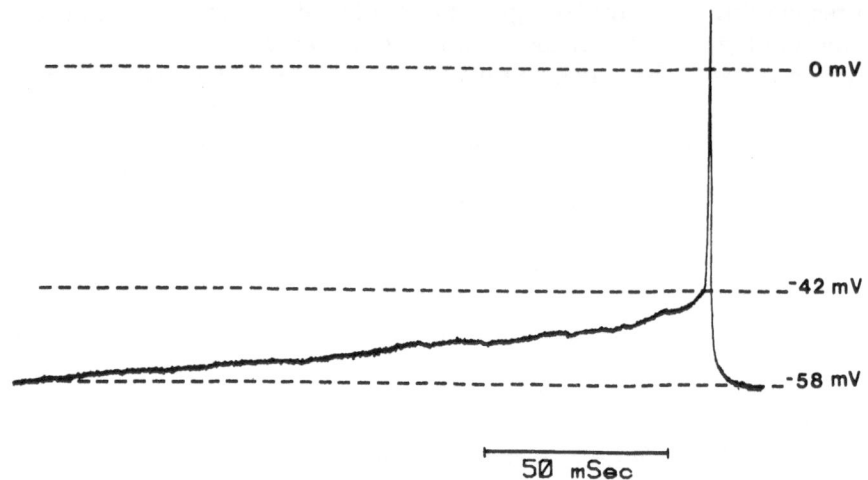

Figure 6. DA cell action potentials were observed to arise from slow depolarizations. The slow depolarization bridges the voltage difference between the resting membrane potential (−58 mV) and the atypically high IS spike threshold (−42 mV) characteristic of DA neurons. The action potential triggered by the slow depolarization is followed by an AHP that brings the membrane potential back to baseline levels prior to the onset of the next slow depolarization.

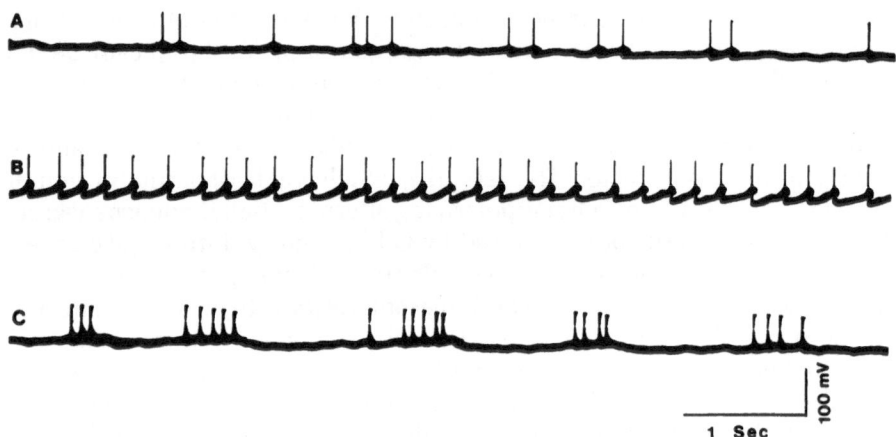

Figure 7. Effects of manipulating intracellular calcium levels on DA cell firing pattern. Recorded intracellularly, DA cells typically fire in a slow, irregular pattern (A). However, if the $I_{K(Ca)}$ is blocked by injecting the calcium chelator EGTA intracellularly, the underlying regular, pacemaker firing pattern mediated by the slow depolarization is revealed (B). Conversely, if calcium is injected intracellularly, the DA cell will change into a rapid burst firing mode (C). Thus, the firing pattern of DA cells appears to be regulated between a pacemaker and a rapid burster by the intracellular levels of calcium.

mean interspike interval of about 70 msec (Fig. 8). Within the burst, spikes show a progressive decrease in amplitude and increase in duration. These bursts differ from those observed in other brain regions in several respects: (1) a long interspike interval (70 msec, versus 5–10 msec observed in the hippocampus, cerebellum, and thalamus); (2) an increase in the interspike interval as the DA cell burst progresses; and (3) an inability of short depolarizing pulses to elicit burst firing. DA neurons can be made to fire in bursts, however, by prolonged depolarization (e.g., with glutamate or cholecystokinin iontophoresis, haloperidol systemic administration, or minutes of constant depolarizing current injection). Also, unlike hippocampal pyramidal cells, which fire prolonged bursts in response to EGTA injection (Johnston et al., 1980), intracellular injection of the calcium chelator EGTA actually prevents depolarization from eliciting burst firing in DA cells. Conversely, intracellular injection of calcium leads to burst firing (Fig. 7c; Grace and Bunney, 1983d, 1984c). Furthermore, blockade of a potassium conductance (by intracellular injection of the potassium channel blocker tetraethylammonium or extracellular iontophoresis of barium) also triggers burst firing. The precise mechanism whereby calcium and potassium regulate burst firing is unknown.

Burst firing may be important in increasing release of DA in postsynaptic target sites, since the interspike interval observed during burst firing is the

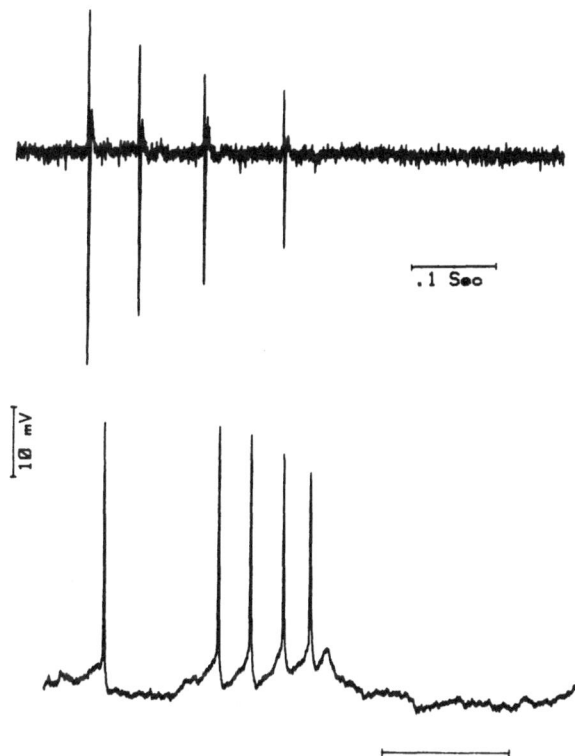

Figure 8. Spontaneously occurring bursts recorded extracellularly and intracellularly in DA neurons. (Top) During extracellular recording, DA cells were observed to spontaneously fire in a bursting pattern consisting of 3–10 spikes of decreasing amplitude and increasing duration. Interspike intervals within the burst were typically near 70 msec, and usually increased as the burst progressed. (Bottom) DA neurons recorded intracellularly were also observed to spontaneously fire in bursts. The spikes within the burst also displayed progressive increases in duration and decreases in amplitude, with similar temporal relationships as observed extracellularly. The burst was also observed to ride on a depolarizing wave which often extended beyond the last spike in the burst before repolarizing (From Grace and Bunney, 1984a, with permission.)

same as that which results in maximal release of DA postsynaptically (Redgrave and Mitchell, 1982), and burst firing has been correlated with a large release of neurohumor in a number of other systems.

2.6. Electrical Coupling

Neighboring DA neurons recorded extracellularly have been shown to occasionally fire in near synchrony with an interspike interval of approximately 2.3 msec (Fig. 9) (Wilson et al., 1977; Grace and Bunney, 1983c). This phenomenon is especially apparent after haloperidol pretreatment. The synchronous firing occurs more often during bursts, with the driven neuron firing with a shorter delay as the burst progresses (Grace and Bunney, 1983c). Such effects have been described in invertebrate systems and appear to result from electrical coupling. However, it is now clear that electrical synapses are quite common in the mammalian nervous system as well.

A direct electrical interaction between DA neurons is further suggested by the fact that intracellular injection of the dye Lucifer yellow into single DA neurons often results in the labeling of adjacent DA neurons. This is

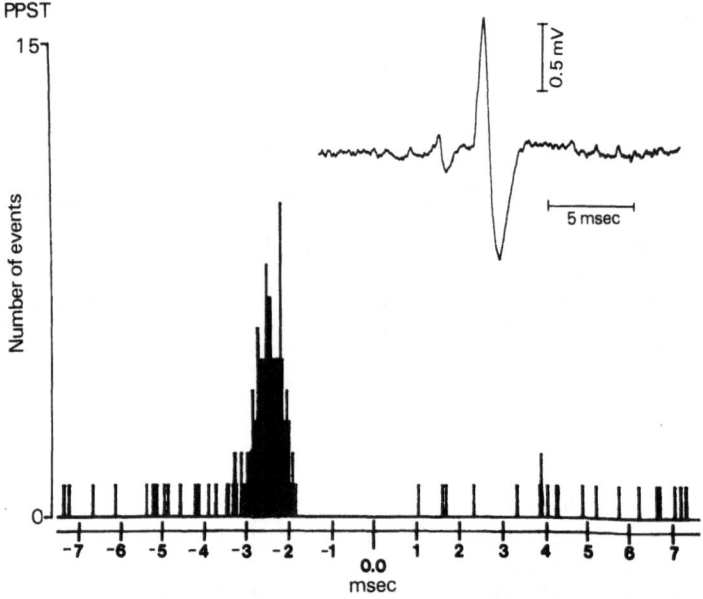

Figure 9. Nearly simultaneously occurring action potentials from two different dopaminergic neurons were commonly observed extracellularly (inset) following haloperidol pretreatment. The cross correlation histogram of a series of 500 paired spikes demonstrates that these two DA cells were firing action potentials separated by a time interval distributed around 2.5 msec. The vertical lines indicate the cumulative interspike intervals between a series of these paired action potentials. The bin width was 30 μsec. (From Grace and Bunney, 1983c, with permission.)

probably due to the ability of Lucifer yellow to cross gap junctions between electrically coupled cells, although the specificity of this technique has been questioned.

Intracellular recording also has provided evidence in favor of electrical coupling between midbrain DA neurons. Thus, when stimulation of DA cell terminal fields fails to produce an antidromic spike, it often results in one or more small (3–15 mV) fast potentials, with the same latency as that observed for antidromic activation. These potentials can be collided with spontaneously occurring small potentials (Grace and Bunney, 1980), but not with directly elicited action potentials. The frequency of the small potential's spontaneous occurrence can also be varied by injection of depolarizing or hyperpolarizing current (Grace and Bunney, 1983c). These small potentials do not have characteristics in common with synaptically mediated events and could reflect electrotonic spread of current from electrically coupled neighboring DA cells that fire spikes in response to antidromic stimulation.

2.7. Autoreceptor Stimulation

DA neurons are known to store DA in their dendrites and release DA in a calcium-dependent manner (Korf et al., 1976; Geffen et al., 1976; Nieoullon et al., 1977). Moreover, nigral DA neurons are very sensitive to their own neurotransmitter and its agonists, being potently inhibited both by systemically administered apomorphine and by iontophoretically administered DA and DA analogs ((Fig. 10; Aghajanian and Bunney, 1977; Bunney et al., 1973). The inhibitory effects of agonists applied directly to DA cells are thought to be due to the presence of DA "autoreceptors" on the cell bodies and dendrites of these neurons. Electrophysiological studies have demonstrated that the autoreceptor is many times more sensitive to DA agonists than is the DA postsynaptic receptor (Skirboll et al., 1979).

A possible behavioral demonstration of the relative difference in sensitivity of autoreceptors and postsynaptic receptors is the finding that low doses of systemically administered DA agonists actually *decrease* the behavioral correlates of dopaminergic influence in the caudate, producing behaviors with some characteristics similar to that of DA antagonists. It is believed that low doses of DA agonists *decrease* the amount of DA reaching postsynaptic sites by preferentially inhibiting the more sensitive DA cells themselves. Dopamine-mediated behaviors can be elicited upon administration of higher doses of the agonist, presumably due to a direct interaction with the postsynaptic DA receptors. Both the electrophysiological (Fig. 10) and behavioral effects of postsynaptically active doses of DA agonists are reversed by intravenously administered DA blockers, such as haloperidol.

The autoreceptor is known to undergo rapid desensitization (tachyphylaxis) with repeated applications of DA agonists. Thus, during the recovery phase from inhibition by intravenously administered apomorphine, additional doses of the drug are much less effective in depressing firing. However,

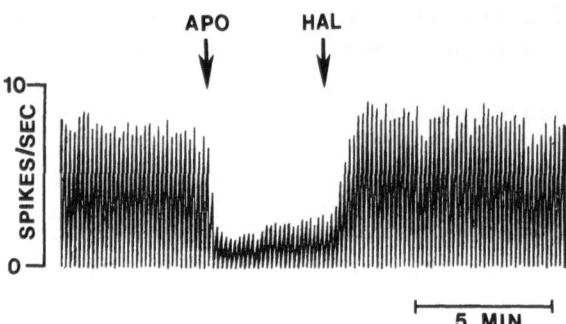

Figure 10. Rate histogram of a spontaneously firing DA neuron showing inhibition by apomorphine (10 μg/kg, i.v., at arrow) and reversal of the inhibition by haloperidol (50 μg/kg, i.v., at arrow). Each vertical line represents a 10-sec epoch, with the height of the line proportional to the firing rate.

once the cell's activity has increased back to baseline levels its original sensitivity to the inhibitory effect of apomorphine returns (Fig. 11). This tachyphylaxis can also be observed with DA iontophoresis.

Intracellular recording studies have demonstrated that low doses of apomorphine have three effects on DA cells (Grace and Bunney, 1983a, 1984a,

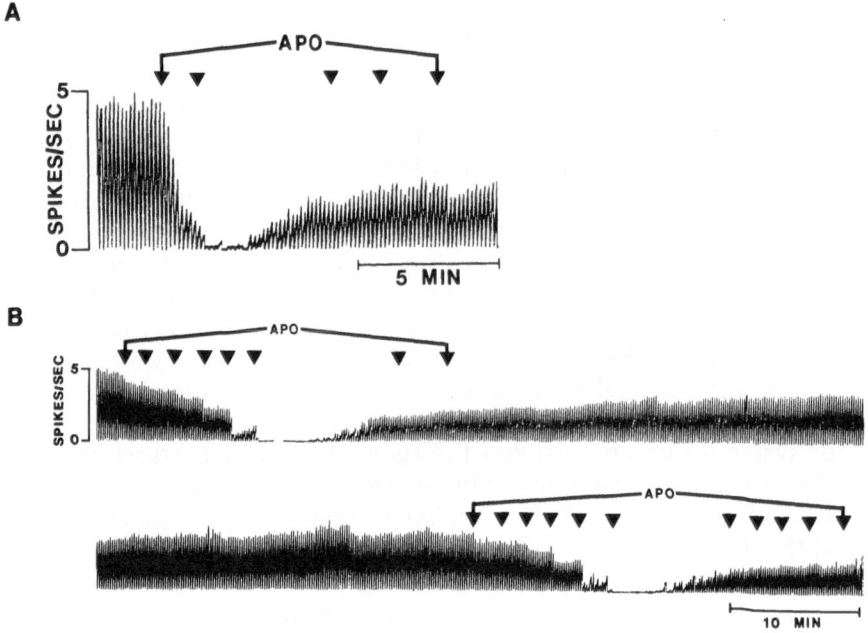

Figure 11. Induction of apomorphine tachyphylaxis in DA cells by prior administration of apomorphine. (A) A DA neuron demonstrating its typical inhibition to i.v. apomorphine will, during the initial stages of recovery, display little sensitivity to the inhibitory effects of this DA agonist and will often fail to respond even to subsequent administration of higher doses of apomorphine (Apomorphine doses in μg/kg = 10,10; 10, 20, 40 administered at arrows). (B) If a DA neuron inhibited by apomorphine is allowed to recover its baseline firing rate, it will also completely recover its sensitivity to inhibition by apomorphine. Subsequent apomorphine doses administered prior to this full recovery display the typical tachyphylactic response. (Apomorphine doses in μg/kg = 1, 1, 2, 4, 8, 16, 32; 1, 1, 2, 4, 8, 16; 4, 8, 16, 32, 64; administered at arrows.)

1985b): (1) inhibition of the slow depolarization that precedes each spike, leading to cessation of spontaneous firing, (2) a small hyperpolarization of the membrane, and (3) an increase in input resistance (Fig. 12). Evidence indicates that this response is actually composed of two subcomponents: a direct effect on the DA cell and an indirect response generated via the feedback pathway originating in the striatum (Grace and Bunney, 1985a). Thus, when the striatonigral feedback pathway is destroyed by a brain lesion, the effect of apomorphine on input resistance is eliminated, although the hyperpolarization is still observed. It appears that the input resistance increase reflects suppression of tonically active GABAergic inputs to DA cells secondary to decreasing DA input to the striatum, whereas the hyperpolarization occurs as a direct result of apomorphine acting on autoreceptors.

2.8. Dopamine Neuron Explants

In addition to investigating the electrophysiology of DA neurons *in vivo* or in *in vitro* slice preparations, extracellular recordings have been made from DA neurons transplanted from fetal rats into adult rat brain ventricles

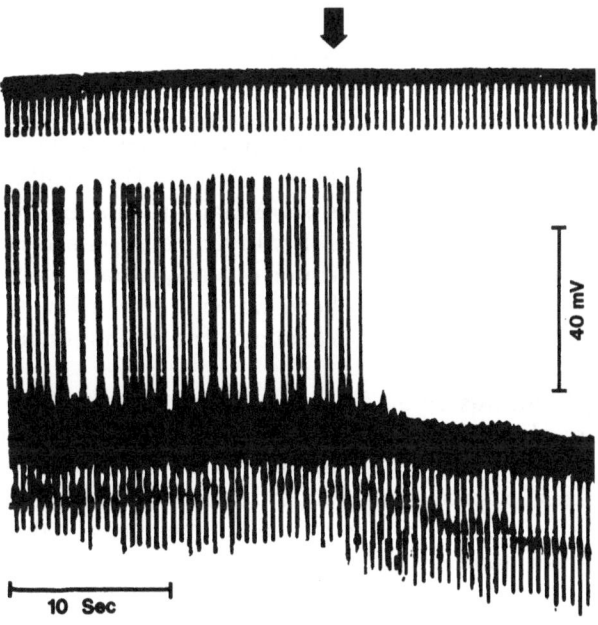

Figure 12. Effects of apomorphine on DA cell electrophysiology during intracellular recording. Intracellular injection of equal amplitude hyperpolarizing current pulses (1.0 nA, top) resulted in membrane deflections proportional to the membrane input resistance (bottom). During intracellular recording, i.v. apomorphine (20 μg/kg, at arrow) resulted in an inhibition of spontaneous firing and a hyperpolarization of the membrane potential. Apomorphine consistently increased DA neuron input resistance, as observed by the increase in the amplitude of the membrane potential deflections. (From Grace and Bunney, 1983a, 1984a, with permission.)

(Wuerthele et al., 1980). These DA neurons were spontaneously active, had spike waveforms similar to those reported in vivo, and could be inhibited by DA agonists. This inhibition was reversed by DA antagonists. Behavioral studies indicate that these transplanted DA neurons can restore function in rats with lesions of DA systems, and there is hope that such transplants may be useful in human disease (Perlow et al., 1979; Freed et al., 1980).

3. POSTSYNAPTIC ACTIONS OF DOPAMINE IN THE CENTRAL NERVOUS SYSTEM

Extracellular recordings have shown dopamine to be inhibitory in a number of brain regions. The following discussion will be limited, however, to those areas where intracellular as well as extracellular recording techniques were used in an attempt to elucidate membrane mechanisms. Despite the similarities in the effects on cell firing, however, intracellular mechanisms differ and a satisfactory understanding of the membrane events underlying the action of DA is still not at hand.

3.1. Striatum

The striatum has been the most intensively investigated target area of DA neurons. Some of the reasons for this interest include: (1) the dense DA innervation of the striatum arising from a circumscribed cell group, (2) the well-characterized behavioral effects of DA manipulation in this system, and (3) the clinical significance of striatal DA in the pathogenesis of Parkinson's disease and dyskinetic syndromes. Unfortunately, to date, electrophysiological studies in the striatum have been rather unrewarding and even the fundamental issue of whether DA is excitatory or inhibitory is strongly contested.

In almost all studies using extracellular recording techniques, spontaneously firing or glutamate-activated striatal cells were inhibited by iontophoretically applied DA or systemically administered DA agonists. Electrical stimulation of the substantia nigra produced similar effects (Moore and Bloom, 1978). In contrast, with intracellular recording some investigators have found excitatory responses to nigral stimulation (Kitai, 1982). However, in each of these studies the latency of striatal cell excitation by nigral stimulation demonstrated that the response was elicited by axons conducting at speeds of at least 1 m/sec or more. DA cell antidromic activation from the striatum, on the other hand, indicates that DA cell axons conduct at velocities of about 0.5 m/sec. (Guyenet and Aghajanian, 1978; Grace and Bunney, 1980). Thus, when synaptic delay is taken into consideration, the excitation of striatal cells by nigral stimulation occurs at velocities about two times faster than the DA cell axons are capable of conducting an impulse to this region. At least three alternative explanations may be proposed for this excitation: (1) the excitation arises via antidromic activation of a striatonigral cell with excitatory connections to the cell under study; (2) the excitation is from direct activation of a non-DA fast-conducting nigrostriatal pathway, as previously described (Guyenet and Crane, 1981); or 3) the excitation is disynaptically mediated or is mediated by fibers passing through the nigra.

Another study (Wilson et al., 1982) attempted to localize the short-latency striatal excitatory response to nigral stimulation using intracellular recording techniques. These authors separated this excitatory response into three components: one that was eliminated by decortication, a second that could be eliminated by thalamic pathway transection, and the last, a long latency excitation that was ascribed to a DA input. Although the *average* latency of inhibition was similar to the conduction velocity of nigral DA neuron axons (without allowing for any synaptic delay), the *range* of latencies for the excitatory response included intervals much too short for even the fastest conducting DA cell axons (over 1 m/sec). Moreover, studies by Feltz and DeChamplain (1972) demonstrated that 6-hydroxydopamine pretreatment was ineffective in decreasing this nigrally mediated striatal excitation. Therefore, the evidence for an excitatory effect of DA in the striatum arising from stimulation of the nigra remains at best controversial.

Studies of the response of striatal neurons to iontophoretically applied DA are also inconclusive. The first experiment was carried out using very short (2–100 msec) pulses of iontophoretic DA (Kitai et al., 1976). Although DA applied in this manner led to excitation of striatal cells, which could be blocked by the DA antagonist (Fig. 13), the results have been questioned on the basis that the current pulses were too short to overcome ionic tip dilution caused by the retaining current (Moore and Bloom, 1978). Moreover, subsequent investigations have failed to replicate this DA effect using similar drug ejection parameters (Bernardi et al., 1978).

A second intracellular recording study suggestive of an excitatory effect of DA on striatal cells was performed by Norcross and Spehlmann (1978). The effects of DA application on the responses of striatal neurons to stimulation of an excitatory afferent were investigated. DA iontophoresis was found to increase the number of evoked spikes, while concurrent administration of the DA antagonists haloperidol, fluphenazine, or chlorpromazine blocked this enhancement. The ionic basis of this increased synaptic efficacy was not further elucidated.

Two electrophysiological investigations combining iontophoresis and intracellular recording found DA to have inhibitory effects on striatal neurons. In both studies DA iontophoresis caused a depolarization of striatal neurons accompanied by a cessation of spontaneous firing (Bernardi et al., 1978; Herrling and Hull, 1980). The basis for this paradoxical effect was suggested by studies in which the distance between recording and iontophoretic pipette was varied. With minimal tip separation some neurons showed an initial hyperpolarization followed by a depolarization. With larger

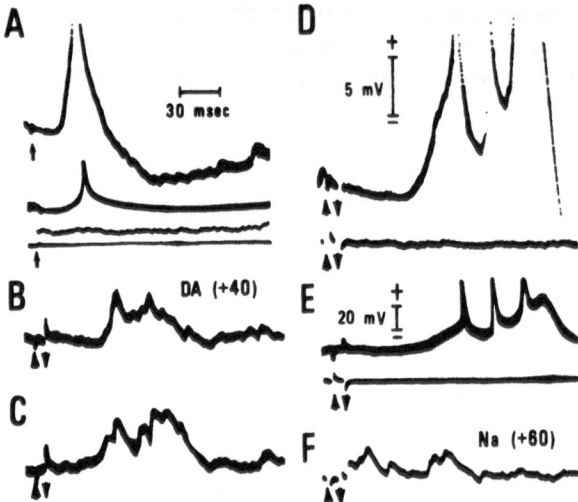

Figure 13. Intracellular recording from caudate neurons. (A) Action potential evoked by substantia nigra stimulation. Top two traces high gain AC and low gain DC record respectively. Bottom two traces, respective extracellular records. (B) Depolarization caused by iontophoretic DA (40 nA, 10 msec). An enhanced effect of successive doses (5 msec) of DA on the same cell is shown in (C) (second dose), (D) (high-gain AC records), and (E) (low gain DC records) (fourth dose). (F) Effect of iontophoretic Na$^+$ on the same neuron. Bottom traces in (D) and (E) are the extracellular control records. (From Kitai et al., 1976, with permission.)

tip separations, only the depolarizing response was observed. It is suggested that the effect of DA at the soma of striatal cells is hyperpolarization, but depolarization occurs when DA reaches distant sites, possibly on dendrites. Fluphenazine blocked both of these responses to DA iontophoresis but did not affect the depolarization and increase in spike frequency obtained by iontophoresis of the excitatory amino acid glutamate, suggesting that both responses reflect an interaction with specific DA receptors. This differential effect of a neurotransmitter, depending on its site of application, has also been observed in the hippocampus with respect to GABA application (see Chapter 2).

In accord with these latter physiological studies, substantial pharmacological evidence confirms that DA has a net inhibitory action on striatal neurons. First, acute and chronic haloperidol administration increases the number of spontaneously active striatal neurons (Filion, 1979; Skirboll and Bunney, 1979). Second, both electrolytic and 6-hydroxydopamine lesions of the nigrostriatal DA pathway increase the spontaneous activity of striatal cells (Arbuthnott, 1976; Filion, 1979; Hull et al., 1974; Ohye et al., 1970; Schultz and Ungerstedt, 1978a,b; Siggins et al., 1976; Steg, 1969; Ungerstedt et al., 1978). These effects can be reversed by systemic administration of apomorphine or L-DOPA (Arbuthnott, 1976; Schultz and Ungerstedt, 1978b). Third, low autoreceptor-specific doses of DA agonists disinhibit striatal cells (i.e., increase their spontaneous activity), whereas higher doses of these drugs inhibit striatal cells (Chiodo and Bunney, 1983; Skirboll et al., 1979). Fourth, intracerebroventricular L-DOPA, which presumably leads to increased DA release, causes a net decrease in striatal cell activity (Shellenberger et al., 1977).

Thus, the majority of evidence indicates that dopamine acts in the striatum in an inhibitory manner. However, given the complexity of DA actions in the striatum, it is probably naïve to attempt to describe DA function in these simple terms. In fact, based upon the ability of L-DOPA and DA agonists to ameliorate the symptoms of Parkinson's disease, a role for DA in the *modulation* of striatal activity is probably more likely.

3.2. Frontal Cortex

Extracellular recordings have shown DA to potently inhibit the firing of neocortical neurons (Krnjevic and Phillis, 1963; Yarbrough et al., 1974). Specific effects of DA are best localized to layers V and VI of the prefrontal cortex (Bunney and Aghajanian, 1976), which are the layers known to contain DA projections and fibers (Berger et al., 1976; Moore and Bloom, 1978). Intracellular recording from neocortical neurons should help elucidate the membrane mechanism underlying this inhibitory action; however, at present the data is fragmentary. Stimulation in the substantia nigra results in the generation of an EPSP/IPSP sequence in cortical neurons (Bernardi et al., 1982). Moreover, 50% of the cells tested with iontophoretic DA (50–200 nA ejection current) responded with depolarization and decreased firing rate with little change in input resistance (Fig. 14). This effect is similar to that

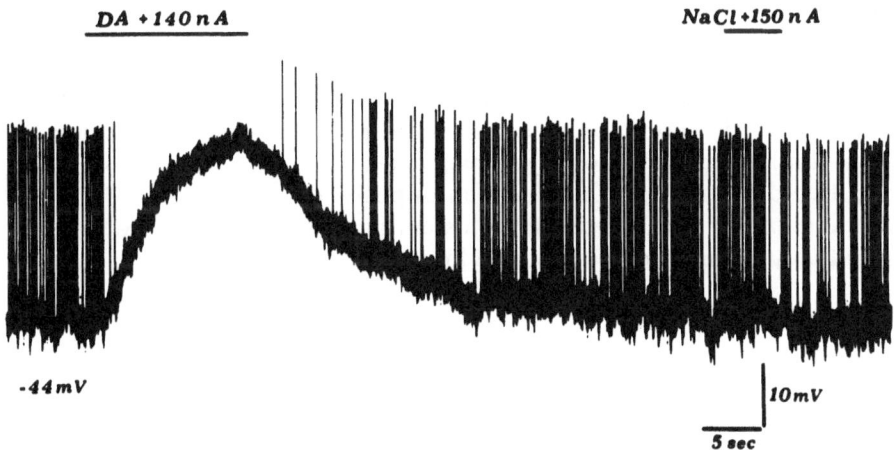

Figure 14. Effect of iontophoretically applied DA on a cortical neuron: 140 nA depolarizes the cell and suppresses spontaneous firing. Same amount of Na$^+$, used for current control, had no effect. (From Bernardi et al., 1982, with permission.)

described by this same group of investigators for the effects of DA on neurons in the striatum (Bernardi et al., 1978). However, in both of these studies spike amplitudes were quite small, suggesting that some damage probably was incurred by the impaled cell.

3.3. Hippocampus

Although there are demonstrated projections from A9 and A10 DA systems (Scatton et al., 1980), a physiologically relevant function for DA in the hippocampus is unclear at present. Iontophoretically administered DA has been shown to inhibit hippocampal neurons recorded extracellularly (Biscoe and Straughan, 1966; Segal and Bloom, 1974). The membrane characteristics of this inhibition have been examined using intracellular recording in vivo and in tissue slices in vitro. In vivo, iontophoretically applied DA elicited a hyperpolarizing response that was accompanied by a large increase in input resistance (Herrling, 1981). However, comparatively high iontophoretic ejection currents were required in this study, raising the possibility that nonspecific effects may have been produced.

In in vitro studies, Benardo and Prince (1982a,b) found that DA hyperpolarized hippocampal pyramidal cells and *decreased* input resistance (Fig. 15). It was suggested that the primary effect of DA was an enhancement of a calcium-activated potassium conductance ($I_{K(Ca)}$). This conclusion was based on three lines of evidence: (1) the reversal potential of the DA effect was near the equilibrium potential for potassium; (2) the afterhyperpolarization following a spike train (believed due to activation of the $I_{K(Ca)}$) was increased in amplitude and duration with DA administration; and (3) both intracellular injection of EGTA (a calcium chelator) and to some extent extracellular application of Mn^{2+} (a calcium blocker) prevented DA-induced hyperpolarization and DA enhancement of the afterhyperpolarization. The DA effect was blocked by the DA antagonists flupenthixol and chlorpromazine and was mimicked by cyclic AMP, lending additional support to the specificity of dopaminergic action. From a functional point of view, potentiation of spike afterhyperpolarization by enhancement of the $I_{K(Ca)}$ could suppress repetitive discharge and thus have an opposite effect to that produced by norepinephrine (see Chapter 8) or histamine (see Chapter 10), which depress the $I_{K(Ca)}$ and thereby promote firing.

3.4. Retina

Some of the most valuable work on the central actions of DA has been carried out in the retina of fish and turtles. Horizontal cells in these species have a well characterized input from dopaminergic interplexiform cells (Dowling and Ehringer, 1978). Moreover, there is a DA-sensitive adenylate cyclase in the retina that is activated by low micromolar concentrations of

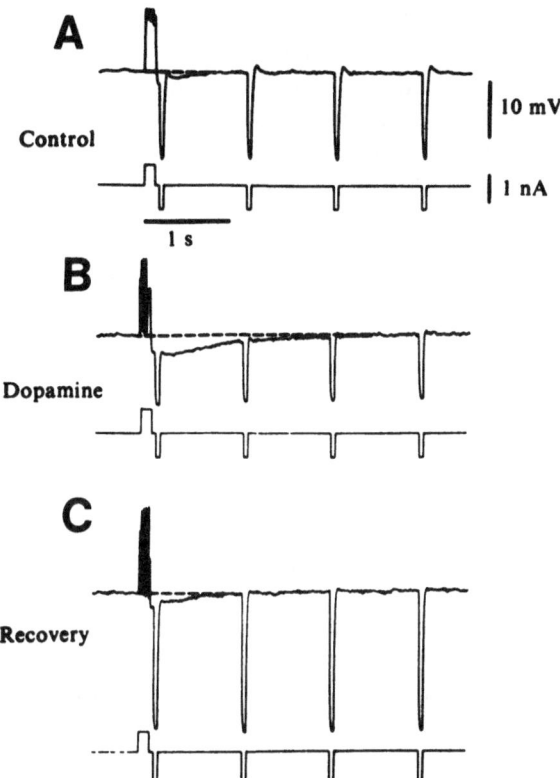

Figure 15. Intracellular recording from a CA₁ hippocampal pyramidal cell showing effect of DA on afterhyperpolarizations (AHPs) induced by depolarizing current pulses. (A) Chart recording of control response to a depolarizing pulse. The AHP lasts 600 msec reaches 2 mV in amplitude, and is associated with a peak decrease in resistance of 11%. (B) Following DA application (10 μM) this cell hyperpolarized (not shown) and input resistance decreased. The membrane was depolarized to the resting potential of (A) and the amplitude of the depolarizing current pulse adjusted to elicit a number of spikes comparable to those of the stimulus in (A). This was necessary because of a decrease in baseline input resistance of 35% compared with the control. In these conditions, AHPs lasted for 2.5 sec, reached 4 mV in amplitude, and were associated with proportionately larger decreases in resistance (peak decrease of 20%). (C) Recovery of AHPs to control duration and amplitude was seen in this same neuron 45–60 min after DA application. (From Benardo and Prince, 1982a, with permission.)

DA and can be blocked by nanomolar concentrations of the DA antagonists haloperidol, fluphenazine and (+)-butaclamol (Watling and Dowling, 1981). In the intact retina, DA was observed to depolarize horizontal cells and decrease the light evoked response (Hedden and Dowling, 1978); however, these studies used relatively high and possibly nonphysiological concentrations of DA. In contrast, isolated carp horizontal cells maintained in tissue culture show no change in membrane potential or input resistance to either DA or cyclic AMP and its membrane permeable analogs, dibutyryl and

8-bromo cyclic AMP (Dowling et al., 1983). This had been interpreted as indicating that the DA-sensitive adenylate cyclase system present in horizontal cells does not mediate direct effects on membrane ionic conductance mechanisms, although it should be noted that tissue-cultured neurons often spontaneously lose their neurotransmitter responsiveness.

More recent studies have uncovered two apparently specific effects of DA in the turtle retina (Piccolino et al, 1982). First, it was observed that low concentrations of DA or the DA agonists epinine, apomorphine, or ADTN will induce a decrease in the receptive field size of horizontal cells. Second, this response is accompanied by a marked reduction in the diffusion of Lucifer yellow dye between adjacent horizontal cells. It is well established that horizontal cells are extensively coupled electrically and that the size of the receptive field of these neurons reflects this coupling. Therefore, both observations have been interpreted in terms of a decrease mediated by DA in the conductance of gap junctions between horizontal cells. In support of this hypothesis is the finding that intraocular injections of 6-hydroxydopamine, which destroy retinal dopaminergic neurons, cause an increase in the receptive field size of horizontal cells (Cohen and Dowling, 1983; Teranishi et al., 1983).

Of particular significance is the observation that both the effect on receptive field size and the diffusion of Lucifer yellow are mimicked by forskolin, a nonspecific activator of adenylate cyclase, and by isobutyl methylxanthine, a phosphodiesterase inhibitor. It has therefore been proposed that dopamine, acting via receptors coupled to adenylate cyclase, causes an increase in the level of intracellular cyclic AMP and this in turn reduces the conductance of gap junctions which interconnect horizontal cells. Ultimately, this results in a reduction in the size of the receptive field of these neurons.

Experiments in the carp retina have provided evidence confirming this view. Application of DA to the intact carp retina decreases the lateral spread of light-evoked hyperpolarizing responses (S potentials) and restricts the diffusion of intracellularly injected Lucifer yellow. Both of these effects are blocked by haloperidol and can be mimicked by dibutyryl cyclic AMP (Teranishi et al., 1983).

As noted in the preceding section, DA neurons in the substantia nigra show presumed electrical interactions more frequently after blockade of DA receptors with haloperidol, suggesting that DA may also be capable of uncoupling electrical synapses in this region as well (Grace and Bunney, 1983c). As in the retina, proof of this action of DA will require a combined biochemical, structural and electrophysiological analysis.

3.5. Interactions with Other Transmitters

In addition to the apparent direct actions of DA on cell firing in the brain areas detailed above, DA has also been shown to modulate the actions of other neurotransmitters on postsynaptic target cells. To date, electrophysiological studies have indicated that DA can interact with GABA and enkephalin, but other interactions are possible.

In the substantia nigra, DA is known to be released locally from DA cell dendrites (see Section 2.7) where it is believed to inhibit neighboring DA neurons (Groves et al., 1975). However, in addition to acting on DA cell autoreceptors, DA may also affect the firing of non-DA-containing zona reticulata neurons. In extracellular iontophoretic studies, DA was demonstrated to specifically decrease GABAergic inhibition of zona reticulata neurons (Waszczak and Walters, 1983). Thus, excitation of zona reticulata neurons by DA (Ruffieux and Schultz, 1980) could be mediated by depression of the inhibition produced by tonically released GABA. The action of DA on zona reticulata neurons has important functional considerations in terms of the integration of basal ganglia output, since it suggests that dopaminergic neurons regulate a major striatal output station (i.e., the zona reticulata nigrothalamic projection) in addition to the striatum itself.

This modulatory effect of DA on GABAergic inhibition has also been demonstrated in the globus pallidus. The globus pallidus receives DA projections from the substantia nigra (Lindvall and Bjorklund, 1979), as well as GABA input from the striatum (Fonnum et al., 1978). A possible interaction between these pathways was suggested by extracellular iontophoretic studies showing DA to excite pallidal neuron firing, apparently by attenuating GABAergic inhibition of pallidal neurons (Bergstrom and Walters, 1984). As yet, the cellular basis underlying the specific modulatory action of DA on GABA-mediated inhibition in the substantia nigra or globus pallidus is unknown.

In addition to interacting with GABA, DA also appears to regulate opioid transmission in the frontal cortex. In this brain region, as in many others, the catecholaminergic innervation is complemented by a prominent enkephalinergic projection (Palmer et al., 1983). Enkephalin iontophoresis inhibits prefrontal neurons. However, this inhibition can be attenuated by blockade of DA receptors or by lesioning the DA input (Palmer and Hoffer, 1980). This evidence suggests that the enkephalin actions in the cortex are dependent on a DA innervation.

Thus, numerous extracellular recording studies have shown DA to be capable of exerting direct effects on DA autoreceptors and postsynaptic cells, as well as modulating the actions of other neurotransmitters.

4. POSTSYNAPTIC ACTIONS OF DOPAMINE IN THE PERIPHERAL NERVOUS SYSTEM

Due to the complexities encountered when attempting to study the actions of DA in the central nervous system, many investigators have turned to the relatively simpler peripheral systems. Three systems have been used:

the superior cervical ganglion, the carotid body, and the dorsal root ganglion. Although these regions may provide a more accessible preparation, the dense sympathetic innervation characteristic of peripheral nervous systems presents problems with regard to distinguishing the effects on DA receptors from those on norepinephrine receptors.

4.1. Superior Cervical Ganglion

Slow postsynaptic potentials in sympathetic ganglia in response to preganglionic stimulation have been known since the investigations of Eccles in 1943. Initial studies attributed these slow potentials to acetylcholine, since atropine was found to specifically block these effects. However, Libet (1970) proposed that the inhibitory component (slow IPSP) of preganglionic stimulation was actually mediated by an excitatory effect of acetylcholine on adrenergic interneurons. The adrenergic transmitter responsible for this resultant inhibition was hypothesized to be DA (Libet and Tosaka, 1970; Tosaka and Libet, 1970). This has now been shown to be incorrect, and the current view is that the slow IPSP is mediated directly by acetylcholine acting on ganglion cells (see Chapter 6).

Despite this setback, there is some evidence that DA does play a role in ganglionic transmission, not as a mediator of the cholinergic potentials, but rather as a modulator to produce a long-lasting enhancement of the slow EPSP and slow IPSP. This alternative view is supported by extracellular recordings from isolated rabbit sympathetic ganglia using the air-gap technique (Fig. 16; Ashe and Libet, 1981). In the presence of an inhibitor of catechol-o-methyltransferase (COMT) to prevent its metabolism, DA produced a prolonged enhancement of the amplitude of both slow muscarinic PSPs, but not the fast nicotinic EPSP. This effect was prevented by the D1 antagonists spiroperidol and butaclamol, but not the D2 antagonists metoclopramide and sulpiride, or the α-antagonist dihydroergotamine. Therefore, the modulation of ganglionic transmission by DA is clearly attributed to activation of D1 receptors; however, it remains to be determined whether this occurs because of the stimulation of adenylate cyclase.

4.2. Carotid Body

The glomus cells of the carotid body are known to be dopaminergic (Bolme et al., 1977; Karasawa et al., 1982) and are believed to modulate the activity of chemo- and baroreceptors by a dopaminergic mechanism (Eyzaguirre and Fidone, 1980). DA has been shown to decrease the rate of chemoreceptor discharge (Zapata, 1975) at a dose of DA too low to cause changes in systemic arterial blood pressure (Llados and Zapata, 1978a). Furthermore, this DA effect can be blocked by DA blockers (spiroperidol, chlorpromazine, haloperidol: Llados and Zapata, 1978b; and flupenthixol:

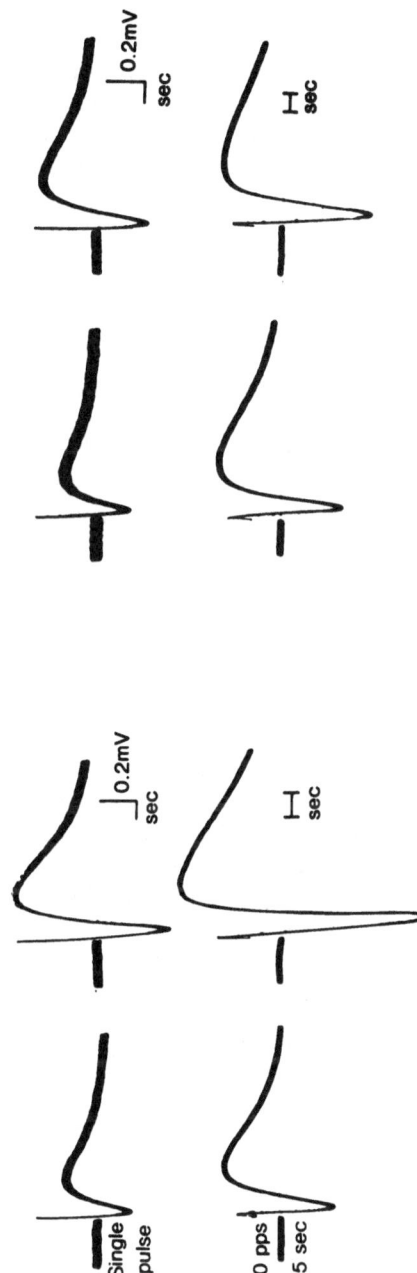

Figure 16. Air-gap extracellular recording from a curarized rabbit superior cervical ganglion demonstrating potentiation of slow EPSP and slow IPSP by DA after pretreatment with an inhibitor of catechol-o-methyltransferase (U-0521). Various stimulation protocols are used to selectively activate the two slow potentials. Top row shows slow EPSP best; bottom row shows slow IPSP best. (A) Left pair, control; right pair, after pretreatment with U-0521 and in the presence of DA (50 μM). (B) Another ganglion, but in the presence of 7 μM (+)-butaclamol. (Adapted from Ashe and Libet, 1981, with permission.)

Docherty and McQueen, 1978); whereas norepinephrine usually causes increases in discharge rates which can be blocked by phenoxybenzamine (Llados and Zapata, 1978b).

In two studies where intracellular recording techniques were used, DA was found to depolarize glomus cells and decrease their rate of discharge (Eyzaguirre and Fidone, 1980; Matsumoto et al., 1982). However, in both cases, rather small resting membrane potentials were reported for the cells investigated.

4.3. Dorsal Root Ganglion

Sensory neurons in dorsal root ganglia isolated from cat respond to DA with a sustained membrane depolarization (Gallagher et al., 1980). This effect seems to be accompanied by a decrease in membrane conductance as determined in experiments where the membrane potential was held constant by passing a continuous hyperpolarizing current through the recording electrode ("manual voltage clamp"). Although rather high concentrations of DA are required to elicit this response (ED_{50} = 0.13 mM), it was specifically antagonized by the DA blockers haloperidol and chlorpromazine without altering the response of the cells to GABA. Apomorphine was at least twice as effective as DA at depolarizing dorsal root ganglion neurons, whereas norepinephrine was much less potent; phentolamine was ineffective at blocking either neurotransmitter. Thus, although high doses of DA were required to produce a response, some pharmacological specificity was demonstrated. The physiological significance of these observations is as yet unknown, although if similar DA receptors are located on terminals of dorsal root ganglia neurons they could serve as targets for spinal cord DA neurons or even DA-containing sensory neurons (see Section 1.2). In line with this idea is the observation that DA depolarizes dorsal root terminals in the isolated toad spinal cord (Phillis and Kirkpatrick, 1979).

5. CONCLUSION

Although DA has been shown to have a net inhibitory effect in most systems examined (Table 1), intracellular recording has shown that this effect can occur via a number of different ionic mechanisms. In contrast to the situation for other transmitters, inhibition of firing caused by DA is, in some cases, associated with a *depolarization* rather than a hyperpolarization. The nature of this depolarizing response is, at present, unclear although in some preparations it seems to occur by an action of DA on distal processes. In other cases, DA-induced inhibition could be consequent to other nonconventional effects, such as extending the inhibitory period following spike activity due to potentiation of a Ca^{2+}-dependent K^+ conductance (as in the

Table 1. Effects of DA Agonists on Central and Peripheral Target Sites

Area	Net effect on neuronal firing	Cyclic AMP mediated	Effect on membrane potential	Effect on input resistance	Proposed mechanism	Reference
Central nervous system						
Substantia nigra, DA cells	Inhibition	No	Hyperpolarization	Negligible increase	Inactivates slow potential	Grace and Bunney (1983a, 1985b)
Striatum, small spiny cells	Inhibition	?	Hyperpolarization	None	?	Herrling and Hull (1980)
Hippocampus, pyramidal cells	Inhibition	Yes	Hyperpolarization	None/increase	Activation of $I_{K(Ca)}$	Benardo and Prince (1982a,b), Herrling (1981)
Prefrontal cortex, pyramidal cells	Inhibition	?	Depolarization	None	?	Bernardi et al. (1978)
Retina, horizontal cells	Inhibition	Yes	None	None	Decreases gap junction conductance	Piccolino et al. (1982)
Peripheral nervous system						
Superior cervical ganglion	n/t[a]	Possible	n/t	n/t	Potentiate slow cholinergic EPSP and IPSP	Ashe and Libet (1981)
Carotid body	Inhibition	?	Depolarization	n/t	?	Eyzaguirre and Fidone (1980), Matsumoto et al. (1982)
Dorsal root ganglion	Inhibition	?	Depolarization	Increase	?	Gallagher et al. (1980)

[a] n/t = not tested.

hippocampus), decreasing electrical coupling interactions (as in the retina and possibly the nigral DA cells), or inhibiting slow pacemaker depolarizations (as in nigral DA neurons). Similar responses to DA application have been described in a variety of invertebrate preparations including activation of a CA^{2+}-dependent K^+ conductance, which causes hyperpolarization in the cockroach salivary gland (Ginsborg et al., 1980) and inhibition of an inward pacemaker potential in *Aplysia* (Wilson and Wachtel, 1978). In the later case the dopamine receptor is pharmacologically different from those present in vertebrates (Gospe and Wilson, 1981).

One important factor in assessing the responses of neurons to DA, as well as to any other neurotransmitter, is specificity of action. This is especially true with respect to the catecholamines, since there is an overlap in the agonist sensitivity of the various catecholamine receptors. Another important consideration is whether DA neurons project to the region under study. Moreover, the actions of locally administered DA must be correlated with synaptic activation of dopaminergic pathways. The slow conduction velocity of all the DA systems studied to date (0.4–0.6 m/sec) can provide a useful additional criterion for establishing a monosynaptic effect produced by stimulation of long pathways. Such stimulation effects should be eliminated by the catecholamine neurotoxin 6-hydroxydopamine. Finally, the pharmacological properties of the putative DA receptor must be characterized with selective DA agonists and antagonists. In no case have all of these criteria been convincingly satisfied, although progress is being made in a number of systems.

An unexpected observation encountered during the analysis of dopamine's cellular actions is its effects on electrical coupling between retinal horizontal cells, which seems to be mediated by the second messenger cyclic AMP. This discovery is the first of a spectrum of potential novel physiological actions of neurotransmitters, pointing out that the conventional electrophysiological measures of membrane potential and ionic conductance are insufficient to fully specify the action of a transmitter.

REFERENCES

Alander, A., Anden, N.-E., and Grabowska-Anden, N. S., 1980, Metoclopramide and sulpiride as selective blocking agents of pre- and postsynaptic dopamine neurons, *Naunyn Schmiedebergs Arch. Pharmacol.* **312**:145–150.

Andén, N. E., 1979, Historical introduction, in: *The Neurobiology of Dopamine* (A. S. Horn, J. Korf, and B. H. C. Westerink, eds.), Academic Press, London, pp. 1–7.

Aghajanian, G. K., and Bunney, B. S., 1977, Dopamine "autoreceptors": Pharmacological characterization by microiontophoretic single unit recording studies, *Nauyn Schmiedebergs Arch. Pharmacol.* **297**:1–7.

Arbuthnott, G. W., 1976, Supersensitivity of dopamine receptors, in: *Biochemistry and Neurology* (P. Bradford and C. D. Marsden, eds.), Academic Press, London, pp. 27–34.

Ashe, J. H., and Libet, B., 1981, Modulation of slow postsynaptic potentials by dopamine in rabbit sympathetic ganglion, *Brain Res.* **217**:93–106.

Bannon, M. J., Reinhard, J. F., Bunney, E. B., and Roth, R. H., 1982, Mesocortical dopamine neurons: Unique response to antipsychotic drugs explained by the absence of terminal autoreceptors, *Nature* **296**:444–446.

Benardo, L. S., and Prince, D. A., 1982a, Dopamine action on hippocampal pyramidal cells, *J. Neurosci.* **2**:415–423.

Benardo, L. S., and Prince, D. A., 1982b, Dopamine modulates a Ca^{2+}-activated postassium conductance in mammalian hippocampal pyramidal cells, *Nature* **297**:76–79.

Berger, B., Thierry, A. M., Tassin, J. P., and Moyne, M. A., 1976, Dopaminergic innervation of the rat prefrontal cortex: A fluorescence histochemical study, *Brain Res.* **106**:133–145.

Bergstrom, D. A., and Walters, J. R., 1984, Dopamine attenuates the effects of GABA on single unit activity in the globus pallidus, *Brain Res.* **310**:23–33.

Bernardi, G., Marciani, M. G., Morocutti, C., Pavone, F., and Stanzione, P., 1978, The actions of dopamine on rat caudate neurons recorded intracellularly, *Neurosci. Lett.* **8**:235–240.

Bernardi, G., Cherubini, E., Marciani, M. G., Mercuri, N., and Stanzione, P., 1982, Responses of intracellularly recorded cortical neurons to the iontophoretic application of dopamine, *Brain Res.* **245**:267–274.

Biscoe, T. J., and Straughan, D. W., 1966, Micro-electrophoretic studies on neurons in the cat hippocampus, *J. Physiol. (Lond.)* **183**:341–359.

Bolme, P., Fuxe, K., Hökfelt, T., and Goldstein, M., 1977, Studies on the role of dopamine in cardiovascular and respiratory control; central versus peripheral mechanisms, *Adv. Biochem. Psychopharmacol.* **16**:281–290.

Bunney, B.S., and Aghajanian, G. K., 1976, Dopamine and norepinephrine innervated cells in the rat prefrontal cortex: Pharmacological differentiation using microiontophoretic techniques, *Life Sci.* **19**:1783–1792.

Bunney, B. S., and Grace, A. A., 1978, Acute and chronic haloperidol treatment: Comparison of effects on nigral dopaminergic cell activity, *Life Sci.* **23**:1715–1728.

Bunney, B. S., Walters, J. R., Roth, R. H., and Aghajanian, G. K., 1973, Dopaminergic neurons: Effect of antipsychotic drugs and amphetamine on single cell activity, *J. Pharmacol. Exp. Ther.* **185**:560–571.

Carlsson, A., 1975, Dopaminergic autoreceptors, in: *Chemical Tools in Catecholamine Research*, Vol. II (O. Almgren, A. Carlsson, and J. Engel, eds.), North-Holland, Amsterdam, pp. 219–225.

Chiodo, L. A., and Bunney, B. S., 1983, Electrophysiological studies on EMD 23 448 (an indole-2-butylamine) in the rat: A putative selective dopamine autoreceptor agonist, *Neuropharmacology* **22**:1087–1093.

Chiodo, L. A., Bannon, M. J., Grace, A. A., Roth, R. H., and Bunney, B. S., 1984, Absense of autoreceptors on a subpopulation of mesocortical dopamine neurons: Electrophysiological and biochemical evidence, *Neuroscience* **12**:1–16.

Cohen, J. L., and Dowling, J. E., 1983, The role of the retinal interplexiform cell: effects of 6-hydroxydopamine on the spatial properties of carp horizontal cells, *Brain Res.* **264**:307–310.

Cooper, J. R., Bloom, F. E., and Roth, R. H., 1982, *The Biochemical Basis of Neuropharmacology*, Third Edition, Oxford University Press, New York, pp. 1–327.

Dahlström, A., and Fuxe, K., 1964, Evidence for the existence of monoamine-containing neurons in the central nervous system, *Acta Physiol. Scand. [Suppl.]* **232**:1–55.

Docherty, R. J., and McQueen, D. S., 1978, Inhibitory action of dopamine on cat carotid chemoreceptors. *J. Physiol. (Lond.)* **279**:425–436.

Dowling, J. E., and Ehringer, B., 1978, The interplexiform cell system. I. Synapses of the dopaminergic neurons of the goldfish retina, *Proc. R. Soc. Lond. B.* **201**:7–26.

Dowling, J. E., Lasater, E. M., Van Buskirk, R., and Watling, K., 1983, Pharmacological properties of isolated fish horizontal cells. *Vision Res.* **23**:421–432.

Eccles, J. C., 1943, Synaptic potentials and transmission in sympathetic ganglion, *J. Physiol. (Lond.)* **101**:465–483.

Eyzaguirre, C., and Fidone, S. J., 1980, Transduction mechanisms in carotid body: Glomus cells, putative neurotransmitters, and nerve endings, *Am. J. Physiol.* **239**:C135–C153.

Feltz, P., and DeChamplain, J., 1972, Enhanced sensitivity of caudate neurons to microiontophoretic injections of dopamine in 6-hydroxydopamine treated cats, *Brain Res.* **43**:601–605.

Filion, M., 1979, Effects of interruption of the nigrostriatal pathway and of dopaminergic agents on the spontaneous activity of globus pallidus neurons in the awake monkey, *Brain Res.* **178**:425–441.

Fonnum, F., Gottesfield, A., and Grofova, I., 1978, Distribution of glutamate decarboxylase, choline acetyltransferase and aromatic amino decarboxylase in the basal ganglia of normal and operated rats. Evidence for striatopallidal, striatoentopeduncular and striatonigral GABAergic fibers, *Brain Res.* **143**:125–128.

Freed, W. J., Perlow, M. J., Karoum, F., Seiger, A., Olson, L., Hoffer, B. J., and Wyatt, R. J., 1980, Restoration of dopaminergic function by grafting of fetal rat substantia nigra to the caudate nucleus. Long-term behavioral, biochemical and histochemical studies, *Ann. Neurol.* **8**:510–519.

Freedman, J. E., Gould, R. J., and Snyder, S. H., 1983, Neuroleptics exhibit noncompetitive effects at dopamine receptors, *Neurosci. Abst.* **9**:32.

Gallagher, J. P., Inokuchi, H., and Shinnick-Gallagher, P., 1980, Dopamine depolarization of mammalian primary afferent neurons, *Nature* **283**:770–772.

Gallego, A., 1971, Horizontal and amacrine cells in the mammal's retina, *Vision Res. (Suppl.)* **3**:33–50.

Geffen, L. B., Jessel, T. M., Cuello, A. C., and Iversen, L. L., 1976, Release of dopamine from dendrites in rat substantia nigra, *Nature* **260**:258–260.

Ginsborg, B. L., House, C. R., and Mitchell, M. R., 1980, On the role of calcium in the electrical responses of cockroach salivary gland cells to dopamine, *J. Physiol. (Lond.)* **303**:325–335.

Gospe, S. M., Jr., and Wilson, W. A., Jr., 1981, Pharmacological studies of a novel dopamine-sensitive receptor mediating burst-firing inhibition of neurosecretory cell R15 in *Aplysia California*, *J. Pharmacol. Exp. Ther.* **216**:368–377.

Grace, A. A., and Bunney, B. S., 1979, Paradoxical GABA excitation of nigral dopaminergic cells: Indirect mediation through reticulata inhibitory neurons, *Eur. J. Pharmacol.* **59**:211–218.

Grace, A. A., and Bunney, B. S., 1980, Nigral dopamine neurons: Intracellular recording and identification using L-DOPA injection combined with fluorescence histochemistry, *Science* **210**:654–656.

Grace, A. A., and Bunney, B. S., 1983a, Intracellular and extracellular electrophysiology of nigral dopaminergic neurons. I. Identification and characterization, *Neuroscience* **10**:301–315.

Grace, A. A., and Bunney, B. S., 1983b, Intracellular and extracellular electrophysiology of nigral dopaminergic neurons. II. Action potential generating mechanisms and morphological correlates. *Neuroscience* **10**:317–331.

Grace, A. A., and Bunney, B. S., 1983c, Intracellular and extracellular electrophysiology of nigral dopaminergic neurons. III. Evidence for electrical coupling, *Neuroscience* **10**:333–348.

Grace, A. A., and Bunney, B. S., 1983d, Single spiking and burst firing in nigral dopamine neurons, *Soc. Neurosci.* **9**:1006.

Grace, A. A., and Bunney, B. S., 1984a, Nigral dopaminergic neurons—extracellular and intracellular electrophysiological characteristics, in: *Proceedings of the 5th International Catecholamine Symposium* (E. Usdin, A. Carlsson, A. Dalkström, and J. Engle, eds.), Alan R. Liss, New York, pp. 323–332.

Grace, A. A., and Bunney, B. S., 1984b, The control of firing pattern in nigral dopamine neurons: Single spike firing, *J. Neuroscience* **4**:2866–2876.

Grace, A. A., and Bunney, B. S., 1984c, The control of firing pattern in nigral dopamine neurons: Burst firing, *J. Neuroscience* **4**:2877–2890.

Grace, A. A., and Bunney, B. S., 1985a, Opposing effects of striatonigral feedback pathways on midbrain dopamine cell activity, *Brain Res.* (in press).

Grace, A. A., and Bunney, B. S., 1985b, Low doses of apomorphine elicit two opposing influences on dopamine cell electrophysiology, *Brain Res.* (in press).

Groves, P. M., Wilson, C. J., Young, S. J., and Rebec, G. V., 1975, Self-inhibition by dopaminergic neurons, *Science* **190**:522–529.

Guyenet, P. G., and Aghajanian, G. K., 1978, Antidromic identification of dopaminergic and other output neurons of the rat substantia nigra, *Brain Res.* **150**:69–84.

Guyenet, P. G., and Crane, J. K., 1981, Non-dopaminergic nigrostriatal pathway, *Brain Res.* **213**:291–305.

Hedden, W. L., and Dowling, J. E., 1978, The interplexiform cell system. II. Effects of dopamine on goldfish retinal neurons, *Proc. R. Soc. Lond. B* **201**:27–55.

Herrling, P. L., 1981, The membrane potential of cat hippocampal neurons recorded *in vivo* displays four different reaction-mechanisms to iontophoretically applied transmitter agonists, *Brain Res.* **212**:331–343.

Herrling, P. L., and Hull, C. D., 1980, Iontophoretically applied dopamine depolarizes and hyperpolarizes the membrane of cat caudate neurons, *Brain Res.* **192**:441–462.

Hornykiewicz, O., 1973, Parkinson's disease: From brain homogenate to treatment, *Fed. Proc.* **32**:183–190.

Hull, C. D., Levine, M. S., Buchwald, N. A., Heller, A., and Browning, R. A., 1974, The spontaneous firing pattern of forebrain neurons. I. The effects of dopamine and non-dopamine depleting lesions on caudate unit firing patterns, *Brain Res.* **73**:241–262.

Johnston, D., Hablitz, J. J., and Wilson, W. A., 1980, Voltage clamp discloses slow inward current in hippocampal burst-firing neurones, *Nature* **286**:391–393.

Juraska, J. M., Wilson, C. J., and Groves, P. M., 1977, The substantia nigra of the rat: A golgi study, *J. Comp. Neurol.* **172**:585–600.

Karasawa, N., Kondo, Y., and Nagatsu, I., 1982, Immunohistochemical and immunofluorescent localization of catecholamine-synthesizing enzymes in the carotid body of the bat and dog, *Arch. Histol. Jpn.* **45**:429–435.

Kebabian, J. W., and Calne, D. B., 1979, Multiple receptors for dopamine, *Nature* **277**:93–96.

Kitai, S. T., 1982, Electrophysiology of the corpus striatum and brain stem integrating systems, in: *Handbook of Physiology, The Nervous System II*, (S. R. Geiger, ed.), Williams & Wilkins, Baltimore, Maryland, pp. 997–1015.

Kitai, S. T., Sugimori, M., and Kocsis, J. D., 1976, Excitatory nature of dopamine in the nigro-caudate pathway, *Exp. Brain Res.* **24**:351–363.

Korf, J., Zieleman, M., and Westerink, B. H. C., 1976, Dopamine release in the substantia nigra, *Nature* **260**:257–258.

Krnjevic, K., and Phillis, J. W., 1963, Actions of certain amines on cerebral cortical neurons, *Br. J. Pharmacol.* **70**:471–490.

Kuhar, M. J., Murrin, L. C., Malouf, A. T., and Klemm, K., 1978, Dopamine receptor binding in vivo: The feasibility of autoradiographic studies, *Life Sci.* **22**:203–210.

Libet, B., 1970, Generation of slow inhibitory and excitatory postsynaptic potentials, *Fed. Proc.* **29**:1943–1956.

Libet, B., and Tosaka, T., 1970, Dopamine as a sympathetic transmitter and modulator in sympathetic ganglia: A different mode of synaptic action, *Proc. Natl. Acad. Sci.* **67**:667–673.

Lindvall, O., and Björklund, A., 1978, Organization of catecholamine neurons in the rat central nervous system, in: *Handbook of Psychopharmacolgy*, Vol. 9 (L. L. Iversen, S. D. Iversen, and S. H. Snyder, eds.), Plenum Press, New York, pp. 139–231.

Lindvall, O., and Björklund, A., 1979, Dopaminergic innervation of the globus pallidus by collaterals form the nigrostriatal pathway, *Brain Res.* **172**:169–173.

Llados, F., and Zapata, P., 1978a, Effects of dopamine analogues and antagonists on carotid body chemoreceptors in situ, *J. Physiol. (Lond.)* **274**:487–499.

Llados, F., and Zapata, P., 1978b, Effects of adrenoceptor stimulating and blocking agents on carotid body chemosensory inhibition, *J. Physiol. (Lond.)* **274**:501–509.

Matsumoto, S., Nakajima, T., Uchida, T., Ozawa, H., and Ushiyama, J., 1982, Effects of sodium cyanide, dopamine and acetylcholine on the resting membrane potential of glomus cells in the rabbit, *Brain Res.* **239**:674–678.

Meech, R. W., 1978, Calcium-dependent potassium activation in nervous tissues. *Annu. Rev. Biophys. Bioeng.* **7**:1–18.

Moore, K. E., and Demarest, K. T., 1982, Tuberoinfundibular and tuberohypophyseal dopaminergic neurons, in: *Frontiers in Neuroendocrinology*, Vol. 7 (W. F. Ganong and L. Martini, eds.), Raven Press, New York, pp. 161–190.

Moore, R. Y., and Bloom, F. E., 1978, Central catecholamine neuron systems: Anatomy and physiology of the dopamine systems, *Annu. Rev. Neurosci.* **2**:129–169.

Nieoullon, A., Cheramy, A., and Glowinski, J., 1977, Release of dopamine *in vivo* from cat substantia nigra, *Nature* **266**:375–377.

Norcross, K., and Spehlmann, R., 1978, A quantitative analysis of the excitatory and depressant effects of dopamine on the firing of caudatal neurons: Electrophysiological support for the existence of two distinct dopamine-sensitive receptors. *Brain Res.* **156**:168–174.

Ohye, C., Bouchard, R., Boucher, R., and Poirieer, L. J., 1970, Spontaneous activity of the putamen after chronic interruption of the dopaminergic pathways. Effects of L-DOPA, *J. Pharmacol. Exp. Ther.* **175**:700–708.

Palacios, J. M., Niehoff, D. L., and Kuhar, M. J., 1981, ³H-Spiperone binding sites in brain: Autoradiographic localization of multiple receptors, *Brain Res.* **213**:277–289.

Palmer, M., and Hoffer, B., 1980, Catecholamine modulation of enkephalin-induced electrophysiological responses in cerebral cortex, *J. Pharmacol. Exp. Ther.* **213**:205–215.

Palmer, M. R., Sieger, A., Hoffer, B. J., and Olson, L., 1983, Modulatory interactions between enkephalin and catecholamines: Anatomical and physiological substrates, *Fed. Proc.* **42**:2934–2945.

Perlow, M. J., Freed, W. J., Hoffer, B. J., Seiger, A., Olson, L., and Wyatt, R. J., 1979, Brain grafts reduce motor abnormalities produced by destruction of nigrostriatal dopamine system, *Science* **204**:643–647.

Phillis, J. W., and Kirkpatrick, J. R., 1979, Action of biogenic amines on the isolated toad spinal cord, *Gen. Pharmacol.* **10**:115–119.

Piccolino, M., Neyton, J., Whitkovsky, P., and Gerschenfeld, H. M., 1982, gamma-Aminobutyric acid antagonists decrease junctional communication between L-horizontal cells of the retina, *Proc. Natl. Acad. Sci. USA* **79**:3671–3675.

Price, J., and Mudge, A. W., 1983, A subpopulation of rat dorsal root ganglion neurons is catecholaminergic, *Nature* **301**:241–243.

Redgrave, P., and Mitchell, I., 1982, Functional validation of projection topography in the nigrostriatal dopamine system, *Neuroscience* **7**:885–894.

Ruffieux, A., and Schultz, W., 1980, Dopaminergic activation of reticulata neurones in the substantia nigra, *Nature* **285**:240–241.

Sanghera, M. K., Trulson, M. E., and German, D. C., 1983, *In vitro* electrophysiological and pharmacological properties of midbrain dopamine neurons in the mouse, *Soc. Neurosci. Abst.* **9**:1005.

Scatton, B., Simon, H., LeMoal, M., and Bischoff, S., 1980, Origin of dopaminergic innervation of the rat hippocampal formation, *Neurosci. Lett.* **18**:125–131.

Schultz, W., and Ungerstedt, U., 1978a, Striatal cell supersensitivity to apomorphine in dopamine-lesioned rats correlated to behavior, *Neuropharmacology* **17**:349–353.

Schultz, W., and Ungerstedt, U., 1978b, Short-term increase and long-term reversion of striatal cell activity after degeneration of the nigrostriatal dopamine system, *Exp. Brain Res.* **33**:159–171.

Seeman, P., 1980, Brain dopamine receptors, *Pharmacol. Rev.* **32**:229–313.

Segal, M., and Bloom, F. E., 1974, Norepinephrine in the rat hippocampus. I. Iontophoretic studies, *Brain Res.* **72**:79–97.

Shellenberger, M. K., Young, D. N., and Levine, M. S., 1977, Effects of intracerebroventricular L-DOPA on caudate unit firing, *Brain Res. Bull.* **2**:273–277.

Siggins, G. R., Hoffer, B. J., Bloom, F. E., and Ungerstedt, U., 1976, Cytochemical and electrophysiological studies of dopamine in the caudate nucleus, in: *The Basal Ganglia* (M. D. Yahr, ed.), Raven Press, New York, pp. 227–248.

Skirboll, L. R., and Bunney, B. S., 1979, The effects of acute and chronic haloperidol treatment on spontaneously firing neurons in the caudate nucleus of the rat, *Life Sci.* **25**:1419–1434.

Skirboll, L. R., Grace, A. A., and Bunney, B. S., 1979, Dopamine auto- and postsynaptic receptors: Electrophysiological evidence for differential sensitivity to dopamine agonists, *Science* **206**:80–82.

Steg, G., 1969, Striatal cell activity during systemic administration of monoaminergic and cholinergic drugs, in: *Third Symposium on Parkinson Disease* (F. Gillingham and I. Donaldson, eds.), Livingstone, Edinberg, pp. 26–29.

Teranishi, T., Negishi, K., and Kato, S., 1983, Dopamine modulates S-potential amplitude and dye-coupling between external horizontal cells in carp retina, *Nature* 301:243–246.

Thierry, A. M., Tassin, J. P., Blanc, G., and Glowinski, J., 1978, Studies on mesocortical dopamine systems, in: *Advances in Biochemical Psychopharmacology*, Vol. 19 (P. J. Roberts, G. N. Woodruff, and L. L. Iversen, eds.), Raven Press, New York, pp. 205–216.

Tosaka, T., and Libet, B., 1970, Additional (adrenergic) synaptic step in sympathetic ganglia, *Fed Proc.* 29:716.

Ungerstedt, U., Ljungberg, T., Hoffer, B., and Siggins, G., 1978, Dopaminergic supersensitivity in the striatum, in: *Advances in Neurology*, Vol. 9, *Dopaminergic Mechanisms* (D. B. Calne, T. N. Chase, and A. Barbeau, eds.), Raven Press, New York, pp. 57–65.

Wagner, H. N., Burns, H. D., Daniels, R. F., Wong, D. F., Langstrom, B., Duefler, T., Frost, J. J., Ravert, H. T., Links, J. M., Rosenbloom, S. B., Lukas, S. E., Kramer, A. V., and Kuhar, M. J., 1983, Imaging dopamine receptors in the human brain by positron tomography, *Science* 221:1264–1266.

Waszczak, B. L., and Walters, J. R., 1983, Dopamine modulation of the effects of gamma-aminobutyric acid on substantia nigra pars reticulata neurons, *Science* 220:218–223.

Watling, K. J., and Dowling, J. E., 1981, Dopaminergic mechanisms in the teleost retina. I. Dopamine-sensitive adenylate cyclase in homogenates of carp retina; effects of agonists, antagonists and ergots, *J. Neurochem.* 36:559–568.

Wilson, C. J., Young, S. J., and Groves, P. M., 1977, Statistical properties of neuronal spike trains in the substantia nigra: Cell types and their interactions, *Brain Res.* 136:243–260.

Wilson, C. J., Chang, H. T., and Kitai, S. T., 1982, Origin of postsynaptic potentials evoked in identified rat neostriatal neurons by stimulation in substantia nigra, *Exp. Brain Res.* 45:157–167.

Wilson, W. A., and Wachtel, H., 1978, Prolonged inhibition in burst firing neurons: synaptic inactivation of the slow regenerative inward current, *Science* 202:772–775.

Wuerthele, S. M., Freed, W. J., Olson, L., Morihisa, J., Spoor, L., Wyatt, R. J., and Hoffer, B. J., 1980, Effects of dopamine agonists and antagonists on the electrical activity of substantia nigra neurons transplanted into the lateral ventricle of the rat, *Exp. Brain Res.* 44:1010.

Yarbrough, G. G., Lake, N., and Phillis, J. W., 1974, Calcium antagonism and its effects on the inhibitory actions of biogenic amines on cerebral cortical neurons, *Brain Res.* 67:77–88.

Zapata, P., 1975, Effects of dopamine on carotid chemo- and baroreceptors *in vitro*, *J. Physiol. (Lond.)* 244:235–251.

10

Histamine

HELMUT L. HAAS

1. INTRODUCTION

1.1. Historical Perspective

Early in this century, histamine (imidazolethylamine) was detected by Sir
Henry Dale and his co-workers as a uterine stimulant in extracts of contam-
inated ergot (Barger and Dale, 1910). In the following years, its potent effects
on smooth muscle and its participation in the allergic response were established. Although originally suspected to be the result of bacterial action
during putrefaction, the compound was later successfully isolated from several types of fresh tissue and was therefore given the name histamine, which
is derived from the Greek word histos for tissue. In 1943, using the guinea
pig ileum as bioassay, Kwiatkowski detected histamine in brain and observed
that there was a higher concentration in the grey than in the white matter.
More sensitive methods for the determination of histamine were subsequently developed, including fluorometric and enzymatic-isotopic assays,
but until very recently it has not been possible to directly visualize histaminergic neurons in brain. Thus, histamine has attracted less attention among
neurobiologists than other biogenic amines, although evidence that it acts
as a neurotransmitter is at least as good (Green, 1970; Green et al., 1978,
Schwartz et al., 1985).

1.2. Regional and Subcellular Distribution

Determination of histamine in small brain samples has provided information regarding its regional localization in brain. The highest levels are

found in the hypothalamus, particularly in the arcuate and suprachiasmatic nuclei in rat (Green, 1970; Brownstein et al., 1974b), and in the mammillary bodies in monkey and man (Snyder and Taylor, 1972; Lipinski et al., 1973). Moderate amounts are found in cortical areas, and low levels are present in cerebellum and spinal cord. Absolute histamine levels in brain average about 50 ng/g, ten times lower than the levels of some other amine transmitters. However, histamine turnover is faster and therefore more histamine may be released per unit time (Dismukes and Snyder, 1974; Pollard et al., 1974).

The histamine-specific biosynthetic enzyme histidine decarboxylase is considered a better marker than the amine itself for histaminergic neurons and their terminals. This enzyme is generally distributed in a parallel fashion to histamine except in the hippocampus, where enzyme activity is high but amine levels are low (Baudry et al., 1973). At the subcellular level, the major portion of histamine is found in the synaptosomal fraction associated with synaptic vesicles, while histidine decarboxylase is found in the cytoplasm. A significant amount of cerebral histamine is contained within the granules of mast cells. The turnover of this nonneuronal histamine is much slower than that of the vesicular histamine (Schwartz, 1975; Schwartz et al., 1985). A mouse mutant lacking mast cells is deficient in as much as 50% of normal brain histamine (Yamatodani et al., 1982; Grzanna and Schultz, 1983).

1.3. Pathways in Brain

Although fluorescent products can be formed by condensation of histamine with aldehydes, it has not been possible to visualize histaminergic neurons with histofluorescence techniques, as is the case for other biogenic amines. Immunohistochemistry using antibodies against a BSA-histamine conjugate or histidine decarboxylase is now providing this missing picture. Histaminergic fibers emanating from the posterior ventral hypothalamus and the mammillary nuclei innervate the whole forebrain in a diffuse manner. Thus, immunoreactive varicose fibers are observed in the diencephalon and telencephalon, with highest densities in the basal hypothalamus and the mammillary region. Two major ascending and a minor descending projection have been described (Wilcox and Seybold, 1982; Watanabe et al., 1983; Panula et al., 1984; Steinbusch and Mulder, 1984).

Prior to the development of immunohistochemical techniques for the visualization of histaminergic neurons, lesion studies had suggested the existence of long histaminergic pathways in the brain. Appropriately placed lesions cause anterograde degeneration of histaminergic neurons resulting in a disappearance of histamine and histidine decarboxylase from target regions. Using this method, a projection pattern similar to the catecholamines and serotonin was revealed (Fig. 1). For example, unilateral lesions of the medial forebrain bundle lead to a fall of histidine decarboxylase activity in the whole ipsilateral forebrain, indicating that histaminergic fibers form a widespread, diffuse projection but do not cross the midline to a significant extent (Garbarg et al., 1974). Quantitating histidine decarboxylase activity

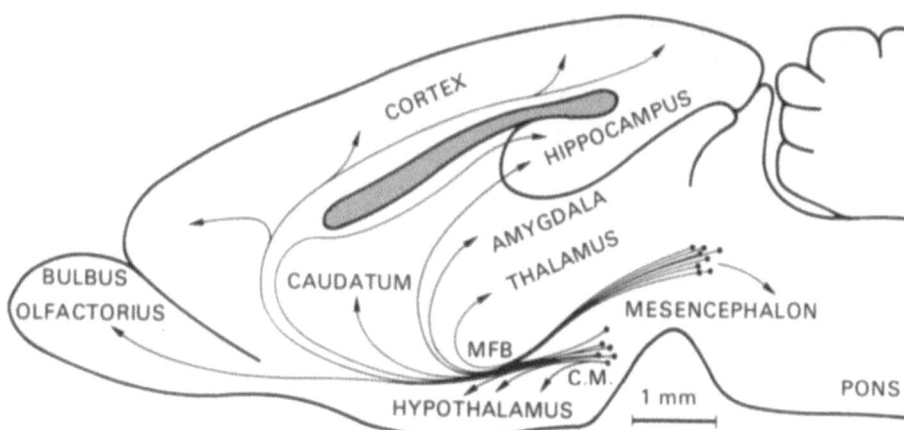

Figure 1. Histaminergic pathways in the mammalian (rat) brain, as determined by lesion experiments and confirmed by immunohistochemistry and electrophysiology. Histaminergic neurons are situated in the mammillary bodies and a supramammillary mesencephalic area. The widespread projection to the whole forebrain is similar to the pattern of other aminergic fibers but is, in contrast to these, largely unilateral.

in the cortex after small lesions at different locations along the midbrain and hypothalamus has allowed a relatively precise localization of the histaminergic neurons in the diencephalon. Thus, lesions caudal to the supramammillary region have no effect on histidine decarboxylase activity, whereas selective destruction of cell bodies in this area by localized injection of kainic acid does reduce enzyme levels (see Schwartz et al., 1985).

The hippocampus receives its afferents through the medial forebrain bundle and fibers enter by both a dorsal (fornix) and a ventral (perforant path) route. Transection of either of these inputs results in about a 50% decrease of histidine decarboxylase, while destruction of both inputs together results in a complete loss of the enzyme. By a similar approach, it has been possible to characterize projections to the striatum, olfactory bulb, thalamus, hypothalamus, the bed nucleus of the stria terminalis, and the amygdala (Ben-Ari et al., 1977; Garbarg et al., 1974) (Fig. 1).

1.4. Metabolism and Release

Histamine is synthesized in brain from histidine by a specific decarboxylase, which is distinct from the aromatic-L-amino acid decarboxylase found in other aminergic neurons. The enzymes differ in kinetics and regional distribution and can be selectively blocked by specific inhibitors (Garbarg et al., 1980; Schwartz, 1975). Histamine synthesis may be regulated by the local availability of its amino acid precursor. The major pathway for histamine degradation is methylation by histamine methyltransferase, which uses S-adenosylmethionine as methyl donor (Snyder and Taylor, 1972). Ox-

idative deamination and dehydrogenation subsequently lead to methylimi-
dazoleacetic acid, which is eventually excreted by the kidney. There is no
high-affinity uptake system for histamine, and therefore methylation could
be the major means of inactivation of the transmitter (Green, 1970).

Endogenous histamine is released by potassium-evoked depolarization
from brain slices in a calcium-dependent fashion. Histamine inhibits its own
release from depolarized slices of rat cerebral cortex by an action on receptors
that are pharmacologically distinct from conventional histamine receptors
(see Section 1.5; Arrang et al., 1983). Reserpine releases histamine along
with other amines, suggesting that they have similar vesicular storage sites.
Lesions in the medial forebrain bundle cause a transient increase in the
histamine content in cortex and hippocampus, which may reflect an interruption of ongoing release. The mast cell degranulator 48/80 also releases
histamine from brain slices, but this histamine comes from the slowly metabolized pool in mast cells (Schwartz et al., 1985).

1.5. Histamine Receptors

The classical antihistamines developed in the 1940s are now classified
as H_1 receptor antagonists, the prototype being pyrilamine (for mepyramine).
At low concentrations, these drugs antagonize most of the actions of histamine on smooth muscle but are ineffective in blocking histamine induced
stimulation of heart rate and gastric secretion. The H_2 receptors mediating
these latter actions were defined in the early 1970s when Black and his
colleagues (Black et al., 1972) synthesized burimamide, metiamide, and cimetidine, substances that antagonized these responses. Highly specific H_2
receptor agonists such as dimaprit and impromidine are now also available.
To date however, all H_1 receptor agonists that have been synthesized, such
as 2-methylhistamine, 2-pyridylethylamine, and 2-thiazolethylamine, have
considerable H_2 agonist activity (Schwartz, 1979).

Histamine H_1-receptors can be labeled in brain membranes with either
[³H]mepyramine (Hill et al., 1978; Chang et al., 1979) or [³H]doxepin, an
antidepressant (Tran et al., 1981). The binding sites display pharmacological
specificity characteristic of histamine H_1 receptors with some differences in
drug selectivity in various brain regions and species. An autoradiographic
study in the rat has revealed high receptor densities in the bed nucleus of
the stria terminalis, the area dentata, the hypothalamus, and the brain stem
(Palacios et al., 1981). A small fraction of these receptors are on vascular
smooth muscle (see Green, 1983; Schwartz, 1979; Schwartz et al., 1985). The
hypothalamus (especially the supraoptic and suprachiasmatic nuclei) and
the hippocampus are particularly rich in H_1 receptors. In guinea pig, however, the highest density is surprisingly in the cerebellum, which seems
devoid of endogenous histamine.

The criteria for specific labeling of the H_2 receptor seem to be met by
[³H]tiotidine (Gajtkowski et al., 1983). High affinity for H_2 receptor binding
was found in hippocampus, cortex and striatum (in this order) while cere-

bellum and pons displayed no significant binding (Norris et al., 1984). Histamine H_2 receptors in brain are coupled to adenylate cyclase, and it has
been possible to demonstrate histamine stimulation of cyclic AMP production in intact tissues (brain slices) as well as cell-free preparations of guinea
pig and rat brain via this receptor (Daly, 1976; Green, 1983; Kanof and
Greengard, 1979). In intact cells, however, the situation is complicated by
the fact that H_1 receptors can modulate the H_2 effect on cyclic AMP accumulation (Palacios et al., 1978). The brain regions richest in histamine-stimulated adenylate cyclase are neocortex and hippocampus. Because the cyclic
AMP response is abolished by intrahippocampal injections of the neurotoxin
kainic acid, it is likely that the histamine-stimulated adenylate cyclase is
present in neurons and not in glial cells.

H_1 receptor antagonists are used clinically because of their antiallergic
and antiemetic actions; their major side effect is sedation. The phenothiazine
and butyrophenone neuroleptics also block H_1 receptors (Green, 1983). On
the other hand, tricyclic antidepressants such as imipramine block H_1 and
H_2 receptors (as well as muscarinic cholinergic receptors), but the highest
affinity is for the H_1 receptor (Schwartz et al., 1981). H_2 receptor antagonists
such as cimetidine and ranitidine are widely used clinically to suppress
gastric acid secretion.

1.6. Histamine Neurons in Invertebrates

Excellent evidence supporting a role for histamine as a neurotransmitter
is provided by studies in invertebrates. Histamine and histidine decarboxylase are present in a number of identified molluscan neurons (Weinreich,
1977; Brownstein et al., 1974a; Turner and Cottrell, 1977), and several types
of excitatory and inhibitory responses to histamine have been reported. Excitatory, depolarizing responses in *Aplysia* and *Onchidium* are mediated by
an H_1 type receptor and act through an increase in sodium conductance
(Carpenter and Gaubatz, 1975; Gotow et al., 1980). A slow hyperpolarization,
mediated by H_2 receptors, seems to be due to an increase in potassium
conductance.

In *Aplysia*, histamine also causes a fast hyperpolarizing response that
is due to chloride ion efflux and is not blocked by H_1 or H_2 antagonists but
is reduced by curare (Gruol and Weinreich, 1979). A pharmacologically
similar chloride-dependent inhibitory response to histamine is present in
neurons of the lobster stomatogastric ganglion (Claiborne and Selverston,
1984). However, Gotow et al. (1980) ascribe the H_2-mediated hyperpolarizing
response in *Onchidium* mainly to stimulation of an electrogenic pump. Excitatory and inhibitory responses to histamine have also been observed in
Helix and *Achatina* but could not be clearly classified.

The best demonstration of histaminergic transmission in any nervous
system is provided by McCaman and Weinreich (1982), who were able to
simultaneously record from a single identified histamine-containing neuron
and its follower cell in the cerebral ganglion of *Aplysia*. Stimulation of the

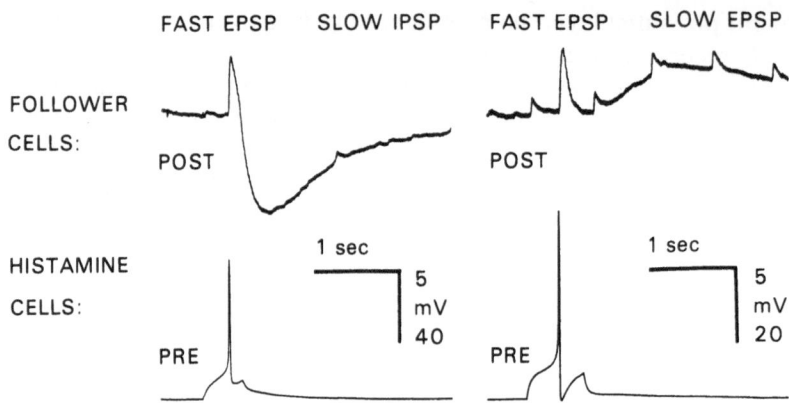

Figure 2. Simultaneous intracellular recording from histamine-containing neurons and their follower cells in *Aplysia*. A single action potential, evoked by intracellular current injection in the histamine cells, causes synaptic potentials in the follower cells. (Courtesy of D. Weinreich.)

presynaptic neuron evoked several histamine mediated synaptic potentials (Fig. 2). IPSPs and hyperpolarizing histamine effects, due to an increase in potassium conductance, were selectively blocked by cimetidine.

2. CENTRAL NERVOUS SYSTEM: STUDIES *IN VIVO*

2.1. Spinal Cord

Lesion and immunohistochemical mapping studies have demonstrated the existence of descending projections of diencephalic histamine neurons to the brain stem and spinal cord. In extracellular recordings in the cat spinal cord it was observed that ionophoretically applied histamine depresses the firing of many spinal interneurons and motoneurons. Early intracellular experiments by Phillis et al. (1968a) revealed that histamine hyperpolarized motoneurons and caused a reduction of synaptic potentials. Later, Engberg et al. (1976) reported that histamine caused an increase in membrane resistance and a decrease in the afterhyperpolarization following the spike. However, the physiological relevance of these observations was questioned by the authors, as a number of phenolic amines, as well as local anesthetics, calcium, and protons, had similar effects.

2.2. Brainstem

In the unanesthetized decerebrate cat, neurons in the medial reticular formation of the medulla, including identified bulbospinal neurons, respond to iontophoretic histamine with a depression of firing. Histamine metabolites have a similar but usually weaker activity (Anderson et al., 1973; Haas et al., 1973). (Imidazoleacetic acid, however, is as strong a depressant as GABA. Since its inhibitory action is blocked by the GABA antagonist bicuculline it may not act at histamine receptors.) Most vestibular neurons are also inhibited by histamine, although some cells are excited. Metiamide selectively blocks the inhibitory response, indicating that it is mediated by H_2 receptors (Satayavivad and Kirsten, 1977). Histamine also depresses dorsal raphe serotonergic neurons in the rat via H_2 receptors (Lakoski et al., 1984).

2.3. Hypothalamus

In contrast to other brain regions, iontophoresis of histamine into the environment of hypothalamic neurons often results in excitation (Haas, 1974). Usually the excitation is prolonged, lasting several seconds, although occasionally it is more rapid. These excitatory effects may be related to H_1 receptors. Depression of firing is found in a variable percentage of cells as well; these responses are mimicked by H_2 agonists and blocked by H_2 antagonists. The catabolite of histamine, tele-methylhistamine, displays actions similar to histamine but is far less potent (Haas and Wolf, 1977).

Specific responses to histamine have been observed in certain functionally or electrophysiologically identified hypothalamic neurons. Vasopressin- and oxytocin-secreting neurons in the supraoptic nucleus can be identified by antidromic invasion from the hypophyseal stalk and by their response to changes in blood osmolarity (Barker et al., 1971). These neurons are excited by histamine (Fig. 3), and the excitation is blocked by the H_1 antagonist mepyramine (Haas et al., 1975; Haas and Wolf, 1977). This is in keeping with experiments showing that local injection of histamine into the supra-

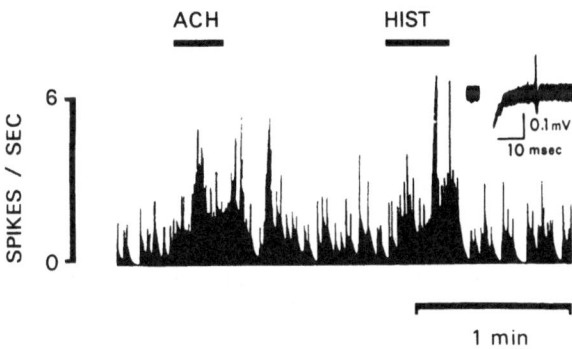

Figure 3. Ratemeter record from a neurosecretory neuron in the cat supraoptic nucleus. Inset shows antidromic action potential after stimulation of the neurohypophysis. Acetylcholine and histamine iontophoretically ejected from a micropipette (60 nA) increase the firing rate.

optic nucleus causes a mepyramine-sensitive antidiuretic effect, presumably due to stimulation of vasopressin release (Bennett and Pert, 1974).

Some thermosensitive neurons in the rostral hypothalamus also respond to histamine (Sweatman and Jell, 1977), as do preoptic-septal neurons projecting to the median eminence and arcuate nucleus (Carette, 1978) and neurons located in the ventromedial nucleus (Renaud, 1976).

2.4. Cortex

Histamine actions have been studied on cortical neurons of the rat, cat, and guinea pig. The firing of most responsive neurons is reduced by iono-tophoretic histamine (Phillis et al., 1968b), and this action seems to be mediated by H_2 receptors (Haas and Bucher, 1975; Phillis et al., 1975; Haas and Wolf, 1977; Haas et al., 1978) but may also involve H_1 receptors (Sastry and Phillis, 1976a). Recordings from unidentified deep cortical neurons and from pyramidal cells projecting to the brainstem or spinal cord have yielded similar results. Specific H_2 agonists (4-methylhistamine, impromidine) mimic the depressant actions, and these effects are blocked by the H_2 antagonists metiamide and cimetidine. Excitatory and dual actions are occasionally observed; however, only the depressant component is reversed by metiamide (Haas and Wolf, 1977). Although there is some suggestive evidence to support the view that the excitatory effects are due to stimulation of H_1 receptors, this cannot be stated with confidence, since truly specific H_1 antagonists are not yet available. The H_1 antagonist mepyramine unfortunately has local anesthetic properties and in iontophoretic studies blocks the actions of histamine (as well as other agents) in a nonspecific fashion.

Evidence for the physiological relevance of H_2 receptor-mediated depressant effects in neocortex is provided by the observation that the H_2 antagonist metiamide seems to specifically block the presumed histaminergic medial forebrain bundle–neocortical pathway (Sastry and Phillis, 1976b; Haas and Wolf, 1977). Electrical stimulation of the medial forebrain bundle produces inhibition of cortical neurons, which is reversed by iontophoretic metiamide. The selectivity of this effect is demonstrated by the finding that the inhibitory pause caused in response to direct cortical stimulation (presumably due to activation of intrinsic inhibitory neurons) is unaffected.

Lesions in the ascending histaminergic pathway to the cortex at the level of the medial forebrain bundle produce an increased sensitivity to iono-phoretic histamine, but not GABA. This supersensitivity parallels the fall in histidine decarboxylase activity and appears only on the side ipsilateral to the lesion (Haas et al., 1978). In studies of the hippocampal histaminergic projection, it was observed that the late component of the IPSP (as judged from peristimulus histograms) produced in response to fimbria stimulation can be specifically reduced by metiamide, suggesting that the inhibition is at least partially mediated by histamine acting via H_2 receptors.

3. CENTRAL NERVOUS SYSTEM: STUDIES *IN VITRO*

3.1. Hypothalamus

3.1.1. Tissue Culture

Tuberal hypothalamic neurons in tissue culture can respond with either excitation or depression to locally applied histamine. About one half of the cells are depressed, one quarter are excited, and the remainder are unaffected. The general pharmacological principles derived from *in vivo* studies seem to apply to these neurons *in vitro*. The antagonists metiamide (H_2) and promethazine (H_1), added to the perfusion fluid, selectively block the inhibitory and excitatory responses to iontophoretic histamine, respectively. Moreover, the H_2 agonist dimaprit causes only depressions, while the partial H_1 agonist 2-pyridylethylamine elicits both effects (Geller, 1976, 1981). The depressions persist in calcium-free medium, indicating a direct postsynaptic effect, and are potentiated by phosphodiesterase inhibitors, supporting a role for cyclic AMP in mediating the response (Geller, 1979).

3.1.2. Tissue Slices

Most hypothalamic nuclei can be easily identified by inspection in unfixed slices. Spontaneously firing cells in several nuclei respond well to locally applied or bath perfused histamine with similar patterns as observed *in vivo*. Intracellular recordings have been obtained from presumed neurosecretory neurons in the paraventricular nucleus. These cells, identified by their location and typical firing pattern, showed a clear excitatory response to bath applied histamine. However, this seemed to result from an increased frequency of EPSPs, rather than a direct postsynaptic action. Therefore in these experiments histamine appeared to activate neighboring cells with excitatory connections to the neurosecretory neurons instead of the endocrine cells themselves (Haas and Geller, 1982).

3.2. Hippocampus

The action of histamine in the hippocampus has been clarified by intracellular recordings in tissue slices. In keeping with the observations from *in vivo* studies, local application of histamine by iontophoresis or pressure ejection depresses the spontaneous or evoked firing of the majority of CA_1 pyramidal and dentate granule cells. This depression of firing is associated with hyperpolarization of the somal membrane and in some cases with a moderate conductance increase (Fig. 4). As in other systems, this hyperpolarization appears to be mediated by H_2 receptors, as it is mimicked by

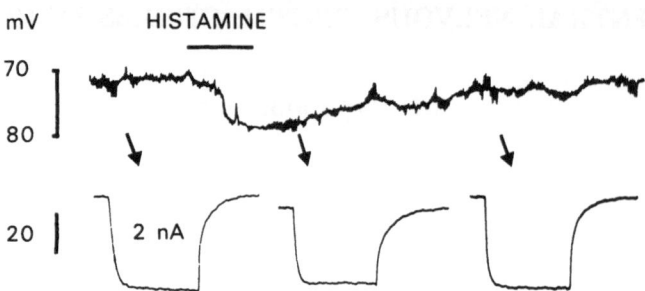

Figure 4. Hyperpolarization of a dentate granule cell in a rat hippocampal slice. Histamine was ejected by pressure from a micropipette during the period indicated by the bar (3 min). Lower traces are the voltage responses to hyperpolarizing current injections (2 nA, 100 msec) illustrating a conductance increase during the histamine effect.

the H_2 agonist impromidine. The hyperpolarizing effect of histamine is due to a direct postsynaptic action as it persists in low calcium/high magnesium or tetrodotoxin-containing media (Haas, 1981).

Application of histamine microdrops to the slice surface can also cause a slow depolarization with no observable conductance change, which is blocked by the H_1 antagonist promethazine (1 mM). In addition, the EPSP, recorded extra- and intracellularly in the CA_1 and the CA_3, area, was found augmented by histamine (Segal, 1980, 1981). These effects are believed to be generated by a *presynaptic* action of histamine because the responsiveness to direct application of glutamate was unaffected and because they could not be demonstrated in low calcium/high magnesium or tetrodotoxin-containing media. Other extra- and intracellular experiments in the CA_1 area, however, showed a reduction or no change in EPSPs, but an enhanced response to glutamate ionophoresis in the presence of histamine (Haas, 1984; Greene and Haas, 1985).

When histamine or the H_2 agonist impromidine are added to the perfusion fluid of hippocampal slices, the population spike in the CA_1 region is increased with no change in the EPSP (Fig. 5A), indicating a postsynaptic action (Haas, 1984). Intracellular recording disclosed a slight membrane depolarization; however, the major effect was on the afterhyperpolarization following a burst of spikes. In CA_1 pyramidal neurons, as in other cell types, the long-lasting (several second) afterhyperpolarization is believed to be due to the activation of a calcium-dependent potassium conductance. [This conductance has been related to a specific membrane current I_{AHP} (Lancaster and Adams, 1984), which may be distinct from the well-known I_C (Brown and Griffith, 1983).] As is the case for norepinephrine (see Chapter 8), histamine depresses amplitude and time course of this afterhyperpolarization (Haas and Konnerth, 1983; Haas, 1984), which results in enhanced repetitive firing (block of "accommodation"; Madison and Nicoll, 1984).

The H_2 agonist impromidine, but not the H_1 agonist thiazolethylamine, mimicks these effects of histamine. Moreover, the H_2 antagonists metiamide and cimetidine block the action of histamine on the afterhyperpolarization, whereas the H_1 antagonist mepyramine and the β-antagonist propranolol do not. These observations provide strong evidence that the effect is due to activation of H_2 receptors.

In the presence of tetrodotoxin, which blocks the sodium component of action potentials, calcium-dependent spikes can be evoked in CA_1 neurons that are of markedly prolonged duration. An afterhyperpolarization occurs following these calcium spikes. Histamine specifically depresses the slow (but not the fast) component of this afterhyperpolarization (Fig. 5C,D). A reduction in the afterhyperpolarization might be secondary to a block of calcium entry as, for example, occurs when cadmium ions eliminate calcium spikes and the resultant afterhyperpolarization. This is unlikely, however, as calcium spikes are actually enhanced and prolonged, rather than reduced by the amine. Blockers of potassium channels such as tetraethylammonium, barium, and intracellular cesium maximize the visibility of calcium spikes. Even under these circumstances the calcium spikes are not reduced by histamine. When calcium currents are blocked by adding cadmium to the medium, histamine still has a depolarizing action, but intracellular EGTA (which chelates calcium ions) prevents it. Furthermore, in calcium-deficient, magnesium-enriched medium where the slow afterhyperpolarization is blocked, histamine (acting through H_2 receptors at concentrations as low as 10 nM) can still produce the depolarization. This depolarizing response has been attributed to depression of a steady potassium conductance and it has been speculated that histamine reduces the intracellular availability of calcium ions leading to a reduction in a resting calcium-activated potassium current (Haas et al., 1984; Haas, 1984).

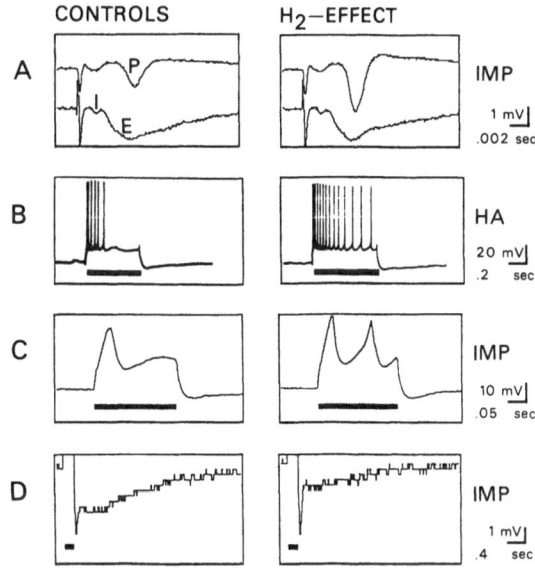

Figure 5. Effect of histamine (HA) and impromidine (IMP) on excitation of CA_1 pyramidal cells in hippocampal slices of the rat. (A) Somatic population spikes (P), input fiber volleys (I), and dendritic extracellular EPSPs (E) after stimulation of str. radiatum. The population spike, but not the EPSP, is significantly increased by 1 μM impromidine. (B, C, D) Responses to intracellular depolarizing current injection, indicated by black bars. (B) Normal medium; 1 μM histamine blocks accommodation of firing. (C, D) Tetrodotoxin-treated slice; 1 μM impromidine facilitates calcium spikes (C) and blocks the long-lasting afterhyperpolarization (D).

As noted in Section 1.5, there is evidence from biochemical studies that H_2 receptors in brain are coupled to adenylate cyclase. The effect of histamine on the afterhyperpolarization can be mimicked by the nonhydrolyzable, lipid-soluble cyclic AMP analog 8-bromo cyclic AMP and the histamine response is potentiated by the phosphodiesterase inhibitor Ro 20-1724 (Haas, 1985). Thus, as for norepinephrine, there is reason to believe that cyclic AMP mediates the effect. Additional evidence in favor of this concept is the observation that only amines that stimulate adenylate cyclase in brain slices (i.e., histamine and norepinephrine; Green, 1983; Etgen and Browning, 1983) produce the effect on the afterhyperpolarization. Dopamine and serotonin are ineffective in either regard.

In addition to an action on pyramidal cells, histamine also seems to affect interneurons in the hippocampal slice. This has been inferred from intracellular recordings in pyramidal cells where there is an increase in the frequency of IPSPs during perfusion with histamine.

4. SYMPATHETIC GANGLIA

Like many other substances, histamine can affect synaptic transmission in sympathetic ganglia. In the rabbit isolated superior cervical ganglion, histamine produces two antagonistic effects, an H_1 receptor-mediated facilitation and an H_2 receptor-mediated depression of ganglionic transmission (Brimble and Wallis, 1973). Moreover, the actual effect of histamine itself depends on the type of ganglionic response involved. Thus, micromolar concentrations of histamine reduce the compound action potential evoked by a single stimulus but facilitate the response to repetitive stimulation. In rat sympathetic ganglia, histamine has also been shown to cause a depression of the compound action potential (Lindl, 1978). Although a dual action of histamine on blood pressure is known, the physiological significance of the ganglionic responses in mediating these effects are uncertain. As in brain, histamine stimulates cyclic AMP accumulation in sympathetic ganglia via an action on H_2 receptors; H_1 receptor activation causes an increase in cyclic GMP levels (Study and Greengard, 1978). However, the role of cyclic nucleotides in mediating ganglionic responses to histamine remains to be elucidated.

5. CONCLUSION

Recordings from brain and spinal cord neurons in conjunction with iontophoresis of histamine, its metabolites, agonists, and antagonists have significantly advanced our understanding of the functional neuropharmacology of central histamine receptors and have provided good circumstantial evidence that histamine serves as a central transmitter. Inhibitory effects of ionophoretically applied histamine have been described for most regions in the central nervous system and are usually mediated by H_2-receptors. At least in the hippocampus, this action seems to reflect membrane hyperpolarization, which involves a conductance increase probably to potassium ions. On the other hand, excitatory responses to histamine, such as occur in the hypothalamus, may be due to H_1 receptor activation, but the underlying membrane mechanisms are unknown.

Perhaps more important than its effects on passive membrane properties in hippocampal neurons is the ability of histamine to cause a decrease in a calcium-activated potassium conductance. This may occur through an interference with intracellular calcium sequestration mediated by H_2 receptors linked to adenylate cyclase. As histamine releases the neurons from an endogenous potassium current, its action could be described as an "intrinsic disinhibition." From a functional point of view, reduction of the spike afterhyperpolarization through a suppression of the calcium-activated potassium conductance allows a powerful facilitation of repetitive firing in response to depolarizing signals. In concert, the hyperpolarizing action of histamine and its potentiation of excitatory stimuli could act to increase the response to strong synaptic inputs while suppressing weaker ones, so that the "signal-to-noise" ratio is increased (see also Chapter 8). Of course, more information is needed to understand how these mechanisms operate naturally.

The widespread distribution of histaminergic neurons suggests that they, like other amine pathways, may influence the functional state of target regions rather than transmit discrete signals. Together with other systems ascending from the reticular formation, histamine neurons may be involved in the regulation of states of awareness, circadian and other biological rhythms, cerebral circulation and energy metabolism, and neuroendocrine and vegetative functions (Gross, 1982; Schwartz et al., 1985). The sedative action of H_1 antagonists has led to speculations of an involvement of histamine in the regulation of sleep and waking. The desynchronization of the EEG by centrally applied histamine (Wolf and Monnier, 1973) and the fluctuation of endogenous brain histamine during the day and night cycle (Schwartz et al., 1985) are in keeping with this possibility.

Histaminergic systems also seem to participate in the regulation of water balance and drinking behavior, in part through an action on the hypothalamic supraoptic and paraventricular neurons that project to the posterior pituitary. Thus, microinjection of histamine into the region of the supraoptic and paraventricular nuclei stimulates vasopressin release via H_1 receptors, and this is probably due to the excitatory effects of histamine on these neurons.

Anterior pituitary functions may also be controlled by histamine neurons in the hypothalamus (Weiner and Ganong, 1978; Roberts and Calcutt, 1983). For example, prolactin secretion is increased by H_1 and decreased by H_2 receptor activation, perhaps explaining the rise in plasma prolactin occurring in some patients receiving cimetidine (see Schwartz et al., 1985).

Histamine neurons may also be involved in the control of autonomic functions. Centrally administered histamine causes a transient increase in blood pressure and heart rate. Interestingly, spontaneously hypertensive rats display increased histamine levels in the hypothalamus. Temperature regulation may also involve histamine neurons as hypothermia can be induced through H_2 receptor activation (Green et al., 1976). H_1 receptor antagonists are well known to have an antiemetic action on the chemoreceptor trigger zone in the area postrema, but the role of histamine neurons in the vomiting reflex is unknown. The recent availability of neuroanatomical maps precisely localizing brain histamine neurons and their projections and the growing understanding of the cellular mechanisms underlying the transmitter actions of histamine should allow clarification of the role of histamine in these diverse behavioral functions.

REFERENCES

Anderson, E. G., Haas, H. L., and Hösli, L., 1973, Comparison of effects of noradrenaline and histamine with cyclic AMP on brain stem neurones, *Brain Res.* **49:**471–475.

Arrang, J.-M., Garbarg, M., and Schwartz, J. C., 1983, Auto-inhibition of brain histamine release mediated by a novel class (H_3) of histamine receptor, *Nature* **302:**832–837.

Barger, G., and Dale, H. H., 1910, Die physiologische Wirkung einer Secalebase und deren Identifizierung als Imidazolaethylamin, *Z. Physiol.* **24:**885–889.

Barker, J. L., Crayton, J. W., and Nicoll, R. A., 1971, Noradrenaline and acetylcholine responses of supraoptic neurosecretory cells, *J. Physiol. (Lond.)* **218:**19–32.

Baudry, M., Martres, M. P., and Schwartz, J. C., 1973, The subcellular localisation of histidine decarboxylase in various regions of rat brain, *J. Neurochem.* **21:**1301–1309.

Ben-Ari, Y., Le Gal la Salle, G., Barbin, G., Schwartz, J. C., and Garbarg, M., 1977, Histamine synthesizing afferents within the amygdaloid complex and bed nucleus of the stria terminalis of the rat, *Brain Res.* **138:**285–294.

Bennett, C. T., and Pert, A., 1974, Antidiuresis produced by injections of histamine into the cat supraoptic nucleus, *Brain Res.* **78:**151–156.

Black, J. W., Duncan, W. A. M., Durant, C. J., Ganellin, C. R., and Parsons, E. M., 1972, Definition and antagonism of histamine H_2-receptors, *Nature* **236:**385–390.

Brimble, M. J., and Wallis, D. I., 1973, Histamine H_1 and H_2-receptors at a ganglionic synapse, *Nature* **246:**156–158.

Brown, D. A., and Griffith, W. H., 1983, Calcium-activated outward current in voltage clamped hippocampal neurones of the guinea-pig, *J. Physiol. (Lond.)* **337:**287–301.

Brownstein, M. J., Saavedra, J. M., Axelrod, J., Zeman, G. H., and Carpenter, D. O., 1974a, Coexistence of several putative neurotransmitters in single identified neurons of aplysia, *Proc. Natl. Acad. Sci. USA* **71:**4662–4665.

Brownstein, M. J., Saavedra, J. M., Palkovits, M., and Axelrod, J., 1974b, Histamine content of hypothalamic nuclei of the rat, *Brain Res.* **77:**151.

Carette, B., 1978, Responses of preoptic-septal neurons to iontophoretically applied histamine, *Brain Res.* **145:**391–395.

Carpenter, D. O., and Gaubatz, G. L., 1975, H_1 and H_2 histamine receptors on aplysia neurones, *Nature* **254:**343–344.

Chang, R. S. L., Tran, V. T., and Snyder, S. H., 1979, Heterogeneity of histamine H_1-receptors: Species variations in (3H) mepyramine binding of brain membranes, *J. Neurochem.* **32:**1653–1663.

Claiborne, B. J., and Selverston, A. I., 1984, Histamine as a neurotransmitter in the stomatogastric nervous system of the spiny lobster, *J. Neurosci.* **4:**708–721.

Daly, J. W., 1976, The nature of receptors regulating the formation of cyclic AMP in brain tissue, *Life Sci.* **18:**1349–1358.

Dismukes, K., and Snyder, S. H., 1974, Dynamics of brain histamine, *Adv. Neurol.* **5:**101–109.

Engberg, I., Flatman, J. A., and Kadzielawa, K., 1976, Lack of specificity of motoneurone responses to microiontophoretically applied phenolic amines, *Acta Physiol. Scand.* **96:**137–139.

Etgen, A. M., and Browning, E. T., 1983, Activators of cyclic AMP accumulation in rat hippocampal slices: Action of vasoactive intestinal peptide (VIP), *J. Neurosci.* **3:**2487–2493.

Gajtkowski, G. A., Norris, D. B., Rising, T. J., and Wood, T. P., 1983, Specific binding of ^{3}H-tiotidine to histamine H_2-receptors in guinea pig cerebral cortex, *Nature* **304:**65–67.

Garbarg, M., Barbin, G., Feger, J., and Schwartz, J. C., 1974, Histaminergic pathway in rat brain evidenced by lesions of the medial forebrain bundle, *Science* **186:**833–835.

Garbarg, M., Barbin, G., Rodergas, E., and Schwartz, J. C., 1980, Inhibition of histamine synthesis in brain by alpha-fluoromethylhistidine, a new irreversible inhibitor: in vitro and in vivo studies, *J. Neurochem.* **35:**1045–1052.

Geller, H. M., 1976, Effects of some putative neurotransmitters on unit activity of tuberal hypothalamic neurons in vitro, *Brain Res.* **108:**423–430.

Geller, H. M., 1979, Are histamine H_2-receptor depressions of neuronal activity in tissue cultures of rat hypothalamus mediated through cyclic adenosine monophosphate? *Neurosci. Lett.* **14:**49–53.

Geller, H. M., 1981, Histamine actions on activity of cultured hypothalamic neurons: Evidence for mediation by H_1 and H_2 histamine receptors, *Dev. Brain Res.* **1:**89–101.

Gotow, T., Kirkpatrick, C. T., and Tomita, T., 1980, Excitatory and inhibitory effects of histamine on molluscan neurons, *Brain Res.* **196:**151–167.

Green, J. P., 1970, Histamine, in: *Handbook of Neurochemistry*, Volume 4 (A. Lajtha, ed.), Plenum Press, New York, pp. 221–250.

Green, J. P., 1983, Histamine receptors in brain, in: *Handbook of Psychopharmacology*, Volume 17 (L. L. Iversen, S. D. Iversen, and S. H. Snyder, eds.), Plenum Press, New York, pp. 385–419.

Green, J. P., and Maayani, S., 1977, Tricyclic antidepressant drugs block histamine H_2-receptors in brain, *Nature* **269:**163–165.

Green, J. P., Johnson, C. L., and Weinstein, H., 1978, Histamine as a neurotransmitter, in: *Psychopharmacology: A Generation of Progress* (A. Lipton, A. Di Mascio, and K. F. Killam, eds.), Raven Press, New York, pp. 319–332.

Green, M. D., Cox, B., and Lomax, P., 1976, Sites and mechanisms of action of histamine in the central thermoregulatory pathways of the rat, *Neuropharmacology* **15:**321–324.

Gross, P. M., 1982, Cerebral histamine: indications for neuronal and vascular regulation, *J. Cereb. Blood Flow Metab.* **2:**3–23.

Gruol, D. L., and Weinreich, D., 1979, Two pharmacologically distinct histamine receptors mediating membrane hyperpolarization on identified neurons of aplysia californica, *Brain Res.* **162:**281–301.

Grzanna, R., and Shultz, L. D., 1982, The contribution of mast cells to the histamine content of the central nervous system: A regional analysis, *Life Sci.* **30:**1959–1964.

Haas, H. L., 1974, Histamine: Action on single hypothalamic neurones, *Brain Res.* **76:**363–366.

Haas, H. L., 1981, Histamine hyperpolarizes hippocampal neurones in vitro, *Neurosci. Lett.* **22:**75–78.

Haas, H. L., 1984, Histamine potentiates neuronal excitation by blocking a calcium dependent potassium conductance, *Agents Actions* **14:**534–537.

Haas, H. L., 1985, Histamine may act through cyclic AMP on hippocampal neurones, *Agents Actions* **16:**234–235.

Haas, H. L., and Bucher, U. M., 1975, Histamine H_2-receptors on single central neurones, *Nature* **255:**634–635.

Haas, H. L., and Geller, H. M., 1982, Electrophysiology of histaminergic transmission in the brain, in: *Advances in Histamine Research, Advances in the Biosciences*, Volume 33, (B. Urnäs and K. Tasaka, eds.) Pergamon Press, Oxford, pp. 81–91.

Haas, H. L., and Konnerth, A., 1983, Histamine and noradrenaline decrease calcium-activated potassium conductance in hippocampal pyramidal cells, *Nature* **302**:432–434.

Haas, H. L., and Wolf, P., 1977, Central actions of histamine, microelectrophoretic studies, *Brain Res.* **122**:269–279.

Haas, H. L., Anderson, E. G., and Hösli, L., 1973, Histamine and metabolites: Their effects and interactions with convulsants on brain stem neurones, *Brain Res.* **51**:269–278.

Haas, H. L., Wolf, P., and Nussbaumer, J. -C., 1975, Histamine: Action on supraoptic and other hypothalamic neurones in the cat, *Brain Res.* **88**:166–170.

Haas, H. L., Wolf, P., Palacios, J. M., Garbarg, M., Barbin, G., and Schwartz, J. C., 1978, Hypersensitivity to histamine in the guinea-pig brain: Microiontophoretic and biochemical studies, *Brain Res.* **156**:275–291.

Haas, H. L., Jefferys, J. G. R., Slater, N. T., and Carpenterr, D. O. 1984, Modulation of low calcium-induced field bursts in the hippocampus by monoamines and cholinominetics, *Pflügers Arch.* **400**:28–33.

Hill, S. J., Young, J. M., and Marrian, D. H., 1978, Specific binding of 3H-mepyramine to histamine H_1-receptors in intestinal smooth muscle, *Nature* **270**:361–363.

Kanof, P. D., and Greengard, P., 1979, Pharmacological properties of histamine sensitive adenylate cyclase from mammalian brain, *J. Pharmacol. Exp. Ther.* **209**:87–96.

Kwiatkowski, H., 1943, Histamine in nervous tissue, *J. Physiol. (Lond.)* **102**:32–41.

Lakoski, J. M., Gallagher, D. W., and Aghajanian, G. K., 1984, Histamine-induced depression of serotonergic dorsal raphe neurons: Antagonism by cimetidine, a reevaluation, *Eur. J. Pharmacol.* **103**:153–156.

Lancaster, B., and Adams, P. R., 1984, Single electrode voltage clamp of the slow AHP current in rat hippocampal pyramidal cells, *Neurosci. Abstr.* **10**:872.

Lindl, T., 1978, Cyclic AMP and its relation to ganglionic transmission. A combined biochemical and electrophysiological study of the rat superior cervical ganglion in vitro, *Neuropharmacology* **18**:227–235.

Lipinski, J. F., Schaumburg, H. H., and Baldessarini, R. J., 1973, Regional distribution of histamine in human brain, *Brain Res.* **52**:403–408.

Madison, D. V., and Nicoll, R. A., 1984, Control of the repetitive discharge of Ca 1 pyramidal neurones in vitro, *J. Physiol. (Lond.)* **354**:319–331.

McCaman, R. E., and Weinreich, D., 1982, On the nature of histamine-mediated slow hyperpolarizing synaptic potentials in identified molluscan neurones, *J. Physiol. (Lond.)* **328**:485–506.

Norris, D. B., Gajtkowski, G. A., and Rising, T. J., 1984, Histamine H_2-binding studies in the guinea pig brain, *Agents Actions* **14**:543–545.

Palacios, J. M., Garbarg, M., Barbin, G., and Schwartz, J. C., 1978, Pharmacological characterization of histamine receptors mediating the stimulation of cyclic AMP accumulation in slices from guinea pig hippocampus, *Mol. Pharmacol.* **14**:971–982.

Palacios, J. M., Wamsley, J. K., and Kuhar, M. J., 1981, The distribution of histamine H_1-receptors in the rat brain: An autoradiographic study, *Neuroscience* **6**:15–37.

Panula, P., Yang, H. -Y. T., and Costa, E., 1984, Histamine containing neurones in the rat hypothalamus, *Proc. Natl. Acad. Sci. USA* **81**:2572–2576.

Phillis, J. W., Tebecis, A. K., and York, D. H., 1968a, Depression of spinal motoneurones by noradrenaline, 5-hydroxytryptamine and histamine, *Eur. J. Pharmacol.* **4**:471–475.

Phillis, J. W., Tebecis, A. K., and York, D. H., 1968b, Histamine and some antihistamines: their actions on cerebral cortical neurones, *Br. J. Pharmacol.* **33**:426–440.

Phillis, J. W., Kostopoulos, G. K., and Odutola, A., 1975, On the specificity of histamine H_2-receptor antagonists in the rat cerebral cortex, *Can. J. Physiol. Pharmacol.* **53**:1205–1209.

Pollard, H., Bischoff, S., and Schwartz, J. C., 1974, Turnover of histamine in rat brain and its decrease under barbiturate anesthesia, *J. Pharmacol. Exp. Ther.* **190**:88–99.

Renaud, L. P., 1976, Histamine microiontophoresis on identified hypothalamic neurons: 3 Patterns of response in the ventromedial nucleus of the rat, *Brain Res.* **115**:339–344.

Roberts, F., and Calcutt, C. R., 1983, Histamine and the hypothalamus, *Neuroscience* **9**:721–739.

Sastry, B. S. R., and Phillis, J. W., 1976a, Depression of rat cerebral cortical neurones by H_1 and H_2 histamine receptors agonists, Eur. J. Pharmacol. **38**:269–273.

Sastry, B. S. R., and Phillis, J. W., 1976b, Evidence for an ascending inhibitory histaminergic pathway to the cerebral cortex, Can. J. Physiol. Pharmacol. **54**:782–786.

Satayavivad, U., and Kirsten, E., 1977, Iontophoretic studies of histamine and histamine antagonists in the feline vestibular nuclei, Eur. J. Pharmacol. **41**:17–26.

Schwartz, J. C., 1975, Histamine as a transmitter in brain, Life Sci. **17**:503–518.

Schwartz, J. C., 1979, Histamine receptors in brain, Life Sci. **25**:895–912.

Schwartz, J. C., Garbarg, M., and Quach, T. T., 1981, Histamine receptors as targets for tricyclic antidepressants, Trends Pharmacol. Sci. **2**:122–125.

Schwartz, J. C., Garbarg, M., and Pollard, H., 1985, Histaminergic transmission in brain, Handbook of Physiology, American Physiological Society, in press.

Segal, M., 1980, Histamine produces a calcium-sensitive depolarization of hippocampal pyramidal cells in vitro, Neurosci. Lett. **19**:67.

Segal, M., 1981, Histamine modulates reactivity of hippocampal CA 3 neurons to afferent stimulation in vitro, Brain Res. **213**:443–448.

Snyder, S. H., and Taylor, K. M., 1972, Histamine in the brain: A neurotransmitter, in: Perspectives in Neuropharmacology (S. H. Snyder, ed.), Oxford University Press, New York, pp. 43–73.

Steinbusch, H. W. M., and Mulder, A. H., 1984, Immunohistochemical localization of histamine in neurons and mast cells in the rat brain, in: Handbook of Chemical Neuroanatomy, Vol. 3 (A. Björklund, T. Hökfelt, and M. J. Kuhar, eds.), Elsevier, Amsterdam, pp. 126–140.

Study, R. E., and Greengard, P., 1978, Regulation by histamine of cyclic mucleotide levels in sympathetic ganglia, J. Pharmacol. Exp. Ther. **207**:767–778.

Sweatman, P., and Jell, R. M., 1977, Dopamine and histamine sensitivity of rostral hypothalamic neurones in the cat: Possible involvement in thermoregulation, Brain Res. **127**:173–178.

Tran, V. T., Lebovitz, R., Toll, L., and Snyder, S. H., 1981, [³H]Doxepin interactions with histamine H_1-receptors and other sites in guinea pig and rat brain homogenates, Eur. J. Pharmacol. **70**:501–509.

Turner, J. D., and Cottrell, G. A., 1977, Properties of an identified histamine containing neurone, Nature **267**:447–448.

Watanabe, T., Taguchi, Y., Hayashi, H., Tanaka, J., Shiosaka, S., Tohyama, M., Kubota, H., Terano, Y., and Wada, H. (1983). Evidence for the presence of a histaminergic neuron system in the rat brain: An immunohistochemical analysis, Neurosci. Lett. **39**:249–254.

Weiner, R. I., and Ganong, W. F., 1978, Role of brain monoamines and histamine in regulation of anterior pituitary secretion, Physiol. Rev. **58**:905–976.

Weinreich, D., 1977, Histamine containing neurons in Aplysia, in: Biochemistry of Characterized Neurons (C. N. N. Osborne, ed.), Pergamon Press, Oxford, pp. 153–175.

Wilcox, B. J., and Seybold, V. S., 1982, Localization of neuronal histamine in rat brain, Neurosci. Lett. **29**:105–110.

Wolf, P., and Monnier, M., 1973, Electroencephalographic, behavioral and visceral effects of intraventricular infusion of histamine in the rabbit, Agents Actions **3**:196.

Yamatodani, A., Maeyama, K., Watanabe, T., Wada, H., and Kitamura, Y., 1982, Tissue distribution of histamine in a mutant mouse deficient in mast cells. Clear evidence for the presence of non mast cell histamine, Biochem. Pharmacol. **31**:305–310.

PART IV
NEUROPEPTIDES

Opioid Peptides: Central Nervous System

RAYMOND DINGLEDINE

1. INTRODUCTION

1.1. Historical Perspective and Overview

Opium derivatives have been in medical use for at least 2000 years, possibly longer than any other class of drugs. Parenteral administration of these compounds results in a multitude of pharmacological effects mediated by the central nervous system (Jaffe and Martin, 1980). The brain regions involved in these actions have been identified in some instances by local microinjection of pmole quantities of opioids. For example, profound analgesia can be elicited by microinjection of morphine into the periaqueductal gray or nucleus reticularis paragigantocellularis, but not into other nearby regions (Yaksh and Rudy, 1978; Akaike et al., 1978). Electrographic seizure activity localized to limbic structures such as the hippocampus and amygdala can be produced by microinjection of opioids into the lateral ventrical (Henricksen et al., 1978; Snead and Bearden, 1982). A primary goal of opioid research is to understand the actions of opioids on integrative activities of the nervous system, both in terms of the circuitry involved and the ionic conductance mechanisms affected by these drugs.

Information relevant to understanding the cellular actions of opioids in the brain began to appear in the early 1970s as microiontophoretic techniques were applied in conjunction with single-unit recording from anesthetized animals. More recently, *in vitro* electrophysiological studies of opiate sensitive neurons have been possible, both with brain slices and with primary tissue cultures. In these studies, the ease of obtaining high-quality intracellular recordings, as well as the more traditional pharmacological advantage of precise control over drug concentrations, have allowed more detailed information to be gathered concerning the cellular actions of opioids. The focus of this chapter is primarily on these in vitro studies. Numerous reviews concerned with the neurochemistry and clinical relevance of opioid peptides and opioid receptors are available (Kosterlitz and Paterson, 1980; Chang and Cuatrecasas, 1981; Frederickson and Geary, 1982). North (1979) has reviewed the effects of opioids on single unit activity in the mammalian brain.

Table 1 presents a survey of the effects of opioids on spontaneous firing and synaptically evoked activity in a number of brain regions. All agonist effects listed in this table were reported to be blocked by naloxone and so were presumably mediated by classical opiate receptors. Two trends emerge. First, in most cases the direction of the drug effect (inhibitory or excitatory) was independent of the agonist. Possible exceptions include dynorphin on hippocampal CA3 pyramidal cells and β-endorphin in several limbic regions, where it could either excite or depress spontaneous firing. Second, in the overwhelming majority of brain regions the naloxone-reversible effect of opioids was inhibition of spontaneous or evoked firing. Apparent exceptions are hippocampal CA1 pyramidal cells, Renshaw cells, neurons in the hypothalamic ventromedian nucleus, and nucleus reticularis paragigantocellularis of the medulla. In the hippocampus, however, the excitatory effect of opioids is most likely achieved by depression of the excitability of inhibitory interneurons (see below). Whether local circuitry plays a similar role in determining the effects of iontophoresed opioids for the other three "exceptions" has not been explored, although to date an unequivocal demonstration of a direct excitatory effect of an opioid on any mammalian CNS neuron is lacking.

1.2. Opioid Peptides

The discovery in 1975 that mammalian brain contains a number of peptides with opiatelike activity accelerated interest in the cellular actions of opioids. It is now clear that at least three structurally related families of opioid peptides exist in the CNS, each coded by a different gene (Cox, 1982; Herbert et al., 1983; Udenfriend and Kilpatrick, 1983). The first precursor sequenced was pre-proopiomelanocortin (POMC), which is proteolytically cleaved into ACTH and the opioid peptide β-endorphin (Fig. 1). Pre-proenkephalin is the second large precursor peptide, from which both methionine- and leucine-enkephalin are derived (Noda et al., 1982). The third member of the group is pre-prodynorphin, which is processed to two related dynorphin sequences and α-neoendorphin, each of which has opioid activity.

The opioid peptides are distributed differently in the brain, attesting to their separate functional roles. Opioid peptides derived from POMC are secreted along with ACTH by the corticotrophs of the pituitary. These peptides are also synthesized by a small group of medio-basal hypothalamic neurons, which send fibers to a number of limbic and midbrain structures such as the septum, locus coeruleus, and amygdala (Bloom et al., 1978). The enkephalins are more widely distributed within the CNS. Enkephalin-containing perikarya are found in large numbers in the substantia gelatinosa and the caudate nucleus, and in many other subcortical nuclei (Pickel et al., 1980; Walmsey et al., 1980; Sumal et al., 1982). Dense terminal synaptic fields of enkephalin fibers are found in the globus pallidus, locus coeruleus, dorsal raphe, substantia gelatinosa, and central amygdaloid nucleus. At the ultrastructural level, enkephalin-containing axon terminals make typical assymmetric synapses with unlabeled dendrites or dendritic spines in the locus coeruleus (Pickel et al., 1979), striatum (Pickel et al., 1980), and substantia gelatinosa of the spinal cord (Hunt et al., 1980; Sumal et al., 1982; Glazer and Bausbaum, 1983). Axo-axonal contacts are extremely rare. The dynorphin family is found principally in the magnocellular neurons of the supraoptic and paraventricular nuclei of the hypothalamus, although dynorphins are also highly concentrated in the granule cells of the dentate gyrus, and in the nucleus parabrachialis and tractus solitarius of the brainstem (Watson et al., 1982, 1983; Weber and Barchas, 1983; McGinty et al., 1983).

The three opioid peptide systems are assumed to have widespread functional significance. Few generalizations are yet possible based on the immunohistochemical mapping studies, although it does seem that most enkephalin-containing neurons are short-axoned and may therefore operate as interneurons, whereas the β-endorphin system consists primarily of long-axoned projection neurons. The potential to be released into the circulation as a neurohormone cannot be ignored. It is likely that each pharmacological action of exogenously administered opioids mimics that of an endogenous system that is called into play under certain conditions. The attempt to understand the physiological functions of the various opioid peptide-containing neurons comprises a growing area of opioid research. Electrophysiological studies have demonstrated two inhibitory pathways in the brain that may use an opioid peptide as a neurotransmitter, based on sensitivity to naloxone. Focal iontophoresis of this opioid antagonist attenuated the brief (20–300 msec) suppression of unit activity in the globus pallidus caused by electrical stimulation of the striatum (Napier et al., 1983), and the very long-lasting (minutes) inhibition of nociceptive neurons in the nucleus reticularis ventralis of the medulla produced by stimulation within the periaqueductal gray (Hill et al., 1983). In both cases nerve fibers that connect the relevant regions have been shown to contain opioid peptides by immunocytochemical methods.

1.3. Opioid Receptors

A large number of synthetic alkaloids and peptides are available that demonstrate opioid agonist activity in a variety of assays. It has been difficult to fit all the data into a single receptor scheme. Potency ratios differ for

Table 1. Effects of Opioids on Activity of CNS Neurons

Region	Agonist[a]	Effect[b]		Reference
		Spontaneous	Evoked	
Cortical Areas				
Neocortex	Mor, Enk	−		Satoh et al. (1976), Palmer et al. (1978)
Hippocampus	Mor, Enk, β-E	+	−(IPSPs)	Zieglgänsberger et al. (1979), Nicoll et al. (1980), Dunwiddie et al. (1980), Dingledine (1981); Gruol et al. (1983)
Cingulate gyrus	Dyn	+, −		French and Siggins (1980), Forney and Klemm (1983)
	Mor, Enk	−		
Olfactory bulb	Enk		−(IPSPs)	Nicoll et al (1980)
Cerebellum	Mor, Enk, β-E	+, −		French and Siggins (1980)
Forebrain/Midbrain				
Caudate nuc.	Mor, Enk, β-E	−		Frederickson and Norris (1976), Nicoll et al. (1977)
Nuc. accumbens	Mor, Enk	−		McCarthy et al. (1977)
Globus pallidus	Mor	−		Huffman and Felpel (1981), Napier et al. (1983)
Amygdaloid nuclei	Enk	−		French and Siggins (1980)
	Mor, β-E	−,+		French and Siggins (1980)
Bed nuc. stria terminalis	Enk	−	−(Stria terminalis)	Sawada and Yamamoto (1981)
Mesen. reticular formation	Mor, Enk	−	−(Noxious pinch)	Hosford and Haigler (1980)
Septum (medial and lateral)	Mor, Enk	−		French and Siggins (1980)
	β-E	−,+		French and Siggins (1980)
Thalamus				
Ventrobasal	Mor	−	−(Noxious pinch, heat)	Guilbaud et al. (1983)
Nuc. lateralis anterior	Enk	−	−(Noxious heat)	Hill and Pepper (1978)
Unidentified	Mor, Enk, β-E	−		Hill et al. (1976), Nicoll et al. (1977)

Region	Peptide	Effect	Stimulus	References
Hypothalamus				
Arcuate nuc.	Enk, β-E, Dyn	–		MacMillan and Clarke (1983)
Periventricular nuc.	Mor, Enk	–		Muehlethaler et al. (1980)
Ventromedian nuc.	Mor, Enk	+		Kerr et al. (1974), Ono et al. (1980)
Lateral hypothalamic area	Mor, Enk	–		Kerr et al. (1974), Ono et al. (1980)
Supraoptic nuc. (oxytocin cells)	Mor, Enk	–		Wakerly et al. (1983)
Anterior preoptic area	Mor	–,+		Baldino et al. (1980)
Medulla/Pons				
Locus coeruleus	Mor, Enk	–		Korf et al. (1974), Pepper and Henderson (1980), Williams et al. (1982); Segal (1979)
Substantia nigra	Mor	–(i.v.)	–(Noxious pinch)	Iwatsubo and Clouet (1977)
Periaqueductal gray	Enk	–		Frederickson and Norris (1976)
Trigeminal nuc. caudalis	Enk	–	–(Noxious tooth pulp stim.)	Andersen et al. (1978)
Inferior olive	Enk	–		Schulman (1981)
Nuc. reticularis paragigantocellularis	Mor, Enk	+		Satoh et al. (1979), Mohrland and Gebhart (1981)
Respiratory center (nuc. tractus solitarius, ambiguous, parabrachialis medialis)	Mor, Enk	–		Denavit-Saubie et al. (1978)
Lateral vestibular nuc.	Enk	–		Chan-Palay et al. (1982)
Spinal Cord				
Substantia gelatinosa	Enk	–		Yoshimora and North (1983)
Motoneurons	Mor, Enk	0	–(Monosynaptic EPSPs)	Zieglgänsberger and Bayerl (1976), Zieglgänsberger and Tulloch (1979)
Dorsal horn interneurons	Mor, Enk	–	–(Noxious heat)	Zieglgänsberger and Bayerl (1976), Duggan et al. (1977), Murase et al. (1982)
Renshaw cells	Mor	+	–(Ventral root[c])	Duggan et al. (1976)

[a]Abbreviations: MOR, morphine or normorphine; ENK, an enkephalin or derivative; β-E, β-endorphin; DYN, dynorphin.
[b]–, reduced activity; +, increased activity; 0, no effect; (i.v.) indicates the effect was reported only for systemic administration. The stimulus used in evoked response studies is indicated in parentheses.
[c]The latency to first spike of a burst evoked by ventral root stimulation was increased.

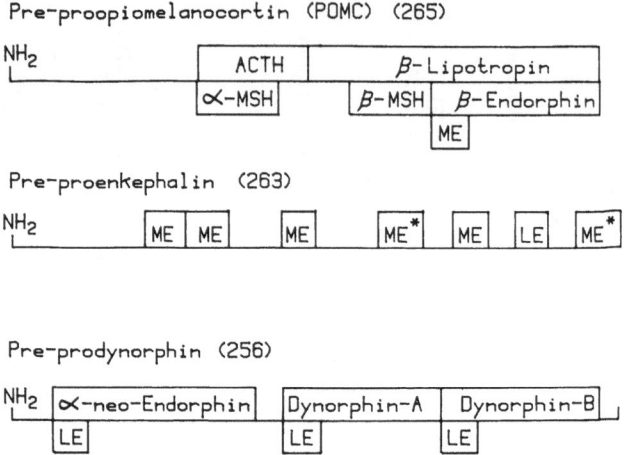

Figure 1. The three families of opioid peptides. The number of amino acid residues is shown in parentheses next to each parent peptide. Abbreviations: ME, methionine-enkephalin (Tyr-Gly-Gly-Phe-Met); LE, leucine-enkephalin (Tyr-Gly-Gly-Phe-Leu); ME*, C-terminally extended ME derivatives. Each propeptide contains several biologically active peptides, some of which are shown in boxes.

agonists in binding assays and bioassays, and naloxone, the classic opioid antagonist, is a weaker antagonist against some agonists than against others (Kosterlitz and Paterson, 1980). Alternative explanations such as different degradation rates for various agonists appear to have been ruled out, and at least three opioid receptor subtypes are proposed to explain the pharmacological data: μ, of which morphine is the prototype agonist; δ, with [D-Ala^2, D-Leu^5]-enkephalin (DADL) as the prototype; and κ, which responds preferentially to certain benzomorphans such as ethylketocyclazocine. The dynorphin family of opioid peptides is thought to interact preferentially with κ receptors (Chavkin et al., 1982). Direct evidence for the existence of multiple opioid binding sites was first provided by Chang and Cuatrecasas (1979), who compared the potency of various agonists in competing for the binding of radiolabeled alkaloids and enkephalins. The alkaloids morphine and normorphine were found to be approximately 8–10 times more potent when inhibiting the binding of tritiated dihydromorphine or naloxone than when competing for radiolabeled [D-Ala^2, D-Leu^5] enkephalin binding, and vice versa for the enkephalins. These results imply the existence of separate binding sites for the alkaloids and enkephalins. Not all opioid receptors fall neatly into the above classification scheme, however, and alternative schemes involving interconvertible μ and δ receptors have been suggested (Bowan et al., 1981). An additional level of complexity was introduced by Cox and Chavkin (1983), who showed that the spare receptor fraction for apparently identical κ receptors was different in different tissues. Thus the possibility of different degrees of receptor reserve for different agonists must be considered as an alternative to the presence of multiple receptor types when potency ratio is used as the only criterion.

Studies to date have provided us with a low-resolution map of opioid receptors in the brain. The three receptor types are differentially distributed throughout the brain, as shown both with binding assays (Chang et al., 1979; Chang and Cuatrecasas, 1981) and, in the case of μ and δ receptors, with light-microscopic autoradiography (Goodman et al., 1980). Mu opioid receptors are clustered in the corpus striatum, periaqueductal gray, certain thalamic and hypothalamic nuclei, the pyramidal cell layer of the hippocampus, and several other regions. Delta receptors are generally more diffusely distributed, but appear to be selectively concentrated in the amygdala, nucleus accumbens, and olfactory tubercle, among other regions. Both μ and δ receptors are found in high density in the substantia gelatinosa, partly on primary afferent nerve terminals. Localizing κ receptors by autoradiography has proved more refractory since it has been difficult to radiolabel this class of binding site selectively.

Figure 2 shows autoradiographs that illustrate the differential distri-

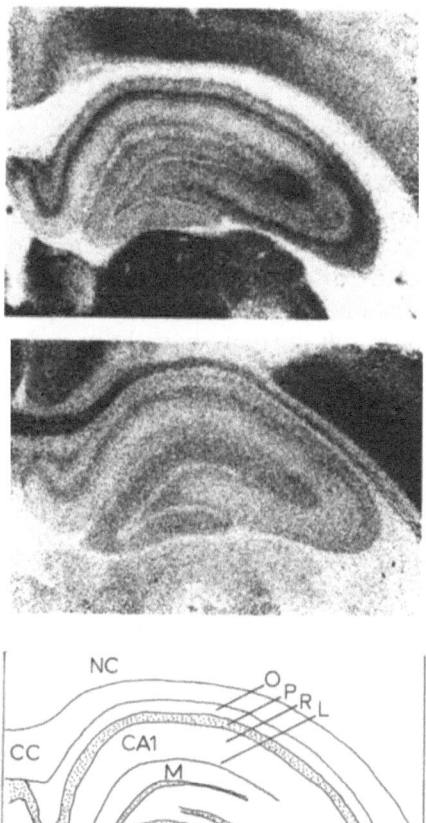

Figure 2. Autoradiographic images of opioid receptor binding in rat hippocampus. Frozen coronal sections were incubated with 0.7 nM ^{125}I-FK-33824 (upper panel) to label μ receptors, or 0.5 nM ^{125}I-DADL (middle panel) to label δ-receptors. In the latter case 1 μM PLO-32, a morphiceptin analog that is a powerful μ agonist, was included in the incubation to suppress the binding of labeled DADL to μ receptors. The sections were washed, pressed against Ultrofilm, and exposed in the dark for three (μ) or six (δ) weeks before developing with D-19. Parallel binding assays performed on tissue sections indicated that 95% of the binding of ^{125}I-FK-33824 was specific (not displaced by an excess of diprenorphine), where 70% of the ^{125}I-DADL binding was specific. Near-background labeling in both cases occurs over the fimbria. A schematic diagram identifying the laminated structures is shown in the lower panel. Abbreviations used are: CC, corpus callosum; NC, neocortex; F, fimbria; T, thalamus; O, stratum oriens; P, stratum pyramidale; R, stratum radiatum; L, stratum lacunosum-moleculare; M, stratum moleculare of the dentate gyrus; CA1 and CA3, hippocampal subfields. (From B. Crain, and J. O. McNamara, unpublished.)

bution of μ and δ opioid receptors in the rat hippocampus. These are bright-field photomicrographs so the silver grains marking receptors appear black on a white background. Mu receptors (upper panel) are concentrated in a sharp band surrounding stratum pyramidale, as well as over stratum lacunosum moleculare of CA_3 at the foot of the hippocampal fissure. Delta receptors (middle panel) are relatively dense in stratum moleculare of the dentate gyrus, in a diffuse layer around stratum pyramidale, and in stratum oriens of CA_3. Regions surrounding the hippocampus are also selectively labeled, with dense δ receptor binding in part of the corpus callosum and neocortex, and heavy μ receptor labeling in the underlying thalamus. Similar information about the regional distribution of μ and δ receptors is now available for the entire brain. Due to the inherently low spatial resolution of film autoradiography, however, the identity of the cells that bear these opioid receptors is still unknown.

2. CELLULAR ACTIONS OF OPIOIDS

2.1. Dorsal Root Ganglia

Action potentials of dorsal root ganglion (DRG) neurons grown in primary cell culture have both sodium and calcium components (Dunlap and Fishbach, 1981; Heyer and MacDonald, 1982). Approximately the first millisecond of the spike is due to sodium current with the remaining broad plateau due to calcium current. The calcium spike can be studied in relative isolation after sodium current has been blocked by tetrodotoxin (TTX), and potassium currents have been reduced by tetraethylammonium (TEA) and the divalent cation Ba^{2+}, which also carries current through calcium channels directly. DRG cells in culture are large, hardy, and easy to impale, a fortunate combination of attributes that allows the study of drug effects in some detail.

The application of several enkephalin derivatives to the medium surrounding DRG neurons quickly reduced both the amplitude and duration of calcium spikes triggered by depolarizing current injection (Mudge et al., 1979; Werz and MacDonald, 1983a; Fig. 3). Calcium spike shortening was observed only in a proportion of cells and resembled that produced by several neurotransmitters (GABA, norepinephrine, serotonin), all of which are thought to reduce calcium conductance in DRG neurons (Dunlap and Fischbach, 1981). The effect of the opioid peptides occurred at submicromolar concentrations and could be blocked by low concentrations of naloxone. Calcium spike shortening by opioids appeared to be especially prominent when TTX, TEA, or Ba^{2+} was present to enhance calcium spikes. No alteration by opioids of membrane potential or passive membrane conductance has been detected. Of special interest was the demonstration that the calcium spike after-hyperpolarization was enhanced by enkephalins even in the face of reduced

Figure 3. Shortening of the DRG neuron somatic calcium spike by Leu-enkephalin. Pressure ejection of a 500-nM solution of Leu-enkephalin near the soma of a DRG neuron for 4 sec (A), or a 5-μM solution for 5 min (B), reduced the duration and amplitude of calcium spikes evoked every 15 sec. In A1, B1, the control spike is shown in (1) and the maximum effect of leu-enkephalin in (2). A2, B2 show gradual recovery 1.5 min (7 in A1) or 2 min (28 in A2) after terminating drug ejection. Note that during prolonged 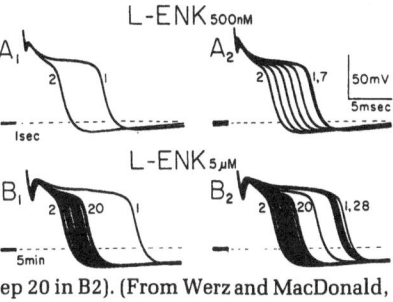 opioid application the drug effect gradually faded (sweep 20 in B2). (From Werz and MacDonald, 1983a, with permission.)

calcium entry (spike duration) (Fig. 3). In contrast, calcium spike shortening caused by Cd^{2+} was accompanied by a concomitant reduction in afterhyperpolarization. This suggests that enkephalins may decrease action potential duration in sensory neurons by activating a potassium conductance. Indeed, blockade of the effect of enkephalin by intracellular injection of Cs^+, a potassium channel blocker, supports this idea (Werz and MacDonald, 1983b). In the same cells, naloxone-sensitive calcium spike shortening produced by 1 μM dynorphin was, however, insensitive to Cs^+ injection (Werz and MacDonald, 1984), and it was proposed that κ receptors may directly regulate calcium conductance.

Both μ and δ opioid receptors are thought to mediate the shortening of somatic calcium-dependent action potentials by enkephalins (Werz and MacDonald, 1983a). Of significance is the finding that the DRG cell population appears to be heterogeneous with respect to the density of μ and δ receptors. Both morphiceptin, an agonist selective for μ opioid receptors, and Leu-enkephalin, a somewhat δ-selective agonist, decreased the duration of the DRG neuron calcium spike in a dose-dependent manner. Both agonists were active over a similar concentration range, approximately 0.1–10 μM. In a low proportion of neurons (approximately 10%), calcium spikes were shortened more by morphiceptin than by equimolar Leu-enkephalin, whereas a majority of the cells responded much better to Leu-enkephalin than to morphiceptin. Naloxone was a much more potent antagonist (against both agonists) for the morphiceptin responders than it was for the Leu-enkephalin responders (Fig. 4). These results imply that individual DRG neurons may possess predominantly μ or δ receptors, although a portion of the DRG neurons have both receptors on their somatic membranes. Most DRG neurons appear to be of the delta type (i.e., relatively insensitive to naloxone). It will be of great interest to determine the factors that regulate the differential expression of μ and δ receptors, whether the same potassium channels are coupled to each receptor, and whether the two cell populations subserve distinct physiological functions. A similar shortening by opioid peptides of calcium action potentials in DRG *terminals* could form the basis for a selective and powerful presynaptic inhibition of sensory transmitter release. Indeed, quantal analysis of EPSPs in synaptically coupled DRG-spinal neu-

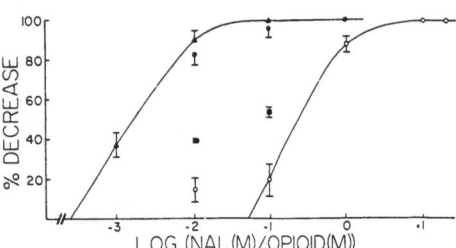

Figure 4. Two populations of DRG neurons based on sensitivity to peptide agonists and naloxone. The ordinate is the percent decrease of response to opioid peptides produced by naloxone. The abscissa is the log of the ratio of naloxone to agonist concentration (1 = a tenfold higher concentration of naloxone over that of the peptide agonist). Shortening of calcium spikes by morphiceptin (MC) was highly sensitive to naloxone antagonism (▲). Leu-enkephalin responses were equally well antagonized by naloxone in the population of DRG neurons that responded well to morphiceptin (MC$^+$, ●); these neurons are considered to have predominantly μ receptors. In contrast, Leu-enkephalin responses in DRG neurons relatively insensitive to morphiceptin (○) were 100-fold less sensitive to naloxone; these cells have predominantly delta receptors. Those neurons responding approximately equally well to Leu-enkephalin and morphiceptin (■) were intermediate in their sensitivity to naloxone; this population presumably contains both μ and δ opioid receptors. [From Werz and MacDonald (1983a) with permission.]

ron cell pairs in culture has provided some evidence for presynaptic inhibition of sensory transmitter release by etorphine (MacDonald and Nelson, 1978).

2.2. Locus Coeruleus

The basis for the depression of firing rate of extracellularly recorded locus coeruleus (LC) neurons by opiates (Korf et al., 1974) has recently been investigated by intracellular recordings from slices of pons containing the LC (Pepper and Henderson, 1980; Williams et al., 1982, 1984). Normorphine, Met-enkephalin, and DADL, when applied by superfusion or pressure ejection from a blunt pipette, hyperpolarized LC neurons in a dose-dependent manner (Fig. 5A), with effective concentrations in the nanomolar to micromolar range. The hyperpolarizations could be elicited in the absence of calcium in the perfusion fluid, implying that the opioids acted directly on LC neurons and not by causing the release of an inhibitory transmitter from a nearby cell.

A good deal of evidence has been presented indicating that the most likely mechanism for the hyperpolarization is an increase in potassium conductance. First, the hyperpolarization was accompanied by a membrane conductance increase and was reversed to a depolarization when the membrane potential was held more negative than approximately -100 mV. Second, the reversal potential for the opioid-induced hyperpolarization varied in a Nernstian fashion when bath potassium concentration was changed (Fig. 5C, D) but was unaffected by manipulations of the chloride equilibrium potential. Third, certain potassium conductance blockers, i.e., externally applied Ba^{2+} or internally applied Cs$^+$, prevented the opioid effect. Opioids also prolonged the spike burst afterhyperpolarization, which is thought to reflect a calcium-dependent potassium conductance in LC neurons. The last two findings are consistent with opioids activating a calcium-dependent potassium channel, although the preservation of opioid effects in the absence of external calcium is a counter-argument. This hypothesis could be retained if the primary effect of opioids was to impair cytoplasmic calcium buffering, in which case the source of calcium could be an intracellular store, or to modify the sensitivity of the potassium channel gating mechanism to membrane potential or cytoplasmic calcium concentration.

The opioid evoked hyperpolarizations in the LC appear to be mediated

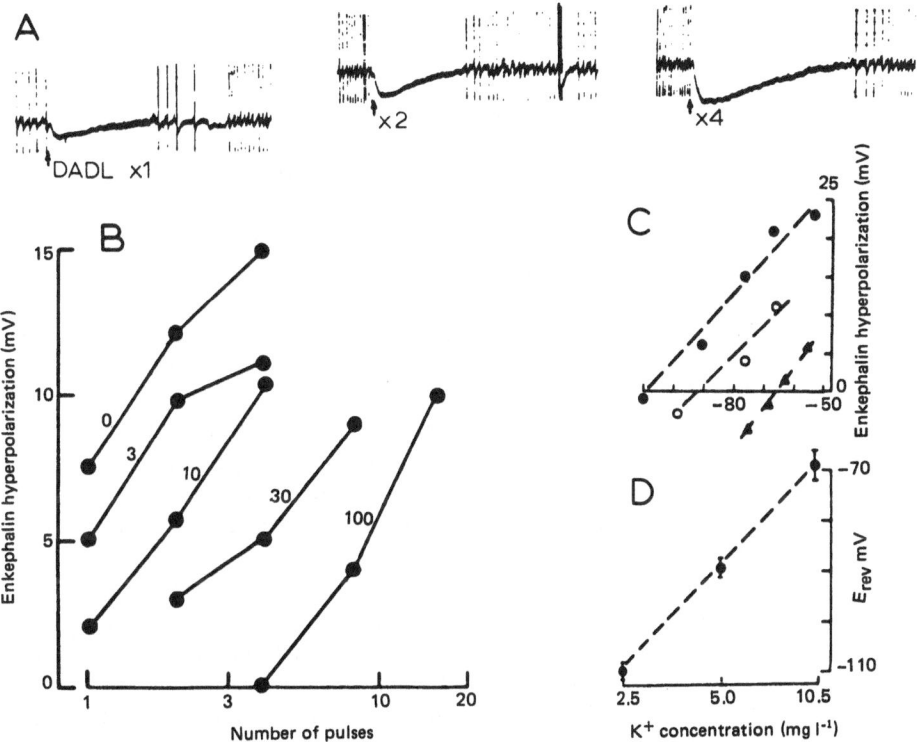

Figure 5. Competitive antagonism by naloxone of potassium-sensitive hyperpolarization of LC neurons by DADL. (A) The opioid peptide was dissolved in perfusion medium and pressure ejected (arrows, 24-msec pulses, number of pulses indicated) near a LC neuron. DADL caused a dose-dependent hyperpolarization and cessation of spontaneous firing. (B) The maximum hyperpolarization by DADL (ordinate) is plotted as a function of the number of pressure pulses (abscissa) in different concentrations of naloxone (nM) applied by perfusion. Naloxone caused a parallel shift to the right in the DADL dose–response curve. The half-maximally effective concentration of naloxone, calculated by a Schild plot, was 1–2 nM, which is consistent with μ receptor mediation of the DADL response. (C) Hyperpolarization evoked by a standard pulse of DADL was plotted as a function of membrane potential in three K^+ concentrations: 2.5 mM (●), 5 mM (○) and 10.5 mM (▲). (D) The reversal potential for DADL-evoked hyperpolarization in different K^+ concentrations agrees well with the Nernst prediction (broken line), indicating that the hyperpolarization is due to a K^+ conductance increase. (Adapted from Williams et al., 1982, with permission.)

by μ receptors. Hyperpolarizations evoked by either the μ-selective agonist normorphine, or by DADL, which has higher affinity for delta than μ receptors, were equally sensitive to blockade by a range of antagonists. μ-Selective antagonists such as naloxone were much more potent than δ receptor antagonists (e.g., the peptide ICI 154129), suggesting mediation by μ opioid receptors. The half-maximally effective concentration of naloxone, determined in Schild plots, was approximately 1.5 nM (Fig. 5B), consistent with mediation by μ receptors. Dynorphin and cyclazocine, κ-receptor agonists, had no effect on membrane potential at concentrations up to 1 μM. The data obtained so far suggest that LC neurons are homogeneous with respect to opioid receptors: the hyperpolarizing response is linked to μ, but not δ or κ, receptors.

2.3. Hippocampus

The hippocampal slice preparation has been used extensively to explore the cellular basis for the epileptiform action of opioid peptides in limbic regions (Nicoll et al., 1980; Lee et al., 1980; Haas and Ryall, 1980; Dingledine, 1981 and references therein). Afferent inputs to hippocampal pyramidal cells are segregated so that virtually all excitatory synapses are made on dendritic spines, whereas GABAergic inhibitory synapses are concentrated around the soma. Inhibitory synapses are, however, also scattered throughout the dendritic layers. Orthodromic stimulation of afferent fibers in the dendritic layers evokes a mixed EPSP-IPSP that can trigger an action potential. The most reproducibly observed effect of opioid peptides in the hippocampus was an enhancement of the synaptic activation of pyramidal cells by orthodromic inputs. Subthreshold EPSPs were increased in amplitude, and stimuli that would normally trigger a single spike evoked a short burst of 2–3 action potentials after exposure of the cells to an opioid peptide (Fig. 6). In extracellular recordings, both in the slice and *in vivo*, the spontaneous firing rate of pyramidal cells was elevated and synaptically driven population spike field potentials were increased in amplitude.

A number of possible modes of action of opioids have been ruled out. A potentiation of excitatory transmitter release is not involved since dendritic field potentials indicative of excitatory postsynaptic current were unchanged and iontophoretic mapping studies localized the site of action of DADL to the cell layer, several hundred microns from the excitatory synapses. Opioid peptides caused no detectable change in the membrane properties of pyramidal cells (membrane potential, input resistance, or voltage threshold for eliciting sodium spikes). Further, enkephalin derivatives neither facilitated calcium spikes nor potentiated depolarizations produced by brief iontophoretic pulses of excitatory amino acids delivered into the excitatory synaptic layers, arguing against a direct action on electrotonically distant pyramidal cell dendrites. The "excitatory" action of opioid peptides appears to be caused by a suppression of GABAergic IPSPs, which leads to

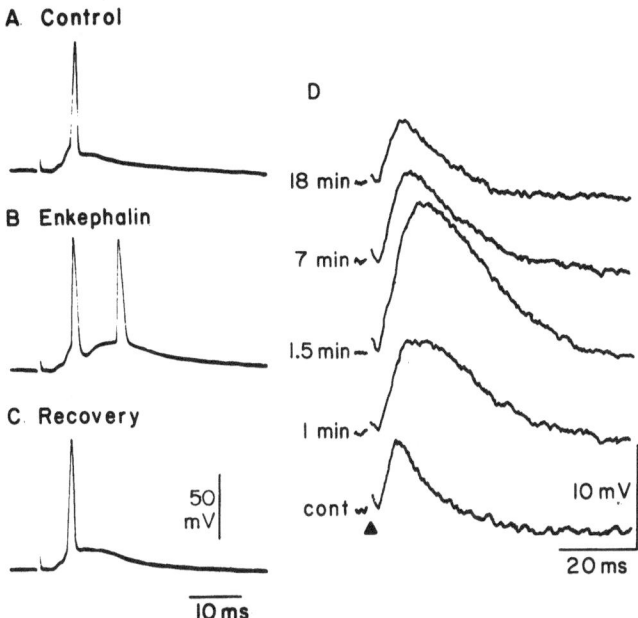

Figure 6. Potentiation of the synaptic activation of hippocampal pyramidal neurons by DADL. (A) Iontophoretic application of DADL (50 nA, 20 sec) increased the number of spikes triggered by a constant orthodromic stimulus from 1 to 2. Recovery occurred by 7 min. (B) Orthodromic stimulation evoked a mixed EPSP/IPSP in control (cont), which was converted to a large depolarizing potential following a droplet of 10 μM DADL applied to the slice surface. Recovery occurred within 18 min. (From Dingledine, 1981, with permission.)

an unmasking of underlying EPSPs. Nicoll et al. (1980) first demonstrated that GABAergic IPSPs could be reduced in amplitude by opioid peptides. Enkephalin derivatives have also been reported to reduce IPSPs in cultured hippocampal neurons (Gähwiler, 1980). Not all IPSPs in the hippocampus are equally sensitive to opioid agonists, however, and an understanding of the actions of these drugs requires a consideration of hippocampal intrinsic circuitry.

GABAergic synaptic inhibition has been demonstrated on both the soma and dendrites of hippocampal pyramidal cells. A mixed soma/dendrite IPSP can be elicited by orthodromic stimulation, whereas somatic IPSPs can be evoked in the near absence of contaminating EPSPs and dendritic IPSPs by selective antidromic stimulation of the pyramidal cell axons grouped together in the alveus. Dendritic IPSPs, as recorded by intrasomatic micropipettes, are difficult to study in isolation since they are often overwhelmed by the much more prominent somatic IPSPs. Whereas the evidence appears strong that opioid peptides can attenuate IPSPs on hippocampal pyramidal cells, it is also clear that a potentiation of EPSPs and population spikes can be observed in the absence of detectable reductions in somatic IPSPs (Haas and Ryall, 1980; Dingledine, 1981; Fig. 7). Bearing in mind that orthodromic stimulation elicits a mixed EPSP/IPSP, more direct evidence supports the hypothesis that the increase in EPSP amplitude is not due to a reduction in size of a somatic IPSP. If this were the case, then hyperpolarizing the pyramidal cell membrane below the apparent reversal potential for antidromically evoked recurrent IPSPs should result in a change in sign of the opioid effect; that is, opioids should then reduce the amplitude of evoked EPSPs. The magnitude of the opioid peptide enhancement of EPSPs was indeed voltage dependent, decreasing as the membrane potential was hyperpolarized, but the membrane potential at which the opioid effect on EPSPs was abolished (approximately -90 mV) was very different from the measured reversal potential for the recurrent IPSP (-75 mV). This result is incompatible with the potentiation of the EPSP being due to a reduction in somatic IPSPs, but is consistent with the idea that opioids block electrically distant, dendritic IPSPs. The selective effect of opioid peptides in the hippocampus is in striking contrast to the actions of the epileptogenic agent penicillin, which invariably attenuated both antidromic and orthodromic IPSPs at concentrations sufficient to enhance EPSPs (Dingledine and Gjerstad, 1980; Dingledine, 1981).

The following hypothesis can be put forward based on the above evidence: Opioid peptides in low concentrations selectively reduce dendritic IPSPs in the hippocampus, the effect of which is to enhance the size and effectiveness of EPSPs. This results in a potentiation of population spikes

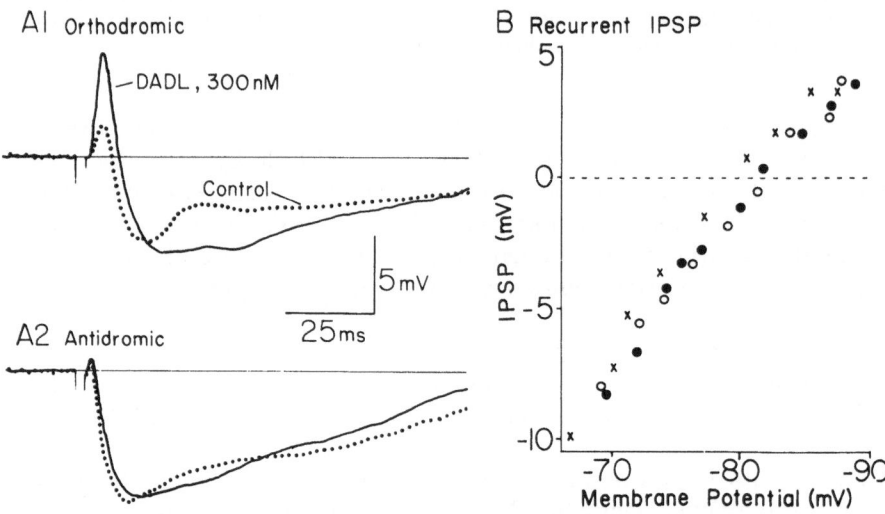

Figure 7. Potentiation of EPSP in hippocampal pyramidal cell by DADL without detectable reduction in IPSPs. (A) Intracellular responses to orthodromic (1) and antidromic (2) stimuli, before (control) and after perfusing slice with 300 nM DADL. The EPSP is enhanced with little reduction of either orthodromic or antidromic IPSPs. Each trace is the average of four sweeps. Subsequent perfusion with DADL plus 500 nM naloxone returned the orthodromic response to its control size (not shown). (B) In the same cell, the recurrent IPSP is plotted as a function of membrane potential in control (●), DADL (○), and DADL plus naloxone (X). No effect of DADL on the recurrent IPSP is seen. (Adapted from Dingledine, 1981, with permission.)

recorded extracellularly and can also lead to evoked burst activity. At higher agonist concentrations, somatic IPSPs may also be attenuated, resulting in more intense epileptiform activity.

What is the mechanism for the reduction in dendritic IPSPs by opioid peptides? It is unlikely to involve a direct blocking action on postsynaptic GABA receptors since opioids had no effect on responses of pyramidal cells to iontophoretically applied GABA. In addition to the lack of any direct opioid effect on pyramidal cell membrane properties, two other experiments indicate that the site of action of opioid peptides in the hippocampus is not directly on pyramidal neurons, but rather on inhibitory interneurons. First, Lee et al. (1980) discovered a population of nonpyramidal cells, the evoked firing of which was suppressed by opioids. These cells had many of the physiological characteristics expected of interneurons. Second, Nicoll et al. (1980) demonstrated that spontaneous IPSPs could be reduced in frequency by opioid peptides. Since the spontaneous IPSPs could also be blocked by tetrodotoxin, it was postulated that they arose from the spontaneous discharge of nearby inhibitory interneurons. It seems reasonable to conclude that opioid effects in the hippocampus are due to a suppression of the firing of a select population of inhibitory interneurons. Indeed, a population of presumed hippocampal interneurons was recently shown to be hyperpolarized by an enkephalin derivative (Nicoll and Madison, 1984). Further progress will require exploration of the inhibitory nature of these cells.

Mu, δ and κ opioid receptors have been demonstrated in hippocampal membranes with binding assays. To determine the receptor types responsible for the pharmacological action of opioids on hippocampal neurons, the potentiation of evoked population spikes was studied (Valentino and Dingledine, 1982; Bostock et al., 1984). Relative potencies for eight agonists are shown in Table 2. The potency rank order agrees well with that reported for the electroencephalographic seizure activity of opioids. Thus the enkephalins are more potent than morphine, and ethylketocyclazocine is virtually inactive.

A good argument can be made for the involvement of μ opioid receptors in this assay, since the highly selective μ agonists morphiceptin and its [N-methyl-Phe^3,D-Pro^4] derivative are too potent to be acting on δ receptors. Indeed, the results of binding assays carried out on hippocampal membranes suspended in physiological saline indicated negligible binding of morphiceptin to δ receptors even at high concentrations (Bostock et al., 1984). In contrast, the dissociation constant of morphiceptin for μ receptors (0.15–1.41 μM; 95% confidence interval) under the same conditions was similar to its EC$_{50}$ in the hippocampal slice (0.5–4.6 μM).

The two most potent peptides tested, DADL and D-Tyr-Ser-Gly-Phe-Leu-Thr (DSLET), are both selective for δ opioid receptors. However, these peptides do not have high selectivity for δ over μ receptors, and in the absence of additional information it is not yet possible to state whether they are acting on δ or μ receptors in the hippocampus. Still unexplained is why the alkaloid morphine and the other nonpeptide opioids are so weak in the hippocampus. It is important to realize that there is no basis for assigning

Table 2. Facilitation of Evoked Firing by Opioids in the Hippocampus

	EC$_{50}$ (nM)[a]	Potency ratio
DADL	68	1.0
Tyr-D-Ser-Gly-Phe-Leu-Thr	330	0.21
[N-Methyl-Phe^3,D-Pro^4]-morphiceptin	~400	~0.17
β-endorphin	450	0.15
Morphiceptin	1600	0.04
Morphine	3000	0.02
Normorphine	~ 3000	~0.02
Ethylketocyclazocine	>10000	<0.007

[a]Concentration required to produce a standard leftward shift in the input-output curve, a quantitative measure of the excitatory effect of opioids in the CA1 region of the hippocampus. Values were interpolated from concentration-response curves. [From Valentino and Dingledine (1982) with permission, and unpublished data.]

the label of partial agonist to the alkaloids. Thus, the maximum response of morphine was the same as that of morphiceptin or DADL, and morphine could not block the effect of morphiceptin. It is possible that the stimulus-response relationship for peptides on μ receptors may be stronger than that for nonpeptide opioids.

A form of tolerance or desensitization develops in the hippocampus during prolonged (hours) continuous exposure to opioid peptides (Dingledine et al., 1983). The magnitude of the opioid effect was measured as the leftward shift in the input–output curve formed by plotting population spike amplitude as a function of the field EPSP (Valentino and Dingledine, 1982). The opioid effect was then monitored by constructing input–output curves every 3–10 min for 5–7 hr during perfusion with opioids. The peak effect for both 1 μM DADL and 10 μM morphiceptin (equipotent concentrations) was achieved within 12–25 min of the start of drug perfusion but then slowly declined. Approximately 50–60% of the peak effect was lost after 4 hr of continuous perfusion with DADL (Fig. 8), or 1 hr with morphiceptin. This form of tolerance developed in the absence of any sign of dependence, since subsequent perfusion with naloxone merely reversed residual agonist effects without causing an "overshoot" of the input–output curve. A significant reduction in the number of δ, but not μ, opioid receptors occurred in slices perfused with DADL for 4 h, as demonstrated by Scatchard plots. In contrast, neither δ nor μ binding was changed by perfusing slices with morphiceptin. The data suggest a fundamental difference in the means by which hippocampal neurons adapt to the continued presence of δ and μ receptor agonists. Desensitization to δ agonists may result from down-regulation of δ receptors, but a different mechanism must be responsible for desensitization to μ agonists.

2.4. Spinal Cord

As in many other regions of the CNS, the most consistent naloxone-sensitive action of opioids in the dorsal horn of the spinal cord is a depression

Figure 8. Slow desensitization of the excitatory effect of DADL in the hippocampal slice. The characteristic response to opioids, as measured with field potentials, is a shift to the left in the sigmoid input-output curve formed by plotting population spike amplitude as a function of field EPSP. Each input-output curve consisted of 50–100 data points. The excitatory response to DADL is measured as the reduction in the field EPSP (input) required to evoke a standard 30% maximum population spike [explained in detail in Valentino and Dingledine (1982)]. This value, the EPSP-30, is plotted as a function of time, each point representing a measurement obtained from a single input-output curve. During the time indicated by the bars, the perfusion fluid contained DADL (1 μM), morphine (20 μM) and naloxone (1 μM). The slice responded well to morphine after partial desensitization to DADL had occurred. After 5 h continuous exposure to opioids, subsequent perfusion with naloxone merely reversed residual agonist effects with no apparent overshoot of the curve. (From Dingledine et al., 1983, with permission.)

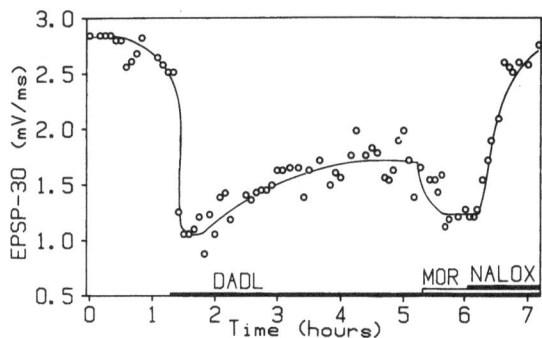

of spontaneous or glutamate-driven firing activity. In addition, opioids applied systemically or iontophoretically depress the activation of lamina V neurons by nociceptive stimuli (Duggan et al., 1977 and references cited therein). Non-noxious inputs to the same cells are much less affected, so the modality specificity is consistent with clinical experience. Many of the projection neurons that transmit sensory information to the brain are located in lamina V, and the assumption is that recordings have been obtained from this population of cells. Duggan's group have applied morphine and enkephalin derivatives locally into various regions of the dorsal horn while recording from lamina V cells in an attempt to localize the site of the analgesic action. When applied into lamina V itself (i.e., the region of the cell bodies), opioids produced only inconsistent and apparently nonspecific effects on neuronal responses to sensory stimulation. When applied directly into the substantia gelatinosa, where most of the nociceptive fibers synapse onto dendrites of lamina V cells, opioids selectively reduced responses to noxious stimuli when compared to other sensory modalities. The inhibitory effect of morphine could be reversed by systemic injection of naloxone and, conversely, naloxone applied directly into the substantia gelatinosa could reverse the effect of systemic morphine on lamina V responses. Thus it seems clear that one site for the analgesic action of morphine is the substantia gelatinosa of the dorsal horn. It is not known, however, whether the selectivity for sensory modality is achieved by presynaptic inhibition of transmitter release from primary afferents, a postsynaptic effect on the dendrites of lamina V cells, or an action on a restricted interneuron population. The known anatomy may favor the latter two interpretations since most enkephalin-containing processes appear to be separated from primary afferent terminals by an intervening dendrite (Sumal et al., 1982). Indeed, Ruda

(1982) has found a select population of spinothalamic neurons in lamina V whose soma and proximal dendrites are heavily invested with enkephalin-containing synaptic terminals. This could provide a morphological substrate for feed-forward postsynaptic inhibition, mediated by enkephalin, on the second order relay neurons for nociceptive transmission. The possibility of diffusion of enkephalin to nearby sensory terminals, where it might directly inhibit transmitter release (Section 2.1), must also be considered.

A detailed intracellular study of the effects of opioids on identified lamina V projection neurons activated by well-defined nociceptive and non-noxious stimuli may help resolve the issue. A start in this direction has been made by Zieglgänsberger and Bayerl (1976), who reported that morphine reduced glutamate-evoked depolarizations, as well as the rate of rise of EPSPs evoked by afferent nerve stimulation. Although most of their observations were on motoneurons, the major findings seemed to hold with the few lamina V cells tested. Interestingly, morphine and enkephalin caused a small hyperpolarization in the majority of cells tested.

Intracellular recordings have also been obtained from neurons situated in the substantia gelatinosa of dorsal horn slices removed from adult rats (Yoshimura and North, 1983). Both normorphine and DADL hyperpolarized a proportion of substantia gelatinosa neurons and caused a fall in input resistance. The hyperpolarization was apparently caused by a rise in potassium conductance since it could be reversed in polarity by hyperpolarizing the membrane, and the measured reversal potential varied as predicted by the Nernst equation when bath potassium concentration was changed. The opioid effect presumably occurred directly on the impaled cell since it persisted when synaptic transmission had been blocked by adjusting divalent ion concentrations. These results suggest that the dense matwork of enkephalin-staining fibers in the substantia gelatinosa may mediate direct synaptic inhibition of a population of neurons resident in this area. The function of the opioid-sensitive neurons in terms of sensory information processing has not been determined.

A myriad of other actions of opioids have been reported in studies of neurons in spinal cord cultures (Gruol and Smith, 1981; Werz and Mac-Donald, 1982 and references therein). Most of the reported effects on cultured spinal cord cells do not appear to be mediated by classically defined opiate receptors since they were insensitive to antagonism by naloxone (even though a small degree of stereoselectivity was usually reported) and required quite high concentrations (e.g., 30–500 μM morphine). These nonspecific effects include antagonism of inhibitory conductance changes evoked by GABA and glycine, and consequent production of seizurelike paroxysmal depolarizations. Interestingly, the nonspecific actions were elicited only by opioid alkaloids such as morphine and levorphanol, but not be enkephalin derivatives. A report that opioids reduce glutamate-evoked depolarization in spinal cord cultures (Barker et al., 1978) has not been confirmed in subsequent studies (Gruol and Smith, 1981; Werz and MacDonald, 1982).

3. SUMMARY AND FUNCTIONAL CONSIDERATIONS

The mechanisms involved in the inhibitory action of opioids on certain CNS neurons are beginning to emerge from recent work employing *in vitro* preparations of various brain regions. In locus coeruleus, substantia gelatinosa, and dorsal root ganglion, evidence is accumulating in favor of the hypothesis that μ and δ receptor activation leads to a rise in an inhibitory potassium conductance. This mode of action would be consistent with the known inhibitory actions of opioids on other opiate-sensitive CNS neurons, including hippocampal inhibitory interneurons. Which of the many potassium conductances resident in mammalian neurons is opioid-sensitive has not been determined. Some type of a calcium-dependent potassium channel might be involved in the LC and DRG, however, since calcium mediated afterhyperpolarizations are potentiated by enkephalins in both cases. The finding that opioids hyperpolarized LC neurons, but not DRG cells, could then reflect the relative amount of calcium-dependent potassium conductance in the two cell types. Direct tests of this hypothesis await the results of voltage-clamp experiments and single-channel recordings from identified potassium channels on opioid-sensitive neurons. Such experiments are ongoing in several laboratories. Whether activation of potassium conductance represents the sole inhibitory action of opioid peptides, or whether other ionic mechanisms may be involved on certain neurons, remains to be determined. For example, Werz and MacDonald (1984) have provided evidence that a population of DRG neurons may contain κ receptors linked to voltage-dependent calcium channels. Opioid peptide modulation of sodium conductances, as first postulated from the sensitivity of opioid agonist binding to Na^+ (Pert and Snyder, 1974), has not been supported by most electrophysiological studies (but see Zieglgänsberger and Bayerl, 1976; Barker et al., 1978). It seems quite reasonable to suppose, however, that multiple opioid receptors are coupled to multiple conductance mechanisms, just as is the case with cholinergic and adrenergic receptors.

One widespread functional consequence of opioid agonist action appears to be inhibition of transmitter release from opioid-sensitive neurons, an action readily explained by potassium conductance increase or calcium spike shortening. Such a modulation of synaptic transmission could account for many findings in the spinal cord and hippocampus, as well as in peripheral sites such as the myenteric plexus, vas deferens, and mesenteric ganglion, where the action of opioids is manifested mainly as a presynaptic inhibition of evoked synaptic potentials (see Chapter 12). Opioid-sensitive neurons employ a variety of transmitter (ACh, norepinephrine, GABA), arguing against a special relationship between opioids and any particular synaptic transmitter.

Although opioid action results in a depression of the release of neurotransmitter in many regions of the nervous system, the term "presynaptic inhibition" may not be entirely appropriate to describe the effect in the CNS. This term was originally used to characterize the situation whereby an axo-axonic synapse depressed transmitter release by an (usually ill-defined) action on the nerve terminal itself. The crux of the definition lies with the location of the receptors for the inhibitory transmitter. Although opioids do appear to act directly on nerve terminals (in a presynaptic inhibitory mode) in the autonomic nervous system (see Chapter 12), the situation in the CNS is not as easily interpreted. Whether endogenous opioid synapses mediate direct synaptic inhibition, presynaptic inhibition, or mixed-mode inhibition, will depend on the anatomical location of the opioid synapses and opioid receptors in each region. A combination of techniques—electrophysiology, EM immunohistochemistry, and receptor autoradiography—will be required to settle the matter in each case.

It seems clear that modulation of transmitter release from nociceptive pathways in the substantia gelatinosa, or of GABA release in limbic regions, might help explain such seemingly diverse effects as the analgesic action of opioids in the spinal cord, on the one hand, and epileptiform limbic seizures, on the other. Pursuing the physiological roles subserved by the three families of opioid peptides has been hampered so far by the lack of highly specific antagonists for the various receptor subtypes. However, predictions based on the known physiology and anatomy can be put forward. The likelihood that opioid peptides and "classical" transmitters reside in the same nerve terminals, as appears to be the case with certain other peptides (Hökfelt et al., 1980), offers intriguing clues to peptide function. For example, it is probable that at least some of the GABAergic (GAD staining) interneurons in the hippocampus also contain an enkephalin, which suggests that opioid autoreceptors may regulate the release of GABA and thereby exert fine control over pyramidal cell activity.

In conclusion, some degree of understanding of the physiological actions of opioid peptides at the cellular and membrane level will undoubtedly contribute to a deeper appreciation of their roles in the integrative functions of the brain.

REFERENCES

Akaike, A., Shibata, T., Satoh, M., and Takagi, H., 1978, Analgesia induced by microinjection of morphine into, and electrical stimulation of the nucleus reticularis paragigantocellularis of rat medulla oblongata, *Neuropharmacology* **17**:775–778.

Andersen, R. K., Lund, J. P., and Puil, E., 1978, Enkephalin and substance P effects related to trigeminal pain, *Can. J. Physiol. Pharmacol.* **56**:216–222.

Baldino, F., Beckman, A. L., and Adler, M. W., 1980, Actions of iontophoretically applied morphine on hypothalamic thermosensitive units, *Brain Res.* **196**:199–208.

Barker, J. L., Neale, J. H., Smith, T. G., and MacDonald, R. L., 1978, Opiate peptide modulation of amino acid responses suggests novel form of neuronal communication, *Science* **199**:1451–1453.

Bloom, F. E., Battenberg, E., Rossier, J., Ling, N., and Guillemin, R., 1978, Neurons containing β-endorphin in rat brain exist separately from those containing enkephalin: Immunocytochemical studies, *Proc. Natl. Acad. Sci. USA* **75**:1591–1595.

Bostock, E., Dingledine, R., Xu, G., Chang, K. J., 1984, Mu opioid receptors participate in the excitatory effect of opiates in the hippocampal slice, *J. Pharmacol. Exp. Ther.* **231**:512–517.

Bowan, W. D., Gentleman, S., Herkenham, M., and Pert, C. B., 1981, Interconverting μ and δ forms of the opiate receptor in striatal patches, *Proc. Natl. Acad. Sci. USA* **78**:4818–4822.

Chan-Palay, V., Ito, M., Tongroach, P., Sakurai, M., and Palay, S., 1982, Inhibitory effects of motilin, somatostatin, [Leu]enkephalin, [Met]enkephalin, and taurine on neurons of the lateral vesticular nucleus: Interactions with gamma-aminobutyric acid, *Proc. Natl. Acad. Sci. USA* **79**:3355–3359.

Chang, K. -J., and Cuatrecasas, 1981, Heterogeneity and properties of opiate receptors, *Fed. Proc.* **40**:2729–2734.

Chang, K. -J., Cooper, B. R., Hazum, E., and Cuatrecasas, P., 1979, Multiple opiate receptors: Different regional distribution in the brain and differential binding of opiates and opioid peptides, *Mol. Pharmacol.* **16**:91–104.

Chavkin, C., James, I. F., and Goldstein, A., 1982, Dynorphin is a specific endogenous ligand of the opioid receptor, *Science* **215**:413–415.

Cox, B. M., 1982, Endogenous opioid peptides: A guide to structures and terminology, *Life Sci.* **31**:1645–1658.

Cox, B. M., and Chavkin, C., 1983, Comparison of dynorphin-selective kappa receptors in mouse vas deferens and guinea pig ileum. Spare receptor fraction as a determinant of potency, *Mol. Pharmacol.* **23**:36–43.

Denavit-Saubie, M., Champagnat, J., and Zieglgänsberger, W., 1978, Effects of opiates and methionine-enkephalin on pontine and bulbar respiratory neurones of the cat, *Brain Res.* **155**:55–67.

Dingledine, R., 1981, Possible mechanisms of enkephalin action on hippocampal CA1 pyramidal neurons, *J. Neurosci.* **1**:1022–1035.

Dingledine, R., and Gjerstad, L., 1980, Reduced inhibition during epileptiform activity in the *in vitro* hippocampal slice, *J. Physiol. (Lond.)* **305**:297–313.

Dingledine, R., Valentino, R. J., Bostock, E., King, M. E., and Chang, K. -J., 1983, Down-regulation of δ but not μ opioid receptors in the hippocampal slice associated with loss of physiological response, *Life Sci.* **33** (sup. I):333–336.

Duggan, A. W., Davies, J., and Hall, J. G., 1976, Effects of opiate agonists and antagonists on central neurons of the cat, *J. Pharmacol. Exp. Ther.* **196**:107–120.

Duggan, A. W., Hall, J. G., and Headley, P. M., 1977, Suppression of transmission of nociceptive impulses by morphine: Selective effects of morphine administered in the region of the substantia nigra, *Br. J. Pharmacol.* **61**:65–76.

Dunlap, K., and Fischbach, G. D., 1981, Neurotransmitters decrease the calcium conductance activated by depolarization of embryonic chick sensory neurones, *J. Physiol. (Lond.)* **317**:519–535.

Dunwiddie, T., Mueller, A., Palmer, U., Stewart, J., and Hoffer, B., 1980, Electrophysiological interactions of enkephalins with neuronal activity in the rat hippocampus. I. Effects on pyramidal cell activity, *Brain Res.* **184**:311–330.

Forney, E., and Klemm, W. R., 1983, Unit activity indicators of a catecholamine role in expression of morphine effects, *Prog. Neuropsychopharmacol. Biol. Psychiat.* **7**:73–82.

Frederickson, R. C. A., and Geary, L. E., 1982, Endogenous opioid peptides: Review of physiological, pharmacological and clinical aspects, *Prog. Neurobiol.* **19**:19–69.

Frederickson, R. C. A., and Norris, F. H., 1976, Enkephalin-induced depression of single neurons in brain areas with opiate receptors-antagonism by naloxone, *Science* **194**:440–442.

French, E. D., and Siggins, G. R., 1980, An iontophoretic survey of opioid peptide actions in the rat limbic system: In search of opiate epileptogenic mechanisms, *Regulatory Peptides* **1**:127–146.

Gähwiler, B. H., 1980, Excitatory action of opioid peptides and opiates on cultured hippocampal pyramidal cells, *Brain Res.* **194**:193–203.

Glazer, E. J., and Basbaum, A. I., 1983, Opioid neurons and pain modulation: an ultrastructural analysis of enkephalin in cat superficial dorsal horn, *Neuroscience* **10**:357–376.

Goodman, R. R., Snyder, S. H., Kuhar, M. J., and Young, W. S., 1980, Differentiation of delta and mu opiate receptor localizations by light microscopic autoradiography, *Proc. Natl. Acad. Sci. USA* **77**:6239–6243.

Gruol, D. L., and Smith, T. G., 1981, Opiate antagonism of glycine-evoked membrane polarizations in cultured mouse spinal cord neurons, *Brain Res.* **223**:355–365.

Gruol, D. L., Chavkin, C., Valentino, R. J., and Siggins, G. R., 1983, Dynorphin-A alters the excitability of pyramidal neurons of the rat hippocampus in vitro, *Life Sci.* **33** (Supp. I):533–536.

Guilbaud, G., Kayser, V., Banoist, J. M., and Gautron, M., 1983, Depressive effects of morphine and of an enkephalinase inhibitor on responses of ventro-basal thalamic neurones to noxious stimuli, *Life Sci.* **33** (Supp. I):545–547.

Haas, H. L., and Ryall, R. W., 1980, Is excitation by enkephalins of hippocampal neurons in the rat due to presynaptic facilitation or to disinhibition? *J. Physiol. (Lond.)* **308**:315–330.

Haigler, H. J., 1976, Morphine: Ability to block neuronal activity evoked by a nociceptive stimulus, *Life Sci.* **19**:841–858.

Henricksen, S. J., Bloom, F. E., McCoy, F., Ling, N., and Guillemin, R., 1978, β-endorphin induces non-convulsive limbic seizures, *Proc. Natl. Acad. Sci. USA* **75**:5221–5225.

Herbert, E., Oates, E., Martens, G., Comb, M., Rosen, H., and Uhler, M., 1983, Generation of diversity and evolution of opioid peptides, *Cold Spring Harbor Symp. Quant. Biol.* **48**:375–384.

Heyer, E. J., and MacDonald, R. L., 1982, Calcium- and sodium-dependent action potentials of mouse spinal cord and dorsal root ganglion neurons in cell culture, *J. Neurophysiol.* **47**:641–655.

Hill, R. G., and Pepper, C. M., 1978, The depression of thalamic nociceptive neurones by D-ala², D-leu⁵-enkephalin, *Eur. J. Pharmacol.* **47**:223–225.

Hill, R. G., Pepper, C. M., and Mitchell, J. F., 1976, Depression of nociceptive and other neurones in the brain by iontophoretically applied met-enkephalin, *Nature* **262**:604–606.

Hill, R. G., Morris, R., and Sofroniew, M. V., 1983, Naloxone reversible inhibition of reticular neurones in the rat caudal medulla produced by electrical stimulation of the periaqueductal grey matter, *Pain* **15**:249–263.

Hökfelt, T., Johansson, O., Ljundahl, A., Lundberg, J. M., and Schultzberg, M., 1980, Peptidergic neurones, *Nature* **284**:515–521.

Hosford, D. A., and Haigler, H. J., 1980, Morphine and methionine-enkephalin: different effects on spontaneous and evoked neuronal firing in the mesencepalic reticular formation, *J. Pharmacol. Exp. Ther.* **213**:355–363.

Huffman, R. D., and Felpel, L. P., 1981, A microiontophoretic study of morphine on single neurons in the rat globus pallidus, *Neurosci. Lett.* **22**:195–199.

Hunt, S. P., Kelly, J. S., and Emson, P. C., 1980, The electron microscopic localization of methionine-enkephalin within the superficial layers (I and II) of the spinal cord, *Neuroscience* **5**:1871–1890.

Iwatsubo, K., and Clouet, D. H., 1977, Effects of morphine and haloperidol on the electrical activity of rat nigrostriatal neurons, *J. Pharmacol. Exp. Ther.* **202**:429–436.

Jaffe, J. H., and Martin, W. R., 1980, Opioid analgesics and antagonists, in: *The Pharmacological Basis of Therapeutics* (A. G. Gilman, L. S. Goodman, and A. Gilman, eds.), MacMillan, New York, pp. 494–534.

Kerr, F. W. L., Triplett, J. N., and Beeler, G. W., 1974, Reciprocal (push-pull) effects of morphine on single units in the ventromedian and lateral hypothalamus and influences on other nuclei: with a comment on methadone effects during withdrawal from morphine, *Brain Res.* **74**:81–103.

Korf, J., Bunney, B. S., and Aghajanian, G. K., 1974, Noradrenergic neurons: Morphine inhibition of spontaneous activity, *Eur. J. Pharmacol.* **25**:165–169.

Kosterlitz, H. W., and Paterson, S. J., 1980, Characterization of opioid receptors in nervous tissue, *Proc. R. Soc. Lond. B* **210**:113–122.

Lee, H. K., Dunwiddie, T., and Hoffer, B., 1980, Electrophysiological interactions of enkephalins with neuronal circuitry in the rat hippocampus. II. Effects on interneuron excitability, *Brain Res.* **184**:331–342.

MacDonald, R. L., and Nelson, P. G., 1978, Specific opiate-induced depression of transmitter release from dorsal root ganglion cells in culture, *Science* **199**:1449–1451.

MacMillan, S. J., and Clarke, G., 1983, Opioid peptides have differential actions on subpopulations of arcuate neurones, *Life Sci.* **33** (Suppl. I):529–532.

McCarthy, P. S., Walker, R. J., and Woodruff, G. N., 1977, Depressant actions of enkephalins on neurones in the nucleus accumbens, *J. Physiol. (Lond.)* **267**:40–41P.

McGinty, J. F., Henricksen, S. J., Goldstein, A., Terenius, T., and Bloom, F. E., 1983, Dynorphin is contained within hippocampal mossy fibers: Immunochemical alterations after kainic acid administration and colchicine-induced neurotoxicity, *Proc. Natl. Acad. Sci. USA* **80**:589–593.

Mohrland, J. S., and Gebhart, G. F., 1981, Effect of morphine administered in the periaqueductal gray and at the recording locus on nociresponsive neurons in the medullary reticular formation, *Brain Res.* **225**:401–412.

Mudge, A. W., Leeman, S. E., and Fischbach, G. D., 1979, Enkephalin inhibits release of substance P from sensory neurons in culture and decreases action potential duration, *Proc. Natl. Acad. Sci. USA* **76**:526–530.

Muehlethaler, M., Gähwiler, B. H., and Dreifuss, J. J., 1980, Enkephalin-induced inhibition of hypothalamic paraventricular neurons, *Brain Res.* **197**:264–268.

Murase, K., Nedeljkov, V., and Randić, M., 1982, The actions of neuropeptides on dorsal horn neurons in the rat spinal cord slice preparation: An intracellular study, *Brain Res.* **234**:170–176.

Napier, T. C., Pirch, J. H., and Strahlendorf, H. K., 1983, Naloxone antagonizes striatally-induced suppression of globus pallidus unit activity, *Neuroscience* **9**:53–59.

Nicoll, R. A. and Madison, D. V., 1984, The action of enkephalin on interneurons in the hippocampus, *Soc. Neurosci. Abst.* **10**:660.

Nicoll, R. A., Siggins, G. R., Ling, N., Bloom, F. E., and Guillemin, R., 1977, Neuronal actions of endorphins and enkephalins among brain regions: A comparative microiontophoretic study, *Proc. Natl. Acad. Sci. USA* **74**:2584–2588.

Nicoll, R. A., Alger, B. E., and Jahr, C. E., 1980, Enkephalin blocks inhibitory pathways in the vertebrate CNS, *Nature* **287**:22–25.

Noda, U., Furutani, Y., Takahashi, H., Toyosato, M., Hiroge, T., Inayama, S., Nakanishi, S., and Numa, S., 1982, Cloning and sequence analysis of cDNA for bovine adrenalproenkephalin, *Nature* **295**:202–206.

North, R. A., 1979, Opiates, opioid peptides and single neurons, *Life Sci.* **24**:1527–1546.

Ono, T., Oomura, Y., Nishino, H., Sasaki, D., Muramoto, K., and Yano, I., 1980, Morphine and enkephalin effects on hypothalamic glucoresponsive neurons, *Brain Res.* **185**:208–212.

Palmer, M. R., Morris, D. H., Taylor, D. A., Stewart, J. M., and Hoffer, B., 1978, Electrophysiological effects of enkephalin analogues in rat cortex, *Life Sci.* **23**:851–860.

Pepper, C. M., and Henderson, G., 1980, Opiates and opioid peptides hyperpolarize locus coeruleus neurons in vitro, *Science* **209**:394–396.

Pert, C. B., and Snyder, S. H., 1974, Opiate receptor binding of agonists and antagonists affected differentially by sodium, *Mol. Pharmac.* **10**:868–879.

Pickel, V. M., Joh, T. H., Reis, D. J., Leeman, S. E., and Miller, R. J., 1979, Electron microscopic localization of substance P and enkephalin in axon terminals related to dendrites of catecholaminergic neurons, *Brain Res.* **160**:387–400.

Pickel, V. M., Sumal, K. K., Beckley, S. C., Miller, R. J., and Reis, D. J., 1980, Immunocytochemical localization of enkephalin in the neostriatum of rat brain: A light and electron microscopic study, *J. Comp. Neurol.* **189**:721–740.

Ruda, M. A., 1982, Opiates and pain pathways: Demonstration of enkephalin synapses on dorsal horn projection neurons, *Science* **215**:1523–1525.

Satoh, M., Zieglgänsberger, W., and Herz, A., 1976, Actions of opiates upon single unit activity in the cortex of naive and tolerant rats, *Brain Res.* **115**:99–110.

Satoh, M., Akaike, A., and Takagi, H., 1979, Excitation by morphine and enkephalin of single neurons of nucleus reticularis paragigantocellularis in the rat: a probable mechanism of analgesic action of opioids, *Brain Res.* **169**:406–410.

Sawada, S., and Yamamoto, C., 1981, Postsynaptic inhibitory actions of catecholamines and opioid peptides on the bed nucleus of the stria terminalis, *Exp. Brain Res.* **41:**264–270.

Schulman, J. A., 1981, Anatomical distribution and physiological effects of enkephalin in rat inferior olive, *Regulatory Peptides* **2:**125–137.

Segal, M., 1979, Serotonergic innervation of the locus coeruleus from the dorsal raphe and its action on responses to noxious stimuli, *J. Physiol. (Lond.)* **286:**401–415.

Snead, O. C., and Bearden, L. J., 1982, The epileptogenic spectrum of opiate agonists, *Neuropharmacology* **21:**1137–1144.

Sumal, K. K., Pickel, V. M., Miller, R. J., and Reis, D. J., 1982, Enkephalin-containing neurons in substantia gelatinosa of spinal trigeminal complex: Ultrastructure and synaptic interaction with primary sensory afferents, *Brain Res.* **248:**223–236.

Udenfriend, S., and Kilpatrick, D. L., 1983, Biochemistry of the enkephalins and enkephalin-containing peptides, *Arch. Biochem. Biophys.* **221:**309–323.

Valentino, R. J., and Dingledine, R., 1982, Pharmacological characterization of opioid effects in the rat hippocampal slice, *J. Pharmacol. Exp. Ther.* **223:**502–509.

Wakerley, J. B., Noble, R., and Clarke, G., 1983, Effects of morphine and D-ala, D-leu enkephalin on the electrical activity of supraoptic neurosecretory cells in vitro, *Neuroscience* **10:**73–81.

Wamsley, J. K., Young, W. S., and Kuhar, M. J., 1980, Immunohistochemical localization of enkephalin in rat forebrain, *Brain Res.* **190:**153–174.

Watson, S. J., Khachaturian, H., Akil, H., Coy, D. H., and Goldstein, A., 1982, Comparison of the distribution of dynorphin systems and enkephalin systems in brain, *Science* **218:**1134–1136.

Watson, S. J., Khachaturian, H., Taylor, L., Fischli, W., Goldstein, A., and Akil, H., 1983, Prodynorphin peptides are found in the same neurons throughout rat brain: Immunocytochemical study, *Proc. Natl. Acad. Sci. USA* **80:**891–894.

Weber, E., and Barchas, J. D., 1983, Immunohistochemical distribution of dynorphin B in rat brain: Relation to dynorphin A and α-neo-endorphin systems, *Proc. Natl. Acad. Sci. USA* **80:**1125–1129.

Werz, M. A., and MacDonald, R. L., 1982, Opiate alkaloids antagonize postsynaptic glycine and GABA responses: correlation with convulsant action, *Brain Res.* **236:**107–119.

Werz, M. A., and MacDonald, R. L., 1983a, Opioid peptides with differential affinity for mu- and delta-receptors decrease sensory neuron calcium-dependent action potentials, *J. Pharmacol. Exp. Ther.* **227:**394–402.

Werz, M. A., and MacDonald, R. L., 1983b, Opioid peptides selective for mu- and delta-opiate receptors reduce calcium-dependent action potential duration by increasing potassium conductance. *Neurosci. Lett.* **42:**173–178.

Werz, M. A., and MacDonald, R. L., 1984, Dynorphin reduces Ca-dependent action potential duration by decreasing voltage-dependent calcium conductance, *Neurosci. Lett.* **46:**185–190.

Williams, J. T., Egan, T. M., and North, R. A., 1982, Enkephalin opens potassium channels on mammalian central neurons, *Nature* **299:**74–77.

Williams, J. T., Henderson, G., and North, R. A., 1984, Locus coeruleus neurons, in: *Brain Slices* (R. Dingledine, ed.), Plenum Press, New York.

Yaksh, T. L., and Rudy, T. A., 1978, Narcotic analgesics: CNS sites and mechanisms of action as revealed by intracerebral injection techniques, *Pain* **4:**299–359.

Yoshimura, M., and North, R. A., 1983, Substantia gelatinosa neurones in vitro hyperpolarized by enkephalins, *Nature* **305:**529–531.

Zieglgänsberger, W., and Bayerl, H., 1976, The mechanism of inhibition of neuronal activity by opiates in the spinal cord of cat, *Brain Res.* **115:**111–128.

Zieglgänsberger, W., and Tulloch, I. F., 1979, The effects of methionine- and leucine-enkephalin on spinal neurones of the cat, *Brain Res.* **167:**53–64.

Zieglgänsberger, W., French, E. D., Siggins, G. R., and Bloom, F. E., 1979, Opioid peptides may excite hippocampal pyramidal neurons by inhibiting adjacent inhibitory interneurons, *Science* **205:**415–417.

Opioid Peptides: Peripheral Nervous System

SHIRO KONISHI

1. INTRODUCTION

1.1. Historical Perspective and Overview

As exemplified by the history of research in classical autonomic physiology, synapses in the peripheral nervous system can serve as excellent experimental models for the identification of transmitter substances and the detailed elucidation of mechanisms of chemical transmission. This has been particularly true in the study of signal transmission associated with peptidergic neurons. Until the early 1970s there was firm evidence supporting only two substances, acetylcholine (ACh) and norepinephrine, as neurotransmitters in the mammalian peripheral nervous system. During the past several years, however, a series of studies on vertebrate autonomic neurons, especially in sympathetic ganglia, have provided good evidence that some neuropeptides, including enkephalins, LHRH-like peptide (see Chapter 16), and substance P (see Chapter 13), serve as neurotransmitters for particular forms of synaptic responses, characterized by their relatively long durations, that modulate cholinergic transmission in the ganglia. This chapter reviews experiments aimed at elucidating the neurotransmitter role of opioid peptides and the cellular mechanisms of their actions in the peripheral nervous system.

Although attempts to identify opioid peptides as neurotransmitters in central nervous system have been hampered by the structural complexity of central circuitry, direct evidence for an inhibitory transmitter role of the opioid peptides has now been provided by experiments in the periphery.

Within the mammalian peripheral nervous system, the prevertebral sympathetic ganglia, in particular the inferior mesenteric and coeliac-superior mesenteric ganglia, have been best studied. A class of neurons containing enkephalin immunoreactivity in the guinea pig spinal cord send their axons into the lumbar splanchnic nerves to terminate in the inferior mesenteric ganglion (Schultzberg et al., 1979; Dalsgaard et al., 1982b). Recent electrophysiological experiments have shown that enkephalins released by stimulation of the lumbar splanchnic nerves act to presynaptically inhibit cholinergic transmission in the ganglia (Konishi et al., 1979a, 1981).

A second form of peptidergic transmission believed to take place in the inferior mesenteric ganglion is that mediated by substance P. Many of the principal sympathetic neurons are densely innervated by visceral afferent fibers containing substance P immunoreactivity (see Dalsgaard et al., 1982a). Activation of these afferent fibers initiates a slow excitatory postsynaptic potential (EPSP) in the ganglion cells that remains unaffected after the blockade of cholinergic transmission (Konishi et al., 1980; Tsunoo et al., 1982), and evidence is now accumulating that substance P released from the visceral afferent terminals mediates this noncholinergic slow EPSP (see Otsuka and Konishi, 1983 and Chapter 13). The noncholinergic slow transmission involving substance P-containing visceral afferents also appears to be under the influence of enkephalinergic presynaptic inhibition (Konishi et al., 1979b, 1980; Jiang et al., 1982).

In other sites of the peripheral nervous system, attempts have been made to explore the functional roles of the opioid peptides. Certain subpopulations of enteric neurons containing enkephalins form widespread networks within the nerve plexuses and muscle layers of the gastrointestinal tract (Schultzberg et al., 1980; Jessen et al., 1980; Furness et al., 1983). Pharmacological and biochemical studies have shown that opiates and opioid peptides inhibit the release of ACh and other neurotransmitters from intramural and extrinsic autonomic neurons that innervate visceral smooth muscles (Paton, 1957; Hughes et al., 1975; Waterfield et al., 1977). Opioid peptides have also been implicated in the regulation of the peristaltic movement of the intestinal muscles (Puig et al., 1977; Kromer and Pretzlaff, 1979; Gintzler and Scalisi, 1982).

Intracellular recordings have attempted to analyze the mode and site of inhibitory action of opioids at autonomic effectors in the gut and vas deferens and in the enteric nervous system. These studies have suggested that opioids act on presynaptic nerve terminals to inhibit the release of neurotransmitters either by suppression of Ca^{2+} entry into nerve endings (Illes et al., 1980; Ito and Tajima, 1980) or hyperpolarization of axon terminals (Morita and North, 1981).

1.2. Distribution of Enkephalin-Containing Neurons

In the mammalian peripheral nervous system, certain sympathetic ganglia contain particularly high concentrations of immunoreactive enkephalins

(Hughes et al., 1977; Yang et al., 1980). Schultzberg et al. (1979) demonstrated that enkephalins occur in dense plexiform networks in the guinea pig prevertebral ganglia, i.e., the inferior mesenteric and coeliac-superior mesenteric ganglia, which innervate the abdominal viscera. Subsequent studies by Dalsgaard et al. (1982b) using combined techniques of retrograde tracing and immunohistochemistry showed that the enkephalin-containing nerve terminals in the inferior mesenteric ganglion originate from neurons that lie in the sympathetic preganglionic nuclei of the lumbar spinal cord. In the superior cervical ganglia, some principal neurons and SIF (small intensely fluorescent) cells have also been shown to contain immunoreactive enkephalins. Localization of opioid peptides in the parasympathetic ganglia is not well described except for the demonstration of enkephalin immunoreactivity in some fibers of the vagus nerve. However, since certain autonomic preganglionic neurons in the cat sacral spinal cord have been shown to contain enkephalin (Glazer and Basbaum, 1980), these neurons are likely to supply the parasympathetic ganglia in the pelvic organs (see Alm et al., 1981).

In the gastrointestinal tract, enkephalins are found in intrinsic neurons of the myenteric plexus, representing a considerable proportion (15–23%) of the total myenteric neurons (Schultzberg et al., 1980; Furness et al., 1983). Within the small and large intestine, processes of the enkephalin-containing neurons ramify widely, projecting to other neurons in the myenteric and submucous plexuses and the circular and longitudinal muscle layers.

Apart from their localization in the autonomic and enteric neurons, opioid peptides are also present in endocrine cells of the adrenal medulla and in the gastrointestinal mucosa (see Yang et al., 1980; Udenfriend and Kilpatrick, 1983). Enkephalin immunoreactivity is also contained in some cells in the cat carotid body (Lundberg et al., 1979) and in rat sinus hair follicles (Merkel cells) (Hartschuh et al., 1979). Although dynorphin is known to occur in the porcine duodenum, there is little information regarding the detailed localization of dynorphins and other opioid peptides in the peripheral nervous system.

1.3. Opioid Receptors

Physiological studies and receptor binding assays in two types of peripheral preparations, the guinea-pig ileum and mouse vas deferens, have revealed the existence of multiple opioid receptors (Lord et al., 1977). Opioid peptides are believed to interact with two pharmacologically distinct receptor types, the μ- and δ-receptors, each of which has a distinct distribution in the peripheral tissues of various species. The prototype preferential agonist for the μ-receptor site is the alkaloid morphine, whereas the endogenous agonists, Met- and Leu-enkephalin, exhibit higher affinity for the δ site than the μ site. β-Endorphin is relatively nonselective for μ- and δ-receptors. The most widely used antagonist for opioid receptors is naloxone, which appears to be about 10 times more potent in blocking the μ-binding site than the δ-binding site. Additional opiate receptor subtypes have also been proposed to explain the pharmacological properties of opioids in the peripheral and central nervous systems (see Chapter 11 and Paterson et al., 1983). However, due to the lack of specific antagonists, the classification of opioid receptors is not as complete as in the case for other peripheral transmitters such as ACh or norepinephrine. Reliable antagonists that can specifically interact with the various receptor subtypes are required before functional differences between these multiple subtypes can be elucidated.

2. AUTONOMIC GANGLIA

Of the mammalian autonomic ganglia, the prevertebral sympathetic ganglia of the guinea pig have been particularly useful for studying peptidergic synaptic mechanisms because of the dense innervation of the ganglia by peptidergic neurons containing enkephalins, substance P, and some other peptides. From a practical point of view, the relative morphological simplicity of the ganglion makes it possible to clearly view single neurons and fibers so that intra- and extracellular microelectrodes for recording, stimulation and drug application can be accurately placed under visual control (see Kuffler, 1980).

2.1. Effects on Cholinergic Excitation

In the periphery, as well as in the CNS (see Chapter 11), a major action of opioid peptides is the presynaptic inhibition of chemical transmission. Cholinergic synapses in the sympathetic ganglia of several species have served as model systems to analyze this effect. Particularly well studied are the prevertebral ganglia, the most accessible of which is the inferior mesenteric ganglion. Principal neurons of this ganglion receive cholinergic synaptic inputs from lumbar splanchnic nerves that originate in the sympathetic preganglionic nuclei of the spinal cord. Stimulation of the preganglionic nerves produces typical cholinergic fast EPSPs in the ganglion cells (Fig. 1B). These EPSPs are markedly inhibited by perfusion of the ganglia with enkephalins (Fig. 1A) (Konishi et al., 1979a) and morphine (Bornstein and Fields, 1979). This effect is not diminished by repeated application or even in the continued presence of the peptides (Fig. 1A). Among enkephalin-related peptides the metabolically stable analog, [D-Ala²]-Met-enkephalin-amide (DAEA), showed the highest potency for the inhibition of the EPSPs. The inhibitory action of the peptides was blocked by the opiate antagonist, naloxone (Fig. 1A, B). The inhibition of the fast EPSPs by opioid peptides was not associated with significant changes in the resting membrane potential or the cell input resistance estimated by the injection of constant current pulses (Fig. 1B). The lack of effects of the peptides on the passive membrane

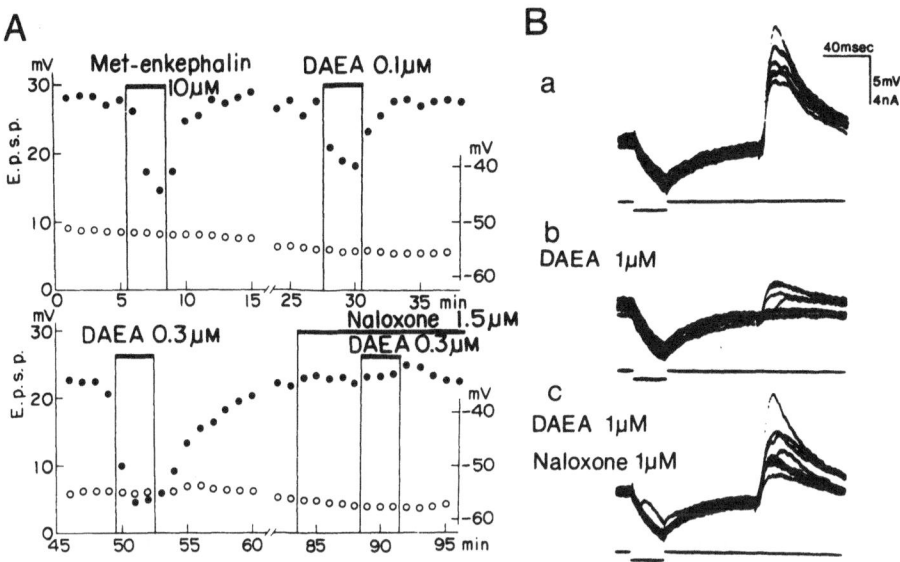

Figure 1. Effects of Met-enkephalin and [D-Ala²]-Met-enkephalinamide (DAEA) on cholinergic fast EPSPs and electrical membrane properties of neurons in the guinea pig inferior mesenteric ganglion. The lumbar splanchnic nerve was stimulated at 1-min intervals for 16 sec at 2.5 Hz to evoke cholinergic fast EPSPs. (A) The amplitude of the EPSPs (solid circles) was determined by averaging 32 successive responses. The resting potential (open circles) was measured from a continuous record displayed on a pen-recorder. The peptides and naloxone were perfused into the bath during the periods indicated. Ordinate: left, amplitude of the averaged EPSPs; right, resting potential. (B) Hyperpolarizing current pulses were passed into a ganglion cell to estimate the membrane resistance (lower trace a–c) followed by preganglionic nerve stimulation to evoke fast EPSPs. Several traces are superimposed in each record. (a) Control; (b) DAEA (1 μM); (c) DAEA plus naloxone (1 μM). Membrane potential, -75 mV. (Modified from Konishi et al., 1979a, with permission.)

properties of the ganglion cells is true even if high concentrations of Met-enkephalin are pressure ejected near the cell surface, although this causes a dramatic reduction in the fast EPSPs. As illustrated in the records in Fig. 1B, a characteristic feature of enkephalin-induced presynaptic inhibition is an increase in the number of failures (zero responses) to suprathreshold nerve stimulation, which suggests that a fraction of the nerve impulses reaching the presynaptic nerve terminals fail to release any transmitter.

Two further approaches have been used to analyze the mechanism of the inhibitory action of enkephalins at ganglionic synapses. The first has been to examine whether the sensitivity of the postsynaptic membrane to ACh is affected by the peptides. Focal application of ACh results in depolarization of ganglion cells, which mimics the fast EPSP evoked by nerve stimulation. The ACh-induced depolarization was not altered by the enkephalin analog DAEA, whereas fast EPSPs recorded from the same neurons were markedly inhibited (Fig. 2A), indicating that enkephalins act on pre-

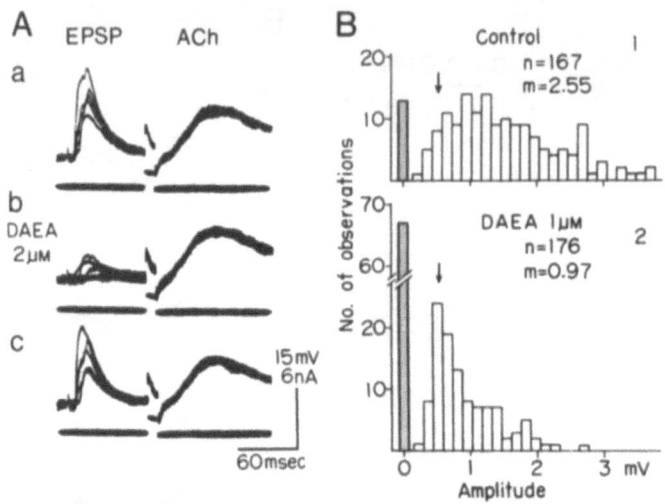

Figure 2. Effects of DAEA on cholinergic fast EPSPs and ACh-induced depolarization of a neuron in the guinea pig coeliac-superior mesenteric ganglion. (A) EPSPs were evoked by stimulation of the greater splanchnic nerve at an interval of 1 min with 16 pulses at 0.5 Hz. ACh was iontophoretically applied to the neuron about 80 msec after each nerve stimulus. Upper traces in (a–c) show superimposed fast EPSPs (left) and ACh-induced potentials (right) and lower traces monitor the intensity of current pulses passed into the ACh-containing micropipette. (a) Control; (b) in DAEA (2 μM); (c) after washing out of DAEA. (B) Amplitude histograms of the EPSPs evoked by the preganglionic nerve stimulation at 2 Hz. (1) Control; (2) in DAEA (1 μM). The mean quantal content, m, was estimated from the numbers of stimulation trials, n, and failures (zero responses, stippled columns). The estimated unit sizes of the EPSPs are shown by arrows. (From Konishi et al., 1979a, with permission.)

synaptic terminals to inhibit the release of ACh but do not affect the ACh sensitivity of the post-synaptic membrane.

Another approach to determining the site of enkephalin action is the use of quantal analysis of transmitter release. The process of ACh release was well characterized at the neuromuscular junction by the experiments of del Castillo and Katz (1954), and their observations resulted in the formulation of the quantal hypothesis of transmitter release: ACh appears to be released from nerve terminals at the neuromuscular junction in multi-molecular packets (or quanta), and the synaptic potentials evoked by nerve impulses fluctuate in amplitude in a stepwise fashion, each response appearing to be an integral multiple of the unit response generated by a single ACh quantum. Based on the quantal hypothesis, the fluctuation of ACh release, i.e., the quantal composition of the synaptic potential, is predicted by Poisson statistics under the condition that the probability of transmitter release is low (see Martin, 1977, for further details). The applicability of this hypothesis has been demonstrated at other chemical synapses including the cholinergic synapses in autonomic ganglia (see Dennis et al., 1971). In the experiment illustrated in Fig. 2B, the method of quantal analysis was applied to test whether the site of the enkephalin-induced inhibition in the coeliac-superior mesenteric ganglia is pre- or postsynaptic. The amplitude distributions of cholinergic fast EPSPs were compared in control medium and in medium containing a low concentration of the opioid peptide DAEA. Preganglionic nerve stimulation in control medium evoked fast EPSPs with a considerable fluctuation in amplitude including occasional failures (Fig. 2B1). In the presence of DAEA, the number of failures was markedly increased (Fig. 2B2). Because of the difficulty in measuring the mean amplitude of spontaneous EPSPs that occur with low frequency at the autonomic ganglion synapses, the mean number of ACh quanta liberated by each stimulus (mean quantal content, m) was estimated indirectly from the total number of stimuli, N, and the observed number of failures, n_o, using the equation $m = \ln N/n_o$. The mean quantal content of the EPSPs estimated in such a way was reduced by DAEA to 40–60% of the control. However, the estimated amplitude of the unit EPSPs was not significantly affected by the peptide (Fig. 2B1 and 2; Konishi et al., 1979a). Similar results were obtained when the mean quantal content was estimated by the coefficient of variation method (S. Konishi, unpublished observations). Morphine has also been shown to inhibit fast EPSPs in the same manner as enkephalins (Bornstein and Fields, 1979), but is approximately 10 times less potent than the peptides. These observations led to the conclusion that enkephalins inhibit cholinergic fast EPSPs in the guinea pig prevertebral ganglia by reducing the amount of ACh released from preganglionic fibers (Konishi et al., 1979a). The presynaptic inhibitory action of Met-enkephalin and the opiates, morphine and etorphine, has been demonstrated by a similar experimental approach at the frog neuromuscular junction and from sensory ganglion cells innervating spinal cord neurons in tissue culture (Macdonald and Nelson, 1978; Bixby and Spitzer, 1983).

In the cat ciliary ganglion, exogenously applied Met-enkephalin hyperpolarizes some of the parasympathetic ganglion cells and inhibits the cholinergic fast EPSPs evoked by preganglionic stimulation (Katayama and Nishi, 1981). Since the ACh-induced depolarization of the ciliary ganglion cells was not changed by the peptide, the site of the enkephalin-induced inhibition of EPSPs in this ganglion appears to be the presynaptic nerve terminal, as in the guinea pig prevertebral ganglia.

2.2. Effects on Synaptic Inhibition

Effects of the opioid peptides on other autonomic ganglia have been examined mainly by extracellular recording using the sucrose-gap method. In the frog paravertebral ganglia and the cat superior cervical ganglion, application of enkephalins or morphine induces a hyperpolarization in the postganglionic nerve bundles and suppresses the slow synaptic inhibition produced by repetitive stimulation of the preganglionic fibers (Wouters and van den Bercken, 1980; Machova and Kvaltinova, 1983). The physiological significance of the hyperpolarization remains to be determined; however, the effect on slow synaptic inhibition probably occurs by a presynaptic mechanism similar to that described above for fast excitatory transmission. Although it was formerly believed that the slow inhibitory postsynaptic potential (IPSP) in the mammalian sympathetic ganglia is generated by dopamine released from interneurons (Libet, 1979), this concept has been seriously challenged and a recent study in the amphibian sympathetic ganglion has indicated that the slow IPSP is mediated directly by ACh acting at inhibitory muscarinic receptors on the principal neurons (see Chapter 6). With reference to the present discussion, it has been observed that Met-enkephalin produces little effect on the hyperpolarization caused by exogenous dopamine, so that if dopamine is involved in synaptic inhibition, the effect of Met-enkephalin is presynaptic (Wouters and van den Berken, 1980). Whatever the mechanism, however, it seems likely that opioid peptides inhibit not only nicotinic fast EPSPs but also muscarinic slow IPSPs in certain autonomic ganglia.

2.3. Effects on Noncholinergic Slow Excitation

Recent experiments in the guinea pig inferior mesenteric ganglion have shown that repetitive stimulation of either pre- or postganglionic fibers evokes a noncholinergic slow EPSP following the cholinergic fast EPSPs in the ganglion cells (see Fig. 3). Compelling evidence has been provided that the noncholinergic slow EPSP results from the transmitter action of substance P released from axon collateral terminals of certain visceral afferent fibers that traverse the inferior mesenteric ganglion on their way from the visceral organs to the dorsal root ganglia (Dalsgaard et al., 1982a; Konishi et al., 1983;

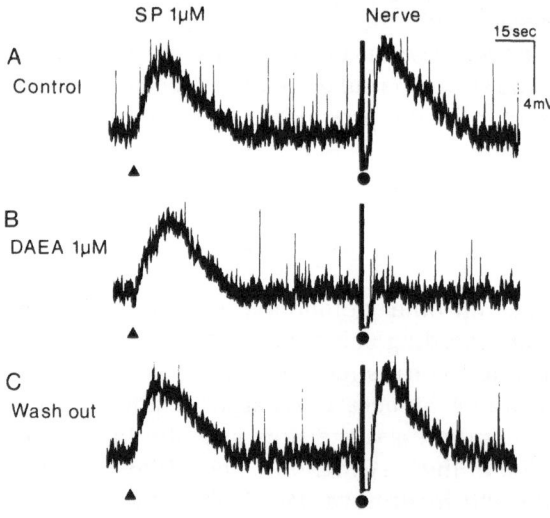

Figure 3. Effects of DAEA on noncholinergic slow EPSP and substance P-induced depolarization recorded from a neuron in the guinea pig inferior mesenteric ganglion. At triangles, substance P (1 μM) was ejected from a micropipette in the vicinity of the neuron by pressure pulses (0.5 sec). At circles, repetitive preganglionic stimulation (20 Hz for 2 sec) was applied to the lumbar splanchnic nerve. (A) In control solution; (B) in DAEA (1 μM); (C) after washing out of DAEA. Tops of the cholinergic fast EPSPs (deflections above the circles) were cut off. (S. Konishi, unpublished observations.)

Otsuka and Konishi, 1983; see Chapter 13). It has been suggested that the substance P-operated synapses in this ganglion are another target for the opioid peptide. As shown in Fig. 3, the Met-enkephalin analog DAEA inhibited the noncholinergic slow EPSP without altering the resting potential of the ganglion cell (Konishi et al., 1979b; Jiang et al., 1982). The mechanism of this inhibition has been explored in two ways. First, substance P, when applied by pressure ejection from micropipettes, produces a depolarization of the ganglion cells that resembles the noncholinergic slow EPSP in amplitude as well as time course. This substance P-induced depolarization was not affected by the opioid peptide (Fig. 3B). Second, biochemical studies using the guinea pig prevertebral ganglia revealed that the amount of substance P released into the incubation medium by high K^+ was reduced by the enkephalin analog DAEA and that this inhibition was reversed by addition of naloxone (Konishi et al., 1980). These observations support a presynaptic nature of the enkephalin-induced inhibition of noncholinergic slow transmission in the ganglion and are consistent with the findings that opioid peptides inhibit the release of substance P from slices of the rat spinal trigeminal nucleus (Jessell and Iversen, 1977) and from the chick spinal ganglion cells in culture (Mudge et al., 1979). Although a similar noncholinergic slow EPSP has been described in the rabbit superior cervical ganglion (Ashe and Libet, 1981), little is known about the chemical identity of the transmitter substance causing this response or about the effects of opioid peptides on it.

2.4. Neurally Evoked Enkephalinergic Inhibition

The pharmacological experiments described in the previous sections have led to the hypothesis that enkephalins function as neurotransmitters for presynaptic inhibition of the cholinergic fast and the noncholinergic slow transmission in the guinea-pig prevertebral ganglia and other autonomic ganglia. A rigorous test of this hypothesis is to determine whether stimulation of the enkephalin-containing fibers that innervate a particular ganglion produces an inhibitory action on ganglionic transmission similar to that observed with exogenously applied enkephalin. Such a test has been carried out in the guinea pig inferior mesenteric ganglion (Konishi et al., 1980, 1981), where the synaptic inputs to ganglionic neurons are derived from separate preganglionic nerve bundles that can be individually stimulated (see Fig. 4A). On the basis of combined retrograde tracing and immunohistochemistry, it has been determined that some of the enkephalin-containing neurons in the spinal cord send axons to the inferior mesenteric ganglion through the preganglionic nerve bundles (Dalsgaard et al., 1982b), providing a rationale for stimulating these fibers to evoke the release of the opioid peptide.

As illustrated in Fig. 4B, test cholinergic fast EPSPs, evoked by stimulation of a single bundle of the preganglionic nerves and recorded from the ganglion cells, were markedly inhibited by conditioning stimulation given

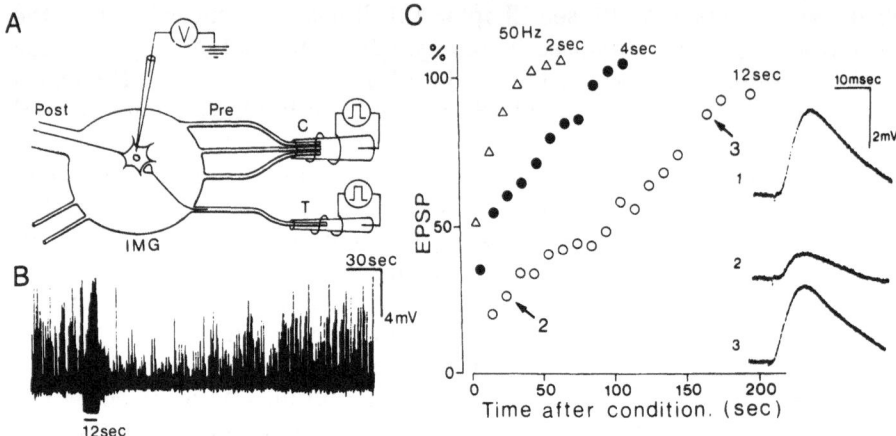

Figure 4. Effect of conditioning preganglionic stimulation on the cholinergic fast EPSPs recorded from a neuron in the inferior mesenteric ganglion (IMG). (A) Experimental arrangement. Intracellular recordings were made in perfused guinea pig IMG. Test stimuli (T) were applied to a single bundle of the lumbar splanchnic nerve to evoke cholinergic fast EPSPs. Conditioning stimulation (C) was applied to the remaining bundles of the lumbar splanchnic nerve. Pre: preganglionic nerves. Post: postganglionic nerves. (B) An example of the inhibitory effect of conditioning stimulation on the test EPSPs. Each upward deflection shows a test EPSP evoked every 10 sec at 1 Hz. Repetitive conditioning stimulation at 50 Hz for 12 sec was given during the period indicated by bar under the record. (C) Time courses of the inhibition of test EPSPs following conditioning stimulation at 50 Hz for 2 (triangles), 4 (solid circles), and 12 (open circles) sec. Ordinate: the amplitude of test EPSPs was determined every 10 sec by averaging eight successive responses and are expressed as a percentage of the mean amplitude of control responses determined for the periods prior to conditioning stimulation. Abscissa: time after the initiation of conditioning stimulation. Each series of observations was repeated at 7-min intervals. Inset records show the signal-averaged responses of test EPSPs. (1) Control response; (2, 3) responses after conditioning stimulation, which were recorded during the 10-sec periods indicated by arrows in the graph. (S. Konishi, A. Tsunoo, and M. Otsuka, unpublished observations.)

to the remaining nerve bundles. The inhibitory effect outlasted the conditioning stimulation and became progressively longer-lasting as the number of conditioning stimuli was increased (Fig. 4C). Addition of naloxone (1–3 μM) abolished the inhibitory effect of conditioning stimulation (Fig. 5A). Several endogenous substances such as noradrenaline, dopamine, and γ-aminobutyric acid, in addition to enkephalins, are known to inhibit cholinergic transmission in the sympathetic ganglia (see Kato and Kuba, 1980). However, naloxone blocked only the inhibitory action of exogenously applied enkephalins without affecting the inhibitory effects of the other substances (Konishi et al., 1981). The fact that the inhibition of the cholinergic EPSPs following conditioning stimulation remained unaffected in the presence of the muscarinic antagonist atropine or the α-adrenoceptor blocker phentolamine indicates that catecholamine-containing interneurons (e.g., SIF cells) are probably not involved in this inhibitory process (see Libet, 1979).

The experiments illustrated in Figs. 5B and 6 addressed the question of whether the mechanism of the neurally evoked inhibition is pre- or postsynaptic. After conditioning stimulation the membrane resistance and ACh sensitivity of ganglion cells were not reduced (Fig. 5Bb, Bc), whereas test cholinergic fast EPSPs recorded in the same neurons were markedly inhibited (Fig. 5Ba). Quantal analysis of test EPSPs showed that conditioning stimulation increased the number of failures (see records in Fig. 6A) and reduced the mean quantal content of the EPSPs (m) to about 40% of the control (Fig. 6Ba, Bb). In contrast, the estimated unit size of EPSPs was not significantly affected by conditioning stimulation, supporting the presynaptic nature of the neurally evoked inhibition of the EPSPs. The effects of conditioning stimulation (i.e., the increase in the number of failures and the decrease of quantal content) were also reversed by naloxone (Fig. 6Ac, Bc). The results demonstrate that electrical stimulation of enkephalinergic fibers in the pre-

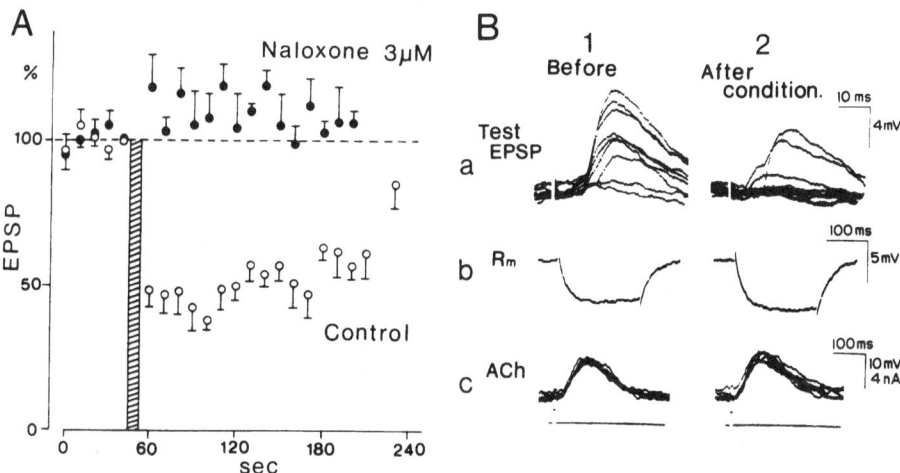

Figure 5. (A) Blockade by naloxone of the inhibitory effect of conditioning preganglionic stimulation on cholinergic fast EPSPs recorded from a neuron of the guinea pig inferior mesenteric ganglion. Conditioning stimulation was applied (as described in the legend to Fig. 4) for 8 sec at 50 Hz during the period indicated by the hatched column. The amplitude of test responses was determined by averaging eight successive test EPSPs at 1 Hz and are expressed as a percentage of the control response recorded immediately before the conditioning stimulation. Each point and vertical bar represent the mean ± S.E.M. determined by three successive trials of conditioning stimulation repeated at 6-min intervals on the same neuron. (open circles) In control solution; (closed circles) in solution containing naloxone (3 μM). (B) Effects of conditioning stimulation on cholinergic test EPSPs, electrotonic potentials, and ACh-induced depolarizations recorded from a single neuron of the inferior mesenteric ganglion. (a) Test EPSPs evoked at 1 Hz. (b) Averaged electrotonic potentials produced by hyperpolarizing current pulses (0.1 nA, 200 msec) injected into the neuron at 1 Hz. (c) Depolarizing potentials (upper traces) produced by ACh applied iontophoretically to the neuron. Current pulses (lower traces) were passed through the ACh-containing micropipette at 0.5 Hz. (1) Responses recorded during the control period. (2) Responses recorded 20–30 sec after the termination of conditioning stimulation (50 Hz for 8 sec). (From Konishi et al., 1981, with permission.)

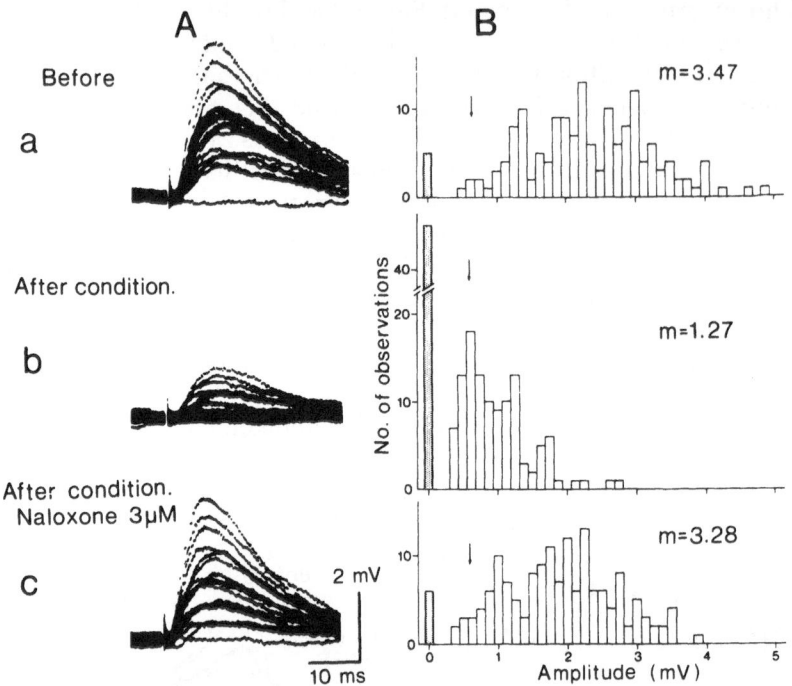

Figure 6. Effects of conditioning stimulation on the amplitude distributions of cholinergic fast EPSPs recorded from a neuron in the inferior mesenteric ganglion. EPSPs were evoked at 1 Hz and conditioning stimulation was applied at 50 Hz for 12 sec. (A) Sample records of superimposed test EPSPs. (B) Amplitude histograms, each of which was compiled from the test EPSPs in successive 160 trials. (a) Test responses recorded during the control period before conditioning stimulation. (b, c) Conditioned test responses recorded during the periods 10–170 sec after the end of conditioning stimulation. (a, b) In control solution; (c) in the solution containing naloxone (3 μM). The mean quantal content, m, was estimated from the proportion of test stimuli ($n = 160$) and failures (stippled columns). Arrows represent the estimated unit size of the EPSPs. (Modified from Konishi et al., 1981, with permission.)

ganglionic nerves evokes presynaptic inhibition of cholinergic fast EPSPs in the ganglia that mimics the action of exogenously applied enkephalins. These findings in conjunction with the morphological evidence suggest that an endogenous opioid peptide acts presynaptically to regulate the release of ACh from the preganglionic fibers (see Fig. 7; Konishi et al., 1980, 1981). Although a peptide that reacts with enkephalin antisera is known to exist in the ganglia, the precise characterization of its structure has not yet been accomplished.

In addition to the effect on nicotinic cholinergic transmission, neurally released opioid peptides in the inferior mesenteric ganglion also appear to act on substance P-containing nerve terminals to inhibit noncholinergic slow transmission. This view is supported by the pharmacological evidence described in the previous section and by a recent study of Jiang et al. (1982)

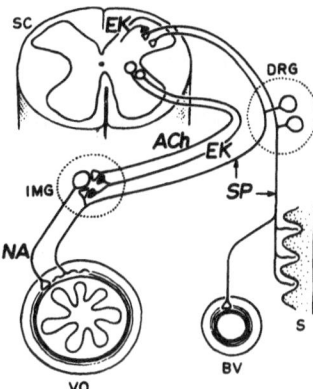

Figure 7. Schematic illustration of functional interrelationships of enkephalin-, ACh-, and SP-containing neurons in the inferior mesenteric ganglion. Connections with somatic and visceral effectors are also shown. ACh, acetylcholine; NA, norepinephrine; EK, enkephalin; SP, substance P; BV, blood vessel; DRG, dorsal root ganglion; IMG, inferior mesenteric ganglion; S, skin; SC, spinal cord; VO, visceral organ. (Modified from Konishi et al., 1980, with permission. For peptidergic synapses in the spinal cord and visceral organs, see, e.g., Jessell and Iversen, 1977; Schultzberg et al., 1980.)

who demonstrated that the noncholinergic slow EPSP evoked by repetitive nerve stimulation is potentiated by the opiate antagonists naloxone or naltrexone. Since the substance P- and enkephalin-containing terminals in the ganglion are respectively derived from the dorsal and ventral roots of lumbar spinal nerves (Fig. 7; see also Dalsgaard et al., 1982a,b; Tsunoo et al., 1982), it should be possible to directly show that stimulation of the ventral root elicits enkephalinergic inhibition of the substance P-mediated slow excitatory transmission.

3. AUTONOMIC NEUROEFFECTOR JUNCTIONS AND THE ENTERIC NERVOUS SYSTEM

3.1. Effects on Adrenergic and Cholinergic Transmission

Autonomic neuroeffector junctions, such as the mouse vas deferens and the guinea pig ileum, are the classical experimental preparations that have been used to study the pharmacology of opiate actions. They have also served as powerful bioassay systems for the survey of endogenous opioid peptides. Most studies with these preparations have focused on the smooth muscle contraction in response to electrical stimulation of the autonomic fibers and have shown that opiates and opioid peptides inhibit stimulation-induced contraction with different rank order of potencies depending upon the preparation and species. These findings underlie the concept of multiple opioid receptor subtypes (see Section 1.3).

On the basis of biochemical experiments showing that opiates and opioid peptides suppress the release of noradrenaline and ACh from presynaptic neurons innervating smooth muscle, it has been suggested that opioids block stimulation-induced muscle contraction by a presynaptic mechanism (Hughes et al., 1975; Waterfield et al., 1977; see also Paton, 1957). More recently these observations have been supported by electrophysiological experiments showing that morphine inhibits neuroeffector transmission without altering the membrane potential, membrane resistance, or action potential threshold of smooth muscle cells in the guinea pig ileum and the mouse vas deferens (Bennett and Lavidis, 1980; Illes et al., 1980; Ito and Tajima, 1980). The opiate-induced inhibition appears to be selective for excitatory junctional transmission, since inhibitory synaptic potentials recorded from circular muscle cells in the guinea pig ileum are not affected by morphine (Ito and Tajima, 1980).

In addition to the relaxing effect of enkephalins on intestinal smooth muscle, the peptides have also been shown to cause contraction of certain smooth muscle cells in the gut wall. Although the cellular mechanisms underlying this action have not been studied thoroughly, experiments on dissociated gastric muscle cells have demonstrated that the opioid-induced contraction is due to a direct action on the smooth muscle cells (Bitar and Makhlouf, 1982). Furthermore, there is evidence that an opioid peptide released by vagal stimulation may cause the contraction of the rat pyloric sphincter (Edin et al. 1980), suggesting that opioid-induced contraction may be of physiological relevance.

3.2. Effects on Nonadrenergic, Noncholinergic Transmission

In the presence of drugs that block adrenergic and cholinergic transmission, stimulation of autonomic nerves (or the intramural plexus in the gut) still produces at least two types of responses in the smooth muscle of the gastrointestinal and respiratory tract (see Burnstock, 1981; Hirst, 1979). One of these "nonadrenergic, noncholinergic" responses is characterized by a hyperpolarizing synaptic potential associated with relaxation of the smooth muscle; the other is a prolonged muscle-contracting response. Substance P has been implicated as a neurotransmitter of the latter response (Björkroth, 1983; Lundberg et al., 1983), and it is believed that the peptide excites both intramural neurons and the smooth muscle cells directly (Katayama et al., 1979; Björkroth, 1983). The inhibitory response in some tissues appears to be insensitive to enkephalins (Cooks and Burnstock, 1979). On the other hand, it is believed that the nonadrenergic, noncholinergic excitatory response is modulated by opioid peptides liberated from intrinsic enteric neurons (Gintzler and Scalisi, 1982). Application of morphine and enkephalin-related peptides inhibits the contraction of the guinea pig ileum evoked by repetitive transmural stimulation. There is, however, no significant effect on smooth muscle contraction induced by exogenous substance P. Moreover, naloxone can enhance the magnitude of the contraction evoked by transmural stimulation, suggesting that opioid peptide-containing neurons in the enteric nervous system interact with other enteric neurons that contain substance P, ACh, or other transmitters (Puig et al., 1977; Gintzler and Scalisi, 1982). A similar naloxone-sensitive process has been shown to operate in the relaxation phase of the peristaltic reflex in the guinea pig small intestine (Kromer and Pretzlaff, 1979). The complex organization of the enteric nervous system has made it difficult to study the specific cellular events responsible for these pharmacological effects although electrophysiological experiments in preparations consisting of individual enteric neurons and muscle cells (see, e.g., Hirst, 1979) may make this possible in the future.

3.3. Direct Effects on Myenteric Neurons

Intracellular recordings from neurons in the isolated guinea-pig ileum myenteric plexus have shown that opioids have two distinct actions on myenteric neurons. The first is a membrane hyperpolarization associated with a fall in input resistance that is evoked by enkephalins and opiates, such as levorphanol, but not the inactive isomer dextrorphan (Sakai et al., 1978; North et al., 1979). The opioid-induced hyperpolarization is likely to result from an increase in the resting K^+ permeability of myenteric neurons. In support of this concept are the observations that the amplitude of the response is dependent on the extracellular K^+ concentration and that the hyperpolarization reversed to a depolarization when the membrane potential was held more negative than the K^+ equilibrium potential (Morita and North, 1982). The K^+ conductance involved in this hyperpolarization is clearly different from the Ca^{2+}-dependent K^+ conductance, since decreasing the extracellular Ca^{2+} concentration actually *increased* the amplitude of the hyperpolarization produced by enkephalin or morphine.

The hyperpolarization and conductance increase recorded in the soma of myenteric neurons is variable from cell to cell. However, it was demonstrated that iontophoretic application of opioids to cell processes could result in a hyperpolarization (recorded at the soma), even when equivalent applications to the soma were without effect (see North and Williams, 1983). These experiments were made possible by the unique structure of the myenteric plexus, a flat two-dimensional lattice of discrete ganglia and interganglionic connectives that contain axons which project between the ganglia. The observation that hyperpolarization can be induced by iontophoretic application of opiates onto the fiber bundles suggests that opiate receptors are present on the axons of myenteric neurons.

The other action of opioids on myenteric neurons is a prolongation of the afterhyperpolarization which follows a burst of action potentials (Tokimasa et al., 1981). This effect occurs at particularly low concentrations of morphine (0.1–10 nM), and is reversibly blocked by naloxone. Since a Ca^{2+}-dependent K^+ conductance is believed to underlie the afterhyperpolarization, opioids could enhance this response either by inhibition of intracellular Ca^{2+} sequestration, by facilitation of Ca^{2+} entry, or by a direct effect on the Ca^{2+}-dependent K^+ conductance *per se*. It has been suggested that, from a functional point of view, prolongation of the afterhyperpolarization could limit the frequency of repetitive discharge in myenteric neurons.

These opioid actions on myenteric neurons have been implicated in

cellular mechanisms responsible for the opioid-induced inhibition of transmitter release in the enteric nervous system (Section 4). It remains, however,
to be determined whether nerve stimulation can produce naloxone-reversible
synaptic potentials in enteric neurons that resemble the pharmacological
actions observed by exogenously applied opioids.

4. CONCLUSIONS

In the peripheral nervous system, opioid peptides appear to be liberated
from intrinsic neurons as well as from neurons that project to the peripheral
ganglia from the CNS. The major role of these opioid-containing neurons
seems to be the regulation of excitatory synaptic transmission through presynaptic inhibition. For example, in the guinea pig inferior mesenteric ganglion, there is little doubt that enkephalins or closely related peptides are
released upon preganglionic nerve stimulation and that these peptides act
on presynaptic nerve terminals to inhibit the release of ACh and substance
P. This prevents the cholinergic and noncholinergic excitation of ganglionic
adrenergic neurons, which ultimately leads to changes in gastrointestinal
motility or suppression of adrenergic stimulation of the cardiovascular systems (see Fig. 7). Nevertheless, the precise circumstances under which opioid
peptide inhibition is called into play are not known. Although effects of
opioids distinct from presynaptic inhibition have been identified, their physiological importance is less clear.

Despite the fact that enkephalin-induced inhibition in many central and
peripheral systems seems to occur by a presynaptic mechanism, there is
little supporting morphological evidence. Examination of enkephalin-containing nerve terminals at the ultrastructural level has only rarely shown
stained endings forming axo-axonic contacts either in the spinal cord (Aronin
et al., 1981) or autonomic ganglia (Kondo and Yui, 1982). However, it is not
clear that morphologically identifiable synaptic junctions are required for
peptidergic transmission and, in fact, there is some evidence that peptide
transmitters can diffuse for a considerable distance to act upon remote target
sites (see Chapter 16; also Barber et al., 1979).

Like other peptide transmitters, enkephalins produce slow and prolonged responses in sympathetic ganglia (see Fig. 4) and at neuroeffector
junctions, but the conductance mechanisms underlying these effects are
poorly understood. This is, of course, in large part due to the difficulty in
recording directly from presynaptic nerve terminals. Indirect experiments
point to two possible mechanisms to explain the inhibitory action of opioids
on transmitter release. First, the Ca^{2+} influx associated with action potential
invasion of the presynaptic nerve terminal might be suppressed by opiates
and opioid peptides. This possibility is suggested by the observation that
morphine-induced inhibition of excitatory junctional transmission can be
overcome by increasing the concentration of Ca^{2+} in the extracellular me-

dium (Bennett and Lavidis, 1980; Illes et al., 1980; Ito and Tajima, 1980). A further support for this notion comes from the analogy provided by experiments on cultured sensory neurons where opioid peptides shorten the duration of the action potential by suppressing the Ca^{2+} current without associated changes in other electrical parameters of the neuronal membrane (Mudge et al., 1979; Werz and Macdonald, 1982).

An alternative explanation for the effects of opioid peptides on transmitter release that has received some experimental support is that opioids block the invasion of the action potential into presynaptic terminals. This is hypothesized to occur by a hyperpolarization of the nerve terminals. Support for this interpretation is provided by the observation that some neurons in the myenteric ganglia are in fact hyperpolarized by opioids due to activation of the K^+ current (Morita and North, 1982). Furthermore, action potentials, evoked by focal stimulation of interganglionic fiber tracts and recorded from myenteric neurons, were blocked by opioids when they were applied at the stimulation site along the course of the cell process (Morita and North, 1981). However, action potentials propagated in the sympathetic nerve trunk innervating the mouse vas deferens were not impaired by morphine (Ito and Tajima, 1980). Moreover, the hyperpolarizing action of enkephalins on myenteric neurons decreases progressively upon repeated application of the peptides (see Morita and North, 1982); whereas the effects on transmitter release do not (see Fig. 1A). Clearly, the evidence in support of either mechanism is incomplete; however, neither is mutually exclusive and both may contribute to a greater or lesser extent to inhibition of transmitter release at ganglionic synapses or neuroeffector junctions. The slowness and long duration of enkephalin-induced inhibition has suggested that intermediate steps may be involved in the transduction of receptor occupancy to synaptic response, but this speculation is as yet unsupported experimentally.

ACKNOWLEDGMENTS. I am indebted to many colleagues for helpful discussions, particularly to Prof. M. Otsuka, and Drs. T. Murakoshi, and A. Tsunoo. Dr. M. A. Rogawski made numerous suggestions that have improved the text markedly; I am grateful for his help and patience. Part of the author's original work was supported by research grants from the Japanese Ministry of Education, Science and Culture.

REFERENCES

Alm, P., Almets, J., Håkanson, R., Owman, Ch., Sjoberg, N. -O., Stjernqvist, M., and Sunder, F., 1981, Enkephalin-immunoreactive nerve fibers in the feline genito-urinary tract, Histochemistry 72:351–355.

Aronin, N., DiFiglia, M., Liotta, A. S., and Martin, J. B., 1981, Ultrastructural localization and biochemical features of immunoreactive Leu-enkephalin in monkey dorsal horn, J. Neurosci. 1:561–577.

Ashe, J. H., and Libet, B., 1981, Orthodromic production of noncholinergic slow depolarizing response in the superior cervical ganglion of the rabbit, *J. Physiol. (Lond.)* **320:**333–346.

Barber, R. P., Vaughan, J. E., Slemmon, J. R., Salvaterra, P. M., Roberts, E., and Leeman, S. E., 1979, The origin, distribution and synaptic relationships of substance P axons in rat spinal cord, *J. Comp. Neurol.* **184:**331–351.

Bennett, M. R., and Lavidis, N. A., 1980, An electrophysiological analysis of the effects of morphine on the calcium dependence of neuromuscular transmission in the mouse vas deferens, *Br. J. Pharmacol.* **69:**185–191.

Bitar, K. N., and Makhlouf, G. M., 1982, Specific opiate receptors on isolated mammalian gastric smooth muscle cells, *Nature* **297:**72–74.

Bixby, J. L., and Spitzer, N. C., 1983, Enkephalin reduces quantal content at the frog neuromuscular junction, *Nature* **301:**431–432.

Björkroth, U., 1983, Inhibition of smooth muscle contractions induced by capsaicin and electrical transmural stimulation by a substance P antagonist, *Acta Physiol. Scand. [Suppl.]* **515:**11–16.

Bornstein, J. C., and Fields, H. L., 1979, Morphine presynaptically inhibits a ganglionic cholinergic synapse, *Neurosci. Lett.* **15:**77–82.

Burnstock, G., 1981, Neurotransmitters and trophic factors in the autonomic nervous system, *J. Physiol. (Lond.)* **313:**1–35.

Cooks, T., and Burnstock, G., 1979, Effects of neuronal polypeptides on intestinal smooth muscle: a comparison with nonadrenergic, noncholinergic nerve stimulation and ATP, *Eur. J. Pharmacol.* **54:**251–259.

Dalsgaard, C. -J., Hökfelt, T., Elfvin, L. -G., Skirboll, L., and Emson, P., 1982a, Substance P-containing primary sensory neurons projecting to the inferior mesenteric ganglion: Evidence from combined retrograde tracing and immunohistochemistry, *Neuroscience* **7:**647–654.

Dalsgaard, C. -J., Hökfelt, T., Elfvin, L. -G., and Terenius, L., 1982b, Enkephalin-containing sympathetic preganglionic neurons projecting to the inferior mesenteric ganglion: Evidence from combined retrograde tracing and immunohistochemistry, *Neuroscience* **7:**2039–2050.

Del Castillo, J., and Katz, B., 1954, Quantal components of the end-plate potential, *J. Physiol. (Lond.)* **124:**560–573.

Dennis, M. J., Harris, A. J., and Kuffler, S. W., 1971, Synaptic transmission and its duplication by focally applied acetylcholine in parasympathetic neurons in the heart of the frog, *Proc. R. Soc. Lond. Ser. B* **177:**509–539.

Edin, R., Lundberg, J., Terenius, L., Dahlström, A., Hökfelt, T., Kewenter, J., and Ahlman, H., 1980, Evidence for vagal enkephalinergic neural control of the feline pylorus and stomach, *Gastroenterology* **78:**492–497.

Furness, J. B., Costa, M., and Miller, R. J., 1983, Distribution and projections of nerves with enkephalin-like immunoreactivity in the guinea-pig small intestine, *Neuroscience* **8:**653–664.

Gintzler, A. R., and Scalisi, J. A., 1982, Effects of opioids on non-cholinergic excitatory responses of the guinea-pig isolated ileum: Inhibition of release of enteric substance P, *Br. J. Pharmacol.* **75:**199–205.

Glazer, E. J., and Basbaum, A. L., 1980, Leucine enkephalin: Localization in and axoplasmic transport by sacral parasympathetic preganglionic neurons, *Science* **208:**1479–1481.

Hartschuh, W., Weihe, E., Buchler, M., Helmstaedter, V., Feurle, G. E., and Forssmann, W. G., 1979, Met-enkephalin-like immunoreactivity in Merkel cells, *Cell Tissue Res.* **201:**343–348.

Hirst, G. D. S., 1979, Mechanisms of peristalsis, *Br. Med. Bull.* **35:**263–268.

Hughes, J., Kosterlitz, H. K., and Leslie, F. M., 1975, Effect of morphine on adrenergic transmission in the mouse vas deferens. Assessment of agonist and antagonist potencies of narcotic analgesics, *Br. J. Pharmacol.* **53:**371–381.

Hughes, J., Kosterlitz, H. W., and Smith, T. W., 1977, The distribution of methionine-enkephalin and leucine-enkephalin in the brain and peripheral tissues, *Br. J. Pharmacol.* **61:**639–647.

Illes, P., Zieglgänsberger, W., and Herz, A., 1980, Calcium reverses the inhibitory action of morphine on neuroeffector transmission in the mouse vas deferens, *Brain Res.* **191:**511–522.

Ito, Y., and Tajima, K., 1980, Action of morphine on the neuroeffector transmission in the guinea-pig ileum and in the mouse vas deferens, *J. Physiol. (Lond.)* **307:**367–383.

Jessen, K. R., Saffrey, M. J., van Noorden, S., Bloom, S. R., Polak, J. M., and Burnstock, G., 1980, Immunohistochemical studies of the enteric nervous system in tissue culture and in situ: Localization of vasoactive intestinal polypeptide (VIP), substance P and enkephalin immunoreactive nerves in the guinea-pig gut, Neuroscience 5:1717–1735.

Jessell, T. M., and Iversen, L. L., 1977, Opiate analgesics inhibit substance P release from rat trigeminal nucleus, Nature 268:549–551.

Jiang, Z. G., Simmons, M. A., and Dun, N. J., 1982, Enkephalinergic modulation of non-cholinergic transmission in mammalian prevertebral ganglia, Brain Res. 235:185–191.

Katayama, Y., and Nishi, S., 1981, Actions of enkephalin on single neurons in ciliary ganglia, in: Advances in Endogenous and Exogenous Opioids (H. Takagi and E. J. Simon, eds.), Kodansha, Tokyo, pp. 205–207.

Katayama, Y., North, R. A., and Williums, J. T., 1979, The action of substance P on neurones of the myenteric plexus of the guinea-pig intestine, Proc. R. Soc. Lond. Ser. B 206:191–208.

Kato, K., and Kuba, K., 1980, Inhibition of transmitter release in bullfrog sympathetic ganglia induced by γ-aminobutyric acid, J. Physiol. (Lond.) 298:271–283.

Kondo, H., and Yui, R., 1982, An electron microscopic study on enkephalin-like immunoreactive fibers in the celiac ganglion of guinea-pig, Brain Res. 252:142–145.

Konishi, S., Tsunoo, A., and Otsuka, M., 1979a, Enkephalins presynaptically inhibit cholinergic transmission in sympathetic ganglia, Nature 282:515–516.

Konishi, S., Tsunoo, A., and Otsuka, M., 1979b, Substance P and noncholinergic excitatory synaptic transmission in guinea-pig sympathetic ganglia, Proc. Jpn. Acad. Ser. B. 55:525–530.

Konishi, S., Tsunoo, A., Yanaihara, N., and Otsuka, M., 1980, Peptidergic excitatory and inhibitory synapses in mammalian sympathetic ganglia: Roles of substance P and enkephalin, Biomed. Res. 1:528–536.

Konishi, S., Tsunoo, A., and Otsuka, M., 1981, Enkephalin as a transmitter for presynaptic inhibition in sympathetic ganglia, Nature 294:80–82.

Konishi, S., Otsuka, M., Folkers, K., and Rosell, S., 1983, A substance P antagonist blocks noncholinergic slow excitatory postsynaptic potential in guinea-pig sympathetic ganglia, Acta Physiol. Scand. 117:157–160.

Kromer, W., and Pretzlaff, W., 1979, In vitro evidence for the participation of intestinal opioids in the control of peristalsis in the guinea pig small intestine, Naunyn Schmiedebergs Arch. Pharmacol. 309:153–157.

Kuffler, S. W., 1980, Slow synaptic responses in autonomic ganglia and the pursuit of a peptidergic transmitter, J. Exp. Biol. 89:257–286.

Libet, B., 1979, Which postsynaptic action of dopamine is mediated by cyclic AMP? Life Sci. 24:1043–1058.

Lord, J. A., Waterfield, A. A., Hughes, J., and Kosterlitz, H. W., 1977, Endogenous opioid peptides: Multiple agonists and receptors, Nature 267:495–499.

Lundberg, J. M., Hökfelt, T., Fahrenkrug, J., Nilsson, G., and Terenius, L., 1979, Peptides in the cat carotid body (glomus caroticum): VIP-, enkephalin-, and substance P-like immunoreactivity, Acta Physiol. Scand. 107:279–281.

Lundberg, J. M., Saria, A., Brodin, E., Rosell, S., and Folkers, K., 1983, A substance P antagonist inhibits vagally induced increase in vascular permeability and bronchial smooth muscle contraction in the guinea pig, Proc. Natl. Acad. Sci. USA 80:1120–1124.

Macdonald, R. L., and Nelson, P. G., 1978, Specific-opiate-induced depression of transmitter release from dorsal root ganglion cells in culture, Science 199:1449–1451.

Machova, J., and Kvaltinova, Z., 1983, The actions of [Leu^5] enkephalin and morphine in cat sympathetic ganglion, Eur. J. Pharmacol. 87:277–282.

Martin, A. R., 1977, Junctional transmission, II. Presynaptic mechanisms, in: Handbook of Physiology, Vol. 1, Cellular Biology of Neurons, Part 1 (E. R. Kandel, ed.), American Physiological Society, Bethesda, pp. 329–355.

Morita, K., and North, R. A., 1981, Opiate and enkephalin reduce the excitability of neuronal processes, Neuroscience 6:1943–1951.

Morita, K., and North, R. A., 1982, Opiate activation of potassium conductance in myenteric neurons: Inhibition by calcium ion. Brain Res. 242:145–150.

Mudge, A. W., Leeman, S. E., and Fischbach, G. D., 1979, Enkephalin inhibits release of substance P from sensory neurons in culture and decreases action potential duration, *Proc. Natl. Acad. Sci. USA* **76:**526–530.

North, R. A., and Williams, J. T., 1983, How do opiates inhibit neurotransmitter release? *Trends Pharmacol. Sci.* **4:**337–339.

North, R. A., Katayama, Y., and Williams, J. T., 1979, On the mechanism and site of action of enkephalin on single myenteric neurons, *Brain Res.* **165:**67–77.

Otsuka, M., and Konishi, S., 1983, Substance P—the first peptide neurotransmitter? *Trends Neurosci.* **6:**317–320.

Paton, W. D. M., 1957, The action of morphine and related substances on contraction and on acetylcholine output of coaxially stimulated guinea-pig ileum, *Br. J. Pharmacol.* **12:**119–127.

Paterson, S. J., Robson, L. E., and Kosterlitz, H. W., 1983, Classification of opioid receptors, *Br. Med. Bull.* **39:**31–36.

Puig, M. M., Gascon, P., Craviso, G. L., and Musacchio, J. M., 1977, Endogenous opiate receptor ligand: Electrically induced release in the guinea pig ileum, *Science* **195:**419–420.

Sakai, K. K., Hymson, D. L., and Shapiro, R., 1978, The mode of action of enkephalins in the guinea-pig myenteric plexus, *Neurosci. Lett.* **10:**317–322.

Schultzberg, M., Hökfelt, T., Terenius, L., Elfvin, L. -G., Lundberg, J. M., Brandt, J., Elde, R. P., and Goldstein, M., 1979, Enkephalin immunoreactive nerve fibers and cell bodies in sympathetic ganglia of the guinea-pig and rat, *Neuroscience* **4:**249–270.

Schultzberg, M., Hökfelt, T., Nilsson, G., Terenius, L., Rehfeeld, J. F., Brown, M., Elde, R., Goldstein, M., and Said, S., 1980, Distribution of peptide-, and catecholamine-containing neurons in the gastro-intestinal tract of rat and guinea-pig: Immunohistochemical studies with antisera to substance P, vasoactive intestinal polypeptide, enkephalins, somatostatin, gastrin/cholecystokinin, neurotensin, and dopamine β-hydroxylase, *Neuroscience* **5:**689–744.

Tokimasa, T., Morita, K., and North, A., 1981, Opiates and clonidine prolong calcium-dependent afterhyperpolarizations, *Nature* **294:**162–163.

Tsunoo, A., Konishi, S., and Otsuka, M., 1982, Substance P as an excitatory transmitter of primary afferent neurons in guinea-pig sympathetic ganglia, *Neuroscience* **7:**2025–2037.

Udenfriend, S., and Kilpatrick, D., 1983, Biochemistry of the enkephalins and enkephalin-containing peptides, *Arch. Biochem. Biophys.* **221:**309–323.

Waterfield, A. A., Smockum, R. W. J., Hughes, J., Kosterlitz, H. W., and Henderson, G., 1977, In vitro pharmacology of the opioid peptides, enkephalins and endorphins, *Eur. J. Pharmacol.* **43:**107–116.

Werz, M. A., and Macdonald, R. L., 1982, Heterogeneous sensitivity of cultured dorsal root ganglion neurones to opioid peptides selective for μ- and δ-opiate receptors, *Nature* **299:**730–733.

Wouters, W., and van den Bercken, J., 1980, Effects of met-enkephalin on slow synaptic inhibition in frog sympathetic ganglion, *Neuropharmacology* **19:**237–243.

Yang, H. -Y. T., Hexum, T., and Costa, E., 1980, Opioid peptides in adrenal gland, *Life Sci.* **27:**1119–1125.

13

Substance P

NAE J. DUN

1. INTRODUCTION

1.1. Historical Perspective

Slightly over half a century ago, while working on the acetylcholine content of tissue extracts, von Euler and Gaddum (1931) obtained an active compound from alcoholic extracts of equine intestine and brain that when injected intravenously, caused a fall in blood pressure in rabbits and a contraction of the isolated rabbit intestine. As these effects were not prevented by atropine, they suspected that the compound was pharmacologically distinct from acetylcholine. This crude extract acquired the term "substance P" from the working description given to the active compound in the laboratory of the original investigators, and this usage has since persisted in the literature.

A crucial step forward in substance P research was achieved when Chang and Leeman (1970) unexpectedly found that a sialogogic peptide purified from bovine hypothalamic tissues exhibited biological activities similar to that of the crude substance P extract characterized earlier by Lembeck and Starke (1968). Subsequently, the amino acid sequence of the sialogogic peptide was determined, and it was found to be an undecapeptide (Chang et al., 1971; Fig. 1). The elucidation of the amino acid sequence of substance P led quickly to its chemical synthesis (Tregear et al., 1971).

Early investigations revealed a remarkably wide spectrum of biological activities of substance P, and a number of important concepts with regard to the action of substance P were discovered during the course of early investigations, even before its chemical structure was known (Lembeck and Zetler, 1962; Pernow, 1963). For example, the hypothesis that substance P

Mammalian tachykinins

    Arg-Pro-Lys-Pro-Gln-Gln-Phe-Phe-Gly-Leu-Met-NH$_2$ Substance P

Molluscan tachykinins

    Glp-Pro-Ser-Lys-Asp-Ala-Phe-Ile-Gly-Leu-Met-NH$_2$ Eledoisin

Amphibian tachykinins

    Glp-Ala-Asp-Pro-Asn-Lys-Phe-Tyr-Gly-Leu-Met-NH$_2$ Physalaemin
    Glp-Ala-Asp-Pro-Lys-Thr-Phe-Tyr-Gly-Leu-Met-NH$_2$ [Lys^5, Thr^6]Physalaemin
    Glp-Pro-Asp-Pro-Asn-Ala-Phe-Tyr-Gly-Leu-Met-NH$_2$ Uperolein
    Glp-------Asn-Pro-Asn-Arg-Phe-Ile-Gly-Leu-Met-NH$_2$ Phyllomedusin
Asp-Val-Pro-Lys-Ser-Asp-Gln-Phe-Val-Gly-Leu-Met-NH$_2$ Kassinin
Asp-Glu-Pro-Lys-Pro-Asp-Gln-Phe-Val-Gly-Leu-Met-NH$_2$ [Glu^2,Pro^5]Kassinin
Asp-Pro-Pro-Asp-Pro-Asp-Arg-The-Tyr-Gly-Met-Met-NH$_2$ Hylambatin

Figure 1. Amino acid sequences of substance P and other naturally occurring tachykinins.

may be the transmitter released at the central terminals of dorsal root fibers was proposed in the early 1950s by Lembeck (1953), who found that the substance P concentration was much higher in the dorsal roots than in the ventral roots.

Substance P was the first "brain-gut" peptide to be extensively studied, particularly with respect to its role in neural functions. In this chapter, the actions of substance P on central and peripheral neurons, as well as its role as a neurotransmitter at several selected synapses, where evidence for such a role is reasonably strong, are discussed.

1.2. Distribution of Substance P Neurons and Fibers

A brief review of the distribution and localization of substance P-containing neurons and fibers is intended here only in the context of providing a morphological basis for latter discussion of the action of substance P on various central neurons and of their possible physiological roles. Comprehensive treatments of this subject are available (Cuello et al., 1982; Hökfelt et al., 1982).

The term substance P-like immunoreactivity (SPLI) will be used here to describe the substance P or cross-reactive peptide detected by the immunohistochemical or radioimmunoassay procedures. In the mammalian central nervous system, SPLI neurons are found in more than 30 areas or nuclei, including many parts of the brain stem and spinal cord (Hökfelt et al., 1977b; Cuello and Kanazawa, 1978; Cuello et al., 1982; Hökfelt et al., 1982).

Dense groups of immunoreactive somata are found in the medial habenular nucleus, the interpeduncular nucleus and in the pontine central gray. Mapping studies utilizing sensitive radioimmunoassay procedures combined with selective lesions have shown a number of well defined SPLI pathways in the CNS (Mroz et al., 1977; Nicoll et al., 1980). A prominent projection involves cells in the anterior stratium whose fibers terminate in the substantia nigra, which contains the highest concentration of SPLI of any microdissected brain region (Mroz et al., 1977). Other areas that show dense SPLI terminals include the medial amygdala and hypothalamus.

In the spinal cord, dense networks of SPLI fibers are observed in the dorsal horns with the highest concentrations in Lissauer's tract and in laminae I and II; the number of SPLI fibers decreases progressively in the ventral direction (Hökfelt et al., 1977b; Cuello and Kanazawa, 1978). The observations that the dorsal half of the spinal cord contains quantitatively higher amount of SPLI than the ventral half in all animals tested and that ligation or section of the dorsal roots results in a marked reduction of SPLI in the ipsilateral dorsal horn are consistent with the notion that some of the substance P-containing fibers in the dorsal horn may derive from dorsal root ganglia (Otsuka et al., 1975, Hökfelt et al., 1977b; Ljungdahl et al., 1978). By means of immunohistofluorescent techniques, SPLI was indeed visualized in some sensory neurons in the dorsal root ganglia comprising not more than 20% of the total population of dorsal root neurons (Hökfelt et al., 1975). The SPLI-containing dorsal root ganglion cells generally have small somata and unmyelinated or thinly myelinated fibers. Moreover, ligation studies show that these fibers project both centrally to the spinal cord and peripherally to the sensory organs (Hökfelt et al., 1975; Cuello and Kanazawa, 1978; Ljungdahl et al., 1978). The finding that dorsal rhizotomy results in only a 50–60% loss of SPLI in the dorsal horn suggests that SPLI in this area is not derived exclusively from dorsal root ganglia; a portion of it is probably contained either in intrinsic neurons or in descending fibers (Cuello and Kanazawa, 1978; Ljungdahl et al., 1978). Conversely, the SPLI fibers in the ventral horn appear to derive mainly from supraspinal neurons as transaction of the spinal cord at the upper thoracic levels results in a nearly total loss of SPLI fibers (Cuello and Kanazawa, 1978; Ljungdahl et al., 1978). That SPLI-containing fibers in the spinal cord may derive from different sources is further suggested by the experiments where capsaicin is found to cause a depletion of SPLI from a portion of the fibers in the dorsal horn, whereas the SPLI in the ventral horn is not appreciably affected (Jancsó et al., 1981). As capsaicin affects only sensory neurons irrespective of the type of transmitter they contain, the SPLI that disappears after capsaicin treatment should be contained in nerve fibers that are sensory in nature (Jancsó et al., 1981).

Within the intestine, SPLI has been found in the muscularis muscosa layers of both the small and large gut (Nilsson et al., 1975; Pearse and Polak, 1975), as well as within intrinsic neurons of the enteric nervous system (Costa et al., 1980). Dense networks of SPLI fibers are seen surrounding the cell bodies of myenteric plexus neurons and extending between bundles of smooth muscles. SPLI is also present in the extrinsic innervation of the gut and has been reported in fibers of vagus as well as in cell bodies of the nodose and jugular ganglia (Lundberg et al., 1978).

In addition to the brain and intestines, peripheral motor and autonomic nerves, salivary glands, and optic nerves have been found to contain moderate to trace amounts of SPLI (Skrabanek and Powell, 1977). Peripheral sympathetic ganglia contain SPLI, the highest amount being in the guinea pig inferior mesenteric ganglia, where it is localized almost exclusively in nerve fibers. A number of studies indicate that the SPLI fibers in guinea pig inferior mesenteric ganglia are collateral branches of peripheral sensory nerve fibers arising from dorsal root ganglia (Dalsgaard et al., 1982a; Dun and Jiang, 1982; Matthews and Cuello, 1982; Tsunoo et al., 1982). In this respect, there is some evidence that the SPLI fibers observed near the vascular bed may also be derived from sensory ganglia (Furness et al., 1982).

An issue of importance is the coexistence and possible corelease of substance P and other putative transmitter(s) from single neurons. In the CNS, SPLI was visualized in a portion of the serotonin-containing neurons in the lower medulla oblongata (Chan-Palay et al., 1978) and cholecystokinin-containing cells in the mesencephalic central grey (Skirboll et al., 1982) and dorsal root ganglia (Dalsgaard et al., 1982b). The situation appears to be even more complex in the medullary raphe nuclei, where immunoreactivity to substance P, serotonin, and thyrotropic-releasing hormone appears to coexist in a small population of neurons (Johansson et al., 1981). In the periphery, SPLI was observed in postganglionic noradrenergic neurons of the rat superior cervical ganglia (Kessler et al., 1981). The observation that substance P and serotonin immunoreactivity is colocalized in dense core granules of certain central nerve terminals raises the possibility that they may be coreleased under appropriate conditions (Pelletier et al., 1981).

It is certain that additional reports concerning the coexistence of SPLI and other putative transmitter(s) in central and peripheral neurons will be forthcoming. In what way and to what degree coexistence and corelease of SPLI and other putative transmitter(s) modify synaptic events at the target cells remains to be investigated.

1.3. Substance P Receptors and Antagonists

Substance P exerts effects on a wide variety of peripheral tissues and on the central nervous system, yet the receptors mediating these responses are as yet poorly defined. Following the structural identification of substance P, a series of analogs was prepared, and structure-activity relationships were examined on a number of biological test systems. The results indicate that the C terminal, but not the N terminal, is essential for biological activity. Moreover, the biological activity and potency is nearly fully retained with C-terminal fragments down to the hexapeptide, substance $P_{(5-11)}$; conversely, removal of the C-terminal amide results in a dramatic loss of potency. These structural requirements for substance P activity appear to hold in all biological test systems.

The study of the structure-activity relationship was considerably facilitated following the discovery that substance P is but one member of a family of closely related peptides known as the tachykinins (Erspamer, 1981; Fig. 1). These peptides all have a very similar amino acid sequence at the carboxy terminus, -Phe-X-Gly-Leu-Met-NH$_2$, which probably accounts for the biological activity they have in common.

When the rank order potencies of tachykinins on a number of biological test systems were examined, Erspamer and collaborators found that there is a clear distinction among the peptides examined and proposed that there are subtypes of substance P receptors in various tissues (Erspamer, 1981). Subsequent studies have confirmed these observations and have suggested the following subclasses of substance P receptors in peripheral tissues: substance P-P receptors (for physalaemin) where all tachykinins, substance P, physalaemin, eledoisin and kassinin are almost equipotent with some preference for physalaemin; and substance P-E receptors (for eledoisin) where the rank order of potency is kassinin > eledoisin >> substance P = physalaemin (Lee et al., 1982).

With respect to central substance P receptors, the rank order potencies of substance P and its fragments in depolarizing spinal motoneurons appears to be similar to that observed in peripheral tissues, i.e., full activity is retained with C-terminal fragments down to the hexapeptide (Otsuka et al., 1975). The observation that substance P, its short chain analogs, and related tachykinins differ with respect to their potencies in competing with [^{3}H]substance P binding in rat brain, i.e., physalaemin being the most potent, is consistent with the possible existence of multiple substance P receptors in the brain (Lee et al., 1982). The development of highly specific substance P agonists and antagonists will be needed to further characterize the substance P receptors in various peripheral and central tissues.

In this regard, the lack of highly specific and potent substance P antagonists in the past few years has been a constant disappointment in substance P research. Baclofen [β-(chlorophenyl)-γ-amino-butyric acid] surfaced briefly as a substance P antagonist (Saito et al., 1975), but its specificity was questioned in a number of subsequent studies (Phillis, 1976). In the past few years, a systematic study of the activity of substituted substance P analogs for possible antagonistic action was carried out by Rosell and Folkers (1982). A number of substance P analogs, notably (D-Pro^2,D-Phe^7,D-Trp^9)-SP and (D-Pro^2,D-Trp^{7,9})-SP appear to exert some antagonistic action to substance P when tested in several systems. Thus, (D-Pro^2,D-Trp^{7,9})-SP effectively and selectively blocked the increase in firing rates of the locus coeruleus neurons induced by substance P, whereas the excitatory effects of glutamate and acetylcholine on these neurons were not affected (Engberg et al., 1981). However, these two analogs are partial agonists, and are generally low in potency (Caranikas et al., 1982). Clearly, the development of highly specific antagonists is a prerequisite for characterizing the physiological role of substance P in various tissues.

2. ACTION IN THE CENTRAL NERVOUS SYSTEM

Since the availability of synthetic substance P, a large number of studies have examined the effects of substance P and related peptides on various central and peripheral neurons. In early experiments, using extracellular recording and iontophoresis, the predominant effect of substance P on central neurons was excitation, although a depressant effect was observed in some neurons, for example, a subpopulation of dorsal horn neurons (Table 1). The situation was different in Renshaw cells, however, where substance P was found to exert an exclusively depressant action on acetylcholine and glutamate-induced cell discharges (Belcher and Ryall, 1977; Krnjević and Lekic, 1977).

One common feature that was observed in nearly all these studies is the slowness in turning on and off the increase or decrease of cell discharges. Generally, a delay of seconds to minutes was noted between the start of iontophoresis and the change of discharge rates, and the effect often outlasted the termination of iontophoresis by several minutes.

Consistent with the data obtained by extracellular recordings, the principal effect of substance P on central and peripheral neurons as revealed by intracellular recording methods is that of depolarization, which is characteristically slow in onset, requiring seconds and prolonged in duration (lasting for seconds to minutes). Although membrane depolarization is the overwhelming response caused by substance P and related peptides, the underlying mechanism appears to be different depending on the type of neuron in question.

2.1. Spinal Motoneurons and Cuneate Neurons

In an effort to further substantiate the hypothesis that the dorsal root peptide was the transmitter released from primary afferent fibers, Otsuka and colleagues examined the effects of synthetic substance P and related peptides on motoneurons of the isolated frog and newborn rat spinal cord *in vitro* (Otsuka et al.,1975; Otsuka and Konishi, 1977). Substance P when applied by superfusion to the isolated rat spinal cord depolarized the motoneurons, and the effect persisted in a low-Ca/high-Mg solution, although it was somewhat attenuated. The depolarization was always associated with a decrease in membrane resistance and the reversal potential as extrapolated from the current-voltage relationship was between 0 and -10 mV, suggesting that the peptide depolarizes spinal motoneurons by increasing membrane permeability, possibly to sodium. Similarly, substance P was found to depolarize the motoneurons of the isolated frog spinal cord *in vitro*, and the depolarization was also consistently accompanied by a decrease of membrane resistance (Nicoll, 1978). However, the decrease in membrane resistance reported in both studies was small, generally not more than 20%.

Table 1. Effects of Substance P on Discharge Rates of Central and Peripheral Neurons

Preparation	Species	Type of discharges	Response	Percent responding	Reference
Cortical Betz cells[a]	Rat	Spontaneous	Increased[c]	94	Phillis & Limacher (1974)
Cuneate neurons[a]	Cat	Spontaneous	Increased[c]	50	Krnjević and Morris (1974)
Dorsal horn neurons[a]	Cat	Noxious heat and mechanical activated	Increased[c]	50–100	Henry (1976), Randić and Miletic (1977)
Dorsal horn neurons[a]	Cat	Low threshold mechanical activated	Decreased[c]	50	Randić and Miletic (1977)
Dorsal horn neurons[a]	Cat	Noxious heat activated	Variable[c]		Davies and Dray (1980)
Renshaw cells[a]	Cat	Spontaneous	No change[c]		Henry et al. (1975)
	Cat	Glutamate activated	Depressed[c]		Henry et al. (1975)
	Cat	ACh activated	Depressed[c]	90	Ryall and Belcher (1977)
Medial preoptic neurons[a]	Rat	Spontaneous	Increased[c]	50	Mayer and MacLeod (1979)
Locus coeruleus[a]	Rat	Spontaneous	Increased[c]	80	Guyenet and Aghajanian (1977)
Medial amygdala and putamen[a]	Rat	Spontaneous and glutamate activated	Increased[c]	50–90	Le Gal LaSalle and Ben-Ari (1977)
Medullary nucleus raphe magnus[a]	Rat	Noxious stimulus	Increased[c]	50	Pomeroy and Behbehani (1980)
Mesencephalic reticular and substantia nigra[a]	Rat	Spontaneous	Increased[c]	90	Walker et al. (1976)
Myenteric neurons[b]	Guinea pig	Spontaneous	Increased[d]	50–100	Katayama et al. (1979)
Retina ganglion cells[b]	Carp	Light activated	Increased[e]	50	Glickman et al. (1982)

[a]In situ preparation.
[b]In vitro preparation.
[c]Substance P was administered by iontophoresis.
[d]Substance P was administered by bath application.
[e]Substance P was administered by spray.

In contrast to its effects on rat and frog spinal motoneurons, substance P when applied iontophoretically to cat cuneate and motoneurons *in situ* elicited a slowly rising and falling depolarization that was consistently associated with an increase in membrane resistance (Krnjević, 1977). In these experiments, the reversal potential of the substance P depolarization was similar to the extrapolated reversal potential of postspike afterhyperpolarization (both varied between -86 and -88 mV), which is presumably close to the potassium equilibrium potential (E_K). The polarity of the substance P depolarization was reversed at membrane potentials more negative than E_K, suggesting that substance P may inactivate K conductance (Krnjević, 1977).

The apparent difference with respect to the mechanism underlying the substance P depolarization in rat and frog motoneurons, on one hand, and cat motoneurons, on the other, cannot be readily resolved. Apart from species difference, experiments were carried out under different conditions, particularly with respect to the mode of peptide administration. Thus, in *in situ* preparations the peptide was administered iontophoretically, whereas, in isolated rat and frog spinal cord, the peptide was applied by superfusion. Apart from these methodological differences, there is unreliability in the determination of membrane resistance and reversal potential using the current-clamp method.

2.2. Mouse Spinal Cord Neurons in Culture

The effects of substance P on dissociated mouse spinal cord neurons grown in culture have been studied in detail by Nowak and MacDonald (1982). A slow depolarization associated with an increase in membrane resistance was observed in some neurons when substance P or related peptides were applied by pressure ejection from micropipettes near the neuronal membrane. Following a brief application of peptide, a long-lasting depolarization developed within 0.5–1.5 sec, which persisted from 30 sec to 3 min.

The electrogenic mechanism underlying the substance P depolarization in cultured spinal cord neurons was analyzed, and the result is compatible with the hypothesis that the peptide inactivates a voltage-dependent K^+ current that is in some respect similar to the M current found in other vertebrate neurons (see Chapter 6 and Brown et al., 1981). In current clamp experiments, the substance P depolarization was associated with an increase in membrane resistance, and the response was increased and decreased by membrane depolarization and hyperpolarization, respectively, suggesting that substance P depolarized the neurons by decreasing either G_K or G_{Cl} or both. The possible involvement of Cl^- ions was excluded by the observation that substance P still caused depolarization when the cells were loaded with Cl^- by using KCl-filled recording electrodes, which should shift the equilibrium potential for Cl^- to a value more positive than the resting potential. The substance P-induced depolarization was not appreciably affected in Na-deficient (5 mM vs 137 mM) solutions, indicating that Na^+ ions were likewise not involved. Therefore, the mechanism underlying substance P depolarization in cultured mouse spinal cord neurons can best be explained by an inactivation of G_K. The observation that the extrapolated reversal potentials of the substance P depolarization varied with extracellular K concentrations is consistent with this hypothesis. However, the substance P depolarization was not inverted at membrane potential levels more negative than E_K (Fig. 2). These findings have been interpreted as indicating that substance P depolarizes mouse spinal cord neurons by blocking a voltage dependent outward K^+ current that is similar to the M current and recent voltage-clamp experiments seem to confirm this (R. L. MacDonald, personal communication).

2.3. Dorsal Horn Neurons

Dorsal horn neurons in the spinal cord are prime targets of substance P-containing fibers, some of which may derive from dorsal root ganglia. Analyzing effects of substance P on dorsal horn neurons is therefore of importance in understanding the role of substance P as a sensory transmitter. Early studies showed that the predominant effect of substance P on dorsal horn neurons *in situ* was a slow membrane depolarization accompanied by no discernible change in membrane resistance (Sastry, 1979; Zieglgänsberger and Tulloch, 1979). This effect might have been caused by a simultaneous increase and decrease of membrane conductance to several ions, resulting

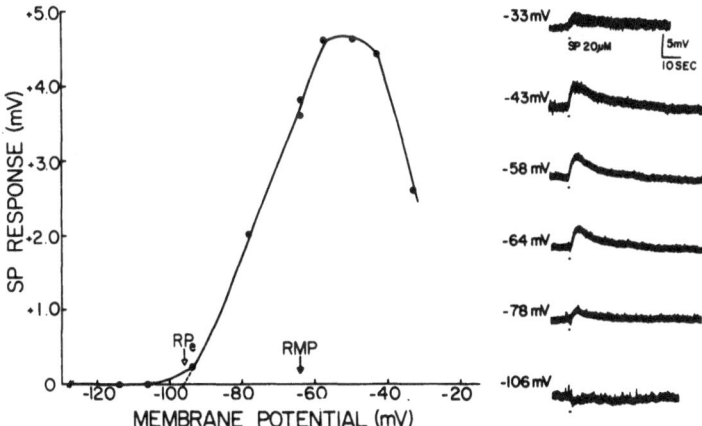

Figure 2. Response of mouse spinal cord neuron in culture to substance P (SP) applied by pressure ejection. The amplitude of the substance P response varied as a function of membrane potential, but the response did not reverse polarity. The response amplitude did not vary as a linear function of membrane potential at potentials less than -50 mV or greater than -95 mV in this neuron. RMP and RPe denote resting membrane potential and extrapolated reversal potential of substance P depolarization, respectively. (From Nowak and MacDonald, 1982, with permission.)

in no net change in membrane resistance. Alternatively, the decrease in membrane conductance might have been masked by coincidental membrane rectification occurring during the depolarization, or the conductance change may have been undetected by the recording electrode, which was separated 100–160 μm from the iontophoretic pipette. Recently, it has been possible to obtain stable intracellular recordings from dorsal horn neurons of the rat neonatal spinal cord in a slice preparation (Murase et al., 1982). Consistent with earlier studies, the most prominent effect of substance P on dorsal horn neurons is a slow membrane depolarization, which in some instances is preceded by a hyperpolarization (Fig. 3). The substance P-induced depolarization was often accompanied by a burst of action potentials and an increase in baseline noise; the latter, as well as the initial hyperpolarization, when it occurred, was abolished in a low-Ca^{2+}/high-Mg^{2+} solution, suggesting that substance P, in addition to directly depolarizing the dorsal horn neurons, may promote transmitter release.

The mechanism underlying the substance P-induced depolarization in dorsal horn neurons appears to be complex. Both an increase and decrease of membrane resistance during the course of the substance P depolarization were observed. Moreover, membrane hyperpolarization increased the amplitude of substance P depolarization in some cells, while decreasing it in

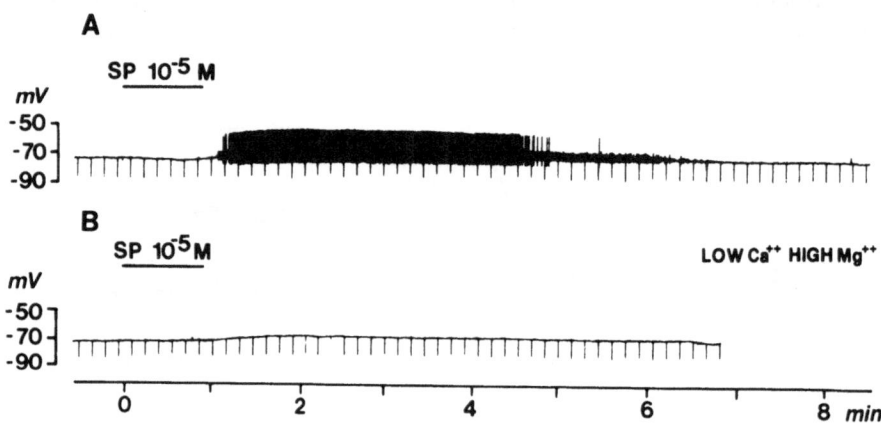

Figure 3. The effects of substance P (SP) on a dorsal horn neuron in a spinal cord slice prepared from a 10-day-old rat. The downward vertical deflections represent membrane responses to constant hyperpolarizing current pulses (300 nA, 50 msec) applied through the recording electrode. (A) Bath application of SP (10 μM) for about a minute causes a depolarization that is accompanied by an increase in the number of synaptic (as evidenced by an increase in baseline noise) and action potentials (action potentials were truncated by the limited frequency response of the pen recorder). Input resistance increased during the depolarizing action of SP. (B) In a low-Ca^{2+}/high-Mg^{2+} solution, the increased synaptic activity and action potential firing are absent, but the depolarization persists although it is reduced slightly in amplitude. (From Murase et al., 1981, with permission.)

others. In the latter cells, membrane hyperpolarization to a level more negative than the extrapolated E_K did not result in a clear reversal of the substance P depolarization. This type of response is in some respect similar to
that seen in cultured mouse spinal cord neurons (Nowak and MacDonald,
1982). The mechanism by which substance P depolarizes dorsal horn neurons remains to be fully investigated.

An effect of substance P on Ca^{2+}-dependent action potentials that appears to be independent of its membrane-depolarizing action was also observed in rat dorsal horn neurons (Murase and Randić, 1984). Depolarizing
current pulses applied to the immature rat dorsal horn neurons bathed in
tetrodotoxin can initiate a slowly rising and falling action potential that
appears to be Ca^{2+} dependent (Murase and Randić, 1982). Substance P effectively shortens the duration of the TTX-resistant spike. The exact mechanism by which this occurs is unclear, inasmuch as it could be due to an
effect on K^+ conductance or to a direct action on Ca^{2+} entry. The effect of
substance P may be similar to that of other transmitter substances on the
calcium spike of embryonic chick dorsal root ganglion cells as described in
other chapters.

2.4. Hypothalamic Neurons

The hypothalamus receives a rich innervation of SPLI-containing fibers.
To examine the role of substance P in this brain region, intracellular recordings have been carried out in guinea pig hypothalamic slices (Ogata and
Abe, 1982). Bath-applied substance P caused a slow depolarization associated with an increase in membrane resistance as seen in other systems. This
effect persisted in Ca^{2+}-free solutions. Occasionally, an initial short-lasting
depolarization accompanied by a decrease in resistance was observed preceding the slow depolarization. The rapid response was abolished in low
Ca^{2+}, suggesting that it may be an indirect, synaptically mediated effect. The
slow substance P depolarization was not affected by Cl^--filled electrodes,
again suggesting that G_K is decreased, although proof of this will require
more detailed experiments.

3. ACTION IN THE PERIPHERAL NERVOUS SYSTEM

3.1 Myenteric Neurons

The most prominent and consistent effect of substance P when applied
to myenteric neurons of the guinea pig ileum in vitro, either by superfusion
in known concentrations or by iontophoresis, is that of membrane depolar-

ization (Katayama and North, 1978; Katayama et al., 1979). Substance P also caused a slow hyperpolarization in a number of cells, however, the nature of this was not determined (Katayama et al., 1979).

The characteristics of the membrane depolarization induced by substance P in myenteric neurons were similar to those of other neurons in terms of time course and amplitude. The electrogenic mechanism underlying this effect was found to be an inactivation of resting G_K (Katayama and North, 1978; Katayama et al., 1979). Accordingly, the depolarization was consistently associated with an increase of membrane resistance (Fig. 4). The effect of substance P was augmented by membrane depolarization and diminished by hyperpolarization. These findings are compatible with the concept that substance P depolarizes the neurons by inactivating either G_K or G_{Cl} or both. Further observations (1) that the substance P depolarization was reversed at the same potential as the spike afterhyperpolarization, (2) that the extrapolated reversal potential of the substance P response varied linearly with the log concentration of extracellular K^+, and (3) that the depolarization was not affected by substitution of extracellular Cl^- with impermeable anions suggest that substance P selectively inactivates resting G_K (Katayama et al., 1979).

More recently, substance P, at concentrations (1 nM) below those causing appreciable membrane depolarization, was found to reduce the amplitude of the slow afterhyperpolarization following the action potential (North et al., 1982). As the slow afterhyperpolarization of myenteric neurons is believed to be due to an increase of G_K triggered by the influx of Ca^{2+} during

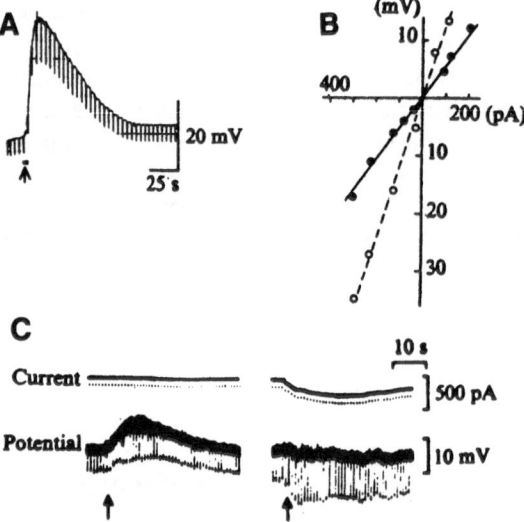

Figure 4. Effects of substance P on a guinea pig myenteric neuron *in vitro*. The peptide was ejected (arrow) from a micropipette positioned close to the soma of the impaled neuron. The neuronal membrane resistance was monitored by hyperpolarizing current pulses applied to the neuron (downward deflections of tracings A and C). (A) Iontophoretic application of substance P caused a large membrane depolarization associated with a substantial increase in neuronal input resistance. (B) Voltage/current relationship before (filled circles) and during the substance P depolarization (open circles). Abscissa: transmembrane current amplitude (pA). Ordinate: steady-state membrane displacement (mV); upwards indicates depolarization. (C) Left panel: substance P caused a depolarization associated with an increase in neuronal input resistance. *Right panel*: the depolarization caused by substance P was annulled by passage of hyperpolarizing current through the recording electrode. Under these conditions, substance P still caused an increase in input resistance. (From Katayama and North, 1978, with permission.)

the action potential (North, 1973), this reduction in the afterhyperpolarization indicates that the peptide closes membrane potassium channels that are gated by intracellular Ca^{2+}.

3.2. Inferior Mesenteric Ganglion Cells

The guinea pig inferior mesenteric ganglion lies in the abdominal cavity and consists of two groups of cells, one on each side of the inferior mesenteric artery, which are interconnected by strands of nerve fibers forming a ring around the artery. The ganglion is associated with a number of nerve trunks, i.e., the splanchnic, the ascending (or intermesenteric), the colonic, and the left and right hypogastric nerves (see Fig. 1 of Dun and Jiang, 1982). Neurons in the inferior mesenteric ganglion send their axons to innervate the distal part of the colon and pelvic viscera.

Following the report that dense networks of SPLI-containing nerve fibers are present in the guinea pig inferior mesenteric ganglia (Hökfelt et al., 1977a), the effects of substance P on these neurons were investigated by two independent groups (Dun and Karczmar, 1979; Dun and Minota, 1981, and Konishi et al., 1979; Tsunoo et al., 1982).

When applied by superfusion, substance P evoked a slow membrane depolarization in most inferior mesenteric ganglion cells. This response was not affected in a low-Ca^{2+}/high-Mg^{2+} solution, suggesting that the peptide depolarizes the neurons directly. A few neurons demonstrated an initial hyperpolarization followed by the more prolonged depolarization (Fig. 5). This latter type of cell was encountered infrequently and it is not known whether the hyperpolarizing response resulted from a direct action of substance P or was indirectly mediated.

The sensitivity of individual inferior mesenteric ganglion cells to substance P (0.5 μM) varied considerably. Membrane depolarization ranging from a few to more than 20 mV were observed in different cells, with a mean of about 10 mV. A common feature of substance P depolarization was the occurrence of high-frequency spike discharges at the peak of depolarization (Fig. 5). The spike discharges were not eliminated in a low-Ca^{2+}/high-Mg^{2+} solution, nor by cholinergic antagonists, indicating that they are probably generated as a result of membrane depolarization rather than being of synaptic origin.

The membrane resistance change during the course of substance P depolarization was studied by manually clamping the membrane potential at the resting potential level of between −50 and −60 mV. In about equal numbers of neurons, substance P caused decrease and increase of membrane resistance; in some neurons, a brief increase occurred prior to the decrease of membrane resistance (Fig. 6). The membrane resistance change, whether increase or decrease, was generally small, usually not more than 20%. However, in a few neurons with relatively high resting membrane potential (> −70 mV), substance P elicited a large depolarization accompanied by a marked

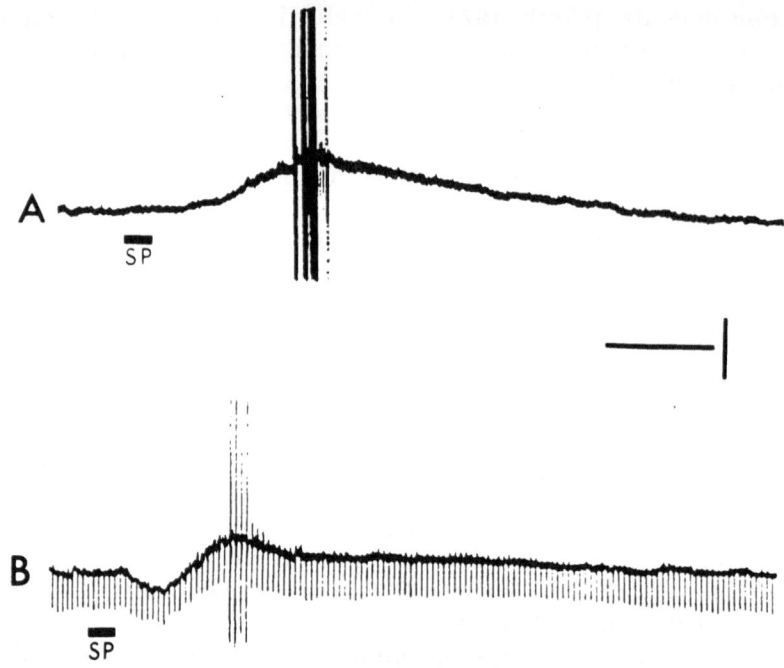

Figure 5. Effects of substance P (SP) on guinea pig inferior mesenteric ganglion neurons. (A) In this cell, SP causes a monophasic depolarization, and the occurrence of spontaneous spike discharges. The resting membrane potential was −56 mV. (B) In a second cell, an initial hyperpolarization was followed by depolarization. Spontaneous spike discharges occurred at the peak of membrane depolarization. Cell resting membrane potential was −54 mV. Downward deflections are electrotonic potentials elicited by hyperpolarizing current pulses of 200-msec duration. Substance P (0.5 μM) was applied by superfusion for 10 sec, as indicated by the bars. Calibration: 10 mV and 40 sec. (From Dun and Minota, 1981, with permission.)

increase in membrane resistance; this was probably due to anomalous rectification as the resistance change was much smaller when membrane potential was clamped at the resting level.

In contrast to the finding in cat cuneate neurons, guinea pig myenteric neurons and mouse spinal cord neurons in culture, membrane hyperpolarization *increased* the substance P depolarization in the large majority of inferior mesenteric ganglion cells tested (Fig. 7). In only a small number of cells did membrane hyperpolarization decrease the substance P response; however, even in these cells, a reversal of the substance P depolarization was not obtained at membrane potentials more negative than the extrapolated E_K. Taken together with the observation that the substance P response was nearly abolished in a Na^+-free solution, but was not affected in a low-Cl^- or low-Ca^{2+} solution, these findings suggest that the ionic mechanism underlying substance P-induced depolarization may involve a combination of G_{Na} activation and G_K inactivation. A similar situation may exist for lutein-

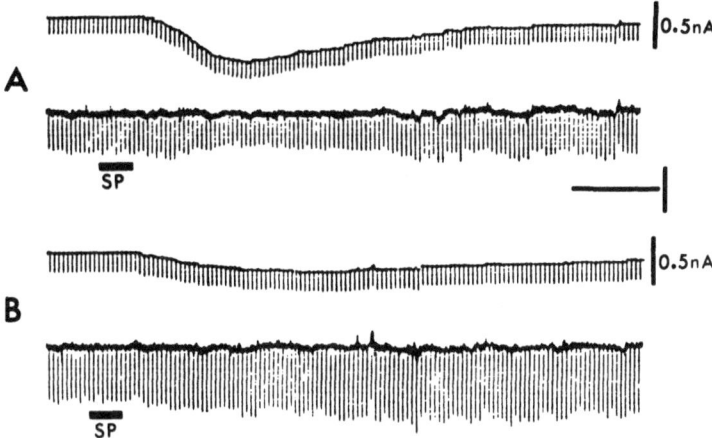

Figure 6. Two types of membrane resistance change induced by substance P (SP) when membrane potential was manually clamped at rest in two different guinea pig inferior mesenteric ganglion cells. (A) Substance P caused a brief, initial increase followed by a decrease of input resistance. (B) Substance P produced a prolonged membrane resistance increase. The resting membrane of these two cells was -55 mV. Electrotonic potentials were elicited by hyperpolarizing current pulses of 200-msec duration. Substance P (0.5 μM) was applied for 15 sec, as indicated by the bars. Calibration: 10 mV and 40 sec. (From Dun and Minota, 1981, with permission.)

izing hormone-releasing hormone (LHRH)-like peptide in the bullfrog sympathetic ganglion (see Chapter 16).

3.3. Bullfrog Sympathetic Neurons

Nishi et al. (1980), in an effort to identify the transmitter responsible for the generation of the noncholinergic late slow EPSP (see Chapter 16), investigated the effects of substance P and related peptides on bullfrog sympathetic neurons. Substance P caused a slow membrane depolarization that persisted in a low-Ca^{2+} solution. The membrane resistance change during the substance P depolarization and the late slow EPSP in a given neuron was found to be similar, suggesting that a similar mechanism may underly these two responses. Furthermore, the late slow EPSP was markedly attenuated following prolonged application of substance P. Later investigators, however, have failed to provide evidence supporting the role of substance P in mediating the late slow EPSP.

The depolarization effect of substance P on bullfrog sympathetic neurons was confirmed recently by Jan and Jan (1982). Nevertheless, cross desensitization between substance P and the late slow EPSP, on one hand, and LHRH (which is the likely transmitter responsible for the late slow EPSP), on the other, was not observed. LHRH, however, readily desensitized the

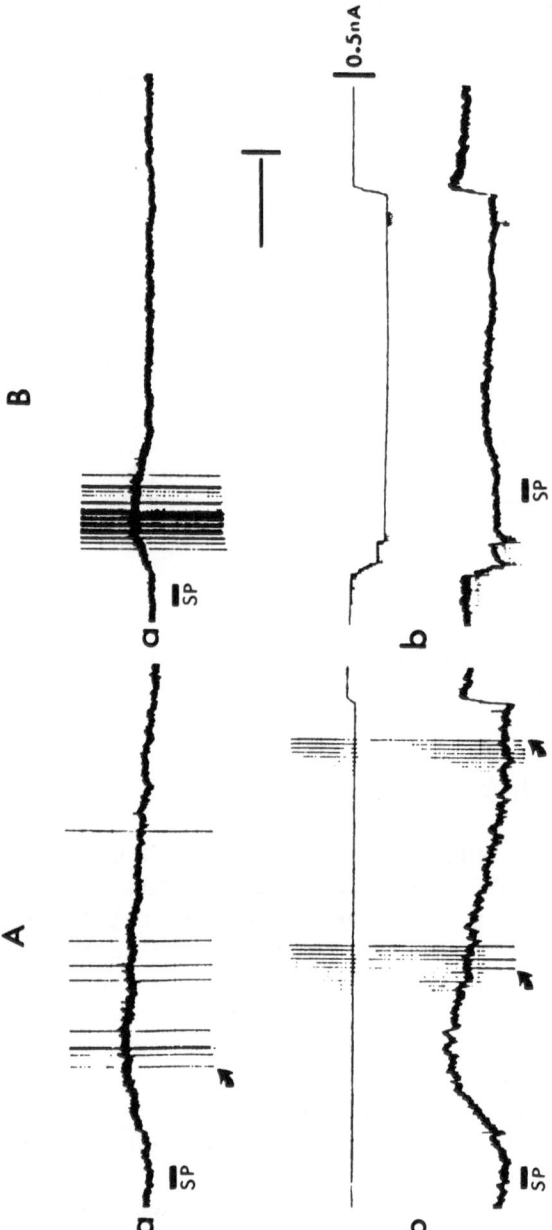

Figure 7. Effects of membrane hyperpolarization on the depolarization induced by substance P (SP) in two different inferior mesenteric ganglion cells. A: (a) SP response elicited in the first cell at resting level of −53 mV. Note that spontaneous spike discharges showed large after-hyperpolarizations (arrow). (b) Membrane potential was increased to −63 mV by passage of a steady DC current (upper trace). The amplitude of the SP depolarization was markedly enhanced (lower trace). The action potentials elicited by intracellular stimulation displayed much smaller afterhyperpolarizations (arrow) as compared to that shown in a. B: (a) Depolarization induced by SP in the second cell at resting level of −54 mV. Spontaneous discharges exhibited large afterhyperpolarizations. (b) The membrane potential was increased to −64 mV by the passage of hyperpolarizing current. In this cell, the substance P depolarization was markedly attenuated. SP (0.5 μM) was applied for 10 sec, as indicated by the bars. Calibration: 10 mV and 40 sec. (From Dun and Minota, 1981, with permission.)

late slow EPSP. The discrepancy between this study and the earlier work of Nishi et al. has not been fully resolved.

Recently, Adams et al. (1983) studied the ionic mechanism underlying the substance P depolarization in bullfrog sympathetic neurons by means of a single-electrode voltage-clamp method and concluded that inhibition of a voltage-dependent potassium current, the M current, can fully account for the depolarization at membrane potentials between -30 mV and -60 mV. Interestingly, in some cells substance P induced an additional inward current (accompanied by an increase in conductance) at membrane potentials more negative than -60 mV; the ionic species responsible for this inward current was not determined. However, in comparison, LHRH has been shown to increase Na^+ and/or Ca^{2+} conductance in addition to inhibition of the M current in a portion of bullfrog sympathetic neurons (Katayama and Nishi, 1982).

By means of immunohistofluorescence techniques, SPLI has been localized to nerve fibers in bullfrog sympathetic ganglia (Jan and Jan, 1982). It remains to be shown whether or not SPLI is released upon appropriate nerve stimulation. In this regard, capsaicin was found to have no appreciable depolarizing effects on bullfrog sympathetic neurons. This drug does seem to release substance P and thereby cause a slow membrane depolarization and subsequent block of the noncholinergic EPSP in guinea pig inferior mesenteric ganglion neurons (see below).

3.4. Actions on Nonneuronal Tissues

In peripheral tissues, substance P exerts a variety of effects including contraction of smooth muscle in the gut, genitourinary tracts, and bronchi, release of histamine from mast cells, vasodilation, and secretagogic activity of the pancreatic and salivary glands (Skrabanek and Powell, 1977). The cellular mechanism underlying the sialagogic effect on parotid acinar cells has been studied in detail using intracellular recording. In these cells, the peptide caused a membrane depolarization associated with a marked decrease in membrane resistance. The membrane potential and conductance changes evoked by substance P on parotid acinar cells were indistinguishable from those elicited by cholinergic or adrenergic stimulation, except that the substance P response was not abolished by muscarinic and α-adrenergic receptor blocking agents, respectively. When the relationship of substance P response and membrane potential was studied, the depolarization was found to reverse at membrane potential levels between -60 and -70 mV. The finding that the reversal potentials for peptidergic, cholinergic, and adrenergic agonists were similar suggested that these three agonists act via a similar ionic mechanism (Gallacher and Petersen, 1980).

Using $^{86}Rb^+$ release from parotid acinar cells as an index of K^+ permeability, Putney (1977) found that substance P, cholinergic, and adrenergic agonists all stimulated $^{86}Rb^+$ efflux. Furthermore, as calcium ionopohores can mimic agonist-induced K^+ release, and as this release is blocked by cobalt, calcium influx appears to be the common cellular substrate that triggers the release of K^+ from parotid acinar cells following activation of the receptors by these three agonists. This is in contrast to the situation in nerve tissue where substance P effects are not blocked by low Ca^{2+}.

4. INTERACTION WITH OTHER TRANSMITTERS

Some evidence suggests that substance P may specifically modify responses to other transmitters. In the spinal cord, substance P has been reported to depress the glutamate-induced firing of Renshaw cells (Belcher and Ryall, 1977). A similar effect was observed in cultured mouse spinal cord neurons, where substance P reversibly depressed the membrane depolarization induced by glutamate in a dose dependent manner (Vincent and Barker, 1979).

Substance P may also specifically block nicotinic, but not muscarinic, responses of Renshaw cells (Krnjević and Lekic, 1977). However, the nicotinic blocking action of substance P was not found in myenteric and inferior mesenteric neurons, as the peptide did not suppress the amplitude of fast cholinergic EPSPs. In fact, in many instances the amplitude of the fast EPSP was enhanced probably as a result of increased membrane resistance following substance P application.

5. SUBSTANCE P AS A SENSORY TRANSMITTER

Over a decade of active research indicates that substance P meets many of the requirements for consideration as a transmitter released by primary sensory neurons, particularly those subserving nociception (see Otsuka and Konishi, 1977; Nicoll et al., 1980). However, the full acceptance of this hypothesis has been hampered by a lack of exact correlation between the effects of exogenous substance P and those of stimulation of specific sensory pathways.

More definitive results, however, have been gathered in the guinea pig inferior mesenteric ganglia to implicate substance P as a sensory transmitter (Dun and Jiang, 1982; Tsunoo et al., 1982). Stimulation of preganglionic nerve fibers to the inferior mesenteric ganglia elicits a fast EPSP lasting about 10–50 msec followed by a slow depolarization lasting 1–2 min (Fig. 8). The fast EPSP is reversibly blocked by nicotinic antagonists and is therefore presumed to be mediated by acetylcholine. The slow depolarization is not blocked by nicotinic or muscarinic antagonists but is reversibly abolished in a low-Ca^{2+}/high-Mg^{2+} solution, indicating that the mediator may be a noncholinergic substance. The slow depolarization is referred to as the "non-

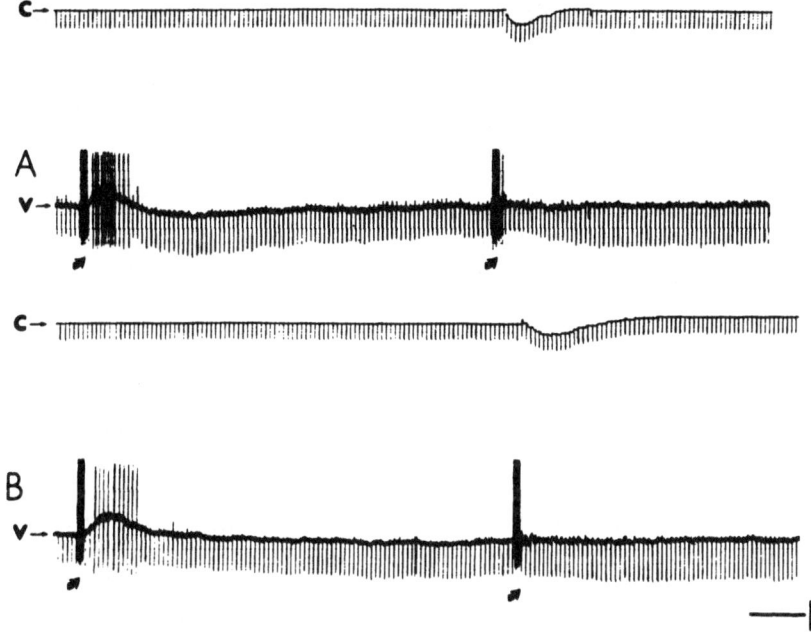

Figure 8. Membrane resistance change during the noncholinergic excitatory potentials elicited in two different guinea pig inferior mesenteric ganglion cells. Electrotonic potentials were induced by hyperpolarizing current pulses of 200-msec duration. In cell A, repetitive stimulation of hypogastric nerves (curved arrow) at a frequency of 30 Hz for 4 sec elicited a burst of action potentials followed by the noncholinergic depolarization. Spontaneous spike discharges occurred at the peak of depolarization. When the membrane depolarization was annulled by the passage of hyperpolarizing current through the recording electrode, membrane resistance showed a small, but persistent decrease followed by an increase. In cell B, repetitive stimulation (curved arrow) elicited a burst of action potentials followed by the noncholinergic potential. Spontaneous spike discharges could also be seen during the depolarization. When the membrane depolarization was nullified, membrane resistance showed a long-lasting increase. The c and v denote current and voltage tracings, respectively. Calibration: 20 mV, 1 nA and 40 sec. (From Dun and Jiang, 1982, with permission.)

cholinergic slow EPSP'' since a muscarinic slow EPSP can be elicited in some of these neurons.

A detectable noncholinergic EPSP can be evoked by stimulation for several seconds at frequencies as low as 1 Hz, and a maximal response can usually be achieved at 20–30 Hz. The threshold for eliciting a noncholinergic EPSP was found to be much higher than that required to induce a fast EPSP, suggesting that they are initiated by different nerve fibers. The latency of the noncholinergic EPSP was estimated to be from 0.5 to 5 sec, which is nearly 1000 times longer than that of the fast EPSP (Dun and Jiang, 1982). On the average, a train of stimuli at 30 Hz for 2–3 sec evoked a noncholinergic EPSP with an amplitude of about 5–10 mV and a duration of 1–2 min. There is a clear similarity between the membrane depolarization induced by substance

P and the noncholinergic EPSP with respect to the time course, latency, and duration.

The evidence that substance P or a similar peptide may be the mediator of noncholinergic EPSPs in the inferior mesenteric ganglia can be summarized as follows: (1) SPLI is present in nerve fibers surrounding majority of ganglionic neurons (Hökfelt et al., 1977a), and it is localized ultrastructurally to dense core granules in the nerve terminals (Kondo and Yui, 1981); (2) SPLI is released from the ganglia by stimulation of dorsal roots or by high-K^+ solution in a Ca^{2+}–dependent manner (Tsunoo et al., 1982); (3) the electrophysiological characteristics of the substance P depolarization closely mimic the noncholinergic EPSP; i.e., there is a parallel change of membrane resistance and of the response to membrane hyperpolarization in a given neuron, suggesting that the underlying ionic mechanisms may be similar (Dun and Jiang, 1982; Tsunoo et al., 1982); (4) there is cross desensitization; i.e., the noncholinergic EPSP is abolished in the presence of substance P, indicating that the transmitter released synaptically and substance P may be acting on the same receptors (Dun and Jiang, 1982; Tsunoo et al., 1982); and (5) the substance P antagonist (D-Pro²,D-Phe⁷,D-Trp⁹)-SP specifically suppresses the noncholinergic EPSP as well as the substance P-induced depolarization (Jiang et al., 1982). In addition, capsaicin, which is known to release substance P (as well as other putative transmitters) from dorsal root ganglia, causes a slow membrane depolarization similar to the noncholinergic EPSP (Dun and Kiraly, 1983). Several lines of evidence suggest that substance P in the inferior mesenteric ganglion derives from sensory neurons in dorsal root ganglia. First, fibers in the inferior mesenteric ganglia can be traced to some SPLI-containing dorsal root ganglion cells using double labeling procedures (Dalsgaard et al., 1982a). Second, the noncholinergic slow EPSP can be evoked in the same neuron by stimulation of the hypogastric as well as the splanchnic nerves (Dun and Jiang, 1982). This may imply that the fibers that release substance P are collaterals of sensory projections passing through the ganglion from the gastrointestinal tract to the dorsal root ganglion (see Fig. 9). Third, ligation of splanchnic, but not hypogastric or colonic, nerves results in a marked loss of SPLI, suggesting that SPLI is transported peripherally (Konishi et al., 1979). Lastly, capsaicin, which seems to act specifically on dorsal root ganglion neurons, depletes SPLI in the inferior mesenteric ganglia (Gamse et al., 1981).

These results collectively support the hypothesis that substance P or a substance P-like peptide is the mediator of the slow excitatory potential in a population of neurons in the guinea pig inferior mesenteric ganglion and that it is released from collateral branches of sensory fibers coursing to the gastrointestinal tract from the dorsal root ganglia. A schematic diagram of the proposed substance P pathways in the prevertebral ganglion is shown in Fig. 9. Activation of sensory fibers in the intestinal tract may excite neurons in the prevertebral ganglia, as well as in the spinal cord, via the release of substance P, thus allowing peripheral reflex modulation of gastrointestinal

Figure 9. Schematic diagram of two possible pathways of substance P-containing fibers in the inferior mesenteric ganglion (IMG) of the guinea pig. Afferent nerve fibers (AN) in the gastrointestinal tract may send collateral endings to neurons in the ganglion. Alternatively, some of the peptide-containing fibers may originate from neurons in the gastrointestinal tract. Although the latter possibility cannot be excluded, the evidence obtained so far appears to indicate that the majority of substance P-containing fibers in

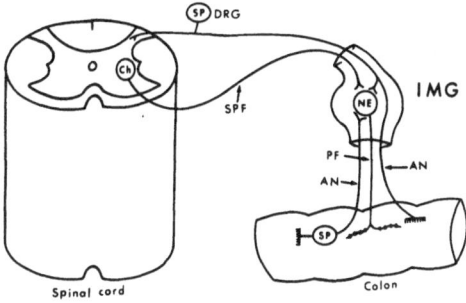

the IMG derive from dorsal root ganglion. The symbols Ch, NE, SP, and DRG denote cholinergic preganglionic neurons, noradrenergic sympathetic neurons, substance P-containing neurons, and dorsal root ganglia, respectively; SPF and PF represent sympathetic preganglionic and postganglionic fibers, respectively. (From Dun and Jiang, 1982; with permission.)

activity independent of the CNS. As yet, however, the specific sensory stimulus that activates substance P neurons is not known.

A noncholinergic EPSP comparable to that observed in neurons of the inferior mesenteric ganglia can be evoked in some neurons of the myenteric plexus by focal stimulation (Katayama and North, 1978; Wood and Mayer, 1979; Johnson et al., 1981). Exogenous substance P induces a comparable response in myenteric neurons (Katayama and North, 1978; Morita et al., 1980); however, whether substance P is the mediator of the slow EPSP in the myenteric plexus is still open to question (see Bornstein et al., 1984).

6. CONCLUSION

The primary action of substance P is to produce a slow membrane depolarization of many neurons in the vertebrate central and peripheral nervous systems. Although, hyperpolarizing effects of substance P are occasionally observed, these *may* be due to indirect, synaptically mediated effects of the peptide.

The characteristics of the membrane depolarization induced by substance P on various central and peripheral neurons are strikingly similar in terms of latency and time course, yet there are marked differences with respect to the electrogenic mechanisms. Thus, depolarizations associated with an increase and/or a decrease of input resistance have been reported in various vertebrate neurons. The mechanisms underlying such disparate actions of substance P are not clear. One possibility is that pharmacologically similar substance P receptors may be coupled to different ionic channels at different sites. Alternatively, there may be subclasses of pharmacologically distinguishable substance P receptors that are coupled to different ionic channels. The development of more specific agonists and antagonists may help to resolve this issue.

Is substance P a sensory transmitter? The evidence accumulated in the past decade indicates that the peptide meets many of the requirements supporting such a role (Otsuka and Konishi, 1977; Nicoll et al., 1980). However, the slowness of the substance P response makes it unlikely to be a transmitter that mediates specific sensory signals. Rather, substance P may play a modulatory role in setting the level of responsiveness of target cells. Two possible mechanisms exist. Substance P could be released conjointly with a rapidly acting transmitter by the same nerve terminal or it may be liberated onto a target cell that receives separate afferent fibers releasing a fast acting transmitter. This latter situation in fact appears to be the case in the inferior mesenteric ganglia, where substance P increases the level of membrane excitability of the postganglionic neurons to the incoming fast-acting ACh.

ACKNOWLEDGMENT. Published and unpublished work carried out in the author's laboratory was supported by NIH grants NS15848 and BRSG RR05368.

REFERENCES

Adams, P. R., Brown, D. A., and Jones, S. W., 1983, Substance P inhibits the M-current in bullfrog sympathetic neurones, *Br. J. Pharmacol.* **79:**330–333.

Belcher, G., and Ryall, R. W., 1977, Substance P and Renshaw cells: a new concept of inhibitory synaptic transmission, *J. Physiol. (Lond.)* **272:**105–119.

Bornstein, J. C., North, R. A., Costa, M., and Furness, J. B., 1984, Excitatory synaptic potentials due to activation of neurons with short projections in the myenteric plexus, *Neuroscience* **11:**723–731.

Brown, D. A., Constanti, A., and Adams, P. R., 1981, Slow cholinergic and peptidergic transmission in sympathetic ganglia, *Fed. Proc.* **40:**2625–2630.

Caranikas, S., Mizrahi, J., D'Orleans-Juste, P., and Regoli, D., 1982, Antagonists of substance P, *Eur. J. Pharmacol.* **77:**205–206.

Chan-Palay, V., Jonsson, G., and Palay, S. L., 1978, Serotonin and substance P coexist in neurons of the rat's central nervous system, *Proc. Natl. Acad. Sci. USA* **75:**1582–1586.

Chang, M. M., and Leeman, S. E., 1970, Isolation of a sialogogic peptide from bovine hypothalamic tissue and its characterization as substance P, *J. Biol. Chem.* **245:**4784–4790.

Chang, M. M., Leeman, S. E., and Niall, H. D., 1971, Amino-acid sequence of substance P, *Nature* **232:**86–87.

Costa, M., Cuello, A. C., Furness, J. B., and Franco, R., 1980, Distribution of enteric neurons showing immunoreactivity for substance P in the guinea-pig ileum, *Neuroscience* **5:**323–331.

Cuello, A. C., and Kanazawa, I., 1978, The distribution of substance P immunoreactive fibers in the rat central nervous system, *J. Comp. Neurol.* **178:**129–156.

Cuello, A. C., Priestley, J. V., and Matthews, M. R., 1982, Localization of substance P in neuronal pathways, in: *Substance P in the Nervous System*, 1982, Ciba Foundation Symposium 91, Pitman, London, pp. 55–79.

Dalsgaard, C.-J., Hökfelt, T., Elfvin, L.-G., Skirboll, L., and Emson, P., 1982a, Substance P-containing primary sensory neurons projecting to the inferior mesenteric ganglion: Evidence from combined retrograde tracing and immunohistochemistry, *Neuroscience* **7:**647–654.

Dalsgaard, C.-J., Vincent, S. R., Hökfelt, T., Lundberg, M. J., Dahlstrom, A., Schultzberg, M.,

Dockray, G. T., and Cuello, A. C., 1982b, Coexistence of cholecystokinin-and substance P-like peptides in neurons of the dorsal root ganglia of the rat, Neurosci. Lett. 33:159–163.

Davies, J., and Dray, A., 1980, Depression and facilitation of synaptic responses in cat dorsal horn by substance P administered into substantia gelatinosa, Life Sci. 27:2037–2042.

Dun, N. J., and Jiang, Z. G., 1982, Non-cholinergic excitatory transmission in inferior mesenteric ganglia of the guinea-pig: Possible mediation by substance P, J. Physiol. (Lond.) 325:145–159.

Dun, N. J., and Karczmar, A. G., 1979, Actions of substance P on sympathetic neurons, Neuropharmacology 18:215–218.

Dun, N. J., and Kiraly, M., 1983, Capsaicin releases a substance P-like peptide in guinea-pig inferior mesenteric ganglia, J. Physiol. (Lond.) 340:107–120.

Dun, N. J., and Minota, S., 1981, Effects of substance P on neurones of the inferior mesenteric ganglia of the guinea-pig, J. Physiol. (Lond.) 321:259–271.

Engberg, H., Svensson, T. H., Rosell, S., and Folkers, K., 1981, A synthetic peptide as an antagonist of substance P, Nature 293:222–223.

Erspamer, V., 1981, The tackykinin peptide family, Trends Neurosci. 4:267–269.

Furness, J. B., Papka, R. E., Della, N. G., Costa, M., and Eskay, R. L., 1982, Substance P-like immunoreactivity in nerves associated with the vascular system of guinea-pigs, Neuroscience 7:447–459.

Gallacher, D. V., and Petersen, O. H., 1980, Substance P increases membrane conductance in parotid acinar cells, Nature 283:393–395.

Gamse, R., Wax, A., Zigmond, R. E., and Leeman, S. E., 1981, Immunoreactive substance P in sympathetic ganglia: Distribution and sensitivity towards capsaicin, Neuroscience 6:437–441.

Glickman, R. D., Adolph, A. R., and Dowling, J. E., 1982, Inner plexiform circuits in the carp retina: effects of cholinergic agonists, GABA and substance P on the ganglion cells, Brain Res. 234:81–99.

Guyenet, P. G., and Aghajanian, G. K., 1977, Excitation of neurons on the nucleus locus coeruleus by substance P and related peptides, Brain Res. 136:178–184.

Henry, J. L., 1976, Effects of substance P on functionally identified units in cat spinal cord, Brain Res. 114:439–451.

Henry, J. L., Krnjević, K., and Morris, M. E., 1975, Substance P and spinal neurons, Can.J. Physiol. Pharmacol. 53:423–432.

Hökfelt, T., Elfvin, L.-G., Schultzberg, M., Goldstein, M., and Nilsson, G., 1977a, On the occurrence of substance P containing fibers in sympathetic ganglia: immunohistochemical evidence, Brain Res. 132:29–41.

Hökfelt, T., Johansson, O., Kellerth, J. O., Ljungdahl, A., Nilsson, G., Nygrads, A., Pernow, B., 1977b, Immunohistochemical distribution of substance P, in: Substance P (U.S. Von Euler and B. Pernow, eds.), Raven Press, New York, pp.217–230.

Hökfelt, T., Kellerth, J. O., Nilsson, G., and Pernow, B., 1975, Substance P: Localization in the central nervous system and in some primary sensory neurons, Science 190:889–890.

Hökfelt, T., Vincent, S., Dalsgaard, C. J., Skirboll, L., Johansson, O., Schultzberg, M., Lundberg, J. M., Rosell, S., Pernow, P., and Jancso, G., 1982, Distribution of substance P in brain and periphery and its possible role as a co-transmitter, in: Substance P in the Nervous System, Ciba Foundation Symposium 91, Pitman, London, pp. 84–100.

Jan, L. Y., and Jan, Y. N., 1982, Peptidergic transmission in sympathetic ganglia of the frog, J. Physiol. (Lond.) 327:219–246.

Jancsó, G., Hökfelt, T., Lundberg, J. M., Kiraly, E., Halasz, N., Nilsson, G., Terenius, L., Rehfeld, J., Steinbusch, H., Verhofstad, A., Elde, R., Said, S., and Brown, M., 1981, Immunohistochemical studies on the effect of capsaicin on spinal and medullary peptide and monoamine neurons using antisera to substance P, gastrin/CCK, somatostatin, VIP, enkephalin, neurotensin and 5-hydroxytryptamine, J. Neurocytol. 10:963–980.

Jiang, Z. G., Dun, N. J., and Karczmar, A. G., 1982, Substance P: A putative sensory transmitter in mammalian autonomic ganglia, Science 217:739–741.

Johansson, O., Hökfelt, T., Pernow, B., Jeffcoate, S. L., White, N., Steinbusch, H. W. M., Verhofstad, A. A. J., Emson, P. C., and Spindel, E., 1981, immunohistochemical support for three putative transmitters in one neuron: Coexistence of 5-hydroxytryptamine, substance

P and thyrotropin releasing hormone-like immunoreactivity in medullary neurons projecting to the spinal cord, *Neuroscience* **6**:1857–1881.

Johnson, S. M., Katayama, Y., Morita, K., and North, R.A., 1981, Mediators of slow synaptic
potentials in the myenteric plexus of the guinea-pig ileum, *J. Physiol. (Lond.)* **320**:175–186.

Katayama, Y., and Nishi, S., 1982, Voltage-clamp analysis of peptidergic slow depolarization
in bullfrog sympathetic ganglion cells, *J. Physiol. (Lond.)* **333**:305–313.

Katayama, Y., and North, R. A., 1978, Does substance P mediate slow synaptic excitation within
the myenteric plexus? *Nature* **274**:387–388.

Katayama, Y., North, R. A., and Williams, J. T., 1979, The action of substance P on neurones
of the myenteric plexus of the guinea-pig small intestine, *Proc. R. Soc. (Lond.) B* **206**:191–208.

Kessler, J. A., Adler, J. E., Bohn, M. C., and Black, I. R., 1981, Substance P in principal sympathetic neurons: Regulation by impulse activity, *Science* **214**:335–336.

Kondo, H., and Yui, R., 1981, An electron microscopic study on substance P-like immunoreactive nerve fibers in the celiac ganglion of guinea pigs, *Brain Res.* **222**:134–137.

Konishi, S., Tsunoo, A., and Otsuka, M., 1979, Substance P and non-cholinergic excitatory
synaptic transmission in guinea pig sympathetic ganglia, *Proc. Jpn. Acad.* **55**:525–530.

Krnjević, K., 1977, Effects of substance P on central neurons in cats, in: *Substance P* (U.S. Von
Euler and B. Pernow, eds.), Raven Press, New York, pp. 217–230.

Krnjević, K., and Lekic, D., 1977, Substance P selectively blocks excitation of Renshaw cell by
acetylcholine, *Can. J. Physiol. Pharmacol.* **55**:958–961.

Krnjević, K., and Morris, M. E., 1974, An excitatory action of substance P on cuneate neurones,
Can. J. Physiol. Pharmacol. **52**:736–744.

Le Gal LaSalle, G., and Ben-Ari, Y., 1977, Microiontophoretic effects of substance P on neurons
of the medial amygdale and putamen of the rat, *Brain Res.* **135**:174–179.

Lee, C. M., Iversen, L. L., Hanley, M. R., and Sandberg, B. E. B., 1982, The possible existence
of multiple receptors for substance P. *Naunyn Schmiedebergs Arch. Pharmakol.* **318**:281–287.

Lembeck, F., 1953, Zur Frage der zentralen Übertragung afferenten Impulse. III. Mitteilung, Das
Vorkommen und die Bedentung der Substanz P in den dorsalen Wurzeln des Ruckenmarks,
Naunyn Schmiedebergs Arch. Pharmakol. Exp. Pathol. **219**:197–213.

Lembeck, F., and Starke, K., 1968, Substanz P and speichelsekretion, *Naunyn Schmiedebergs
Arch. Pharmakol.* **259**:275–285.

Lembeck, F., and Zetler, G., 1962, Substance P: A polypeptide of possible physiological significance, especially within the nervous system, *Int. Rev. Neurobiol.* **4**:159–215.

Ljungdahl, A., Hökfelt, T., and Nilsson, G., 1978, Distribution of substance P-like immunoreactivity in the central nervous system of the rat I. Cell bodies and nerve terminals,
Neuroscience **3**:861–943.

Lundberg, J. M., Hökfelt, T., Nilsson, G., Terenius, L., Rehfeld, J., Elde, R., and Said, S., 1978,
Peptide neurons in the vagus splanchnic and sciatic nerves, *Acta. Physiol. Scand.* **104**:499–501.

Matthews, M. R., and Cuello, A. C., 1982, Substance P-immunoreactive peripheral branches of
sensory neurons innervate guinea pig sympathetic neurons, *Proc. Natl. Acad. Sci. USA*
79:1668–1672.

Mayer, M. L., and MacLeod, N. K., 1979, The excitatory action of substance P and stimulation
of the stria terminalis bed nucleus on preoptic neurons, *Brain Res.* **160**:206–210.

Morita, K., North, R. A., and Katayama, Y., 1980, Evidence that substance P is a neurotransmitter
in myenteric plexus, *Nature* **287**:151–152.

Mroz, E. A., Brownstein, M. J., and Leeman, S. E., 1977, Distribution of immunoassayable
substance P in the rat brain: evidence for the existence of substance P-containing tracts,
in: *Substance P* (U.S. Von Euler and B. Pernow, eds.), Raven Press, New York, pp. 147–154.

Murase, K., and Randic, M., 1982, Electrophysiological properties of rat spinal dorsal horn
neurones in vitro: Calcium-dependent action potentials. *J. Physiol. (Lond.)* **334**:141–153.

Murase, K., and Randic, M., 1984, Actions of substance P on rat spinal dorsal horn neurones,
J. Physiol.(Lond.) **346**:203–217.

Murase, K., Nedeljkov, V., and Randic, M., 1982, The actions of neuropeptides on dorsal horn
neurons in the rat spinal cord slice preparation: An intracellular study, *Brain Res.* **234**:170–176.

Nicoll, R. A., 1978, The action of thyrotropin releasing hormone, substance P, and related
peptides on frog spinal motoneurons, *J. Pharmacol. Exp. Ther.* **207**:817–824.

Nicoll, R. A., Schenker, C., and Leeman, S. E., 1980, Substance P as a transmitter candidate, *Annu. Rev. Neurosci.* **3**:227–268.

Nilsson, G., Larsson, L. T., Hakanson, R., Brodin, E., Pernow, B., and Sundler, F., 1975, Localization of substance P-like immunoreactivity in the mouse gut, *Histochemistry* **43**:97–99.

Nishi, S., Katayama, Y., Nakamine, J., and Ushijima, H., 1980, A candidate substance for the chemical transmitter mediating the late slow epsp in bullfrog sympathetic ganglia, *Biomed. Res.* **1**:(Supp.)144–148.

North, R. A., 1973, The calcium-dependent slow, after-hyperpolarization in myenteric plexus neurones with tetrodotoxin-resistant action potentials, *Br. J. Pharmacol.* **49**:709–711.

North, R. A., Morita, K., and Tokimasa, T., 1982, Peptide actions on autonomic nerves, in: *Systemic Role of Regulatory Peptides* (S. R. Bloom, J. M. Polak, and E. Lindenlaub, eds.) F. K. Schattauer Verlag, Stuttgart, pp. 77–88.

Nowak, L. M., and MacDonald, R. L., 1982, Substance P: Ionic basis for depolarizing responses of mouse spinal cord neurons in cell cultures, *J. Neurosci.* **2**:1119–1128.

Ogata, N., and Abe, H., 1982, Substance P decreases membrane conductance in neurons of the guinea pig hypothalamus in vitro, *Neuropharmacology* **21**:187–189.

Otsuka, M., and Konishi, S., 1977, Electrophysiological and neurochemical evidence for substance P as a transmitter of primary sensory neurons, in: *Substance P* (U.S. Von Euler and B. Pernow, eds.), Raven Press, New York, pp. 207–214.

Otsuka, M., Konishi, S., and Takahashi, T., 1975, Hypothalamic substance P as a candidate for transmitter of primary afferent neurons, *Fed. Proc.* **34**:1922–1928.

Pearse, A. G., and Polak, J. M., 1975, Immunocytochemical localization of substance P in mammalian intestine, *Histochemistry* **1**:373–375.

Pelletier, G., Steinbusch, H. W. M., and Verhofstad, A. A. J., 1981, Immunoreactive substance P and serotonin present in the same dense-core vesicles, *Nature* **293**:71–72.

Pernow, B., 1963, Pharmacology of substance P, *Ann. N.Y. Acad. Sci.* **104**:393–402.

Phillis, J. W., 1976, Is β-(4-chlorophenyl)-GABA a specific antagonist of substance P on cerebral cortical neurons? *Experientia* **32**:593–594.

Phillis, J. W., and Limacher, J. J., 1974, Substance P excitation of cerebral cortical Betz cells, *Brain Res.* **69**:158–163.

Pomeroy, S. L., and Behbehani, M. M., 1980, Response of nucleus raphe magnus neurons to iontophoretically applied substance P in rats, *Brain Res.* **202**:464–468.

Putney, J. W., 1977, Muscarinic, alpha-adrenergic, and peptide receptors regulate the same calcium influx sites in the parotid gland, *J. Physiol. (Lond.)* **268**:139–149.

Randić, M., and Miletic, V., 1977, Effect of substance P in rat dorsal horn neurones activated by noxious stimuli, *Brain Res.* **128**:164–169.

Rosell, S., and Folkers, K., 1982, Substance P antagonists: A new type of pharmacological tool, *Trends Pharmacol. Sci.* **3**:211–212.

Ryall, R. W., and Belcher, G., 1977, Substance P selectively blocks nicotinic receptors in Renshaw cells: A possible synaptic inhibitory mechanism, *Brain Res.* **137**:376–380.

Saito, K., Konishi, S., and Otsuka, M., 1975, Antagonism between Lioresal and substance P in rat spinal cord, *Brain Res.* **97**:177–180.

Sastry, B. R., 1979, Substance P effects on spinal nociceptive neurones, *Life Sci.* **24**:2169–2178.

Skirboll, L., Hökfelt, T., Rehfeld, J., Cuello, A. C., and Dockray, G. J., 1982, Coexistence of substance P-and cholecystokinin-like immunoreactivity in neurons of the mesencephalic periaqueductal gray, *Neurosci. Lett.* **28**:35–39.

Skrabanek, P., and Powell, D., 1977, *Substance P*, Vol. 1, Eden Press, Inc. Montreal.

Tregear, G. W., Niall, H. D., Potts, J. T., Leeman, S. E., and Chang, M. M., 1971, Synthesis of substance P, *Nature* **232**:87–88.

Tsunoo, A., Konishi, S., and Otsuka, M., 1982, Substance P as an excitatory transmitter of primary afferent neurons in guinea-pig sympathetic ganglia, *Neuroscience* **7**:2025–2037.

Vincent, J. D., and Barker, J. L., 1979, Substance P: Evidence for diverse roles in neuronal function from cultured mouse spinal neurons, *Science* **205**:1409–1412.

Von Euler, U.S., and Gaddum, J. H., 1931, An unidentified depressor substance in certain tissue extracts, *J. Physiol. (Lond.)* **72**:74–87.

Walker, R. J., Kemp, J. A., Yajima, H., Kitagawa, K., Woodruff, G. N., 1976, The action of substance P on mesencephalic reticular and substantia nigra neurones of the rat, *Experientia* **32**:214–215.

Wood, J. D., and Mayer, C. J., 1979, Serotonergic activation of tonic-type enteric neurons in guinea-pig small intestine, *J. Neurophysiol.* **42**:582–593.

Zieglgänsberger, W., and Tulloch, F., 1979, Effects of substance P on neurones in the dorsal horn of the spinal cord of the cat, *Brain Res.* **166**:273–282.

Somatostatin

JOHN R. DELFS and MARC A. DICHTER

1. INTRODUCTION

1.1. Overview

Somatostatin (somatotropin release-inhibiting factor, SRIF) is a 14-amino-acid cyclic polypeptide originally isolated from extracts of ovine hypothalamus (Brazeau et al., 1973) on the basis of its ability to inhibit the release of growth hormone (somatotropin) from rat pituitary cells in culture. Somatostatin is now known to be widely distributed throughout the body of vertebrates including in the extrahypothalamic nervous system, pancreas, stomach, intestine, thyroid, and kidney. The original concept of somatostatin as primarily an inhibitor of growth hormone release has been considerably expanded. It is now known to have a major role in regulating the secretion of thyrotropin-releasing hormone, glucagon, and insulin and in modulating many aspects of gut function, and it probably functions as a neuroactive substance in both the peripheral and central nervous systems.

Somatostatin has been found to have a potent influence on animal behavior in several different paradigms (Plotnikoff et al., 1974; Prange et al., 1978; Kastin et al., 1978; Rezek et al., 1977; Ioffe et al., 1978), and it may play a role in several neurological diseases. In Alzheimer's dementia (Davies et al., 1980; Rossor et al., 1980) and in the dementia associated with Parkinson's disease (Epelbaum et al., 1983) the levels of somatostatin appear to be selectively diminished in cerebral cortex and hippocampus (the other major deficiency in Alzheimer's being in the levels of cholinergic markers), while in Huntington's disease, levels of somatostatin have been found to be selectively elevated in basal ganglia (Aronin et al., 1983). An examination of the evidence suggesting the probable importance of somatostatin as a neurotransmitter or neuromodulator forms the major subject matter for this chapter. The availability of several reviews was most helpful in the writing of this chapter and are excellent sources for further reading in the role of somatostatin in other systems (Reichlin, 1982, 1983; Gerich, 1981; Arimura and Fishback, 1981).

Somatostatin is believed to be derived, like most neuropeptides, from a larger prohormone and is probably best considered as one of a family of related peptides derived from a common precursor molecule, or "prepro-hormone" (Fig. 1). The originally described carboxy-terminal somatostatin molecule is therefore often designated somatostatin-14. Since virtually all physiological studies have been carried out with somatostatin-14, we will, unless otherwise noted, use the term "somatostatin" to mean this 14-amino-acid molecule.

1.2. Distribution of Somatostatin in Nervous System

Somatostatin is found throughout both the peripheral and central nervous systems. It has been best characterized in the tuberoinfundibular system of the hypothalamus, but somatostatin has also been found throughout the nonhypothalamic brain and spinal cord. In addition, it is found in sensory fibers of dorsal root ganglia, in both sympathetic and parasympathetic nerves, in the auditory nerve, and in the retina. Somatostatin may also be associated with cholinergic systems, both in the peripheral and central nervous systems.

The vast majority of the data on the distribution of somatostatin comes, as it does with all the peptides, from radioimmunoassay and immunohistochemistry, which are by nature indirect. Other methodologies, especially chromatography, have been used in many studies to confirm that the detected molecule is also physically similar to somatostatin, but, ultimately, sequencing is necessary to have certain identification of a molecule from any particular tissue.

1.2.1. Central Nervous System

1.2.1a. Hypothalamus. Neurons in the anterior periventricular nucleus form the predominant somatostatin system. These project to the median eminence as part of the tuberoinfundibular system to exert inhibitory control on the release of growth hormone and TRH from the anterior pituitary. The medial division of the paraventricular nucleus is also rich in somatostatin-containing neurons and may be the source of the somatostatinergic innervation of the posterior pituitary. Somatostatinergic neurons in many different nuclei of the hypothalamus appear to give off fiber tracts that project between hypothalamic nuclei, as well as to the median eminence, spinal cord, and brainstem. Somatostatinergic hypothalamic neurons also project to the ventral amygdala-hypothalamic pathway of the stria terminalis, the cortico-medial amygdala, and the arcuate and ventral premammillary nuclei (Krisch, 1978).

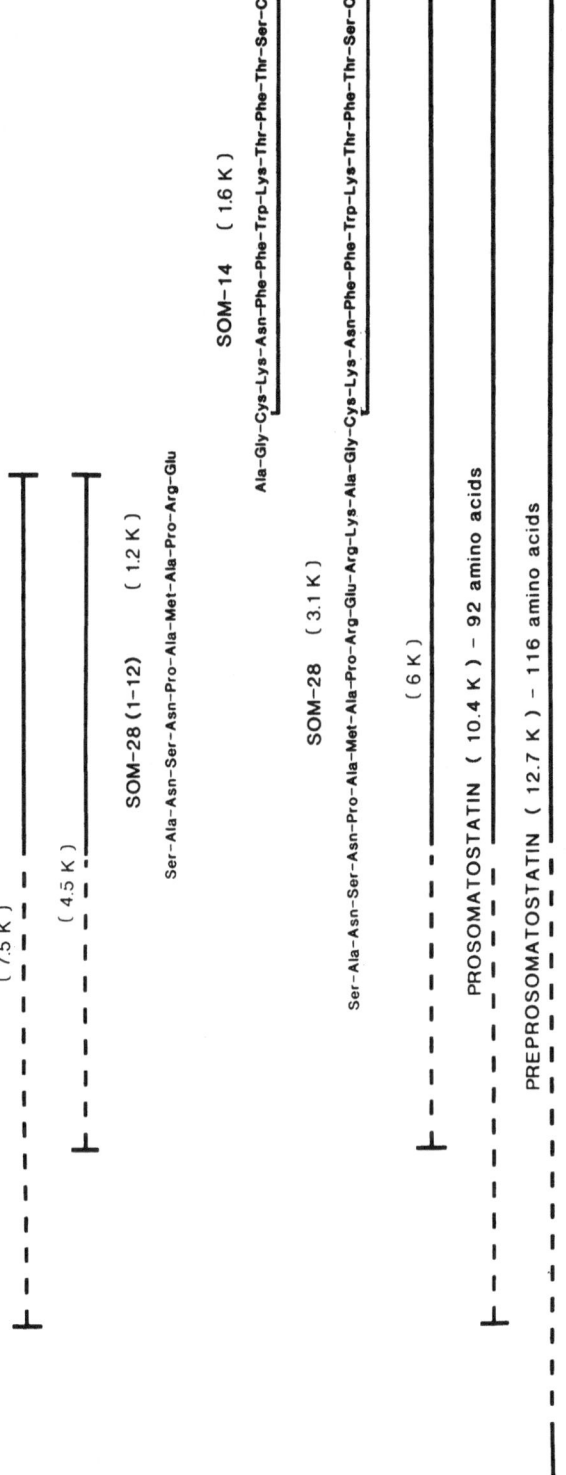

Figure 1. Different molecular forms of somatostatin. Diagram illustrating the different molecular forms derived from preprosomatostatin. The structures of the peptides are now completely characterized for the rat (Goodman et al., 1983). The solid lines represent identical sequences in the larger forms. The molecular weights are noted in parentheses. (Adapted from Benoit et al., 1982, with permission.)

1.2.1b. Extrahypothalamic Brain. Immunoreactive somatostatin has been detected in significant amounts by radioimmunoassay in virtually every area of the nonhypothalamic brain. Somatostatinergic neuronal cell bodies have been reported in cerebral cortex, hippocampus, caudate-putamen, claustrum, accumbens, stria terminalis, and several divisions of the amygdala (Pelletier, 1980; Elde et al., 1978; Bennett-Clarke et al., 1980).

There is conflicting evidence relating to the possibility that the amygdala is a source of extrahypothalamic somatostatinergic projections to the median eminence. Lechan and colleagues (1980) found no retrograde labeling of amygdala after horseradish peroxidase labeling of the median eminence, but Crowley and Terry (1980) found a reduction in median eminence SOM after lesions in the medial-basal amygdala, and others have reported that electrical simulation of the amygdala resulted in orthodromic impulses in tuberoinfundibular neurons (Layton et al., 1981) and an inhibition of growth hormone secretion. It may be more likely that the amygdala projects to tuberoinfundibular neurons through limbic pathways, rather than projecting directly to the median eminence.

The cerebral cortex, predominantly because of its bulk, contains a larger total amount of somatostatin than any other region of the nervous system, including the hypothalamus (Patel and Reichlin, 1978). Somatostatin in the cerebral cortex does not come from hypothalamus (Brownstein et al., 1977; Epelbaum et al., 1977), nor is the influence of the hypothalamus necessary for somatostatin production by cortical neurons (Delfs et al., 1980). In addition, somatostatin-containing cells of the cortex have been shown to differ morphologically from those of the hypothalamus, with the neurons of the cortex containing granules of approximately 65 nm and those of the hypothalamus having granules of about 90–120 nm (Krisch, 1980).

Somatostatinergic neurons are found in all cortical regions and appear to include all or most cellular morphologies, including pyramidal, bipolar, and multipolar types. While neuronal cell bodies containing somatostatin are found in cortical layers II through VI, they are mainly concentrated in layers II, III, and VI (Bennett-Clarke et al., 1980; Krisch, 1980). There has been no description of the extracortical projection of somatostatinergic fibers, suggesting that somatostatinergic neurons may be a predominantly intrinsic system within the cerebral cortex.

In hippocampus, somatostatinergic neurons are present in most regions and include pyramidal, basket, and multipolar neurons, but not the granule cells of the dentate gyrus (Feldman et al., 1982). These observations indicate that somatostatin may be present both in inhibitory interneurons and in excitatory pyramidal neurons, as well as in other hippocampal neurons, suggesting a complex role for somatostatin in this region.

In the visual system, immunoreactive somatostatin fibers have been found in the optic nerve, the lateral geniculate nucleus, superior colliculus, and visual cortex of various vertebrates (Laemle et al., 1981). In the retina it can be localized to several types of cells in the inner plexiform layer (Eriksen and Larsson 1981; Yamada et al., 1980; Krisch and Leonhardt, 1979).

Besides the previously mentioned hypothalamic-brainstem somatostatinergic pathways, somatostatinergic neurons are found intrinsic to the brainstem with cell bodies located in the lateral lemniscus, the reticular formation, the nucleus of the solitary tract, the locus ceruleus, and the spinal trigeminal nucleus, with staining being essentially identical using antisera against somatostatin-14 and against somatostatin-28 (4-14) (Finley et al., 1982; Morley, 1985). Somatostatinergic sensory fibers from the trigeminal nerve and from the hypoglossal nerve terminate in the nucleus of cranial nerve V and in the nucleus propositus hypoglossai and the solitary nuclear complex (Krisch, 1981). In addition, several auditory areas have been found to contain somatostatin in discrete subgroups of perikeria and terminals, suggesting the existence of specific somatostatin-containing auditory pathways (Morley, 1985).

Somatostatin has been anatomically associated with other neuroactive substances in the brain. Somatostatin-immunoreactivity has been reported to coexist in some forebrain neurons with avian pancreatic polypeptidelike immunoreactivity (Vincent et al., 1982). Neurons containing immunoreactivity for both these peptides have been observed in neocortex, hippocampus, striatum, and other areas. Recently, a subpopulation of mammalian cerebral neurons in cell culture have been shown to contain both somatostatin-immunoreactivity and acetylcholinesterase activity (Fig. 2), a finding that may suggest an association between somatostatinergic neurons and the cholinergic system in the central nervous system (Delfs et al., 1984). This latter finding raises the possibility of a specific pathophysiological association between the somatostatinergic and cholinergic systems in Alzheimer's dementia.

The use of increasingly specific antibodies directed toward various forms of somatostatin has allowed delineation of the distribution of somatostatin-14 and several related forms. These studies suggest that while somatostatin-14 is the predominant form of somatostatin in the nonhypothalamic rat brain (Benoit et al., 1982), it is somatostatin-28 (1-12) that predominates in neuronal axons and terminals, suggesting the possibility that this latter form might have the major role in cortical synaptic functioning (Morrison et al., 1983).

1.2.1c. Spinal Cord. The spinal cord contains a system of intrinsic somatostatin neurons and fibers (Burnweit and Forssman, 1979). Local circuit somatostatin fibers appear to interdigitate with descending hypothalamic somatostatin fibers (of periventricular origin) and with the terminals of somatostatinergic sensory afferents (Krisch, 1981).

1.2.2. Peripheral Nervous System

1.2.2a. Sensory Ganglia. Somatostatinergic neurons within dorsal root ganglia give rise to small unmyelinated C-fiber sensory afferents of the type generally associated with perception of pain and temperature. These fibers project centrally to terminate in the substantia gelatinosa of the dorsal root entry zone (Hökfelt et al., 1975; Lundberg et al., 1978). Somatostatinergic

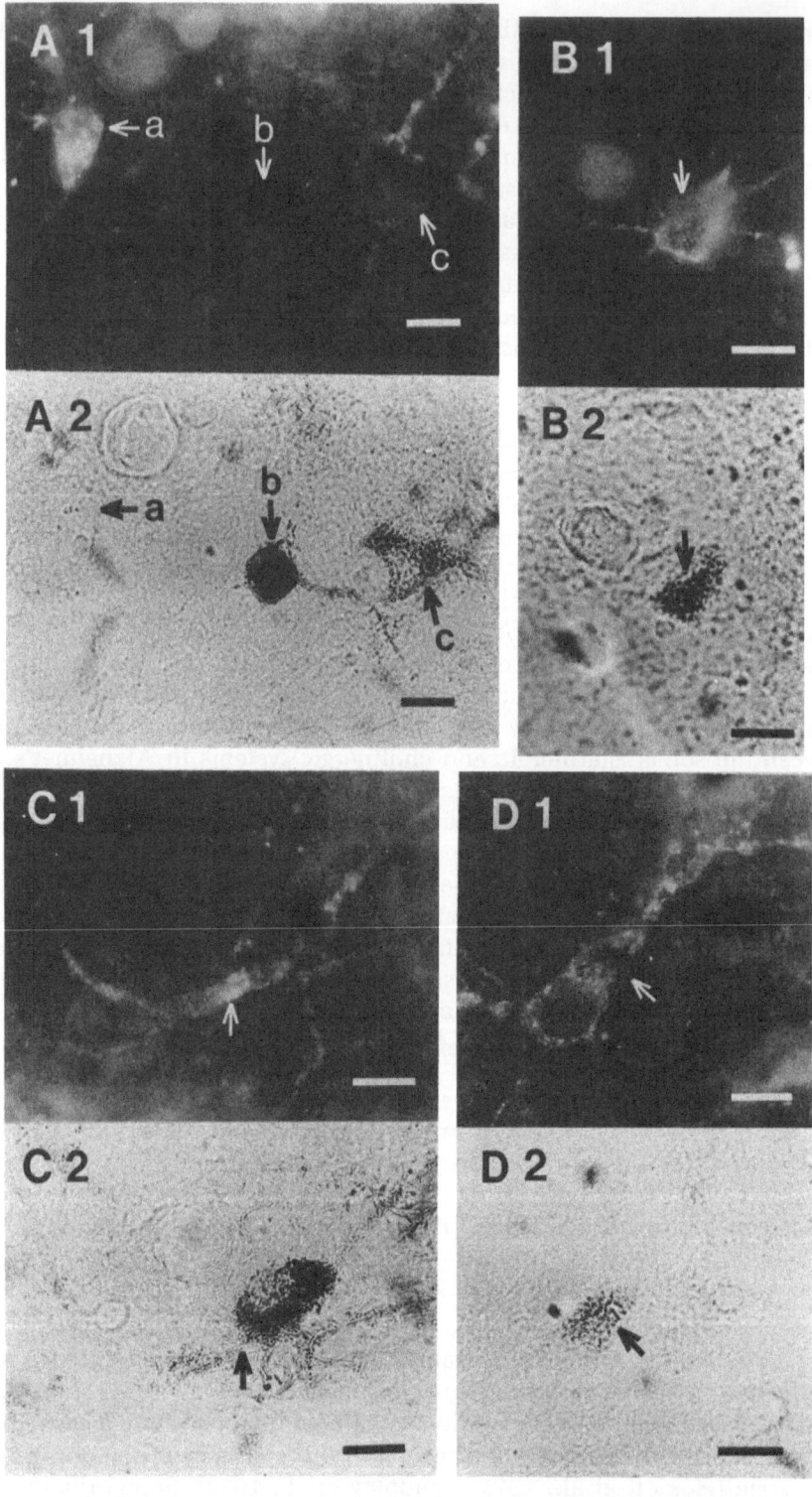

sensory afferents analogous to the spinal afferents are also found in the trigeminal nerve ganglion and in the auditory nerve.

1.2.2b. Autonomic Ganglia. Somatostatinergic neurons are found throughout the autonomic nervous system, including in the superior cervical and celiac superior mesenteric ganglia (sympathetic nervous system) (Lundberg et al., 1978; Hökfelt et al., 1977; Hökfelt et al., 1980), in sacral ganglia (Lowe et al., 1981), and in the nodose ganglia of the vagus nerve (parasympathetic nervous system) (Eriksen and Larsson, 1981). There is also the possibility that some of the somatostatinergic neurons in sympathetic ganglia are part of an afferent system within the sympathetic nerves (Krisch, 1981). The gut is innervated by somatostatinergic neurons from both the submucosal plexus and from extrinsic neurons from the vagus nerve (Sundler et al., 1980). Within sympathetic ganglia, many of the somatostatin-containing neurons are now known to be noradrenergic neurons, the first demonstration of the coexistence of a neuropeptide and a conventional neurotransmitter (Hökfelt et al., 1977). Somatostatin has also been found to be contained in and released from cholinergic nerves in the heart of the toad (Campbell et al., 1982).

1.3. Neurochemistry of Somatostatin

1.3.1. Somatostatin Biosynthesis

In addition to the 14-amino-acid molecule (somatostatin-14), somatostatin can exist as an amino-terminal extended molecule of 28 amino acids (somatostatin-28) (Pradayrol et al., 1980), as the first 12 amino acids of this C-terminal peptide (somatostatin-28 [1-12]) (Benoit et al., 1982), and also in at least four other larger forms (Benoit et al., 1982), probably most of which are secreted (Reichlin, 1983) (Fig. 1). The sequences of somatostatin-14 as

←
_____

Figure 2. Coexistence of somatostatin and acetylcholinesterase in cultured cortical neurons. Fluorescence photomicrographs (top photograph of each set) showing staining for somatostatin-like immunoreactivity (SOM-LI) and the corresponding bright-field micrographs (bottom of each set) showing staining for acetylcholinesterase activity (AChE). (A1) and (A2) demonstrate three populations of neurons definable by these two methods of staining. Neuron *a* stains positively for SOM-LI, but there is no staining for AChE. Neuron *b* stains darkly for AChE, but there is no staining for SOM-LI. Neuron *c* stains positively for AChE and also stains for SOM-LI, which can be seen in the fluorescence photomicrograph to be particularly prominent in the periphery of the perikaryal cytoplasm and out in the neuronal processes. (B1) and (B2) show a multipolar or stellate neuron that has SOM-LI staining in the cell body and out several processes and prominent staining for AChE in the neuron's cell body. (C1) and (C2) show a large bipolar neuron with SOM-LI staining predominantly in its processes and staining for AChE in the perikaryon and, to a lesser extent, out the neuronal processes. In (B) and (C) arrows point to an identical location on the same neuron in both the fluorescent and the bright-field photomicrographs. In each case the calibration bar represents 20 μm. (From Delfs et al., 1984, with permission.)

well as the 116-amino acid pre-prohormone and the 92-amino-acid prohormone have now been fully determined by recombinant DNA techniques (Goodman et al., 1980; Hobart et al., 1980; Goodman et al., 1983), and a molecule that is probably somatostatin has been synthesized in a cell-free system using rat hypothalamic RNA (Joseph-Bravo et al., 1980). At least three molecular forms of somatostatin have physiological activity in some systems, but the relative potencies of these molecules may differ. In each tissue there may be a proportionate distribution of the various forms of somatostatin according to their functional importance. In gut mucosa, somatostatin-28 predominates (Patel et al., 1981), while in neural tissues, such as the sciatic nerve, cerebral cortical cells grown in tissue culture, and extracts of extra-hypothalamic brain, the predominant form is somatostatin-14 (Patel et al., 1981; Benoit et al., 1982). As described earlier, recent histochemical studies suggest a predominance of somatostatin-28 (1-12) in nerve processes and terminals in cerebral cortex (Morrison et al., 1983).

It is assumed that processing of the largest molecular weight somatostatin (preprosomatostatin) takes place in a sequential fashion to obtain smaller and smaller forms of somatostatin within the endoplasmic reticulum and that the final hormone molecule is then translocated in the Golgi apparatus for final processing and assembly into granules (Chertow, 1981; Habener, 1981), which then move to nerve terminals by fast axoplasmic transport (Rasool et al., 1981).

1.3.2. Somatostatin Release

Throughout the nervous system, somatostatin is localized to nerve endings in secretory granules (Pelletier, 1980; Berelowitz et al., 1978). Depolarization of somatostatin-containing neurons by any method always results in the release of somatostatin, and this release is calcium-dependent (Reichlin, 1983). Spontaneous neuronal release of somatostatin is blocked by tetrodotoxin, indicating that sodium action potentials play a necessary role (Robbins et al., 1982b).

A number of neurotransmitters and other neuropeptides appear to influence neuronal release of somatostatin, most consistent of which is the effect of γ-amino-butyric acid (GABA) to suppress release (Games et al., 1980). In cultures of neurons from rat cerebral cortex, acetylcholine has been demonstrated to be a powerful releaser of somatostatin (Robbins et al., 1982a), although, interestingly, this effect of acetylcholine was not seen in perfused hypothalamic slices (Terry et al., 1980), perhaps suggesting regionally specific effects of acetylcholine on somatostatin release.

1.3.3. Somatostatin Receptors

1.3.3a. Binding Studies. Specific somatostatin binding was first characterized in cultured rat pituitary cells by Schonbrunn and Tashjian (1978). Somatostatin binding sites have now been described in whole brain synaptosomal preparations (Mehler et al., 1980; Reubi et al., 1981), and in rat cerebral cortex (Srikant and Patel, 1981a; Czernik and Petrack, 1982). There appears to be some correlation between regional binding capacity and endogenous levels of somatostatin (Epelbaum et al., 1982).

Specific binding sites for somatostatin have been found to have very high affinities, with half maximal binding typically occurring in the high picomolar range (1.25×10^{-10} M in membrane preparations from rat cerebral cortex [Srikant and Patel, 1981a]). Somatostatin binding sites in the pituitary and in the brain have somewhat different affinities for several analogs, suggesting that there may be more than one class of somatostatin receptor (Srikant and Patel, 1981b). Receptor binding studies recently reported using a stable analogue of somatostatin, SMS 201-995, have shown that only about 75 percent of the somatostatin-14 high affinity binidng sites in rat cerebral cortical membranes were recognized by the analogue (Reubi, 1984). This latter finding suggests the presence of more than one population of somatostatin receptors in the cerebral cortex.

1.3.3b. Antagonists. Since the elucidation of the somatostatin structure, hundreds of somatostatin analogs have been synthesized, but until recently all of these were reported to be either general agonists or agonists with relative selectivity for inhibition of either growth hormone, insulin, or glucagon release (Brown et al., 1976). However, Fries and colleagues (1982), using as a starting point a heptapeptide somatostatin agonist, cyclo(Pro-Phe-D-Trp-Lys-Thr-Phe), were able to synthesize a somatostatin antagonist. This molecule, cyclo[7-aminoheptanoyl-Phe-D-Trp-Lys-Thr(Bzl)] cmpletely blocks the inhibitory effects of exogenous somatostatin on growth hormone, insulin, and glucagon release in rats.

1.3.4. Termination of Action

Somatostatin degrading activity is present in both particulate and supernatant fractions of brain (Griffiths et al., 1977), but it is not known what role these peptidases play in the physiological inactivation of somatostatin. As yet, no specific peptidases have been described, nor are there reports of active uptake systems. Tachyphylaxis, which will be discussed in a later section of this chapter, could play a role in the termination of action of somatostatin on neurons (Delfs and Dichter, 1983).

1.4. Nonneuronal Actions of Somatostatin

1.4.1. Endocrine System

Somatostatin, released from the terminals of hypothalamic neurons into the hypothalamic-hypophyseal portal venous circulation, is a prompt and potent inhibitor of release from the pituitary of both growth hormone and thyroid-stimulating hormone (TSH) (Reichlin, 1982). In the pancreas, somatostatin is present in a subpopulation of cells in the Islets of Langerhans (D cells) as well as in nerve terminals and appears to be locally active on other islet cells to inhibit the release of both insulin and glucagon. Some of the effects may be species specific, however, as somatostatin *increases* the release of glucagon in ducks (Strosser et al., 1980).

Some studies have suggested that somatostatin might act in endocrine cells by altering membrane conductance to calcium or to potassium, but there is no consensus on this issue (Wollheim et al., 1978). Pace and Tarvin have shown in cultured pancreatic islet beta cells that somatostatin inhibits glucose-induced insulin release, increases ^{86}Rb efflux (a marker for potassium conductance), hyperpolarizes the membrane, and inhibits glucose-induced spike activity. All of these effects are reversed by the potassium channel blockers tetraethylammonium (TEA) or quinine. These workers have therefore suggested that somatostatin is acting in this system primarily by increasing potassium conductance (Pace and Tarvin, 1981).

1.4.2. Gastrointestinal System

In the gut, somatostatin is present in the terminals of extrinsic autonomic neurons, in intrinsic nerve plexuses, and in epithelial cells, but the major contribution appears to be non-neuronal. Somatostatin has been found to inhibit many processes, including gastric and intestinal motility, intestinal absorption, and gastric acid secretion. Somatostatin in the gut may act via local cell-cell influences and by its effect after being released into the lumen, as well as acting as a true hormone.

2. ACTIONS IN THE PERIPHERAL NERVOUS SYSTEM

2.1. Dorsal Root Ganglia

Somatostatin is contained in primary afferent neurons in dorsal root ganglia, with projections both to the periphery and into the spinal cord dorsal horn. Little is known about the possible role of somatostatin or other peptides in the peripheral fibers projecting to the skin and other tissues. Several studies, however, address the possible role of somatostatin at its point of release in the dorsal horn of spinal cord. Studies in spinal cord preparations will be discussed further in this chapter, and tend to suggest an excitatory or facilitory action on spinal neurons. On the other hand, somatostatin has been observed to decrease the duration of calcium action potentials in neurons cultured from chick dorsal root ganglia (Mudge et al., 1979). If similar effects of somatostatin on calcium conductance mechanisms were to occur at axon terminals, then one role of somatostatin could be as a presynaptic inhibitor of the release of transmitter from other neurons within the dorsal horn of the spinal cord.

2.2. Autonomic Neurons

The majority of studies show that somatostatin inhibits the response to autonomic nerve stimulation in both adrenergically and cholinergically innervated peripheral effector tissues including the vas deferens (Kastin et al., 1978; Magnan et al., 1979; Zetler, 1977), ileum and colon (Guillemin, 1976; Cohen et al., 1978; Furness and Costa, 1979), and pancreas. However, somatostatin does not block the effects of exogenously applied acetylcholine or norepinephrine, suggesting that the peptide acts by interfering with the release of transmitter from autonomic nerve fibers.

The actions of somatostatin may be more complex than simply inhibition of transmitter release however. For instance, an additional action of somatostatin in the gut is a relaxation of intestinal smooth muscle. This response is blocked by tetrodotoxin, suggesting that somatostatin may *stimulate* inhibitory neurons (Furness and Costa, 1979). In addition, somatostatin has a dual action on gut peristalsis that seems dependent on the preexisting frequency of contractions (Kromer and Woinoff, 1981).

It has recently been demonstrated that somatostatin increases the activity of the catecholamine-synthesizing enzyme tyrosine hydroxylase in rat superior cervical ganglia explants and cultures, suggesting that it may have a role in modulating sympathetic catecholaminergic function (Kessler et al., 1983). Other studies have shown that somatostatin can inhibit catecholamine secretion from adrenal medulla (Role et al., 1981) and acetylcholine-induced release of norepinephrine from cultures of isolated bovine adrenal medullary cells (Mizobe et al., 1979).

2.3. Myenteric Neurons

The particular response of myenteric neurons to somatostatin may depend to a large extent on the method of application of the peptide. Katayama and North (1980) recorded intracellularly from myenteric plexus neurons while applying somatostatin by two different techniques. They found that a minority of the myenteric neurons were responsive to somatostatin, and that bath perfusion resulted predominantly in a membrane hyperpolarization, while iontophoretic application of somatostatin more often gave a depolarizing response (Fig. 3). Occasionally, both of these responses could be produced in the same neuron by the appropriate method of application. Both of these responses were preserved in zero-calcium, high-magnesium solutions, suggesting a postsynaptic locus of action. It is not known whether these different effects are on the basis of differences in dose or time course of effect or

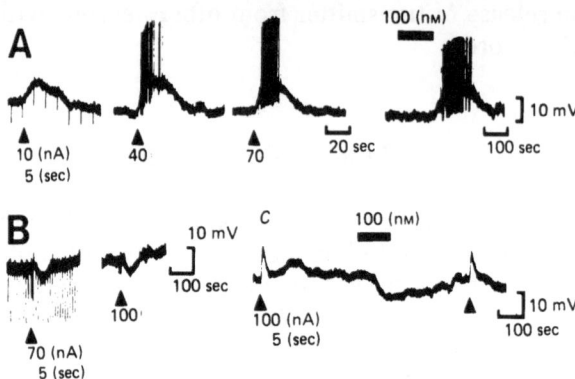

Figure 3. Effects of somatostatin on myenteric neurons. The effect of somatostatin iontophoresis and perfusion on three myenteric neurons. Iontophoresis was made at the time indicated by triangles and perfusion was made during the periods indicated by filled bars. (A) Somatostatin caused a dose-dependent depolarization leading to neuronal firing. Iontophoretic pulse duration was 5 sec; currents were 10, 40, and 70 nA. The right-most panel shows that perfusion of somatostatin (100 nM) had a similar effect to iontophoresis on the same neuron. The amplitude of action potentials was reduced by the pen recorder. (B) Hyperpolarization of another neuron by iontophoresis of somatostatin. Left panel, 70 nA for 5 sec; right panel, 100 nA for 5 sec. The hyperpolarization was associated with a slight decrease in membrane resistance. (C) perfusion of somatostatin (100 nM) caused a hyperpolarization while iontophoresis of somatostatin (100 nA, 5 sec) evoked depolarization. (From Katayama and North, 1980, with permission.)

because different regions of the neuronal membrane may be affected differentially by the somatostatin.

3. ACTIONS IN THE CENTRAL NERVOUS SYSTEM

3.1. Extracellular Studies *in Vivo*

Within the CNS, somatostatin has been shown to have a variety of effects in different regions. Experiments using extracellular field potential recordings and extracellular unit recordings have utilized *in vivo* and *in vitro* preparations from various vertebrate species. These studies have not resulted in any consensus on the effects of somatostatin in either spinal cord (Table 1) or in brain (Table 2), with individual studies showing either predominantly excitation or predominately inhibition of firing. In spinal cord, these differences may be region specific, with somatostatin increasing ventral root potentials (Nicoll, 1978; Padjen, 1977) and depressing the firing of dorsal horn neurons activated by noxious stimuli (Randić and Miletic, 1978). The one study in brainstem showed a predominantly depressant effect on firing rate (Chan-Palay et al., 1982).

In brain (Table 2), while an early report suggested a predominantly depressant action on the firing of cortical neurons (Renaud et al., 1975), more recent studies have observed an excitatory effect as the predominant response to somatostatin application (Iofee et al., 1978; Olpe et al., 1980). A possible reason for the discrepancy may be that different cortical neuronal populations could respond differently to somatostatin. Thus, in one study, somatostatin was found to have an activating effect on virtually all antidromically identified cortical spinal neurons, but a depressant effect on the firing of almost a third of the noncorticospinal neurons (Phillis and Kirkpatrick, 1980).

3.2. Studies in Hippocampal Slice

Even intracellular studies in nearly identical systems have produced what at first glance appear to be contradictory results. Two such studies (Fig. 4) were performed with in vitro hippocampal slices and both involved intracellular recordings from CA_1–CA_2 pyramidal cells. In one study, application by microiontophoresis, by pressure ejection, or by droplet of a 3 mM solution of somatostatin, produced a membrane depolarization and an increase in the number of action potentials per depolarizing ramp of current, with no accompanying change in membrane resistance (Fig. 4A) (Dodd and Kelly, 1978). In the second study, somatostatin applied by bath perfusion (120 nM to 1.2 μM) produced a membrane hyperpolarization, a reduced number of spontaneous and evoked action potentials, and a decrease in membrane resistance (Fig. 4B) (Pittman and Siggins, 1981). It seems likely that the contradictory results were due either to differences in methods of application or in the concentrations of the applied somatostatin. Table 3 shows data from these and several other intracellular studies on the effects of somatostatin on central neurons, including one study (Delfs and Dichter, 1983) which showed both excitatory and inhibitory effects of somatostatin in the same neuronal system.

3.3. Cortical Neurons in Culture

Recent studies utilizing mammalian CNS neurons in dissociated cell culture and a controlled method for somatostatin application have extended our understanding of somatostatin's effects and may at least partially explain the origin of some of the discrepant results using other preparations (Delfs and Dichter, 1983). The neurons in culture possess membrane characteristics resembling neurons in vivo, have both spontaneous and evoked action potentials, and form functioning excitatory and inhibitory synaptic connections (Dichter, 1978). Somatostatin is produced and secreted by a subpopulation of the neurons in these cultures (Delfs et al., 1980).

When applied directly to cortical neurons by a microperfusion technique at controlled concentrations, somatostatin produces a small membrane de-

Table 1. Effects of Somatostatin on CNS Neurons: Extracellular Studies in Spinal Cord and Brainstem

Preparation	Method of application	Concentration	Effects	Proportion of cells responding	Reference
Ventral root of frog spinal cord (sucrose gap recording)	Bath	10 µM	(1) Hyperpolarization (2) Enhancement of polysynaptic excitation of motor neurons	Not stated	Nicoll (1978)
Ventral root of frog spinal cord (sucrose gap recording)	Bath	1–10 µM	(1) Increased ventral root potentials (2) Depression of glutamate-evoked responses	Not stated	Padjen (1977)
Dorsal horn neurons in transected cat spinal cord	Iontophoresis	Unknown	Decreased firing in neurons activated by noxious stimuli	15/16 (94%)	Randić and Miletic (1978)
Lateral vestibular nucleus in anesthetized rabbits	Iontophoresis	Unknown	Decreased firing rate	7/7 (100%)	Chan-Palay et al. (1982)

Table 2. Effects of Somatostatin on CNS Neurons: Extracellular Studies in Brain

Preparation	Method of Application	Concentration	Effects	Proportion of cells responding	Reference
Cerebrum, cerebellum, and hippocampus in anesthetized rats	Iontophoresis	Unknown	Decreased firing rate	44/60 (73%)	Renaud et al. (1975)
Sensorimotor cortex in awake rabbits	Iontophoresis	Unknown	Increased firing rate (and Potentiation of L-glutamate-induced firing)	35/60 (58%)	Ioffe et al. (1978)
Cortex, striatum, and hippocampus in anesthetized rats	Iontophoresis	Unknown	Increased firing rate	140/320 (44%)	Olpe et al. (1980)
Motor cortex in anesthetized rats	Iontophoresis	Unknown	Increased firing rate	27/28 (96%) (corticospinal) 27/64 (42%) (other neurons)	Phillis and Kirkpatrick (1980)
			Decreased firing rate	0/28 (0%) (corticospinal) 21/64 (33%) (other neurons)	

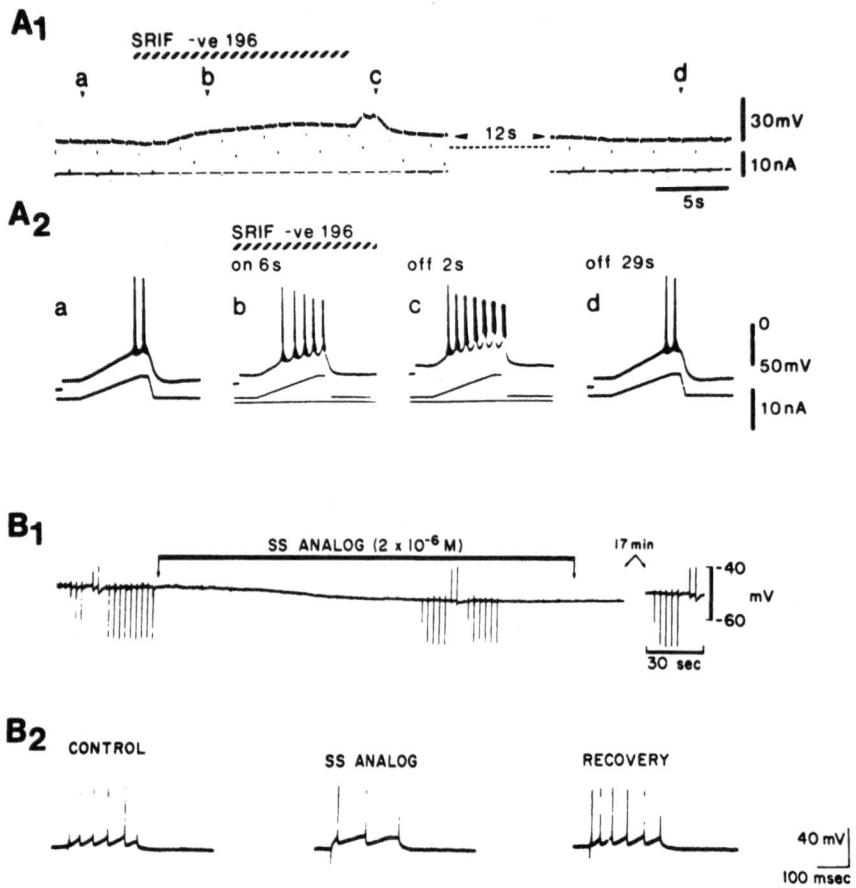

Figure 4. Comparison of two different intracellular studies of the effects of somatostatin on CA₁ pyramidal neurons in rat hippocampal slice preparations. (A) Somatostatin applied into the cell layer by microiontophoresis. (A₁) Somatostatin causes a membrane depolarization of 21 mV. (A₂) Somatostatin increases the number of action potentials evoked by a depolarizing ramp of current, at times denoted in (A₁) as a, b, c, and d. Hatched bar in (A₁) represents the period of somatostatin application and the number of nanoamps used. (From Dodd and Kelly, 1978, with permission.) (B) Somatostatin analog applied by bath prefusion. (Similar results were reported with somatostatin.) (B₁) Somatostatin analog causes membrane hyperpolarization. (B₂) Somatostatin analog causes a decrease in the number of action potentials evoked by a depolarizing current pulse. (From Pittmann and Siggins, 1981, with permission.) In both studies, these effects were reproducible in other neurons and reversible. Resting membrane potentials are −75 and −50 mV respectively.

Table 3. Effects of Somatostatin on CNS Neurons: Intracellular Studies

Preparation	Method of Application	Concentration	Effects	Proportion of cells responding	Reference
Spinal neurons of mouse in dispersed cell culture	Microperfusion	3 nM-300 nM	(1) Depolarization (2) Decreased membrane conductace (either g_K or g_{Cl}) (3) Increased synaptic activity	Not stated	MacDonald and Nowak (1981)
Hippocampal slice (CA_1 neurons) from rat	Iontophoresis and microperfusion	3 mM (unknown at level of neuron)	(1) Depolarization (2) Increased number of evoked action potentials	15/15 (100%)	Dodd and Kelly (1978)
Hippocampal slice (CA_1 neurons) from rat	Bath perfusion	120 nM-1.2 μM (unknown at level of neuron)	(1) Hyperpolarization (2) Decreased number of evoked and spontaneous action potentials	9/9 (100%)	Pittman and Siggins (1981)
Cerebral cortex of awake rabbits	Iontophoresis	Unknown	(1) Depolarization (2) Decreased heights of action potentials	7/17 (41%)	Iofee et al. (1978)
Cerebral cortical neurons from rat in dispersed cell culture	Microperfusion	100 pM-1 μM	(1) Depolarization and excitation (2) Increased synaptic activity (3) Occasional inhibition, possibly dose-related	30/87 (34%) 45/78 (58%)	Delfs and Dichter (1983)

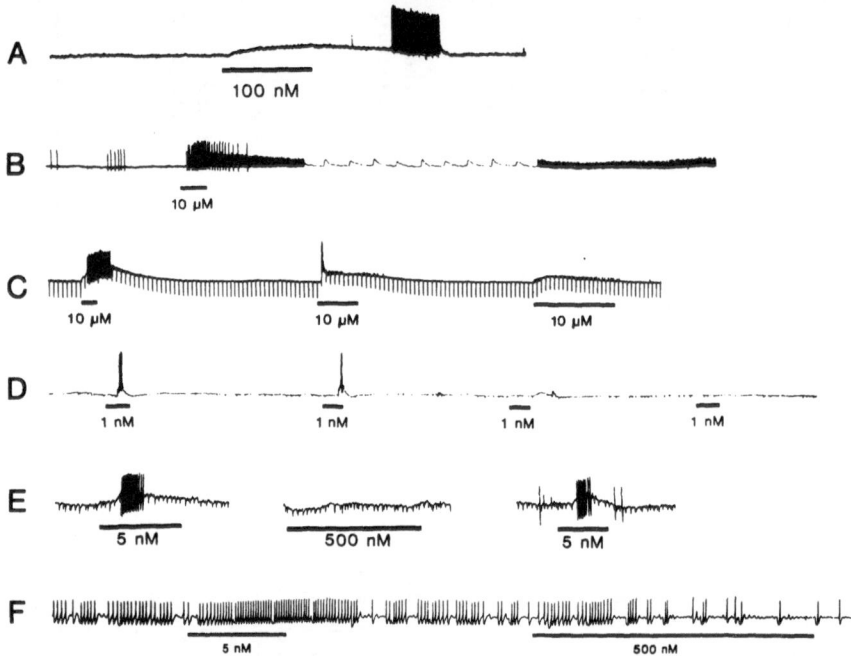

Figure 5. Effects of somatostatin on cerebral cortical neurons in culture. All tracings are from intracellular recordings. Somatostatin was applied to the vicinity of the neuron cell body by pressure microperfusion from glass pipettes. (A) Depolarization. Application of 100 nM somatostatin causes the rapid (latency of less than one second) onset of an 8-mV depolarization. A delayed volley of action potentials occurs in the recovery phase. (B) Increased synaptic activity. Application of 10 μM somatostatin results in no detectable direct membrane effect, but with a latency of 2–3 sec there is the onset of a volley of excitatory postsynaptic potentials (EPSPs), which are initially obscured by a secondary increase in action potentials. When the chart speed is increased, the basis of the response is clearly seen to be the EPSPs. (C and D) Tachyphylaxis, the progressive diminution of the neuronal response to repeated applications of somatostatin. (C) The initial application of somatostatin to this neuron causes a 20-mV depolarization and a 5-sec burst of action potentials, while successive applications of the same dose, even with increased periods of application, result in progressively smaller responses. (D) Somatostatin application initially results in an 8-mV depolarization and burst of action potentials, while successive applications are associated with a progressively diminished response until with the fourth application there is no detectable response at all. (E) Larger response of a neuron to the application of the lower of two concentrations of somatostatin. The initial application of 5 nM somatostatin to a neuron with spontaneous IPSPs causes significant depolarization and a burst of action potentials. Fifteen seconds later the application of a 500-nM concentration causes only a small increase in IPSP frequency, but 10 sec later a repeat application of 5 nM results in a significant depolarization and burst of action potentials. (F) Dose-dependent excitation and inhibition by somatostatin. In a neuron with ongoing firing of spontaneous action potentials, the application of 5 nM somatostatin results in an increased firing rate, while the application of 500 nM somatostatin is associated with an inhibition of spontaneous firing. Resting membrane potentials are -68, -72, -68, -65, -50, and -54 mV, respectively. Time calibrations can be determined by the length of the initial perfusion of somatostatin in each of the neuronal recordings, which were 16.5 sec, 6.4 sec, 3 sec, 2 sec, 3.1 sec, and 5 sec, respectively.

polarization in approximately 40% of the cells (Fig. 5A). The depolarization is associated with either no change or a slight increase in membrane resistance. In other neurons, somatostatin increases the number of action potentials per depolarizing current pule or the rate of spontaneous action potential generation even without a direct depolarization or change in resistance. The depolarizing effect of somatostatin has an unusual dose-response relationship. Responses occur at concentrations as low as 100 pM and maximal effects are seen in the range 5–50 nM. The response then *declines* at higher concentrations. This implies that application of somatostatin in concentrations commonly used may miss relevant responses by virtue of being to the right of an inverted U-shaped dose-response curve. At much higher concentrations (10 μM to 1 mM), a qualitatively different depolarizing response is sometimes seen. This response is often large and irreversible and may be a toxic response.

Somatostatin may also produce an increase in the frequency of ongoing excitatory or inhibitory synaptic potentials (Fig. 5B). In fact, this is the most commonly observed result of somatostatin application in the cortical cultures. This effect is abolished by tetrodotoxin, suggesting that it results from stimulation of action potentials in neurons presynaptic to the cell being studied. Whether the increase in synaptic activity is simply the consequence of the depolarizations noted in a smaller number of neurons or is due to a direct effect on presynaptic terminals has not yet been determined.

The response to somatostatin is often complex. While it is most often excitatory, somatostatin sometimes causes a diminished neuronal excitability or a decrease in the frequency of synaptic activity. Both the qualitative nature and the quantitative magnitude of responses seen in individual neurons are related to the concentration of the applied somatostatin and the prior history of somatostatin exposure. With repeated application of somatostatin, all the responses noted above serially decreased until a given response was no longer observable (Fig. 5C,D). This tachyphylaxis, or desensitization, could occur with as few as two or three applications of low concentrations of somatostatin. After a relatively long interval (often minutes) the response would return. Tachyphylaxis has also been described in cortical neurons *in situ*, as well as *in vitro*, and in the guinea pig ileum and myenteric plexus.

Somatostatin may also produce qualitatively different responses in a single neuron, depending on the concentration applied. A larger depolarizing or excitatory response is often seen with the lower of two successively applied doses of somatostatin, as would be expected from the inverted U-shaped dose-response relationship (Fig. 5E). In some neurons, a lower concentration produced an excitatory response, while a higher dose produced a frank inhibitory response (Fig. 5F). Such a result with studies of a single neurons suggests that somatostatin is activating two different receptors, perhaps a high-affinity receptor that mediates an excitatory response and a lower-affinity receptor that mediates an inhibitory response. To date, no low-affinity somatostatin receptor has been identified in brain. The inhibitory response could also represent a cross reaction with a high-affinity receptor site for some other ligand.

These studies utilizing intracellular recordings from single neurons and localized applications of carefully controlled concentrations of somatostatin therefore indicate several unusual physiological properties of the somatostatin response that may begin to explain the seemingly disparate results of the slice or *in situ* physiological studies. In order to understand the effects of somatostatin at the cellular level, the target cell identity, concentration of somatostatin (and dose range), the method of application, the history of prior exposure, and the time course of the exposure need to be specified.

3.4. Spinal Neurons in Culture

In similar studies carried out on mouse spinal cord neurons in culture, Macdonald and Nowak (1981) found that the predominant action of somatostatin was to increase synaptic activity. In addition, they also noted that somatostatin application was sometimes associated with a membrane depolarization associated with a decreased membrane conductance. Based on extrapolations of the reversal potential for the depolarization and on the observation that somatostatin evoked an inward current at resting membrane potential, they suggest that there is a decrease in conductance for either potassium or chloride.

3.5. Interactions with Other Transmitter Systems

3.5.1. Effects on Transmitter Release

Somatostatin performs a well-characterized role in inhibiting the release of numerous hormonal and other secretory factors throughout the body. The peptide might also serve a similar function in the nervous system to regulate the release of transmitters or other neuroactive substances. Several of the electrophysiological studies described above provide indirect evidence that somatostatin may modulate the release of transmitter substances both in the peripheral and central nervous systems.

Although this issue has been examined in biochemical studies, no consistent picture has emerged. Gothert (1980) reported that somatostatin selectively inhibits the evoked release of norepinephrine from rat hypothalamic neurons in slice preparations, while not affecting the release of norepinephrine from cortical slices nor the release of dopamine or serotonin from either tissue. On the other hand, Tanaka and Tsujimoto (1981) have shown that somatostatin facilitates the evoked release of serotonin from rat hypothalamus, cerebral cortex, and hippocampal slices, and the evoked release of norepinephrine from slices of rat cerebral cortex; (Tsujimoto and

Tanaka, 1981) and Chesselet and Reisine (1983) have shown somatostatin to increase the spontaneous release of dopamine from slices of cat striatum and *in vivo* in cat caudate and substantia nigra. Despite seemingly contradictory results, these studies do suggest that somatostatin could play a role in the presynaptic modulation of neurotransmitter release.

3.5.2. Modulation of Glutamate Response

It has been suggested that somatostatin might modulate the excitatory effects of L-glutamate, although there have been reports both of facilitation and of inhibition of the glutamate response (see Tables 1 and 2). Preliminary studies in rat cortical cell cultures indicate that somatostatin may facilitate or enhance both the presynaptic effect of glutamate to activate synaptic activity, and its postsynaptic depolarizing effect, although these actions occurred at relatively high doses (Dichter and Delfs, 1981). Ioffe has also noted an augmentation by somatostatin of glutamate excitations in rabbit sensorimotor cortex (Ioffe et al., 1978).

In cortical synaptosomes, somatostatin augments the glutamate-associated enhancement of calcium accumulation (see Chapter 5; Tan et al., 1977). Since in the absence of glutamate somatostatin did not influence calcium influx, these findings raise the possibility that somatostatin might specifically modulate the actions of the excitatory neurotransmitter.

3.6. Metabolic Actions in Nervous Tissue

In numerous studies in the pituitary and pancreas, somatostatin has been shown to reduce the concentration of cyclic AMP, but this metabolic change does not appear to be primarily responsible for the inhibitory effect of somatostatin on hormone release (Reichlin, 1982). It could be expected that somatostatin may have similar effects on cells within neural tissues, and in fact somatostatin may decrease the activity of adenylate cyclase and concomitantly increase the activity of guanylate cyclase, resulting in an increase in levels of cyclic GMP and a decrease in levels of cyclic AMP, but whether these changes in cyclic nucleotides have any direct relation to the primary or acute effects of somatostatin on neurons is not known.

Vesely (1980) has reported that the effects of somatostatin on cyclic nucleotide production may be quite dependent on the particular concentration of somatostatin used. In the picomolar and nanomolar range, somatostatin may enhance the activity of guanylate cyclase in many tissues including rat cerebrum, but in the micromolar range it can have the opposite effect. These findings are of particular interest in view of the physiological observation (see above) that somatostatin can have opposite effects on neurons depending on the concentration applied.

4. CONCLUSIONS AND FUNCTIONAL SIGNIFICANCE

The greatest amount of agreement regarding the actions of somatostatin as a neuroactive substance is in the peripheral nervous system, where it is believed that the somatostatin inhibits autonomic activity by blocking the release of acetylcholine and norepinephrine. Even in this system, however, there are conflicting reports and suggestions of a considerable complexity in the neuronal response to somatostatin.

In the central nervous system, there is less agreement. Studies in spinal cord and hippocampus, often using similar preparations, have shown conflicting results. One possible resolution of this dilemma is that somatostatin may have different effects within the same system, depending on the concentration or method of application.

In cerebral cortex, various studies have also shown both inhibitory and excitatory effects. Recent intracellular studies in dissociated cortical cell cultures have shown both postsynaptic effects of depolarization and excitation, as well as presynaptic effects on transmitter release. The precise locus of this latter action, i.e., on somata or nerve terminals, is as yet unclear.

The response to somatostatin may indeed be complex, perhaps involving acute presynaptic and postsynaptic effects, and, in addition, longer-term metabolic effects. If this is the case, it will be important to take into account such factors as tachyphylaxis, unusual dose-response characteristics, the critical nature of the functional state of the experimental preparation, and the importance of rigorously controlled sites of application in further efforts to produce meaningful data.

Somatostatin has a number of profound behavioral effects in the central nervous system, and has demonstrable physiological effects on neurons in numerous *in vitro systems*. The widespread distribution of somatostatin throughout all parts of the peripheral and central nervous system and in neurons of many types suggests a major role in neuronal function. The available evidence indicates that somatostatin acts to regulate synaptic release and modulate the excitability of target cells, rather than serve as a conventional neurotransmitter.

ACKNOWLEDGMENTS. We thank Diane Kilday for help in the preparation of the manuscript and Seymour Reichlin for his encouragement and for his making available to us several prepublication manuscripts for use in preparing this chapter. This work was supported in part by NIH Grants NS15362 and NS00608, and NIH Core Grant HD06276.

REFERENCES

Arimura, A., and Fishback, J. B., 1981, Somatostatin: Regulation of secretion, *Neuroendocrinology* 3:246–256.

Aronin, N., Cooper, P. E., Lorenz, L. J., Bird, E. D., Sagar, S. M., Leeman, S. E., and Martin, J. B., 1983, Somatostatin is increased in the basal ganglia in Huntington disease, Ann. Neurol. 13:519–526.

Bennett-Clark, C., Romagnano, M. A., and Joseph, S. A., 1980, Distribution of somatostatin in the rat brain: telencephalon and diencephalon, Brain Res. 188:473–486.

Benoit, R., Ling, N., Alford, B., and Guillemin, R., 1982, Seven peptides derived from pro-somatostatin in rat brain, Biochem. Biophys. Res. Commun. 107(3):944–950.

Berelowitz, M., Matthews, J., Pimstone, B. L., Kronheim, S., and Sacks, H., 1978, Immunoreactive somatostatin in rat cerebral cortical and hypothalamic synaptosomes, Metabolism 27(Suppl.1):1171–1173.

Brazeau, P., Vale, W., Burgus, R., Ling, N., Butcher, M., Rivier, J., and Guillemin, R., 1973, Hypothalamic polypeptide that inhibits the secretion of immunoreactive pituitary growth hormone, Science 179:77–79.

Brown, M., Rivier, J., and Vale, W., 1976, Somatostatin analogs with selected biologic activities, Metabolism 25(11):1501–1503.

Brownstein, M. J., Arimura, A., Fernandez-Durango, R., Schally, A. V., Palkovits, M., and Kizer, J. S., 1977, The effect of hypothalamic deafferentation on somatostatin-like activity in the rat brain, Endocrinology 100:246–249.

Burnweit, C., and Forssmann, W. G., 1979, Somatostatinergic nerves in the cervical spinal cord of the monkey, Cell Tissue Res. 200:83–90.

Campbell, G., Gibbons, I. L., Morris, J. L., Furness, J. B., Costa, M., Oliver, J. R., Beardsley, A. M., and Murphy, R., 1982, Somatostatin is contained in and released from cholinergic nerves in heart of the toad Bufo marinus, Neuroscience 7:2013–2023.

Chan-Palay, V., Ito, M., Tongroach, P., Sakurai, M., and Palay, S., 1982, Inhibitory effects of motilin, somatostatin, [Leu]enkephalin, [Met]enkephalin, and taurine on neurons of the lateral vestibular nucleus: Interactions with gamma-aminobutyric acid, Proc. Natl. Acad. Sci. U.S.A. 79:3355–3359.

Chertow, B. S., 1981, The role of lysosomes and proteases in hormone secretion and degradation, Endocrine Rev. 2:137–173.

Chesselet M-F., and Reisine, T. D., 1983, Somatostatin regulates dopamine release in rat striatal slices and cat caudate nuclei, J. Neurosci. 3:232–236.

Cohen, M., Rosing, E., Wiley, K., and Slater, I., 1978, Somatostatin inhibits adrenergic and cholinergic neurotransmission in smooth muscle, Life Sci. 23:1659–1664.

Crowley, W. R., and Terry, L. C., 1980, Biochemical mapping of somatostatinergic systems in rat brain: effects of periventricular hypothalamic and medial basal amyglaloid lesions on somatostatin-like immunoreactivity in discrete brain nuclei, Brain Res. 200:283–291.

Czernik, A. J., and Petrack, B., 1983, Somatostatin receptor binding in rat cerebral cortex. Characterization using a nonreducible somatostatin analog, J. Biol. Chem. 258:5525–5530.

Davies, P., Katzman, R., and Terry, R. D., 1980, Reduced somatostatin-like immunoreactivity in cerebral cortex from cases of Alzheimer disease and Alzheimer senile dementia, Nature 288:279–280.

Delfs, J. R., and Dichter, M. A., 1983, Effects of somatostatin on mammalian cortical neurons in culture: Physiological actions and unusual dose-response characteristics, J. Neurosci. 3:1176–1188.

Delfs, J., Robbins, R., Connolly, J., Dichter, M., and Reichlin, S., 1980, Somatostatin production by rat cerebral neurones in dissociated cell culture, Nature 283:676–677.

Delfs, J. R., Zhu, C-H., and Dichter, M. A., 1984, Coexistence of acetylcholinesterase and somatostatin-immunoreactivity in neurons cultured from rat cerebrum, Science 223:61–63.

Dichter, M. A., 1978, Rat cortical neurons in cell culture: Culture methods, cell morphology, electrophysiology, and synapse formation, Brain Res. 149:279–293.

Dichter, M. A., and Delfs, J. R., 1981, Somatostatin and cortical neurons in cell culture, Adv. Biochem. Psychopharmacol. 28:145–157.

Dodd, J., and Kelly, J. S., 1978, Is somatostatin an excitatory transmitter in the hippocampus? Nature 273:674–675.

Elde, R., Höfkelt, T., Johansson, O., Schultzberg, M., Efendic, S., and Luft, R., 1978, Cellular localization of somatostatin, *Metabolism* **27**(9):1151–1159.

Epelbaum, J., Willoughby, J. O., Brazeau, P., and Martin, J. B., 1977, Effects of brain lesions and hypothalamic deafferentation on somatostatin distribution in the rat brain, Endocrinology **101**:1495–1502.

Epelbaum, J., Arancibia, L. T., Kordon, C., and Enjalbert, A., 1982, Characterization, regional distribution, and subcellular distribution of ^{125}I-Tyr$_1$-somatostatin binding sites in rat brain, *J. Neurochem.* **38**:1515–1523.

Epelbaum, J., Ruberg,M., Moyse, E., Javoy-Agid, F., Dubois, B., and Agid, Y., 1983, Somatostatin and dementia in Parkinson's disease, *Brain Res.* **278**:376–379.

Eriksen, E. F., and Larsson, L. I., 1981, Neuropeptides in the retina: Evidence for differential topographical localization, *Peptides* **2**:153–157.

Feldman, S. C., Dreyfus, C. F., and Lichtenstein, E. S., 1982, Somatostatin neurons in the rodent hippocampus: An *in vitro* and *in vivo* immunocytochemical study, *Neurosci. Lett.* **33**:29–34.

Finley, J. C. W., Maderdrut, J. L., Roger, L. J., and Petrusz, P., 1982, The immunocytochemical localization of somtostatin-containing neurons in the rat central nervous system, *Neurosci.* **6**:2173–2192.

Fries, J. L., Murphy, W. A., Sueiras-Diaz, J., and Coy, D. H., 1982, Somatostatin antagonist analog increases GH, insulin, and glucagon release in the rat, *Peptides* **3**:811–814.

Furness, J. B., and Costa, M., 1979, Actions of somatostatin on excitatory and inhibitory nerves in the intestine, *Eur. J. Pharmacol.* **56**:69–74.

Gamse, R., Vaccaro, D., Gamse, G., DuPage, M., Fox, T. O., and Leeman, S. F., 1980, Release of immunoreactive somatostatin from hypothalamic cells in culture: Inhibition by gamma-amino-butyric acid, *Proc. Natl. Acad. Sci. USA* **77**:5552–5556.

Gerich, J. E., 1981, Somatostatin and diabetes, *Am J. Med.* **70**:619–626.

Goodman, R. H., Jacobs, J. W., Chin, W. W., Lund, P. K., Dee, P. C., and Habener, J. F., 1980, Nucleotide sequence of a cloned structural gene coding for a precursor in pancreatic somatostatin, *Proc. Natl. Acad. Sci. USA* **77**:5869–5873.

Goodman, R. H., Aron, D. C., and Roos, B. A., 1983, Rat preprosomatostatin: structure and processing by microsomal membranes, *J. Biol. Chem.* **258**(9):5570–5573.

Gothert, M., 1980, Somatostatin selectively inhibits noradrenaline release from hypothalamic neurones, *Nature* **288**:86–88.

Griffiths, E. C. Jeffcoate, S. L., and Holland, D. T., 1977, Inactivation of somatostatin by peptidases in different areas of the rat brain, *Acta Endocrinologia KBH* **85**:1–10.

Guillemin, R., 1976, Somatostatin inhibits the release of acetylcholine induced electrically in the myenteric plexus, *Endocrinology* **99**:1653–1654.

Habener, J. F., 1981, Principles of peptide-hormone biosynthesis, *Adv. Biochem. Psychopharmacol.* **28**:21–43.

Hobart, P., Crawford, R., Shen, L. P., Pictet, R., and Rutter, W. J., 1980, Cloning and sequence analysis of cDNAs encoding two distinct somatostatin precursors found in the endocrine pancreas of angler fish, *Nature* **288**:137–141.

Hökfelt, T., Elde, R., Johansson, O., Luft, R., and Arimura, A., 1975, Immunohistochemical evidence for the presence of somatostatin, a powerful inhibitory peptide, in some primary sensory neurons, *Neurosci. Lett.* **1**:231–235.

Hökfelt, T., Elfvin, L. G., Elde, R., Schultzberg, M., Goldstein, M., and Luft, R., 1977, Occurrence of somatostatin-like immunoreactivity in some peripheral sympathetic noradrenergic neurons, *Proc. Natl. Acad. Sci. USA* **74**:3587–3591.

Hökfelt, T., Johansson, O., Ljungdahl, A., Lundberg, J. M., and Schultzbert, M., 1980, Peptidergic neurons, *Nature* **284**:515–521.

Ioffe, S., Havlicek, V., Friesen, H., and Chernick, V., 1978, Effect of somatostatin (SRIF) and L-glutamate on neurons of the sensorimotor cortex in awake habituated rabbits, *Brain Res.* **153**:414–418.

Joseph-Bravo, P., Charli, J. L., Sherman, T., Boyer, H., Bolivar, F., and McKelvy, J. F., 1980, Identification of a putative hypothalamic nRNA coding for somatostatin and of its product in cell-free translation, *Biochem. Biophys. Res. Commun.* **94**:1004–1012.

Kastin, A. J., Coy, D. H., Jacquet, Y., Schally, A. V., and Plotnikoff, N. P., 1978, CNS effects of somatostatin, *Metabolism* **27**:1247–1252.

Katayama, Y., and North, R. A., 1980, The action of somatostatin on neurones of the myenteric plexus of the guinea-pig ileum, *J. Physiol. (Lond.)* **303**:315–323.

Kessler, J. A., Adler, J. E., and Black, I. B., 1983, Substance P and somatostatin regulate sympathetic noradrenergic function, *Science* **221**:1059–1061.

Krisch, B., 1978, Hypothalamic and extrahypothalamic distribution of somatostatin-immunoreactive elements in the rat brain, *Cell Tissue Res.* **195**:499–513.

Krisch, B., 1980, Differing immunoreactivities of somatostatin in the cortex and the hypothalamus of the rat, *Cell Tissue Res.* **212**:457–464.

Krisch, B., 1981, Somatostatin-immunoreactive fiber projections into the brain stem and the spinal cord of the rat, *Cell Tissue Res.* **217**:531–552.

Krisch, B., and Leonhardt, H., 1979, Demonstration of a somatostatin-like activity in retinal cells of the rat, *Cell Tissue Res.* **204**:127–140.

Kromer, W., and Woinoff, R., 1981, Dual action of somatostatin upon pristalsis in the guinea pig isolated ileum, *Neuroendocrinology* **33**:136–139.

Laemle, L. K., Feldman, S. C., and Lichenstein, E., 1981, Somatostatin-like immunoreactivity in the rodent visual system, *Soc. Neurosci. Abstr.* **7**:761.

Layton, B. S., Lafontaine, S., and Renaud, L. P., 1981, Connections of medial preoptic neurons with the median eminence and amygdala, *Neuroendocrinology* **33**:235–240.

Lechan, R. M., Nestler, J. L., Jacobson, S., and Reichlin, S., 1980, *Brain Res.* **195**:13–27.

Lowe, I., Blais, D., Ronnekleiv, O., Morgan, C., Nadelhaft, I., and de Groat, W., 1981, Immunohistochemical studies of the distribution of Substance P, somatostatin and cholecystokinin in relation to the sacral parasympathetic nucleus of cat, *Soc. Neurosci. Abstr.* **7**:101.

Lundberg, J. M., Hökfelt, T., Nilsson, G., Terenius, L., Rehfeld, J., Elde, R., and Said, S., 1978, Peptide neurons in the vagus, splanchnic and sciatic nerves, *Acta Physiol. Scand.* **104**:499–501.

Macdonald, R., and Nowak, L., 1981, Somatostatin has excitatory actions on murine spinal cord neurons in primary dissociated cell culture, *Soc. Neurosci. Abstr.* **7**:429.

Magnan, J., Regoli, D., Quirion, R., Lemaire, S., St.-Pierre, S., and Rioux, F., 1979, Studies on the inhibitory action of somatostatin in the electrically stimulated vas deferens, *Europ. J. Pharmacol.* **55**:347–354.

Mehler, P. S., Sussman, A. L., Maman, A., Leitner, J. W., and Sussman, K. E., 1980, Role of insulin secretogogues in the regulation of somatostatin binding by isolated rat islets, *J. Clin. Invest.* **66**:1334–1338.

Mizobe, F., Kozousek, V., Dean, D. M., adn Livett, B. G., 1979, Pharmacological characterization of adrenal paraneurons: Substance P and somatostatin as inhibitory modulators of the nicotinic response, *Brain Res.* **178**:555–566.

Morley, B. J., 1985, The localization and origin of somatostatin-containing fibers in an auditory brainstem nucleus, *Peptides* (in press).

Morrison, J. H., Benoit, R., Magistretti, P. J., and Bloom, F.E., 1983, Immunohistochemical distribution of pro-somatostatin-related peptides in cerebral cortex, *Brain Res.* **262**:344–351.

Mudge, A. W., Leeman, S. E., and Fischbach, G. D., 1979, Enkephalin inhibits release of substance P from sensory neurons in culture and decreases action potential duration, *Proc. Natl. Acad. Sci. USA* **76**(1):526–530.

Nemeth E. F., and Cooper, J. R., 1979, Effect of somatostatin on acetylcholine release from rat hippocampal synaptosomes, *Brain Res.* **165**:166–170.

Nicoll, R. A., 1978, Peptide receptors in the CNS: Neurophysiologic studies in neurobiology of peptides, *Neurosci. Res. Prog. Bull.* **16**:272–285.

Olpe, H.-R., Balcar, V. J., Bittiger, H., Rink, H., and Sieber, P., 1980, Central actions of somatostatin, *Eur. J. Pharmacol.* **63**:127–133.

Pace, C. S., and Tarvin, J. T., 1981, Somatostatin: Mechanism of action in pancreatic islet B-cells, *Diabetes* **30**:836–842.

Padjen, A. L., 1977, Effects of somatostatin on frog spinal cord, *Soc. Neurosci. Abstr.* **3**:411.

Patel, Y. C., and Reichlin, S., 1978, Somatostatin in hypothalamus, extrahypothalamic brain, and peripheral tissues of the rat, *Endocrinology* **102**:523–530.

Patel, Y. C., Wheatley, T., and Ning, C., 1981, Multiple forms of immunoreactive somatostatin: Comparison of distribution in neural and nonneural tissues and portal plasma of the rat, *Endocrinology* **109**:1943–1949.

Pelletier, G., 1980, Immunohistochemical localization of somatostatin, *Prog. Histochem. Cytochem.* **12**:1–41.

Phillis, J. W., and Kirkpatrick, J. R., 1980, The actions of motilin, luteinizing hormone releasing hormone, cholecystokinin, somatostatin, vasoactive intestinal peptide, and other peptides on rat cerebral cortical neurons, *Can. J. Physiol. Pharmacol.* **58**:612–623.

Pittman, Q. J., and Siggins, G. R., 1981, Somatostatin hyperpolarizes hippocampal pyramidal neurons *in vitro*, *Brain Res.* **121**:402–408.

Plotnikoff, N. P., Kastin, A. J., and Schally, A. V., 1974, Growth hormone release inhibiting hormone: Neuropharmacologic studies, *Pharmacol. Biochem. Behav.* **2**:693–696.

Prange, A. J., Breese, G. R., Jahnke, G. D., Martin, B. R., Cooper, B. R., Cott, J. M., Wilson, I. C., Alltop, L. B., Lipton, M. A., Bissette, G., Nemeroff, C. B., and Loosen, P. T., 1978, Modification of pentobarbital effects by natural and synthetic polypeptides: Dissociation of brain and pituitary effects, *Life Sci.* **16**:1907–1914.

Pradayrol, L., Jornvall, H., Mutt, V., and Ribet, A., 1980, N-terminally extended somatostatin: the primary structure of somatostatin-28, *FEBS Lett.* **109**:55–58.

Randić, M., and Miletić, V., 1978, Depressant actions of methionine-enkephalin and somatostatin in cat dorsal horn neurones activated by noxious stimuli, *Brain Res.* **152**:196–202.

Rasool, C. G., Schwartz, A. L., Bollinger, J. A., Reichlin, S., and Bradley, W. G., 1981, Somatostatin distribution and axoplasmic transport in rat peripheral nerve, *Endocrinology* **108**:996–1001.

Reichlin, S., 1982, Somatostatin, in: *Brain Peptides* (D. T. Krieger, M. Brownstein, and J. B. Martin, eds.), John Wiley and Son, Inc., New York, pp. 712–752.

Reichlin, S. 1983, Somatostatin, *N. Engl. J. Med.* **309**:1495–1501, 1556–1563.

Renaud, L. P., Martin, J. B., and Brazeau, P., 1975, Depressant action of TRH, LH-RH and somatostatin on activity of central neurones, *Nature* **255**:233–235.

Reubi, J-C., Perrin, M. H., Rivier, J. E., and Vale, W., 1981, High affinity binding sites for a somatostatin-28 analog in rat brain, *Life Sci.* **28**:2191–2198.

Reubi, J. C., 1984, Evidence for two somatostatin-14 receptor types in rat brain cortex, *Neurosci. Lett.* **49**:259–263.

Rezek, M., Havlicek, B., Hughes, K. R., and Friesen, H., 1977, Behavioral and motor excitation and inhibition induced by the administration of small and large doses of somatostatin into the amygdala, *Neuropharmacology* **16**:157–162.

Robbins, R. J., Sutton, R. E., and Reichlin, S., 1982a, Effects of neurotransmitters and cyclic AMP on somatostatin release from cultured cerebral cortical cells, *Brain Res.* **234**:377–386.

Robbins, R. J., Sutton, R. E., and Reichlin, S., 1982b, Sodium-and calcium-dependent somatostatin release from dissociated cerebral cortical cells in culture, *Endocrinology* **110**:496–499.

Role, L. W., Leeman, S. E., and Perlman, R. L., 1981, Somatostatin and substance P inhibit catecholamine secretion from isolated cells of guinea-pig adrenal medulla, *Neuroscience* **6**:1813–1821.

Rossor, M. N., Emson, P. C., Montjoy, C. Q., Roth, M., and Iversen, L. L., 1980, Reduced amounts of immunoreactive somatostatin in the temporal cortex in senile dementia of Alzheimer type, *Neurosci. Lett.* **20**:373–377.

Schonbrunn, A., and Tashjian, A. H., Jr., 1978, Characterization of functional receptors for somatostatin in rat pituitary cells in culture, *J. Biol. Chem.* **253**:6473–6483.

Srikant, C. B., and Patel, Y. C., 1981a, Somatostatin receptors: Identification and characterization in rat brain membranes, *Proc. Natl. Acad. Sci. USA* **78**(6):3930–3934.

Srikant, C. B., and Patel, Y. C., 1981b, Somatostatin analogs. Dissociation of brain receptor binding affinities and pituitary actions in the rat, *Endocrinology* **108**:341–343.

Strosser, M. T., Cohen, L., Harvey, S., and Mialhe, P., 1980, Somatostatin stimulates glucagon secretion in ducks, *Diabetologia* **18**:319–322.

Sundler, F., Hakanson, R., and Leander, S., 1980, Peptidergic nervous systems in the gut, *Clin. Gastroenterol.* **9**:517–543.

Tan, A. T., Tsang, D., Renaud, L. P., and Martin, J. B., 1977, Effect of somatostatin on calcium transport in guinea pig cortex synaptosomes, *Brain Res.* **123**:193–196.

Tanaka, S, and Tsujimoto, A., 1981, Somatostatin facilitates the serotonin release from rat cerebral cortex, hippocampus and hypothalamus slices, *Brain Res.* **208**:219–222.

Terry, L. C., Rorstad, O. P., and Martin, J. B., 1980, The release of biologically and immunologically reactive somatostatin from perifused hypothalamic fragments, *Endocrinology* **107**:794–800.

Tsujimoto, A., and Tanaka, S., 1981, Stimulatory effect of somatostatin on norepinephrine release from rat brain cortex slices, *Life Sci.* **28**:903–910.

Vesely, D. L., 1980, The interrelationship of somatostatin and guanylate cyclase activity, *Mol. Cell. Biochem.* **32**:131–134.

Vincent, S. R., Skirboll, L., Hökfelt, T., Johansson, O., Lundberg, J. M., Elde, R. P., Terenius, L., and Kimmel, J., 1982, Coexistence of somatostatin and avian pancreatic polypeptide (APP)-like immunoreactivity in some forebrain neurons, *Neuroscience* **7**:439–446.

Wollheim, C. B., Blondel, B., Kikuchi, M., and Sharp, G. W. G., 1978, Inhibition of insulin release by somatostatin: No evidence for interaction with calcium, *Metabolism* **27**:1303–1307.

Yamada, T., Marshak, D., Basinger, S., Walsh, J., Morley, J., and Stell, W., 1980, Somatostatin-like immunoreactivity in the retina, *Proc. Natl. Acad. Sci. U.S.A.* **77**:1691–1695.

Zetler, G., 1977, Effects of Substance P and other peptides on the field-stimulated guinea pig vas deferens, in: *Substance P* (U.S. von Euler and B. Pernow, eds.), Raven Press, New York, pp. 97–116.

Reference

15

Oxytocin and Vasopressin

MICHEL MÜHLETHALER, MARIO RAGGENBASS,
and J. J. DREIFUSS

1. INTRODUCTION

1.1. Historical Perspective and Overview

Toward the end of the 19th century, the functions of most endocrine glands were revealed by a combination of surgical removal and of injection of crude extracts. In particular, the intravenous injection of a crude pituitary extract yielded a clear-cut and measurable rise in blood pressure. In 1898, it was shown that this effect was due to components present only in the posterior ("nervous") subdivision of the gland. In little more than a decade, other actions of posterior pituitary extracts were revealed: the contraction of uterine smooth muscle in late pregnancy and the stimulation of milk ejection during lactation. An effect of the extract on urine output was also noticed at an early date; however, it took several years until it was recognized that the physiological effect was to induce an antidiuresis (for historical references, see Heller, 1974). Vasopressin has been shown in recent years to exert several endocrine actions in addition to its classical antidiuretic and hypertensive effects. Thus, for example, it promotes glycogen breakdown by the liver, acts on spermatogenesis, causes platelet aggregation, and raises the level of antihemophilic globulin in blood.

Regarding the link between the hypothalamus and the posterior pituitary gland, a majority of authors held for many years that the secretory product was manufactured in the pituitary gland and carried to the hypothalamus. This opinion was challenged by Ernest Scharrer in the 1930s, who provided histological evidence that the secretions were produced in the hypothalamus and then transported to the pituitary. This controversy was settled in favor of Scharrer's views after German workers had succeeded in impregnating the entire hypothalamo-neurohypophysial system with Gomori's stain and had shown an accumulation of secretory product in the hypothalamic stump of the sectioned pituitary stalk (Bargmann and Scharrer, 1951). The Gomori method stains compounds having disulfide bridges and therefore reacts with oxytocin, vasopressin, and the neurophysins, but also with other sulfur-rich compounds.

1.2. The Neurohypophysial Peptides

The chemical nature of the hormones of the hypothalamo-neurohypophysial system was investigated during the same period. In the early 1950s, Du Vigneaud and co-workers were able to announce, first, that all known effects of posterior pituitary extracts in mammals could be ascribed to two compounds, oxytocin and vasopressin; second, that both are closely related cyclic nonapeptides with seven common amino acid residues; and third, that the vasopressin in the pig and related species differs from that of other mammals by containing a lysine residue instead of an arginine in position 8 of the molecule. They succeeded in synthesizing the three mammalian posterior pituitary hormones, as well as vasotocin, a structural intermediate of vasopressin and oxytocin known to be present in most nonmammalian species.

The establishment of the formulas of these hormones and their full synthesis represented a major achievement for which Du Vigneaud (1956) was awarded a Nobel Prize in Chemistry. The structure of the nonapeptides is as follows:

arginine-vasopressin   Cys-Tyr-<u>Phe</u>-Gln-Asn-Cys-Pro-<u>Arg</u>-GlyNH$_2$

lysine-vasopressin   Cys-Tyr-<u>Phe</u>-Gln-Asn-Cys-Pro-<u>Lys</u>-GlyNH$_2$

oxytocin   Cys-Tyr-<u>Ile</u>-Gln-Asn-Cys-Pro-<u>Leu</u>-GlyNH$_2$

arginine-vasotocin   Cys-Tyr-<u>Ile</u>-Gln-Asn-Cys-Pro-<u>Arg</u>-GlyNH$_2$

It was soon discovered that within hypothalamo-neurohypophysial neurons, the hormones are associated with other, functionally inactive compounds: the neurophysins. In the early sixties, it was shown that neurohypophysial hormones and their associated neurophysins were produced as parts of a common precursor. The putative precursors were first detected in the course of pulse-chase studies, and, more recently, the nucleotide sequence of a DNA encoding the bovine vasopressin/neurophysin II precursor has been reported (for references, see Brownstein, 1983). The oxytocin/neurophysin I precursor is similar in internal sequence to provasopressin, except that it lacks the C-terminal glycopeptide (Fig. 1).

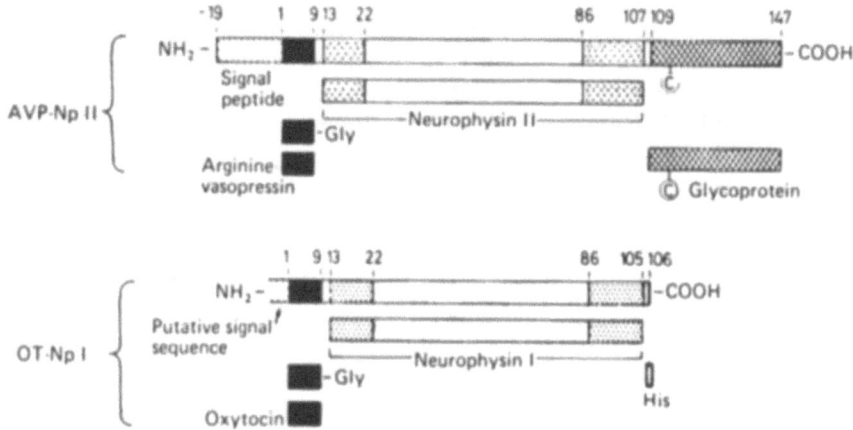

Figure 1. Schematic comparison of the arginine-vasopressin (AVP) and the oxytocin (OT) precursors. The negative number shows the beginning of the signal sequence, the positive numbers refer to the amino acid residues of the prohormones and indicate significant peptides within the precursors. Amino acid sequences between residues 22 and 86 show perfect homology in the two neurophysins (Np I, Np II). C, Carbohydrate chain; His, histidine; Gly, glycine. (From Ivell et al., 1983, with permission.)

Biosynthesis takes place in the hypothalamic perikarya of separate oxytocin-containing and vasopressin-containing neurons. From the endoplasmic recticulum, the prohormones make their way to the Golgi apparatus and are then packaged into secretory granules. During hypothalamo-neurohypophysial transport of the granules, the prohormones are enzymatically cleaved to yield vasopressin, oxytocin, neurophysin I and II, and glycopeptide. These compounds are released into the circulation when the nerve endings in the posterior pituitary are depolarized by incoming action potentials, even though neurophysins and glycopeptide have no known endocrine function.

1.3. Vasopressin and Oxytocin Receptors

Since the relative potency of vasopressin derivatives in raising blood pressure does not parallel their antidiuretic efficacy, it is apparent that vasopressin exerts its various effects by interacting with more than one type of receptor. Moreover, while the antidiuretic effect of vasopressin is associated with an accumulation of cyclic AMP in the renal tubular cells, the glycogenolytic response in hepatocytes is not, but is linked to an increase in membrane phosphatidylinositol turnover and in the concentration of intracellular free calcium. Michell and co-workers (1979) therefore proposed that vasopressin exerts its effects on the liver (and on vascular smooth muscle) by binding to a V_1 receptor whose intracellular signal is carried by calcium, whereas the antidiuretic effect would result from binding to a V_2

receptor linked to an adenylate cyclase. This view has been corroborated by studies on the binding of tritiated vasopressin to cells in kidney, liver and vascular smooth muscle (Jard, 1983).

Oxytocin elicits the contraction of uterine smooth muscle and of mammary myoepithelial cells. High-affinity binding sites for tritiated oxytocin were demonstrated in both tissues, half-maximal binding being achieved at concentrations of 0.5–3.0 nM. Myometrial binding sites are specific inasmuch as various structural analogs compete with tritiated oxytocin in proportion to their oxytocic activity in the uterus (Soloff et al., 1977).

Vasopressin and oxytocin are not only neurohypophysial hormones carried by a vascular route to affect renal, liver, muscle, and other cells, but they also have neural functions. This view is based on the demonstration of their presence in and release from the synaptic endings of extrahypophysial pathways, as well as on their electrophysiological effects in the brain and spinal cord. Recently the availability of high-specific-activity [³H]vasopressin has allowed the direct demonstration of binding sites for neurohypophysial peptides in membranes from mammalian brain (Barberis, 1983). These sites have been localized using an autoradiographic approach at the light microscopic level (Van Leeuwen and Wolters, 1983; Biegon et al., 1984).

1.4. Hypothalamo-Extrahypophysial Systems

1.4.1. Distribution of Vasopressin and Oxytocin Neurons and Their Extrahypophysial Pathways

The existence of extrahypophysial neurosecretory pathways was suspected as early as the 1950s. In studies using the Gomori stain to impregnate the hypothalamo-neurohypophysial system, the existence of an hypothalamo-epithalamic pathway was incidentally observed. Later, other investigators identified extensive extrahypophysial Gomori-positive pathways in the brain (Barry, 1961). From some of these regions of the brain extracts were obtained that possessed biological activities attributable to neurohypophysial peptides. These results went a long way towards establishing the concept of hypothalamo-extrahypophysial systems. However, their significance remained in doubt, because of the nonspecificity of the Gomori stain.

During the 1970s, specific antibodies directed against vasopressin, oxytocin, and neurophysins became available, and their use in immunocytochemical studies and for the radioimmunoassay of homogenates of punched areas from the brain allowed confirmation of the above-mentioned findings. In addition, chromatography of the extracts indicated the presence of compounds that migrate like authentic oxytocin and vasopressin. With specific anti-oxytocin and specific anti-vasopressin sera, a differential distribution for these two peptides was demonstrated: projections towards the limbic system are predominantly vasopressinergic, whereas those directed caudally tend to be oxytocinergic. These findings, originally obtained in the rat brain are valid in many other species as well, including man. Table 1 summarizes the major projection areas revealed from immunocytochemical studies.

There is at present still some uncertainty as to the nuclear origin of these extrahypophysial fiber tracts (De Vries and Buijs, 1983). The parvocellular division of the paraventricular nucleus is considered to be a major source, although a contribution from other nuclei to the vasopressinergic innervation of the brain is not excluded (Fig. 2). The extrahypophysial pathways that originate from the paraventricular nucleus derive mostly from small neurons different from the larger oxytocin and vasopressin neurons that project to the posterior pituitary. Only a very small percentage of neurons project both to the neurohypophysis and to the brain (for references, see Sofroniew and Weindl, 1981).

A projection from the parvocellular division of the paraventricular nucleus to various nuclei in the brainstem and to the spinal cord had been demonstrated even before the introduction of immunocytochemical methods. Using antibodies directed against oxytocin or vasopressin, a predominance of oxytocin- over vasopressin-containing fibers was observed in these territories. The injection of retrogradely transported dyes into the dorsal vagal complex or into the spinal cord demonstrated however that only about 20% of the neurons that were retrogradely filled in the paraventricular nucleus could be stained for either oxytocin or vasopressin. This indicates that these caudally-directed pathways also contain other neurotransmitters (Swanson and Sawchenko, 1983, for a review).

In 1961, Barry demonstrated that in the target fields of extrahypophysial

Table 1. Distribution of Vasopressin and Oxytocin
Fibers in Brain and Spinal Cord[a]

Forebrain	Midbrain (cont.)
Hippocampus (mostly ventral)	N. interpeduncalis
Frontal cortex	N. cuneiformis
N. accumbens	N. parabrachialis (mostly dorsalis)
N. tractus diagonalis Broca	Locus coeruleus
Lateral septum	N. raphe pontis
N. interstitialis stria terminalis	Hindbrain
Amygdala (mostly medial)	N. raphe magnus
Mediodorsal thalamus	N. raphe obscurus
Lateral habenula	N. tractus solitarius
Posterior periventricular hypothalamus	N. dorsalis nervi vagi
N. supramammillaris	N. reticularis lateralis
Midbrain	Substantia gelatinosa trigemini
Substantia nigra pars compacta	Spinal cord
Ventral tegmental area	Laminae I–III
Central gray area	Lamina X
N. raphe dorsalis	N. intermediolateralis

[a]From Sofroniew (1983).

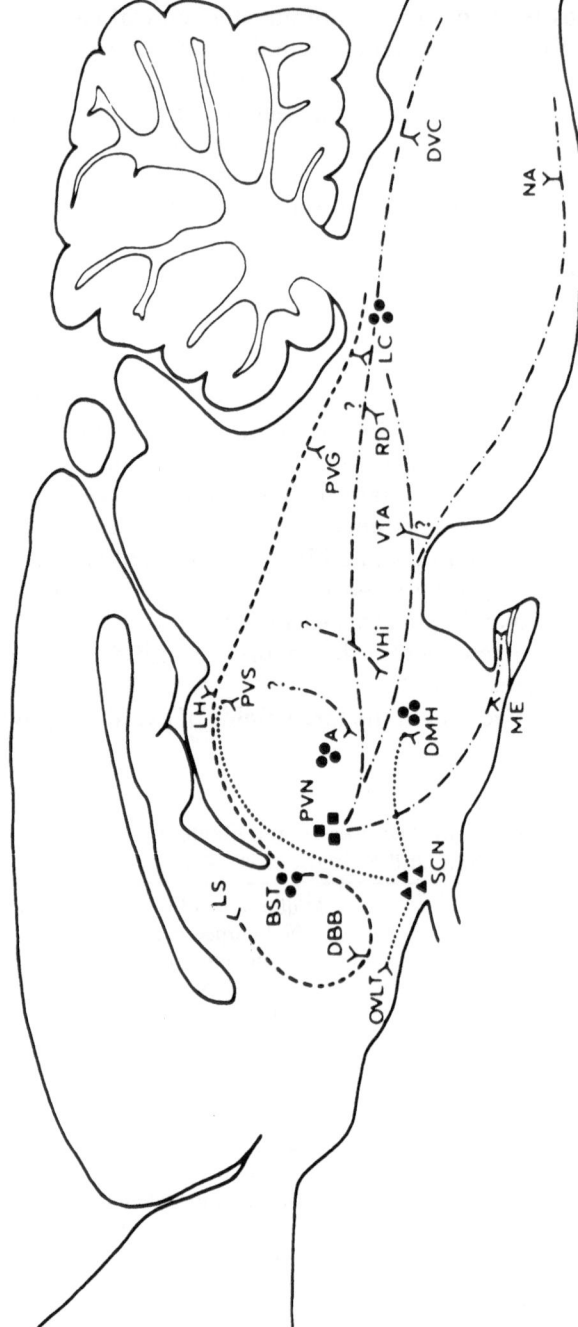

Figure 2. Vasopressin (AVP) pathways in the rat brain (sagittal plane). Pathways from the paraventricular nucleus (PVN; squares) are indicated by dashed-dotted lines (- · - · -) and pathways from the suprachiasmatic nucleus (SCN; triangles) are indicated by dotted lines (· · · · ·). The AVP cell groups found only after colchicine treatment are indicated by large black dots, while the pathways of the bed nucleus of the stria terminalis (BST) are indicated by dashed lines (- - - -). A question mark indicates that the source of the AVP innervation in this area is still unknown. Abbreviations: A, amygdala; DBB, diagonal band of Broca; DMH, dorsomedial nucleus of the hypothalamus; DVC, dorsal vagal complex; LC, locus coeruleus; LH, lateral habenula; LS, lateral septum; ME, median eminence; OVLT, organum vasculosum of the lamina terminalis; PVG, periventricular grey; PVS, periventricular nucleus; RD, dorsal raphe nucleus; VHi, ventral hippocampus; VTA, ventral tegmental area. (From Buijs, 1983, with permission.)

pathways, Gomori-positive terminals are in close contact with neuronal cell bodies and proposed that neurohypophysial peptides might act there as transmitters. The nature of these contacts was resolved only much later by immunoelectron microscopy. In the rat limbic system, Buijs and Swaab (1979) observed presynaptic structures containing vesicles that had reacted with antibodies directed against oxytocin or vasopressin (Fig. 3). The synaptic contacts were mostly axodendritic and the vesicles were 80–100 nm

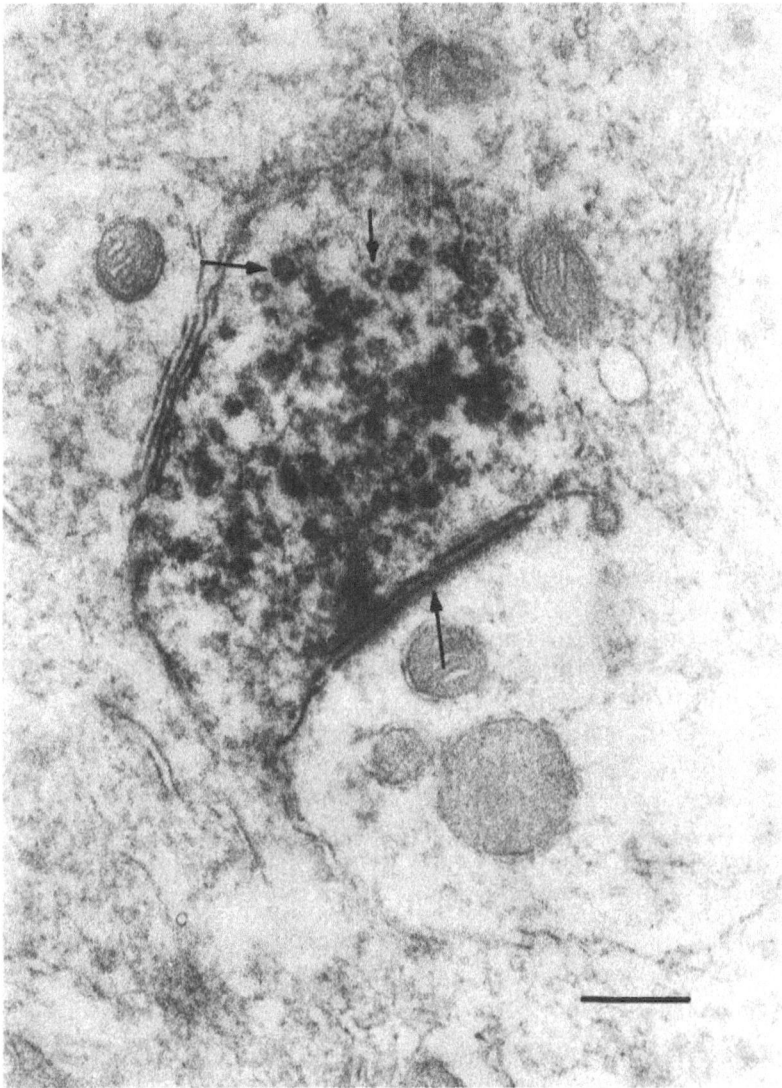

Figure 3. Vasopressin positive terminal forming synapse (long arrow) with unlabeled dendrite in lateral habenula. Note the diaminobenzidine reaction product around vesicles (short arrows). Bar = 0.25 μm. (From Buijs and Swaab, 1979, with permission.)

in diameter, which contrasted with the larger granules found in the posterior pituitary. Vasopressin synapses were absent in Brattleboro rats, a strain which is genetically unable to synthesize hypothalamic vasopressin.

1.4.2. Release of Vasopressin and Oxytocin from Brain Slices

The release of vasopressin and oxytocin from brain slices was studied by Buijs and Van Heerikhuize (1982), who showed that the rate of secretion of both peptides was significantly increased following depolarization with potassium or veratridine. The release process was calcium-dependent. Nevertheless, the amounts present in and released from brain slices were small, approximately 1000 times less than from the posterior pituitary. An indication that stimulated release occurred from axon terminals was provided by the observation that depolarization does not induce the release of vasopressin and oxytocin from the cut axons of hypothalamo-neurohypophysial neurons in the slices.

2. CELLULAR ACTIONS IN THE CENTRAL NERVOUS SYSTEM

Over the last decade or so, a number of studies have explored the effects of iontophoresis of vasopressin and oxytocin onto neurons located in various areas of the brain and spinal cord. A summary of these studies using in situ extracellular recording is shown in Table 2. It is apparent that oxytocin and vasopressin can exert both excitatory and inhibitory effects, the predominant action being different depending upon the brain region. Caution is required in interpreting these data, however, since none of these studies used antagonists or inactive structural analogs to prove a specificity of the response.

In contrast to experiments performed in vivo, detailed pharmacological data regarding the actions of oxytocin and vasopressin on the firing of single neurons in various regions of the brain and spinal cord has been accumulated using in vitro slice preparations. This experimental system has the advantage that the tissue can be perfused with media of known composition. In the following sections, we focus on the cellular actions of neurohypophysial peptides in such slice preparations, with emphasis on those regions where vasopressin and oxytocin pathways are known to terminate.

2.1. Hippocampus

Using extracellular recording techniques in the CA_1 area of rat hippocampal slices, Mühlethaler et al. (1982) and Tiberiis et al. (1983) found a population of neurons which were consistently excited by low concentrations of the neurohypophysial peptides (Fig. 4). When oxytocin and vasopressin were compared, oxytocin was found to be more potent, its threshold

Table 2. Effects of Iontophoretically Applied Neurohypophysial Peptides

Area in rat brain	Peptide(s)[a]	Excited	Percentage of neurons unaffected	Inhibited	Reference
Supraoptic nucleus	LVP	12	38	50	Nicoll and Barker (1971)
Paraventricular nucleus	AVP	0	85	15	Moss et al. (1972)
Paraventricular nucleus	OT	76	24	0	Moss et al. (1972)
Hippocampus and septum	AVP, OT	57	43	0	Joëls and Urban (1982)
Locus coeruleus	AVP, LVP	87	13	0	Olpe and Baltzer (1981)
Brainstem reticular nucleus	AVT	45	55	0	Normanton and Gent (1983)
Caudal medulla	OT	7	23	70	Morris et al. (1980)
Cervical spinal cord	AVP, OT	13	22	65	Gilbey et al. (1982)

[a]Abbreviations: AVP, arginine-vasopressin; AVT, arginine-vasotocin; LVP, lysine-vasopressin; OT, oxytocin.

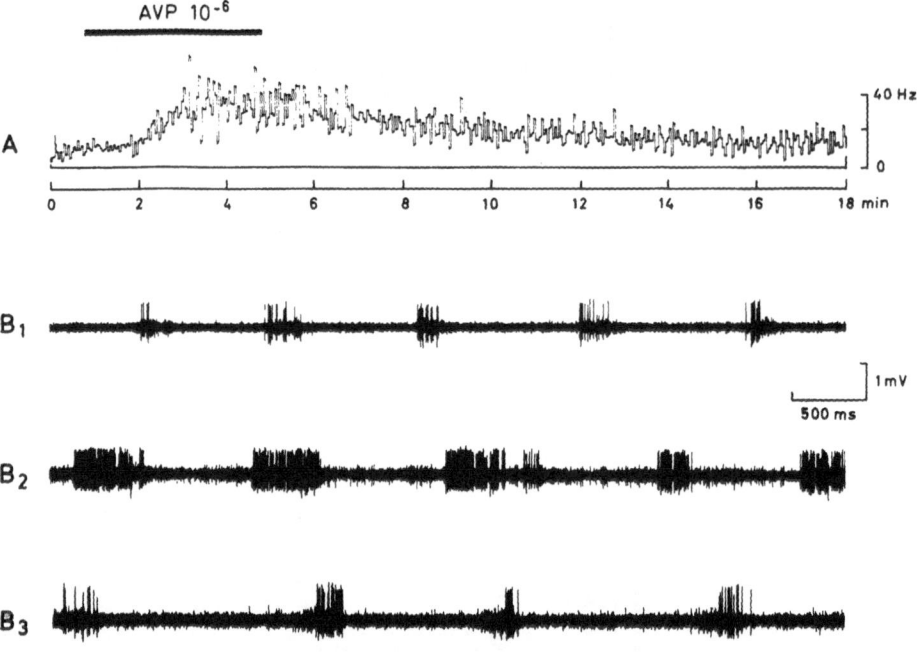

Figure 4. Effect of vasopressin on the rate of firing of a CA_1 neuron in a hippocampal slice. (A) Rate-meter record; arginine vasopressin (AVP), 1 μM, was added to the perfusion medium during the period indicated by the thick bar. (B) Oscilloscope tracings of the activity of this same neuron before (B_1), during (B_2), and after (B_3) AVP application. (From Mühlethaler et al., 1982, with permission.)

concentration being around 10^{-9} M and its stimulatory effect maximal at approximately 10^{-6} M. The dose-response curves ran in parallel (Fig. 5).

A number of structural analogs of oxytocin and vasopressin possessing known endocrine effects (Sawyer et al., 1981) also excited these neurons (Mühlethaler et al., 1983). These compounds include arginine vasotocin, as well as four synthetic structural analoges. Their respective activities as stimulants of uterine contractions are given along the abcissa of Fig. 6; the compound d[Tyr(Me)²]VDAVP is thus devoid of any oxytocic activity (it is actually an antagonist), whereas HO[Thr⁴,Gly⁷]OT is a powerful and specific oxytocic agonist. The potency of each compound in the hippocampus correlated with its activity as an oxytocic agonist in the isolated uterus (Fig. 6); in contrast, no correlation was obtained with either antidiuretic or vasopressor activities. Among the structural analogs tested, the compound acting as an antagonist in the uterus also reversibly blocked the response to oxytocin in the hippocampus (Fig. 7).

Taken together, these observations support the view that the hippocampal response to oxytocin and vasopressin is due to binding of the peptides

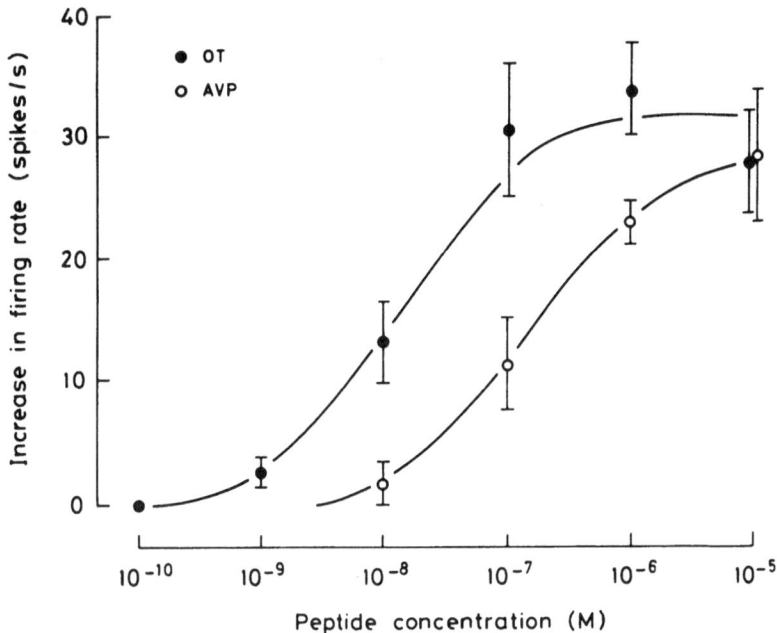

Figure 5. Effects of oxytocin (OT) and arginine vasopressin (AVP) applied at various concentrations on the firing of nonpyramidal neurons. Each point shows mean increase (± S.E.M., n = 5 except for OT, 1 μM, where n = 13, and AVP, 1 μM, where n = 23) in firing rate at the concentration of peptide indicated. (From Mühlethaler et al., 1983, with permission.)

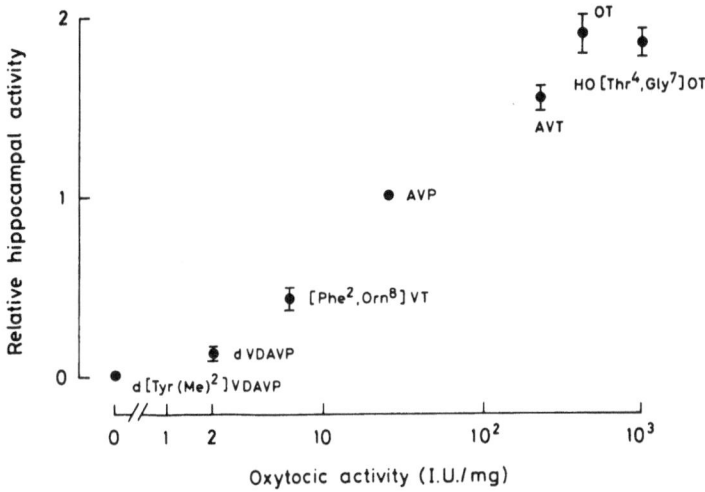

Figure 6. Correlation between oxytocic activity and "relative hippocampal activity" of OT, AVP, arginine vasotocin (AVT) and of four synthetic structural analogs. The mean (± S.E.M., n ≥ 5) increase in hippocampal firing is expressed relative to the effect of AVP 1 μM (ordinate). The logarithm of oxytocic activity, determined on isolated rat uterine horns and expressed as international units (I.U.) per milligram of peptide, is plotted on the abcissa.

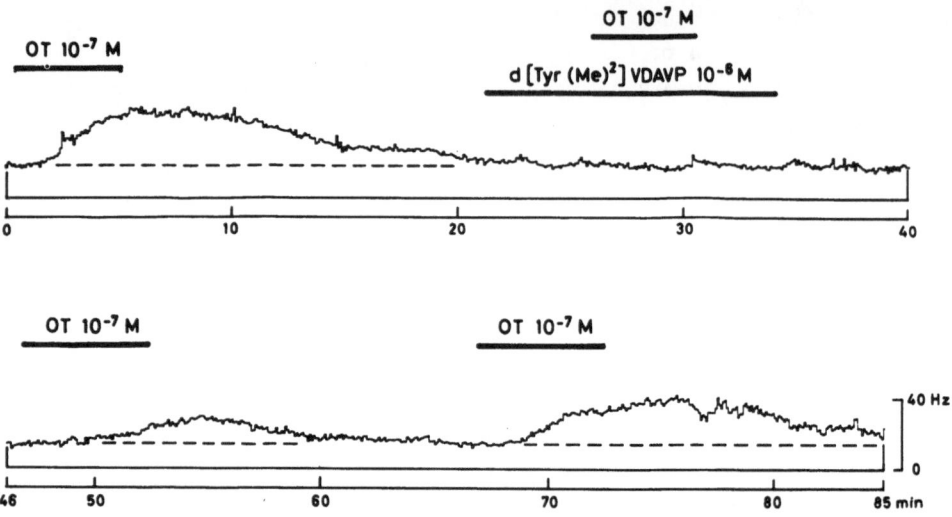

Figure 7. Reversible antagonism of oxytocin (OT) effect on a CA$_1$ neuron by a synthetic structural analog that is an oxytocic and vasopressor antagonist. OT, 0.1 μM, was applied to the bath (during the periods indicated by thick lines) before, during, and after application of the antagonist, d[Tyr(Me)^2]VDAVP, 1 μM. Continuous rate-meter record, except for 6-min deletion. (From Mühlethaler et al., 1983, with permission.)

with a class of receptors for oxytocin similar to those present on uterine cells.

The spontaneously active neurons excited by oxytocin and vasopressin represent only a small percentage of the total number of cells present in the CA$_1$ area of hippocampal slices. Their short duration and low amplitude action potentials, as well as their high rate of spontaneous activity suggested that they are nonpyramidal neurons. The effect of oxytocin and vasopressin on these cells was shown to be postsynaptic, since it persisted in low-calcium, high-magnesium media known to block synaptic transmission (Mühlethaler et al., 1984a).

In contrast, pyramidal neurons were either unaffected or inhibited by oxytocin and vasopressin (Fig. 8A,B). This inhibitory effect was most likely mediated indirectly since neurohypophysial peptides increased the rate of occurrence of spontaneous inhibitory postsynaptic potentials in these cells (Fig. 8C), in addition to causing membrane hyperpolarization. These postsynaptic potentials are due to the release of GABA from inhibitory interneurons. In the hippocampus, such interneurons are few in number, but each has an axon with extensive local ramifications. Thus, although the density of fibers immunoreactive to vasopressin or oxytocin is moderate, interneurons endowed with receptors for oxytocin could transynaptically modulate the activity of a great number of pyramidal neurons.

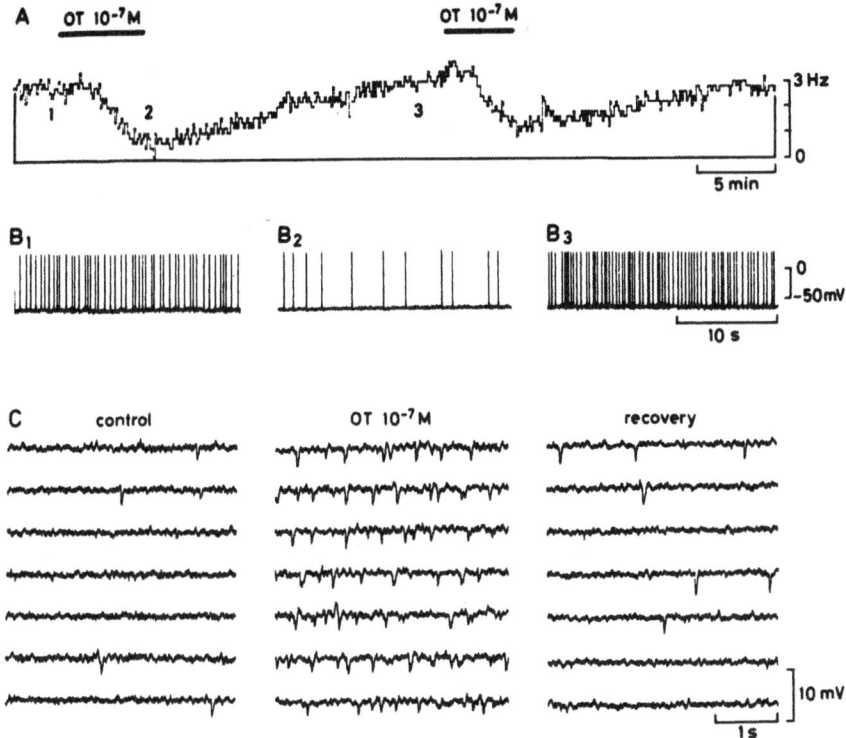

Figure 8. Effects of oxytocin (OT) on the rate of firing and rate of occurence of spontaneous inhibitory postsynaptic potentials (IPSPs) in two pyramidal neurons recorded intracellularly. (A) Rate-meter record of a spontaneously active pyramidal neuron; OT at 0.1 μM, applied to the bath during the periods indicated by thick horizontal lines caused a reversible decrease in firing. (B1–B3) Oscilloscope tracings of action potentials of the same cell at times indicated by numbers in (A). (C) Effect of OT on the rate of occurrence of IPSPs in another hippocampal pyramidal neuron, which had no spontaneous action potentials. Oscilloscope traces are shown before (left panel), during (middle panel) and following (right panel) bath application of OT, 0.1 μM.

2.2. Dorsal Motor Nucleus of the Vagus Nerve

Electrophysiological actions of vasopressin and oxytocin have been assessed in slices from the rat brainstem, in particular in the dorsal motor nucleus of the vagus, which contains the cell bodies of parasympathetic preganglionic neurons.

Neurons whose localization in the dorsal motor nucleus was verified by extracellular staining responded to oxytocin and vasopressin by an increase in firing rate (Fig. 9) Oxytocin was always more potent than vasporessin; the specific oxytocic agonist, HO[Thr⁴,Gly⁷]OT, was as effective as oxytocin; and

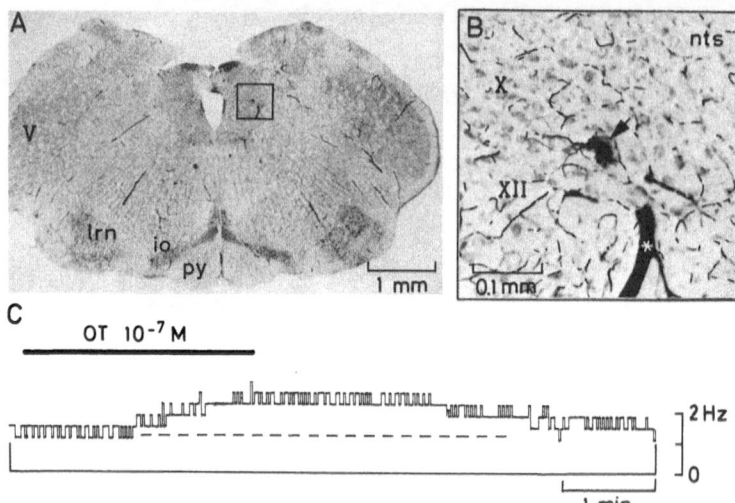

Figure 9. Neuron located in the dorsal motor nucleus of the vagus (X) and its response to oxytocin (OT) added to the perfusion medium. The experiment was performed in a slice of the brainstem and used extracellular unit recording and horseradish peroxidase (HRP) labeling of the recording site. Following recording, HRP was ejected by microiontophoresis and the slice then processed for diaminobenzidine histochemistry and counterstained with cresyl violet (A). Region outlined in square in A, printed at higher magnification in B, shows site of recording (arrow) to be within confines of X. (C) Rate-meter record to show reversible effect of OT, 0.1 μM, on unit's firing rate. Abbreviations: io, inferior olive; lrn, lateral reticular nucleus; nts, nucleus of the solitary tract; py, pyramidal tract; V, trigeminal nucleus; XII, hypoglossal nucleus; *, blood vessel. (From Charpak et al., 1984, with permission.)

an antagonistic structural analog, d[Tyr(Me)²]VDAVP, blocked the excitatory effect of oxytocin (Charpak et al., 1984). These data suggest that similar receptors for neurohypophysial peptides are present in both the hippocampus and the vagal complex.

2.3. Spinal Cord

Fibers immunoreactive for neurohypophysial peptides (mainly oxytocin) are present in laminae I–III and in the central grey matter at all levels of the spinal cord. In addition, at thoracic and lumbar levels, oxytocin fibers are also found in the intermediolateral cell column. Gilbey and co-workers (1982) applied oxytocin and vasopressin by iontophoresis onto antidromically identified preganglionic sympathetic cells located in this cell column. Both peptides exerted inhibitory effects on neurons that were also inhibited by stimulating the area of the paraventricular nucleus. Therefore, descending spinal projections from hypothalamic neurons containing oxytocin and vasopressin might be involved in modulating autonomic function.

In addition to these autonomic effects, it has been shown in isolated spinal cords from neonatal rats that vasopressin and oxytocin, at low concentrations, induce a marked membrane depolarization of motoneurons (Suzue et al., 1982).

2.4. Supraoptic Magnocellular Neurons

In 1964, Kandel obtained intracellular recordings from neurons of the preoptic nucleus of the goldfish, a structure equivalent to the supraoptic and paraventricular nuclei in mammals. He found that antidromically conducted action potentials induced by stimulation of the pituitary stalk were followed by a membrane hyperpolarization of synaptic origin. This phenomenon, and an equivalent one seen in mammals, suggested that axon collaterals of magnocellular neurons might form a recurrent inhibitory pathway. It followed that vasopressin (or vasotocin in fishes), in addition to its release from the posterior pituitary gland, might be released in the supraoptic nucleus where it could mediate hyperpolarization of magnocellular neurons. These considerations led some groups to assess effects of vasopressin in the supraoptic nucleus (for references, see Dyball and Paterson, 1983). However, despite the attractiveness of the hypothesis, vasopressin is probably not the transmitter of recurrent inhibition, since the latter was found to be present in homozygous Brattleboro rats, which are incapable of producing vasopressin.

Using coronal slices from the guinea pig hypothalamus, Abe et al. (1983) recently recorded intracellularly from supraoptic neurons and showed that lysine-vasopressin added to the bath at concentrations of 0.1–2.0 μM, produced a concentration-dependent membrane depolarization (Fig. 10). No change in membrane conductance was observed. The depolarization induced by vasopressin persisted in the absence of synaptic transmission and was not dependent upon the external concentration of K^+, Ca^{2+} or Cl^-. However, when the external Na^+ concentration was lowered, the amplitude of the depolarizing response was reduced, although not markedly, possibly indicating that the effect is due to activation of a sodium conductance.

Since vasopressin binding to V_2 receptors in kidney is associated with a stimulation of adenylate cyclase, the authors reasoned that a similar mechanism might apply in the supraoptic nucleus. As expected, the depolarizing response to vasopressin on supraoptic neurons was mimicked by dibutyryl cyclic AMP and was potentiated in the presence of phosphodiesterase inhibitors. Moreover, the content of cyclic AMP in the slices was increased by vasopressin, although it is not known that this occurs in the magnocellular neurons. Finally, oxytocin was found to be 100 times less potent than vasopressin, the same relative potency ratio for the effects of the peptides on peripheral vasopressin receptors. These results suggest that the effects of vasopressin on supraoptic neurons may be mediated by its binding to a V_2-type receptor.

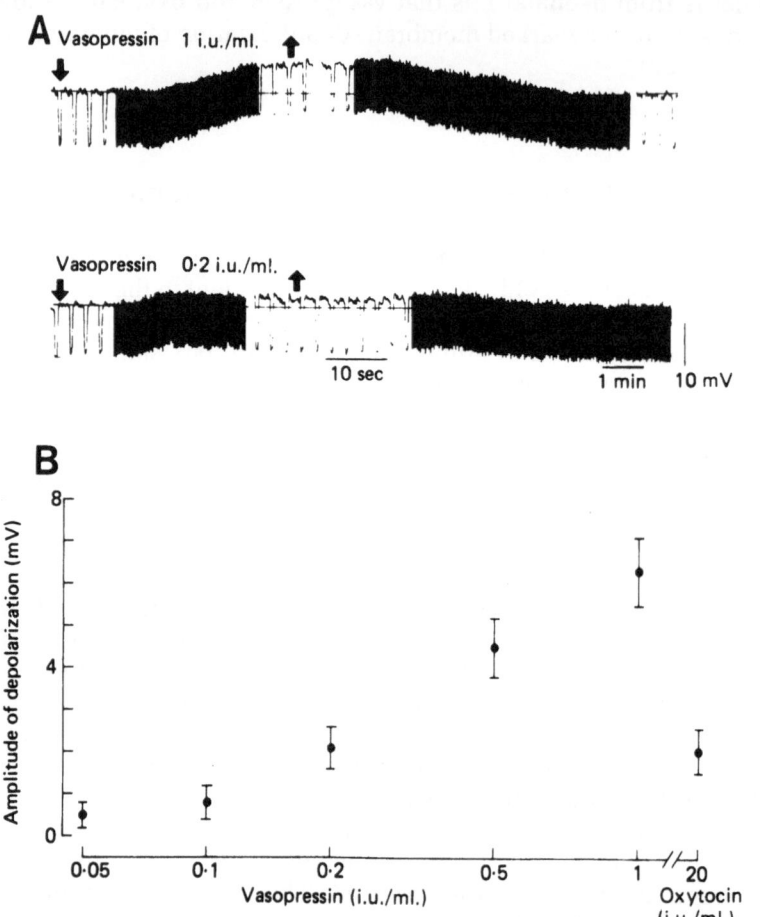

Figure 10 Effect of various concentrations of vasopressin on the membrane potential of supraoptic neurons recorded with intracellular electrodes in hypothalamic slices. (A) Membrane
depolarization induced by lysine vasopressin at 2 μM (1 I.U./ml, upper trace) and 0.4 μM (0.2
I.U./ml, lower trace). Downward deflections reflect potential changes to hyperpolarizing current
injections and show that vasopressin applied during the time indicated by arrows did not affect
membrane conductance. (B) Dose–response relationship for membrane depolarization produced
by vasopressin. The mean membrane potential change induced by 40 μM (20 I.U./ml) oxytocin
is also illustrated. (Adapted from Abe et al., 1983, with permission.)

3. CELLULAR ACTIONS OF VASOPRESSIN AND OXYTOCIN IN INVERTEBRATES

In invertebrate ganglia, electrophysiological investigations of vasopressin and oxytocin action are made easier by the large size of "identified"
neurons. Two large neurosecretory neurons involved in egg laying (cell 11

in the land snail *Otala lactea*) and in the regulation of water balance (cell R15 in the sea mollusc *Aplysia californica*) have been extensively studied (see Barker, 1977; Mühlethaler et al., 1984b, for review).

In dormant *Otala*, intracellular recordings from cell 11 show either no spiking activity or a random activity without bursting pacemaker potentials. Lysine-vasopressin initiated intermittent bursts of action potentials (Fig. 11). The whole structure of the vasopressin molecule is needed to produce this effect, since either the cyclic part alone or the linear part alone or vasopressin deprived of its glycinamide terminal were inactive. On the other hand, oxytocin was as potent as vasopressin.

Using voltage-clamp techniques, Barker and Smith (1976) found that exogenous vasopressin alters the shape of the current–voltage relation by inducing a region with a negative slope. On the basis of ionic substitution experiments they deduced that this effect was due to peptide activation of a voltage-dependent sodium current having a slow inactivation time. It was concluded that this conductance accounts for the initiation of the bursting pacemaker potential. Vasopressin was also found, by analysis of tail currents, to alter the amplitude and kinetics of a voltage-dependent potassium conductance, which is believed to reverse the depolarization.

Levitan and co-workers (1979) addressed the question of the intracellular mechanisms mediating these effects. They observed that bursting pacemaker potentials could be elicited in cell R15 of *Aplysia* and in cell F1 of *Helix pomatia* by phosphodiesterase inhibitors that increase the intracellular levels of both cyclic AMP and cyclic GMP. Neither cyclic AMP alone nor cyclic GMP alone was able to induce oscillatory activity. They also found that vasopressin, oxytocin, as well as ganglionic extracts, were able to increase the level of cyclic nucleotides in *Aplysia* and *Helix* ganglia. They therefore proposed that an endogenous vasopressinlike compound present in invertebrate ganglia increases the levels of both cyclic AMP and cyclic GMP and thereby induces bursting activity.

The endogenous compound that produces vasopressinlike effects was

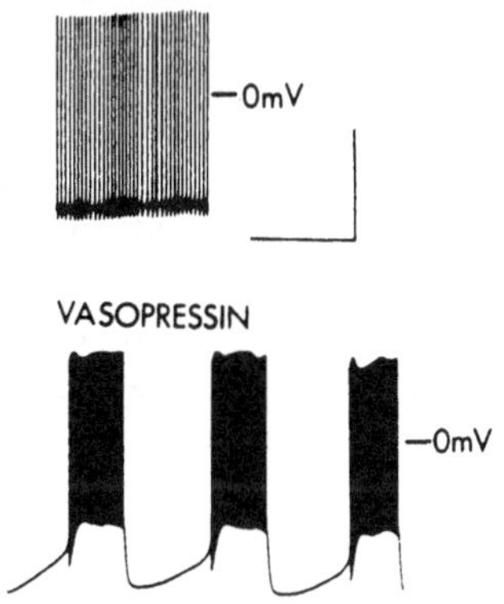

Figure 11 Effect of vasopressin on cell 11 from the snail *Otala lactea*. Cell activity is shown before and during application of vasopressin, 1 μM. Vasopressin caused the cell, which was beating regularly, to adopt a bursting pattern of activity. Calibrations: 50 mV, 20 sec. (Adapted from Barker and Smith, 1976, with permission.)

found, in recent studies to be arginine vasotocin (AVT). In *Aplysia* abdominal ganglia, synthetic AVT, perfused at concentrations as low as 1 pM, induced bursting activity in cell R15 but decreased the activity of cells L3–L7 in the same ganglion. The decrease in activity of cell L7, a central gill motoneuron, is of interest since AVT inhibits a reflex withdrawal of the gill after siphon stimulation (Thornhill et al., 1981). Since AVT also accelerated the rate of habituation, this reflex could serve as a model for studying the effects of neurohypophysial peptides on the electrophysiological correlates of a specific behavior.

4. CONCLUSION AND FUNCTIONAL CONSIDERATIONS

Although oxytocin and vasopressin were the first neuropeptides to be isolated and synthesized, it is only recently that their role as neurotransmitters has been seriously investigated. Studies to date have demonstrated a predominantly excitatory action of the peptides on neurons that is mediated by uterine smooth muscle-type oxytocin receptors, but the cellular mechanisms underlying this action are as yet unknown. On the other hand, there is a suggestion that the depolarizing effect of vasopressin in the basal hypothalamus is mediated by kidney-type (V_1) vasopressin receptors linked to adenylate cyclase. Inhibitory effects that may be physiologically relevant also occur, such as on cells in the intermediolateral cell column of the spinal cord.

Although little is known about the functional role of neurohypophysial peptides as central neurotransmitters, the data obtained from experiments performed in brainstem and spinal cord suggest that oxytocin- and vasopressin-containing neurons could regulate neuroendocrine and autonomic activities. It is also tempting to speculate that the central actions of neurohypophysial peptides complement their endocrine effects, with vasopressin, for example, acting in both the CNS and periphery to achieve an integrated response to changes in the internal milieu.

Many years ago it was proposed that vasopressin may affect the retention of conditioned avoidance tasks in rats (for review, see De Weid, 1980). Other studies suggest that neurohypophysial peptides play a role in the expression of behaviors related to reproduction. Acting as an hormone, oxytocin is involved in parturition and lactation, whereas, acting centrally, it facilitates maternal behavior (Pedersen et al., 1982) and the milk-ejection reflex (Freund-Mercier and Richard, 1981). It therefore seems to participate at various levels in an integrated system aimed at insuring the birth and the survival of the newborn mammal.

ACKNOWLEDGMENT. Supported in part by Swiss NSF grant No. 3.560.083.

REFERENCES

Abe, H., Inoue, M., Matsuo, T., and Ogata, N., 1983, The effects of vasopressin on electrical activity in the guinea-pig supraoptic nucleus in vitro, *J. Physol. (Lond.)* **337**: 665–685.

Barberis, C., 1983, [³H] vasopressin binding to rat hippocampal synaptic plasma membrane. Kinetic and pharmacological characterization, *FEBS Lett.* **162**:400–405.

Bargmann, W., and Scharrer, E., 1951, The site of origin of the hormones of the posterior pituitary, *Am. Sci.* **39**:255–259.

Barker, J. L., 1977, Physiological roles of peptides in the nervous system, in: *Peptides in Neurobiology* (H. Gainer, ed.) Plenum Press, New York, pp. 295–343.

Barker, J. F., and Smith, T. C., 1976, Peptide regulation of neuronal membrane properties, *Brain Res.* **103**:167–170.

Barry, J., 1961, Recherches morphologiques et expérimentales sur la glande diencéphalique et l'appariel hypothalamo-hypophysaire, *Annales Scientifiques de l'Université de Besanfon, Zoologie et Physiologie*, 2ᵐᵉ série, fasc. 15, 135 pp.

Biegon, A., Terlou, M., Voorhuis, T. D., and de Kloet, E. R., 1984, Arginine-vasopressin binding sites in rat brain: A quantitative autoradiographic study, *Neurosci. Lett.* **44**:229–234.

Brownstein, M. J., 1983, Biosynthesis of vasopressin and oxytocin, *Annu. Rev. Physiol.* **45**: 129–135.

Buijs, R. M., 1983, Vasopressin and oxytocin—their role in neurotransmission, *Pharmacol. Ther.* **22**:127–141.

Buijs, R. M., and Swaab, D. R., 1979, Immuno-electron microscopical demonstration of vasopressin and oxytocin synapses in the limbic system of the rat, *Cell Tissue Res.* **204**:353–365.

Buijs, R. M., and Van Heerikhuize, J. J., 1982, Vasopressin and oxytocin release in the brain—a synaptic event, *Brain Res.* **252**:71–76.

Charpak, S., Armstrong, W. E., Mühlethaler, M., and Dreifuss, J. J., 1984, Stimulatory action of oxytocin on neurones of the dorsal motor nucleus of the vagus nerve, *Brain Res.* **300**:83–89.

De Vries, G. J., and Buijs, R. M., 1983, The origin of the vasopressinergic and oxytocinergic innervation of the rat brain, with special reference to the lateral septum, *Brain Res.* **273**: 307–317.

De Wied, D., 1980, Behavioural actions of neurohypophysial peptides, *Proc. R. Soc. Lond. B.* **210**:183–195.

Du Vigneaud, V., 1956, Trails of sulfur research: From insulin to oxytocin, *Science* **123**:967–974.

Dyball, R. E. J., and Paterson, T., 1983, Neurohypophysial hormones and brain function: The neurophysiological effects of oxytocin and vasopressin, *Pharmacol. Ther.* **20**:419–443.

Freund-Mercier, M. J., and Richard, P., 1981, Excitatory effects of intraventricular injections of oxytocin on the milk-ejection reflex in the rat, *Neurosci. Lett.* **23**:193–198.

Gilbey, M. P., Coote, J. H., Fleetwood-Walker, S., and Peterson, D. F., 1982, The influence of the paraventriculo-spinal pathway, and oxytocin and vasopressin on sympathetic preganglionic neurones, *Brain Res.* **251**:283–296.

Heller, H., 1974, History of neurohypophysial research, in: Handbook of Physiology, Section 7, Endocrinology, vol. IV, part 1, (E. Knobil and W. H. Sawyer, eds.) American Physiological Society, Washington, D.C., pp 103–116.

Ivell, R., Schmale, H., and Richter, D., 1983, Vasopressin and oxytocin precursors as model preprohormones, *Neuroendocrinology* **37**:235–239.

Jard, S., 1983, Vasopressin isoreceptors in mammals: Relation to cyclic AMP-dependent and cyclic AMP-independent transduction mechanisms, *Curr. Top. in Membr. Trans.* **19**:255–285.

Joëls, M., and Urban, I. J. A., 1982, The effect of microiontophoretically applied vasopressin and oxytocin on single neurones in the septum and dorsal hippocampus of the rat, *Neurosci. Lett.* **33**:79–84.

Kandel, E., 1964, Electrical properties of hypothalamic neuroendocrine cells, *J. Gen. Physiol.* **47**:691–717.

Levitan, I. B., Harmar, A. J., and Adams, W. B., 1979, Synaptic and hormonal modulation of a neuronal oscillator: A search for molecular mechanisms, *J. Exp. Biol.* **81**:131–151.

Michell, R. H., Kirk, C. J., and Billah, M. M., 1979, Hormonal stimulation of phosphatidylinositol breakdown with particular reference to the hepatic effects of vasopressin, *Biochem. Soc. Trans.* **7:**86–89.

Moss, R. L., Dyball, R. E. J., and Cross, B. A., 1972, Excitation of antidromically identified neurosecretory cells of the paraventricular nucleus by oxytocin applied iontophoretically, *Exp. Neurol.* **34:**95–102.

Morris, R., Salt, T. E., Sofroniew, M. V., and Hill, R. G., 1980, Actions of microiontophoretically applied oxytocin, and immunohistochemical localisation of oxytocin, vasopressin and neurophysin in the rat caudal medulla, *Neurosci. Lett.* **18:**163–168.

Mühlethaler, M., Charpak, S., and Dreifuss, J. J., 1984a, Contrasting effects of neurohypophysial peptides on pyramidal and non-pyramidal neurones in the rat hippocampus, *Brain Res.* **308:**97–107.

Mühlethaler, M., Dreifuss, J. J., and Gähwiler, B. H., 1982, Vasopressin excites hippocampal neurons, *Nature* **296:**749–751.

Mühlethaler, M, Raggenbass, M., and Dreifuss, J. J., 1984b, Peptides related to vasopressin in invertebrates, *Experientia* **40:**777–782.

Mühlethaler, M., Sawyer, W. H., Manning, M. M., and Dreifuss, J. J., 1983, Characterization of a uterine-type oxytocin receptor in the rat hippocampus, *Proc. Natl. Acad. Sci. USA* **80:** 6713–6717.

Nicoll, R. A., and Barker, J. L., 1971, The pharmacology of recurrent inhibition in the supraoptic neurosecretory system, *Brain Res.* **35:**501–511.

Normanton, J. R., and Gent, J. P., 1983, Comparison of the effects of two "sleep" peptides, delta sleep-inducing peptide and arginine-vasotocin, on single neurones in the rat and rabbit brain stem, *Neuroscience* **8:**107–114.

Olpe, H. R., and Baltzer, V., 1981, Vasopressin activates noradrenergic neurones in the rat locus coeruleus: A microiontophoretic investigation, *Eur. J. Pharmacol.* **73:**377–378.

Pedersen, C. A., Ascher, J. A., Monroe, Y. L., and Prange, A. J., Jr., 1982, Oxytocin induces maternal behavior in virgin female rats, *Science* **216:**648–650.

Sawyer, W. H., Grzonka, Z., and Manning, M., 1981, Neurohypophysial peptides, Design of tissue specific agonists and antagonists, *Mol. Cell. Endocrinol.* **22:**117–134.

Sofroniew, M. V., 1983, Morphology of vasopressin and oxytocin neurons and their central and vascular projections, in: *The Neurohypophysis: Structure Function and Control*, Progress in Brain Research, Vol. 60 (B. A. Cross and G. Leng, eds.) Elsevier, Amsterdam, pp. 101–114.

Sofroniew, M. V., and Weindl, A., 1981, Central nervous system distribution of vasopressin, oxytocin and neurophysin, in: *Endogenous Peptides and Learning and Memory Processes* (J. L. Martinez, R. A. Jensen, R. B. Messing, H. Rigter, and J. L. McGaugh, eds.) Academic Press, London, pp. 327–369.

Soloff, M. S., Schroeder, B. T., Chakraborthy, J., and Pearlmutter, A. F., 1977, Characterization of oxytocin receptors in the uterus and mammary gland, *Fed. Proc.* **36:**1861–1866.

Suzue, T., Yanaihara, N., and Otsuka, M., 1981, Actions of vasopressin, gastrin-releasing peptide and other peptides on neurons of newborn rat spinal cord *in vitro*, *Neurosci. Lett.* **26:** 137–142.

Swanson, L. W., and Sawchenko, P. E., 1983, Hypothalamic integration: organization of the paraventricular and supraoptic nuclei, *Ann. Rev. Neurosci.* **6:**269–324.

Tiberiis, B. E., McLennan, H., and Wilson, N., 1983, Neurohypophysial peptides and the hippocampus. II. Excitation of rat hippocampal neurones by oxytocin and vasopressin applied in vitro, *Neuropeptides* **4:**73–86.

Thornhill, J. A., Lukowiak, K., Cooper, K. E., Veale, W. L., and Edström, J. P., 1981, Arginine vasotocin, an endogenous neuropeptide of Aplysia, suppresses the gill withdrawal reflex and reduces the evoked synaptic input to central gill motor neurons, *J. Neurobiol.* **12:** 533–544.

Van Leeuwen, F. W., and Wolters, P., 1983, Light microscopic autoradiographic localization of [^{3}H]arginine-vasopressin binding sites in the rat brain and kidney, *Neurosci. Lett.* **41:**61–66.

16

Luteinizing Hormone-Releasing Hormone

YUH NUNG JAN and LILY YEH JAN

1. INTRODUCTION

1.1. Overview

Luteinizing hormone-releasing hormone (LHRH), originally isolated from mammalian hypothalami, has well-established functions in mediating hypothalamic control of pituitary hormone release (Blackwell and Guillemin, 1973; Schally et al., 1973). Parvicellular hypothalamic neurons that contain LHRH project to portal vessels originating in the median eminence. The LHRH peptides released into the portal capillaries are carried to the anterior pituitary by the hypophyseal portal circulation to trigger the release of luteinizing hormone and follicle-stimulating hormone. Besides functioning as a neuroendocrine hormone, LHRH-like peptides may serve other functions in the central nervous system and in the periphery. Detailed analyses of LHRH action at the cellular level have been possible in the peripheral nervous system (sympathetic ganglia) because of its easy access to experimentation. For this reason, much of the attention concerning the cellular action of LHRH will be directed to studies of the peripheral nervous system, while knowledge concerning the distribution and function of LHRH at the central nervous system will only be summarized briefly in this chapter.

1.2. LHRH-like Peptide

The chemical structure of LHRH in mammals was characterized in the early seventies (Matsuo et al., 1971; Burgus et al., 1972). It is a decapeptide

459

of the sequence pGlu-His-Trp-Ser-Tyr-Gly-Leu-Arg-Pro-Gly-NH$_2$. Recently the primary structure of a teleost LHRH has been determined (Sherwood et al., 1983). It differs from the mammalian LHRH by two amino acids. The seventh amino acid in the mammalian peptide tryptophane, is replaced by leucine and the eighth amino acid, leucine, is replaced by arginine. In the bullfrog nervous system, two LHRH-like peptides have been found; one is identical to mammalian LHRH in amino acid composition, while the other one is immunologically and chromatographically distinct from mammalian LHRH (Eiden and Eskay, 1980; Eiden et al., 1982; Rivier et al., 1981; King and Millar, 1982b).

In mammalian reproductive organs, the LHRH-like peptide was also found to be different from the decapeptide from mammalian hypothalami (McCann, 1982; Sharpe et al., 1981). The fact that more than one LHRH-like peptide are found in the same animal raises the interesting possibility that a family of structurally related LHRH-like peptides may be differentially expressed in different tissues for different functions.

1.3. Distribution of LHRH-like Peptide in the Central Nervous System

Extrapituitary actions of LHRH in the central nervous system have been implicated because LHRH-positive neurons and terminals are found in many extrahypothalamic sites (for review, see Elde and Hökfelt, 1979; Krey and Silverman, 1983). LHRH-positive neurons have been found in septal nuclei, diagonal bands of Broca, the preoptic region, the anterior and medial basal hypothalami, the hippocampus, the prepiriform and the cingulate cortex, the main and the accessory olfactory bulbs, and the amygdala. In most cases, LHRH-positive fibers are found in close contact with ventricular or vascular structures. However, LHRH-positive nerve terminals that form asymmetric synaptic contacts with other neurons have been observed in the accessory olfactory bulb of male hamsters, suggesting that LHRH may play a role in neuronal signaling (Phillips et al., 1982). In the gold fish, LHRH-positive neurons in the olfactory nerve project to the retina and may have physiological effects on ganglion cells (Stell et al., 1984). Possible physiological functions of LHRH in the central nervous system, as indicated from its anatomical distribution, its behavioral effects, and its known physiological effects, will be discussed in Section 4.

1.4. Receptors for LHRH

The pharmacology of the LHRH receptor in mammalian pituitary has been extensively studied (Vale et al., 1977; Schally and Coy, 1977). Literally hundreds of LHRH analogs have been synthetized and a number of potent agonists and antagonists have been found. Some of the most potent ("super") agonists have the glycine at the position 6 replaced by D-amino acids, the glycine at position 10 eliminated, and an ethylamide attached to proline at position 9. These analogs are more resistant to degradation and may also have higher receptor affinity (Vale et al., 1977). More recently, several super antagonists have been generated, which involve amino acid substitutions at the first, second, and third position, plus the afore-mentioned modifications used for generating super agonists (e.g., see Rivier and Vale, 1978). Some of these analogs have been radiolabeled and used in receptor binding assays to quantify receptor levels in the pituitary, in the brain, and in the gonads.

2. LHRH-LIKE PEPTIDE IN FROG SYMPATHETIC GANGLIA: THE LATE SLOW EPSP

In sympathetic ganglia of the bullfrog, an LHRH-like peptide most likely mediates a slow synaptic potential lasting for several minutes (Jan et al. 1979; 1980a,b; Jan and Jan, 1982). In this chapter, we first review the evidence for the LHRH-like peptide to be a neurotransmitter in sympathetic ganglia and then discuss some features of this peptidergic transmission.

2.1. The Late Slow EPSP

Since the late 1930s, acetylcholine has been generally accepted as the excitatory transmitter contained in preganglionic fibers of sympathetic ganglia. In subsequent years, cholinergic fibers were found to initiate, directly or indirectly, three types of synaptic responses (see Chapter 6): (1) the nicotinic fast excitatory postsynaptic potential (EPSP), which last for about 30–50 msec and generally give rise to conducted impulses (Nishi and Koketsu, 1960); (2) the muscarinic slow EPSP, lasting 30–60 sec; and (3) the slow inhibitory postsynaptic potential of 1–2 sec duration, which are also blocked by muscarinic blockers (Nishi and Koketsu, 1968; Tosaka et al. 1968). In 1968, a fourth synaptic potential was discovered and named the "late slow EPSP," which lasts for 5–10 min and is not blocked by cholinergic blockers (Nishi and Koketsu, 1968). Examples of the four types of synaptic potentials are given in Fig. 1.

With a time course about 10,000 times slower than that of the fast EPSP, the late slow EPSP might serve functions quite different from those of the well-known fast EPSP. In order to study the function and underlying mechanism of this slow synaptic potential, we first attempted to identify its transmitter. So far, results from physiological, pharmacological and immunological studies indicate that the transmitter for the late slow EPSP is a peptide that resembles luteinizing hormone-releasing hormone (LHRH).

Slow noncholinergic synaptic potentials that are likely mediated by peptides have been detected in several autonomic nervous systems, such as

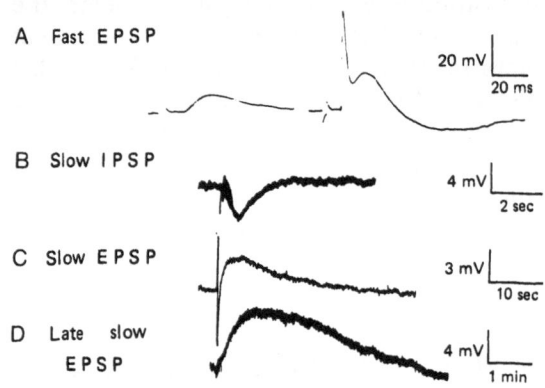

Figure 1. Four types of synaptic responses in the bullfrog tenth sympathetic ganglion recorded with intracellular electrodes. (A) Single nerve stimulus initiates a subthreshold EPSP (left); with stronger stimulation (right), a second larger EPSP produces an action potential. (B) Slow EPSP on stimulation of central portions of 7th and 8th spinal nerves (13 stimuli at 20 Hz). In this record, the fast EPSP was blocked by 1 μM dihydro-β-erythroidine. (C) Four stimuli at 50 Hz to sympathetic chain above the seventh ganglion result in a slow EPSP lasting about 30 sec. The initial rapid deflections are four large conducted impulses. (D) Late slow EPSP (300-sec duration) on stimulation of the seventh and eighth spinal nerves (50 stimuli at 10 Hz). Note different time scales. (From Jan et al., 1979, with permission.)

the guinea pig's inferior mesenteric ganglion (Tsunoo et al., 1982 and myenteric plexes (Katayama and North, 1978) (see Chapter 13). Sympathetic ganglia of the bullfrog have been particularly useful in the study of peptidergic transmission because the chain of ganglia are contained in a thin sheet of connective tissue membrane and can be viewed with Nomarski differential interference optics during electrophysiological experiments, thus making it possible to apply various chemicals iontophoretically or via pressure through micropipettes near the cell surface at precise locations. Also, sympathetic neurons in the frog do not have dendrites; presynaptic nerve terminals form synapses on the cell soma. Consequently, synaptic potentials are recorded without much attenuation and their dependence upon membrane potential may be reliably determined. As will be described later, this simple anatomy has been crucial in the analysis of peptide action.

2.2. Presence and Distribution of LHRH-like Peptides

2.2.1. Radioimmunoassays

Radioimmunoassays using an antiserum highly specific for LHRH revealed that the bullfrog sympathetic ganglia contained a high level of a LHRH-like substance (Jan et al., 1979). The LHRH-like immunoreactivity was not affected by heating in a boiling water bath but was totally destroyed by α-chymotrypsin. If the ganglion extract was passed through a Sephadex G-25 column and the various fractions were assayed for LHRH-like immunoreactivity, the LHRH-like substance was eluted at roughly the same effluent volume as LHRH. Thus, the LHRH-like substance has a molecular weight of around 1000 and is probably a peptide. As described later, although this

LHRH-like peptide is structurally similar to mammalian LHRH, it is not identical to mammalian LHRH.

2.2.2. Immunohistochemical Localization

To directly examine the possibility that the LHRH-like substance is contained in presynaptic elements, we localized the LHRH immunoreactivity in sympathetic ganglia by using various rabbit antisera specific for LHRH and the peroxidase-anti-peroxidase technique of Sternberger. LHRH immunoreactivity was indeed found in numerous nerve terminals around sympathetic neurons. This staining was totally abolished if the primary rabbit antisera were preadsorbed with LHRH (Jan et al., 1980a).

2.2.3. Effect of Denervation

Previous physiological and anatomical studies have shown that 5 days after the preganglionic fibers were cut, synaptic transmission had failed and nerve terminals of cut axons had degenerated. At this time sprouting and regrowth of preganglionic fibers had not yet taken place. Nevertheless, the ganglion cells retained their membrane potentials and gave impulses. Since preganglionic fibers that give rise to the late slow EPSP in the ninth and tenth sympathetic ganglia are known to be contained in the seventh and eighth spinal nerves (see below, Fig. 2), we can remove these preganglionic fibers selectively and test whether the LHRH-like peptide is removed at the same time. Five days after ipsilateral preganglionic axons were cut, 95% of the immunoassayable LHRH-like substance disappeared from the ninth and tenth ganglia, while the LHRH immunoreactivity tripled in the seventh and eighth spinal nerves proximal to the cut region (Jan et al., 1979). A concurrent loss of immunohistochemical staining of LHRH-positive terminals was also seen 5 days after cutting the seventh and eighth nerves (Jan et al., 1980a), suggesting that the LHRH-like substance is contained in the appropriate preganglionic fibers.

2.3. Release

If the LHRH-like substance contained in presynaptic nerve terminals is the transmitter for the late slow EPSP, it should be released either by stimulation of the preganglionic fibers or by raising the external potassium concentration. Further, since the late slow EPSP could be evoked only if solutions contained Ca^{2+}, one would expect the release of the LHRH-like substance to depend on external calcium. Indeed, about 0.6% of the LHRH-like material within ganglia can be collected from the perfusate after 30 min of incubation in isotonic KCl containing 3.2 mM Ca^{2+}. This release is abolished in isotonic KCl solutions containing magnesium, but no calcium (Jan et al., 1979). Similar release of the LHRH-like sustance was also seen after stimulating those

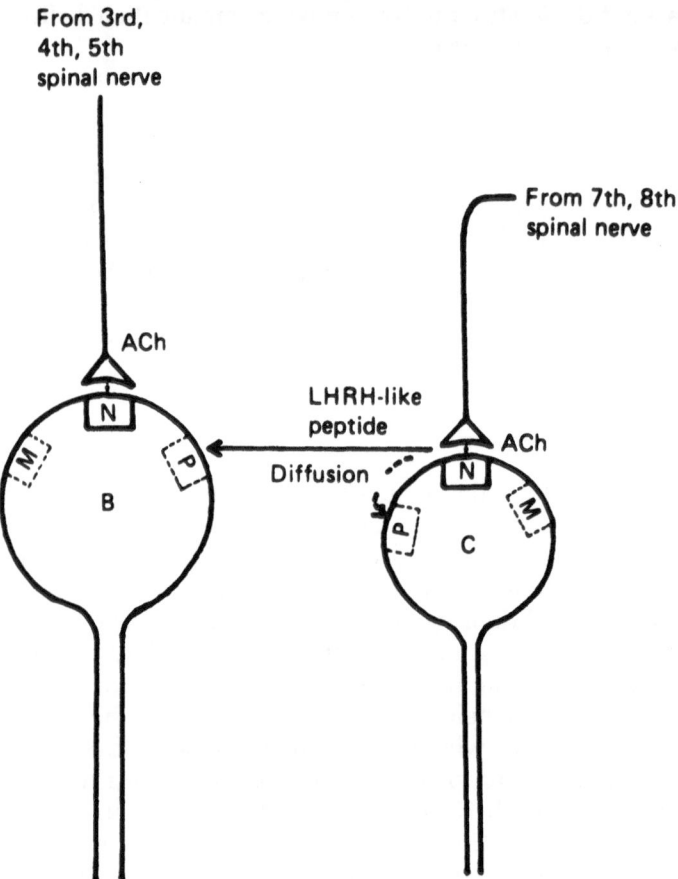

Figure 2. Scheme of innervation of neurons in ninth or tenth bullfrog sympathetic ganglia, the last two ganglia in the sympathetic chain. B cells are larger, whereas C cells are smaller. Cholinergic axons for B neurons arise from the third, fourth, and fifth spinal nerves, whereas preganglionic fibers for C cells come through the seventh and eighth spinal nerves. LHRH-positive nerve terminals are present only on C cells. Most likely, both the LHRH-like peptide and acetylcholine are contained and released from the same preganglionic fibers for C cells. N denotes nicotinic cholinergic receptors; M, muscarinic cholinergic receptors; P, LHRH receptors. Of the three types of receptors only the nicotinic cholinergic receptors have been localized. They are situated in opposition to the synaptic boutons. (From Jan and Jan, 1982, with permission.)

nerves that initiate late slow EPSPs in sympathetic neurons (Jan and Jan, 1982).

2.4. Cellular Actions of LHRH: Mimicry of the Late Slow EPSP

The physiological effects of the late slow EPSP can be mimicked by applying LHRH to the surface of sympathetic neurons: A depolarizing response in sympathetic neurons is induced by synthetic LHRH, when applied either in the bath or locally from a micropipette via a brief pulse of pressure. This depolarizing response persists in media devoid of calcium, indicating that LHRH acts directly on sympathetic neurons. The LHRH-induced depolarization resembles the late slow EPSP in considerable detail (Jan et al., 1979, 1980b; Jan and Jan, 1982; Katayama and Nishi, 1982; Kuffler and Sejnowski, 1983): (1) both are associated with similar conductance changes; (2) their amplitudes vary in parallel as the membrane potential is shifted over a wide range, suggesting that similar ionic mechanisms are involved; (3) both responses increase the excitability of the neurons; and (4) the responses interact with the cholinergic responses in a parallel manner. The similarity between physiological changes during the LHRH-induced depolarization and those during the late slow EPSP suggest that LHRH acts on the same receptors as the natural transmitter for the late slow EPSP.

2.5. Pharmacological Antagonism

Several analogs of LHRH (e.g. [D-pGlu^1,DPhe^2,D-Trp^{3,6}]- LHRH; [Ac-Δ^3-Pro^1, D-Phe^2, DTrp^{3,6}]-LHRH; [Ac-Δ^3-Pro^1,pF-D-Phe^2,D-Trp^{3,6}]- LHRH), that function as LHRH antagonists in mammalian anterior pituitary (Rivier and Vale, 1978), also block the LHRH-induced depolarization of frog sympathetic neurons. Furthermore, these antagonists also block the nerve-evoked late slow EPSP without affecting the resting membrane potential, membrane resistance, or the cholinergic synaptic potentials (Jan and Jan, 1982; Jan et al., 1980b) Fig. 3). Therefore, pharmacologically the receptor for the late slow EPSP behaves like a LHRH receptor.

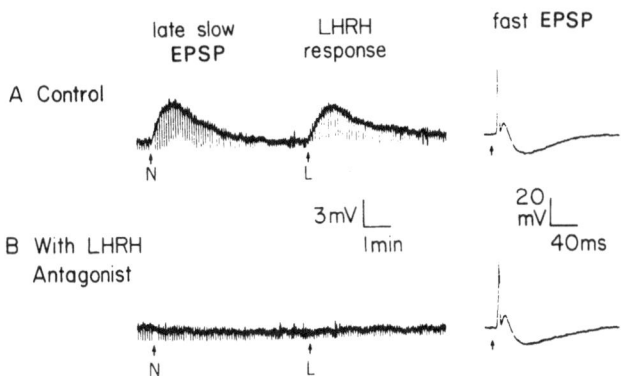

Figure 3. Effect of bath application of an antagonist of LHRH on the late slow EPSP (N), the LHRH-induced response (L), and the cholinergic fast EPSP. Applying an antagonist, [D-pGlu], D-Phe^2, D-Trp^{3,6}]-LHRH, to the bathing medium to a final concentration of 10^{-5} M had no effect on the membrane potential, the membrane resistance, or the cholinergic fast EPSP, but completely blocked both the late slow EPSP and the LHRH-induced response. (From Jan and Jan, 1982, with permission.)

Based on the above four criteria, there seems to be very little doubt that an LHRH-like peptide is the transmitter mediating the late slow EPSP. However, several issues are yet to be resolved completely. These are discussed below.

2.6. The Identity of the LHRH-like Peptide

The LHRH-like transmitter in frog sympathetic ganglia is immunologically and chromatographically similar to, but not identical to, mammalian LHRH (Jan et al., 1979; Eiden and Eskay, 1980). To date, three forms of LHRH have been described in the hypothalami of three different species: mammals, chicken, and fish (King and Millar, 1982a,b; Miyamoto et al., 1982; Sherwood et al., 1983). A recent report suggested that fish LHRH is immunologically and chromatographically most similar to the frog ganglion peptide (Eiden et al., 1982). The relative physiological potencies of mammalian, chicken, and fish LHRH have been examined on frog ganglion cells. Fish LHRH is much more potent than mammalian LHRH, which is much more potent than chicken LHRH. The threshold for a detectable depolarization produced by mammalian LHRH is about 10^{-6} M, while the threshold for fish LHRH is about 10^{-7} M. Fish LHRH-derived antagonists and super agonists are also more potent than mammalian analogs (Jan et al., 1983; Jones et al., 1984). By contrast, it has been reported that fish LHRH is only 2–3% as potent as mammalian LHRH in mammalian assay systems (Sherwood et al., 1983). The relative potency of fish LHRH in the frog ganglion supports the idea that fish LHRH is more similar than mammalian LHRH to the ganglion LHRH-like peptide. However, caution must be used in drawing conclusion about the structure of the ganglion peptide. Fish LHRH differs from mammalian LHRH at positions 7 and 8. Fish LHRH is Trp^7, Leu^8, while mammalian LHRH is Leu^7, Arg^8. It has been found that the Leu^7, Trp^8 analog, which is extremely difficult to distinguish from fish LHRH, even by HPLC (Sherwood et al., 1983), is approximately equapotent with fish LHRH on frog ganglion cells (Jan et al., 1983). Determination of the structure of the frog ganglion LHRH-like peptide must await direct determination of its amino acid sequence.

2.7. Removal of the LHRH-like Peptide after Release

In the classical picture of synaptic transmission, transmitter molecules are quickly removed after release either by enzyme degradation or by an efficient reuptake system. This does not seem to be the case for the LHRH-like peptide. As will be discussed later, the LHRH-like peptide appears to have a half life of many seconds after it is released, indicating that there are no efficient removal systems. In fact, whether removal mechanisms other than diffusion are operative at all is not yet clear.

2.8. The Ionic Basis of the Late Slow EPSP

It was first demonstrated that the late slow EPSP in bullfrog sympathetic ganglia is due to decreased potassium conductance by Shulman and Weight (1976). Adams, Brown and their colleagues later deduced from voltage-clamp studies that a particular voltage-dependent potassium conductance was affected, and that this was the same as the muscarine-sensitive potassium current, known as the M current, that is turned off during the muscarinic slow EPSP (see Chapter 6; Adams and Brown, 1980; Adams et al., 1982). In addition to its sensitivity to transmitters, the M current is distinct from other potassium currents in bullfrog sympathetic neurons in that it is activated at potentials between rest and the spike threshold, i.e., more depolarized than -60 mV, and is noninactivating. It has been possible to show using the single-electrode voltage-clamp that in the same neuron the M current is potently inhibited by fish LHRH and during the late slow EPSP evoked by stimulation (Fig. 4; Jones et al., 1984).

Although the M channel probably is an important component in generating the late slow EPSP, it cannot fully account for the ionic basis of the late slow EPSP. In addition to the M current, at least one more ionic current must be involved, because the late slow EPSP and the LHRH-induced depolarization usually persist at the potassium equilibrium potential (Jan and Jan, 1982; Katayama and Nishi, 1982; Kuffler and Sejnowski, 1983). Katayama and Nishi (1977) first classified the physiological responses of ganglion neurons into two categories. The "Type I" response is associated with a decrease in conductance, while the "Type II" response is associated with an increase in conductance. Both types of responses are often found in the same neuron. As shown in Fig. 5, at membrane potentials more positive than -60 mV, the response is mainly associated with an apparent decrease in conductance, and the response grows larger upon depolarization. At membrane potentials more negative than -60 mV, however, the response grows larger with hyperpolarization, and there is an apparent *increase* in conductance (Katayama and Nishi, 1982). The increased conductance involves mainly Na^+ permeability because replacing external Na^+ with choline eliminated the "Type II" response associated with the conductance increase (Fig. 6). Moreover, in cells with little "Type II" response (Kuffler and Sejnowski, 1983), or in cases where the Type II response was eliminated after Na^+ removal (Katayama and Nishi, 1982), a residual response associated with a conductance decrease could still be seen at membrane potentials more negative than -60 mV and this response reverses at the potassium equilibrium potential. Therefore, the conductance changes involved in the late slow EPSP probably include (1) a decrease in the voltage-dependent K^+ conductance that gives rise to the M current, (2) a decrease in the "resting" K^+ conductance that remains activated near the potassium equilibrium potential, and (3) an increase in a Na^+ conductance.

Adams and Brown (1980) suggested that LHRH acts on the same voltage-sensitive potassium current (the M current) in frog sympathetic neurons as

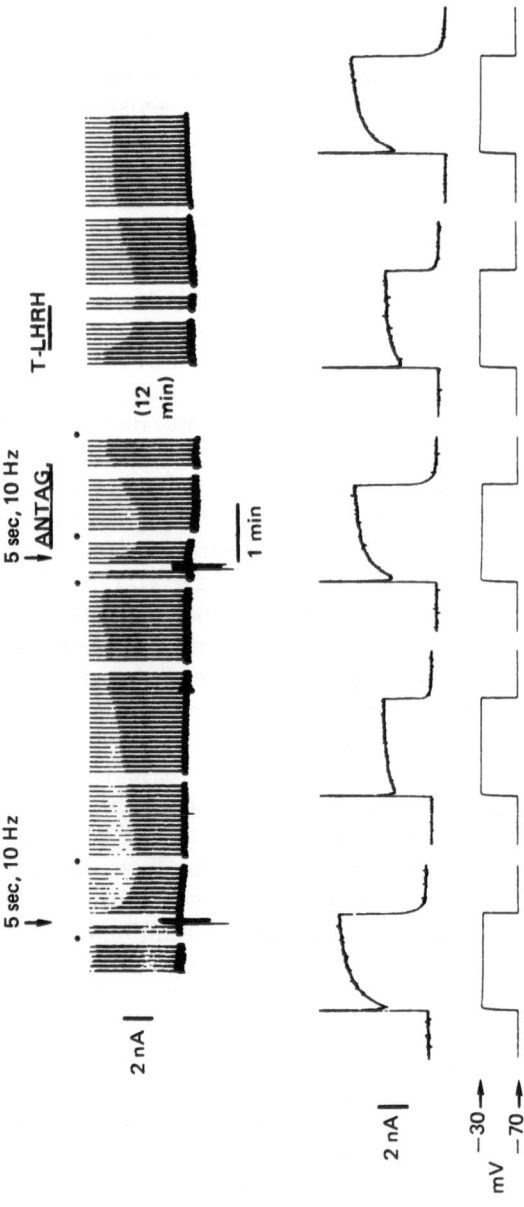

Figure 4. Single-electrode voltage-clamp recording from a bullfrog sympathetic neuron, showing inhibition of the M current during the late slow EPSP and by exogenous fish LHRH (T-LHRH). (Top) Current records for steps from −70 to −32 mV, showing the time course of the response to a train of preganglionic stimuli or to T-LHRH(25μM). During the period marked by the bar labeled ANTAG., 27 μM D-pGlu¹,D-Phe²,D-Trp³,⁶-LHRH, an LHRH antagonist, was applied. (Bottom) Records of currents (at a faster time base) evoked during voltage steps at the times marked by asterisks in top trace. The steps are 1 sec in duration. Note inhibition of slow, outward M current during LHRH. Similar inhibition of M current occurred during T-LHRH. The ganglion was bathed in atropine and d-tubocurarine to block cholinergic responses. (From Jones et al., 1984, with permission.)

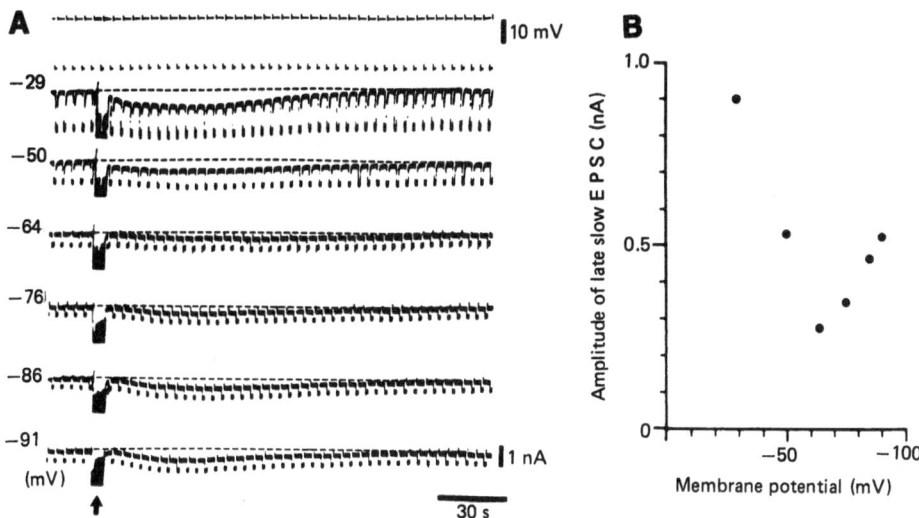

Figure 5. Voltage-clamp recording from a bullfrog sympathetic neuron in the presence of nicotine and atropine to block cholinergic synaptic potentials, showing both Type I and Type II noncholinergic responses to preganglionic stimulation. (A) The late slow excitatory postsynaptic current (EPSC) in response to supramaximal preganglionic stimulation (10 Hz for 5 sec, at arrow) at various holding potentials. Conductance was determined by repeated 1–sec hyperpolarizing steps (voltage shown on the top trace). (B) Peak amplitude of each current response in (A). (From Katayama and Nishi, 1982, with permission.)

muscarinic agonists. Although it is now apparent that LHRH affects inward sodium currents in addition to the effect on potassium currents, it is quite possible that both LHRH and muscarinic agonists act on the same potassium channels. In fact, the muscarinic slow EPSP was greatly reduced when it was initiated during the LHRH-induced or the nerve-evoked responses, even when currents were injected into the cell to counteract the effect of the peptide on the membrane potential (Jan et al., 1980b; Jan and Jan, 1982; Kuffler and Sejnowski, 1983). Such interaction between peptidergic and muscarinic responses cannot be accounted for by changes in the membrane potential or resistance, but may arise because both responses involve the same ionic channels.

3. FEATURES OF PEPTIDERGIC TRANSMISSION IN FROG SYMPATHETIC GANGLIA

Given that a peptide can function as a transmitter for a slow synaptic potential, our next question is: Do peptide transmitters serve functions qualitatively different from those of "classical" transmitters? One striking difference is that the peptidergic responses in autonomic neurons are $10–10^4$

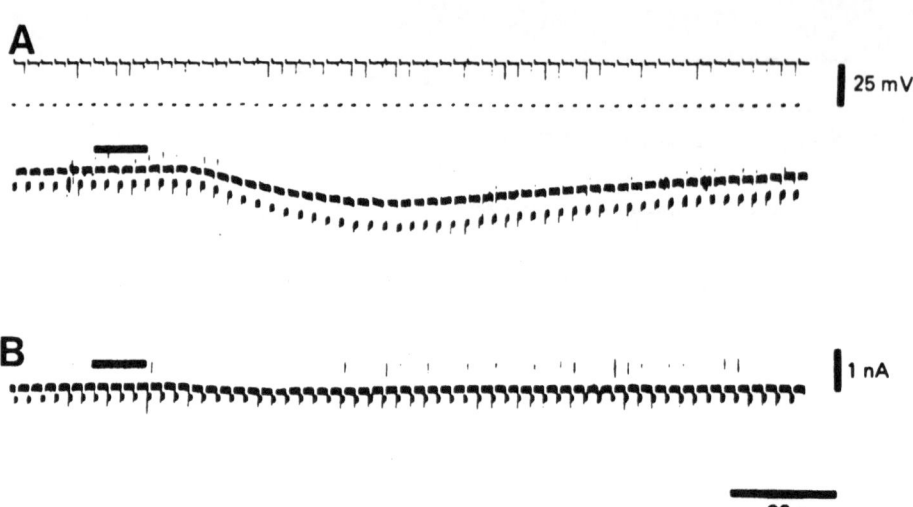

Figure 6. Voltage-clamp recording from a bullfrog sympathetic neuron, showing the effect of removal of sodium on the Type II LHRH current elicited at −50 mV. (A) Control Ringer solution. Note the increase in membrane conductance during the response to LHRH (10 μM; bar). (B) In bathing solution with choline chloride substituted for sodium chloride. The LHRH response is virtually eliminated, however a small Type I (decreased-conductance, inward current) response does remain. (From Katayama and Nishi, 1982, with permission.)

times slower than cholinergic responses (Jan et al., 1979). In frog ganglia, the slow time course of the late slow EPSP is partially due to the long lifetime of the nerve-released peptide transmitter (Jan and Jan, 1982).Further, the LHRH-like peptide appears to be contained in and released from the same preganglionic fibers as acetylcholine (Jan and Jan, 1983). While acetylcholine acts presumably only synaptically, the LHRH-like peptide can diffuse and activate sympathetic neurons that are not in synaptic contact with LHRH-positive nerve terminals. Experimental results in support of the above statements are reviewed in the following sections.

3.1. Coexistence and Corelease of LHRH-like Peptide and Acetylcholine

In the last two ganglia of the lumbar chain, the ninth and tenth ganglia, there are two classes of sympathetic neurons: the larger B cells are in synaptic contact with preganglionic B fibers arising from the third, fourth, and fifth spinal nerves, while the smaller C cells are in synaptic contact with preganglionic C fibers arising from the seventh and eighth spinal nerves. As summarized in Fig. 2, stimulating the third, fourth, and fifth spinal nerves generates cholinergic synaptic potentials in B cells only. On the other hand, stimulating the seventh and eighth spinal nerves generates the late slow EPSP in both B cells and C cells, as well as cholinergic responses in C cells. This raises the following question: Does the same preganglionic C fiber generate both cholinergic responses and the peptidergic late slow EPSP? In other words, does the same preganglionic C fiber contain and release both acetylcholine and the LHRH-like peptide?

In the absence of any known specific markers for acetylcholine or choline-acetyltransferase in frog sympathetic ganglia, we have approached this question with indirect means. In double-labeling experiments, we marked all terminals of preganglionic C fibers with horseradish peroxidase, or a monoclonal antibody specific for a 65,000-dalton vesicle membrane protein (Matthew et al., 1981), and the appropriate fluorescein-labeled second antibodies. The same terminals were then treated with rabbit antibodies against LHRH and rhodamine-labeled second antibodies that bind rabbit antibodies so that we could estimate the proportion of preganglionic C fiber terminals that contain the LHRH-like peptide. It was found that almost all terminals of preganglionic C fibers contained the LHRH-like peptide (Jan and Jan, 1983) as shown in Fig. 7. Since some of these terminals must also contain acetylcholine, which generates in C cells the fast EPSP of only 1–2 msec latency, at least some of the terminals of preganglionic C fibers must contain both acetylcholine and the LHRH-like peptide. Morphologically, terminals of preganglionic C fibers for conventional synaptic contacts with C cells and are uniform in appearance under an electron microscope. Therefore, conceivably all terminals of preganglionic C fibers may contain both acetylcholine and the LHRH-like peptide.

Physiological experiments indicate that each preganglionic C fiber probably releases both acetylcholine and the LHRH-like peptide. A sympathetic C neuron typically receives several cholinergic inputs with different thresholds for stimulation, so that one may raise the stimulation strength gradually to recruit cholinergic preganglionic fibers one by one. In doing so, it was found that each time a cholinergic fiber is recruited, repetitive stimulation at that stimulation strength also resulted in a larger late slow EPSP, indicating that the peptidergic inputs to a C cell have thresholds similar to the thresholds of its cholinergic inputs (Jan and Jan, 1983). These observations suggest that the same preganglionic fibers are responsible for both the cholinergic fast EPSP and the peptidergic late slow EPSP, thus providing evidence that coexistent transmitters can both exert postsynaptic actions on target cells through corelease.

3.2. Diffusion of LHRH-like Peptide

Although stimulating preganglionic C fibers arising from the seventh and eighth spinal nerves generates the late slow EPSP in both B cells and C cells, preganglionic C fibers were found to make synaptic contacts on C cells exclusively. Therefore, the late slow EPSP recorded in B cells must be due

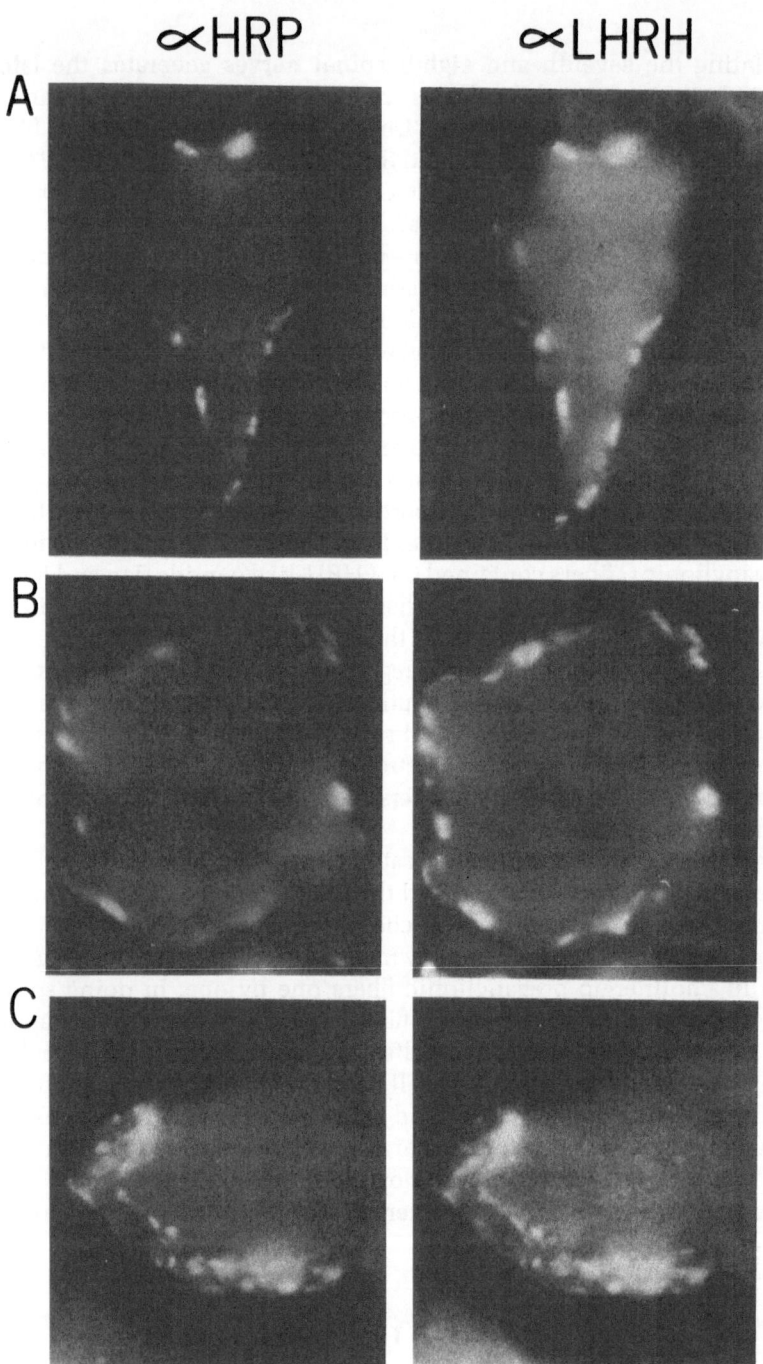

Figure 7. Double labeling of the same terminals of preganglionic C fibers with antibodies to LHRH and horseradish peroxidase (HRP). Preganglionic C fibers were first filled with HRP, then treated with fluorescein-coupled goat antibodies to HRP, rabbit antibodies to LHRH, and rhodamine-labeled goat antibodies to rabbit antibodies. Note that all terminals filled with HRP contain the LHRH-like peptide. (From Jan and Jan, 1983, with permission.)

to peptide transmitters released from preganglionic C fibers that are at a distance from B cells. Evidence in support of these statements is reviewed as follows:

3.2.1. Absence of Synaptic Contacts between C Fibers and B Cells.

If all preganglionic B fibers are destroyed by cutting the sympathetic chain between the sixth and seventh ganglion and allowed 5–10 days for their terminals to degenerate, no synaptic boutons can be seen on the larger B cells by electron microscopy, even though many synaptic boutons are present on smaller C cells. Similarly, filling the remaining preganglionic C fibers with horseradish peroxidase marked 30–50 nerve terminals around each C cell, but no terminals at all on the larger B cells (Jan et al., 1980a). These observations correlate well with immunohistochemistry, which showed that LHRH-positive terminals are found on smaller C cells, but not on the larger B cells (Jan et al., 1980a, Jan and Jan, 1982). Taken together, they showed that no synaptic contacts exist between preganglionic C fibers and B cells.

3.2.2. Nonsynaptic Actions of the Peptide Transmitter

If all preganglionic B fibers arising from the third, fourth, and fifth spinal nerves are cut as described in the preceding paragraph, recordings from neurons in the denervated ganglia 5–10 days after the operation, demonstrated an absence of cholinergic synaptic potentials in B cells with nerve stimulation. However, the late slow EPSP was still generated in those B cells with stimulation of the preganglionic C fibers arising from the seventh and eighth spinal nerves. Three of those B cells that showed the late slow EPSP, but no longer the cholinergic synaptic potentials, were serial sectioned. Electron microscopy revealed no synaptic boutons on the surface of these B cells (Jan et al., 1980a). Therefore, the late slow EPSP recorded in these B cells must be generated by preganglionic C fibers that are not in synaptic contact with their cell surface.

A late slow EPSP normally lasts for several minutes, as shown in Figs. 4 and 6. Thirty seconds after its initiation, applying an antagonist of LHRH through a micropipette caused the response to be truncated (Jan and Jan, 1982) (Fig. 8), suggesting that the LHRH analog can compete with the peptide transmitter for receptor binding 30 sec after it is released. This is probably due to the long lifetime of the peptide transmitter after release, rather than prolonged release of peptide transmitters after nerve stimulation, because applying antagonists 30 sec after a brief pulse of LHRH also caused the LHRH-induced response to be truncated (Jan and Jan, 1982). Thus, the slow time course of the late slow EPSP is partly caused by the long lifetime of the peptide transmitter. As expected, the rise time and duration of the late slow EPSP in B cells are on the average greater than those of the late slow EPSP in C cells (Jan and Jan, 1982).

In summary, an LHRH-like peptide is most likely the transmitter me-

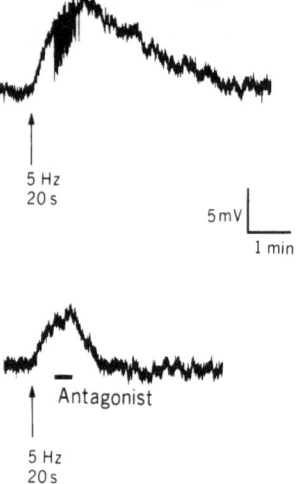

5 Hz
20 s

5 mV

1 min

Antagonist

5 Hz
20 s

Figure 8. Effect of an antagonist of LHRH on the late slow EPSP. After a late slow EPSP was initiated by stimulating the seventh and eighth spinal nerves at 5 Hz for 20 sec, pressure application of [Ac-3-Pro$_1$, pF-D-Phe$_2$, D-Trp^{3,6}]-LHRH, an antagonist of LHRH (1 lb/sq in, 25 sec), reduced both the amplitude and the duration of the late slow EPSP. The antagonist by itself has no effect on the membrane potential of this cell. Notice that the spontaneously occurring action potentials during the late slow EPSP were also eliminated. (From Jan and Jan, 1982, with permission.)

diating the late slow EPSP in the frog sympathetic ganglion, which is composed of two cell types, B cells (30–70 μm in diameter) and C cells (20–45 μm in diameter). LHRH-positive preganglionic C fibers make synaptic contacts exclusively with C cells but are capable of generating late slow EPSPs in B cells. This nonsynaptic activation of B cells is possible because the LHRH-like peptide transmitter remains active for at least 30 sec after release and can diffuse some distance before activating receptors and generating the late slow EPSP. Since B cells and C cells are juxtaposed within the ganglion and most of the LHRH-positive synaptic boutons are clustered around the axon hilloc region of C cells, the LHRH-like peptide probably has to diffuse for tens of microns before reaching the surface of B cells. On the other hand, although almost every B cell tested responded to LHRH with a depolarization, B cells from different regions of a sympathetic ganglion often showed late slow EPSPs of vastly different rise time and amplitude. Most likely the peptide transmitter does not diffuse for distances comparable to the diameter of the ganglion (~1 mm). The action of this peptide transmitter is thus analogues to that of paracrine hormones.

4. ACTIONS OF LHRH IN THE CENTRAL NERVOUS SYSTEM

The involvement of CNS LHRH in the control of reproductive behaviors has been a topic of intense interest (Shivers et al., 1983). Applying exogenous LHRH to specific sites in the CNS potentiates mating behavior (Moss, 1977; 1979). This action of LHRH persists in hypophysectomized and ovariectomized animals, implying an extrapituitary, CNS action of LHRH. Does LHRH function as a neurotransmitter in the CNS pathways involved in mating behavior? Exogenously applied LHRH is known to alter the pattern of action potentials in certain CNS neurons (Moss, 1977; Kelly and Renaud, 1978). Moreover, anti-LHRH antibodies infused into the 3rd ventricle decreased sexual receptivity of estrogen-progesterone-primed, ovariectomized rats (Koslowski and Hostetter, 1979), suggesting that endogenous LHRH is involved in nervous control of mating behavior. Further physiological studies at the cellular level are crucial for an assessment on the possible transmitter role of LHRH in these areas of the central nervous system.

In the goldfish, LHRH-positive neurons in the olfactory nerve project to the inner nuclear and inner plexiform layers of the retina (Stell et al., 1984). Furthermore, bath-applied teleost LHRH has physiological effects at micromolar concentrations on both red-ON-center and red-OFF-center double-color-opponent ganglion cells. Red-OFF-center double-color-opponent ganglion cells, for instance, are normally excited by red center or green surround at light-OFF and inhibited at light-ON. These cells are also excited by green center or red surround at light-ON and inhibited at light-OFF. Fish LHRH increases spontaneous firing rates and reduces the inhibition of firing induced by light stimuli. It further enhances the periodic, pulsatile activity induced by either light-ON or light-OFF. Interestingly, these same physiological effects can also be elicited by another peptide, FMRF-amide, and FMRF-amide-immunoreactive materials are found in the same neurons that contain LHRH immunoreactivity and project to the retina. The effect of FMRF-amide is calcium dependent, suggesting that it acts on cells that are presynaptic to the ganglion cells. Thus, it appears that both LHRH and FMRF-amide could function as transmitters and augment the response of ganglion cells to color contrast (Stell et al., 1984).

5. SUMMARY

Luteinizing hormone-releasing hormone and related peptides have been found in vertebrate hypothalami as well as other regions of the central and peripheral nervous system, and also in peripheral reproductive tissues. Besides serving as a releasing hormone controlling pituitary function, LHRH may act as a central nervous system transmitter with a role in mating behavior, retinal function and undoubtedly other CNS functions.

The physiological actions of LHRH can be studied in detail in the pheripheral nervous system. The structural simplicity of bullfrog sympathetic ganglia has allowed the demonstration that: (1) a LHRH-like peptide is the transmitter for the late slow EPSP; (2) this LHRH-like peptide probably coexists with acetylcholine in the same nerve terminals; and (3) although the peptide transmitter is most probably released together with acetylcholine from the same terminals that form conventional morphological synaptic contacts with sympathetic neurons, it can diffuse a far greater distance than acetylcholine and can act on cells nonsynaptically.

REFERENCES

Adams, P. R., and Brown, D. A., 1980, Luteinizing hormone-releasing factor and muscarinic agonists act on the same voltage-sensitive K^+ current in bull frog sympathetic neurons, Br. J. Pharmacol. **68**:353–355.

Adams, P. R., Brown, D. A., and Constanti, A., 1982, Pharmacological inhibition of the M-current, J. Physiol. (Lond.) **332**: 223–262.

Blackwell, R. E., and Guillemin, R., 1973, Hypothalamic control of adenohypophyseal secretion, Am. Rev. Physiol. **35**:357–390.

Burgus, R., Butcher, M., Amoss, M., Ling, N., Monahan, M., River, J., Fellows, R., Blackwell, R., Vale, W., and Guillemin, R., 1972, Primary structure of the hypothalamic luteinizing hormone-releasing factor (LRF) of ovine origin, Proc, Natl. Acad. Sci. USA **69**:278–282.

Eiden, L. E., and Eskay, R. L., 1980, Characterization of LRF-like immunoreactivity in the frog sympathetic ganglia: Nonidentity with LRH decapeptide, Neuropeptides **1**:29–37.

Eiden, L. E., Loumaye, E., Sherwood, N., and Eskay, R. L., 1982, Two chemically and immunologically distinct forms of luteinizing hormone-releasing hormone are differentially expressed in frog neural tissue, Peptides **3**:323–327.

Elde, R., and Hökfelt, T., 1979, Localization of hypophysiotrophic peptides and other biologically active peptides within brain, Annu. Rev. Physiol. **41**:587–602.

Jan, L. Y., and Jan Y. N., 1982, Peptidergic transmission in sympathetic ganglia of the frog, J. Physiol. (Lond.) **327**:219–246.

Jan, L. Y., Jan, Y. N., and Brownfield, M. S., 1980a, Peptidergic transmitters in synaptic boutons of sympathetic ganglia, Nature **288**: 380–382.

Jan, Y. N., and Jan, L. Y., 1983, Coexistence and corelease of cholinergic and peptidergic transmitters in frog sympathetic ganglia, Fed. Proc. **42**:2929–2933.

Jan, Y. N., Jan, L. Y., and Kuffler, S. W., 1979, A peptide as a possible transmitter in sympathetic ganglia of the frog, Proc. Natl. Acad. Sci. USA **76**:1501–1505.

Jan, Y. N., Jan, L. Y, and Kuffler, S. W., 1980b, Further evidence for peptidergic transmission in sympathetic ganglia, Proc. Natl. Acad. Sci. USA **77**:5008–5012.

Jan, Y. N., Bowers, C. W., Branton, D., Evans, L., and Jan, L. Y., 1983. Peptides in neuronal function: Studies using frog autonomic ganglia, in: Cold Spring Harbor Symp. Quant. Biol. **48**:363–374.

Jones, S. W., Adams, P. R., Brownstein, M. J., and Rivier, J. E., 1984, Teleost luteninizing hormone-releasing hormone: action on bullfrog sympathetic ganglia is consistent with role as neurotransmitter, J. Neurosci. **4**:420–429.

Katayama, Y., and Nishi, S., 1977, The ionic mechanism of the late slow EPSP in amphibian sympathetic ganglion cells, Proc Int. Union Physiol. Sci. **13**:371.

Katayama, Y., and North, R. A., 1978, Does substance P mediate slow sympathetic excitation within the myenteric plexus? **274**:387–388.

Katayama, Y., and Nishi, S., 1982, Voltage-clamp analysis of peptidergic slow depolarization in bullfrog sympathetic ganglion cells, J. Physiol. (Lond.) **333**:305–313.

Kelly, J. S., and Renaud, L. P., 1978, Pharmacology of the hypothalamic neurons, in: Pharmacology of the Hypothalamus (Cox, Morris, and Weston, eds.) University Park Press, Baltimore, pp. 63–104.

King, J. A., and Millar, R. P., 1982a, Structure of chicken hypothalamic luteinizing hormone-releasing hormone. I. Structural determination on partially purified material, J. Biol. Chem. **25**:10722–10728.

King, J. A. and Millar, R. P., 1982b, Structure of chicken hypothalamic luteinizing hormone-releasing hormone. II. Isolation and characterization, J. Biol. Chem. **25**:10729–10732.

Koslowski, G. P., and Hostetter, G., 1979, Cellular and subcellular localization and behavioral effects of gonadotropin-releasing hormone in the rat, in: Central Nervous System Effects of Hypothalamic Hormones and Other Peptides, 1st ed., Raven Press, New York, pp. 138–153.

Krey, L. C., and Silverman, A. J., 1983, Leuteinizing hormone releasing hormone, in: Brain

Peptides (D. T. Krieger, M. J. Brownstein, J. B., Martin, eds.), John Wiley and Sons, New York, pp. 687–709.

Kuffler, S. W., and Sejnowski, T. J., 1983, Peptidergic and muscarinic excitation at amphibian sympathetic synapses, *J. Physiol. (Lond.)* **341:**257–278.

Matsuo, H., Baba, Y., Nair, R., Arimura, A., and Schally, A., 1971. Structure of the procine LH- and FSH-releasing hormone. I. Proposed amino acid sequence, *Biochem Biophys. Res. Commun.* **43:**1334–1339.

Matthew, W., Tsaveler, L., and Reichardt, L. I., 1981. Identification of a synaptic vesicle specific membrane protein that is widely distributed in neuronal and neurosecretory tissue, *J. Cell Biol.* **91:**257–269.

McCann, S. M., 1982, Physiology and pharmacology of LHRH and somatostatin: *Annu. Rev. Pharmacol. Toxicol.* **22:**491–515.

Miyamoto, K., Hasegawa, Y., Minegishi, T., Nomura, M., Takahashi, Y., Igarashi, M., Kanagawa, K., and Matsuo, H., 1982. Isolation and characterization of chicken hypothalamic luteinizing hormone-releasing hormone, *Biochem, Biophys. Res. Commun.* **107:**820–827.

Moss, R. L., 1977, Role of hypophysiotropic neurohormones in mediating neural and behavioral events, *Fed. Proc.* **36:**1978–1983.

Moss, R. L., 1979, Actions of hypothalamic-hypophysiotropic hormones on the brain, *Annu. Rev. Physiol.* **41:**617–631.

Nishi, S., and Koketsu, K., 1960, Electrical properties and activities of single sympathetic neurons of frogs, *J. Cell Comp. Physiol.* **55:**15–30.

Nishi, S., and Koketsu, K., 1968, Early and late after discharges of amphibian sympathetic ganglion cells, *J. Neurophysiol.* **31:**717–728.

Phillips, H. S., Ho, B. T., and Linner, J. G., 1982. Ultrastructural localization of LH-RH-immunoreactive synapses in hamster accessory olfactory bulb, *Brain Res.* **246:**193–204.

Rivier, J., and Vale, W., 1978. [D-pGlu^1, D-Phe^2, Trp^{3,6}]-LRF. A potent luteinizing hormone releasing factor antagonist *in vitro* and inhibitor of ovulation in the rat, *Life Sci.* **23:**869–876.

Rivier, J., Rivier, C., Branton, D., Millar, R., Spiess, J., and Vale, W., 1981, HPLC purification of ovine CRF, rat extra hypothalamic brain somatostatin and frog brain GnRH, in: *Proceedings of the Seventh American Peptide Symposium* (D. H. Rich and E. Gross, eds.), pp. 771–776.

Schally, A. V., Arimura, H., and Kostin, A. J., 1973, Hypothalamic regulatory hormones, *Science* **179:**341–350.

Schally, A. V., and Coy, D. H., 1977, Stimulatory and inhibitory analogs of luteinizing hormone releasing hormone (LHRH), in: *Hypothalamic Peptide Hormones and Pituitary Regulation* (J. C. Porter, ed.), Plenum Press, New York, pp. 99–121.

Sharpe, R. M., Fraser, H. M., Cooper, I., and Romerts, F. F., 1981. Sertoli-Leydig cell communication via an LHRH-like factor, *Nature* **290:**785–787.

Sherwood, N., Eiden, L., Brownstein, M., Spiess, J., Rivier, J., and Vale, W., 1983, Characterization of a teleost gonadotropin-releasing hormone, *Proc. Natl. Acad. Sci. USA* **80:**2794–2798.

Shivers, B. D., Harlan, R. E., and Pfaff, D. W., 1983. Reproduction: The central nervous system role of luteinizing hormone releasing hormone, in: *Brain Peptides* (D. T. Krieger, M. J. Brownstein, and J. B. Martin, eds.), John Wiley and Sons, New York, pp. 389–412.

Shulman, J. A., and Weight, F., 1976, Synaptic transmission: Long-lasting potentiation by a postsynaptic mechanism, *Science* **194:**1437–1439.

Stell, W. K., Walker, S. E., Chohan, K. S., and Ball, A. K., 1984, The goldfish nervus terminalis: A luteinizing hormone-releasing hormone and molluscan cardioexcitatory peptide immunoreactive olfactoretinal pathway, *Proc. Natl. Acad. Sci. USA* **81:**940–944.

Tosaka, T., Chichibu, S., and Libet, B., 1968, Intracellular analysis of slow inhibitory and excitatory postsynaptic potentials in sympathetic ganglia of the frog, *J. Neurophysiol.* **31:**396–409.

Tsunoo, A., Konishi, S., and Otsuka, M., 1982, Substance P as an excitatory transmitter of primary afferent neurons in guinea-pig sympathic ganglia, *Neurosci.* **7:**2025–2037.

Vale, W., Rivier, C., Brown, M., and Rivier, J., 1977. Pharmacology of thyrotropin releasing factor (TRF), luteinizing hormone releasing factor (LRF), and somatostatin in *Hypothalamic Peptide Hormones and Pituitary Regulation* (J. C. Porter, Ed.), Plenum Press, New York, pp. 123–156.

PART V
ADENOSINE AND ATP

17

Adenosine and ATP

DONALD A. McAFEE and BARBARA K. HENON

1. INTRODUCTION

1.1. Historical Perspective and Overview

Previous chapters in this volume have dealt with substances whose roles as signal molecules are well established. Purines, on the other hand, are well known, not as signal molecules, but as elements of genetic material and molecules fundamental to the processes of energy metabolism. Only recently has it become generally acknowledged that purines could also function to carry out, or at least modulate, communication between excitable cells.

Purine is an unsaturated heterocyclic amine, and it is the parent for a large number of derivatives (see Fig. 1). A single amine substitution in the 6 position results in the base—adenine. The N-9 ribosyl derivative of adenine forms the nucleoside—adenosine. Phosphorylation at the 5' carbon of adenosine forms variously adenylic acid (adenosine monophosphate, AMP), cyclic 3', 5' adenosine monophosphate (cyclic AMP), adenosine diphosphate (ADP), and adenosine triphosphate (ATP). As we shall demonstrate below, the physiologic effects of these molecules can be quite distinct despite their similarity in structure.

More than 50 years ago, Drury and Szent-Gyorgyi (1929) found that simple extracts of tissues, when injected intravenously, produced profound cardiovascular effects: principally, bradycardia and hypotension. The primary active agent in these tissue extracts was adenylic acid. However, they demonstrated that adenosine had even more potent actions and went on to describe the effects of these agents on a variety of physiological systems.

These studies pointed to the pharmacological and perhaps physiological actions of purines but do not indicate a neurotransmitter role. The idea that

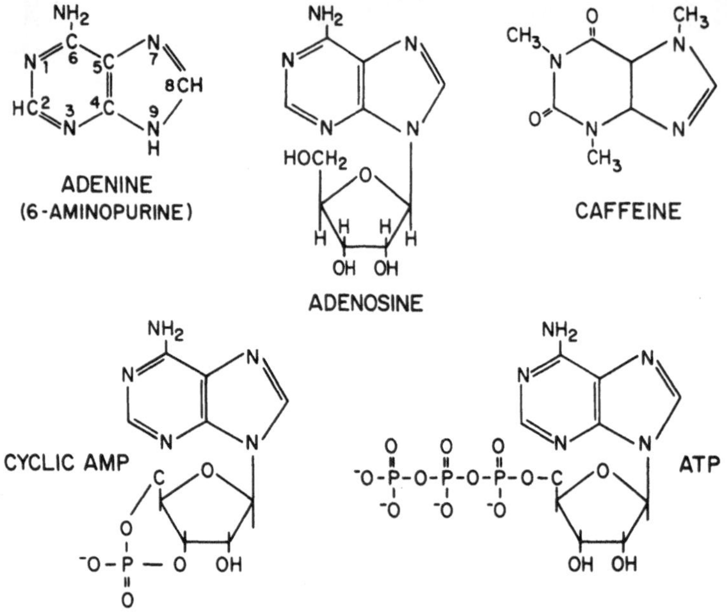

Figure 1. Structure of selected purine compounds having biological significance.

ATP might function as a neurotransmitter was first suggested by Holton and Holton (1954) on the basis of their isolation of a vasodilator substance from spinal roots. They reasoned that since the action of intra-arterially injected ATP mimicked nerve stimulation, ATP might be the neurotransmitter mediating reflex vasodilation. It is now clear that many substances can cause vasodilation. Mimicry of synaptic action by itself is insufficient evidence to conclude that a given substance is a neurotransmitter, and nearly twenty years passed before serious consideration was again given to the idea that purines could function as neurotransmitters. Geoffrey Burnstock has marshalled evidence from many different approaches suggesting that both ATP and adenosine are good candidates for neurotransmitters (Burnstock, 1981).

1.2. Defining a Neurotransmitter Role for Purines

There are a number of criteria by which to judge a substance as a neurotransmitter. The substance must be synthesized and stored in nerve terminals, released with nerve stimulation, and exogenous application must mimic the synaptic response. There should be mechanisms to inactivate the compound and pharmacologic agents that alter the synaptic response by specifically affecting various neurotransmitter mechanisms such as synthesis, release, reception, and inactivation. However, it is not clear that conventional ideas of neurotransmission always apply to purines. For instance, in addition to acting alone as neurotransmitters, they also may be stored and released simultaneously with other neurotransmitters, and, regardless of how released, function to *modulate* the action of the other neurotransmitters. In addition, ATP and adenosine can be released from tissues other than nervous tissue and may subsequently act like a hormone on adjacent tissues.

Burnstock's studies of purines grew out of observations that the relaxing effects of nerve stimulation on smooth muscle in guinea pig *taenea coli* were blocked by neither adrenergic nor cholinergic antagonists (Bennett et al., 1963). He and his colleagues (Burnstock et al., 1970) postulated the existence of enteric nerves that were nonadrenergic and noncholinergic, but utilized another transmitter. Purines were proposed as likely candidates based upon the following evidence: (1) they mimicked the effect of nonadrenergic, noncholinergic nerve stimulation; (2) ATP and adenosine were released during stimulation of nonadrenergic, noncholinergic nerves in a variety of tissues; (3) the responses to exogenous purines and to nonadrenergic, noncholinergic nerve stimulation were both blocked by certain pharmacological antagonists; and (4) blockers of adenosine uptake, such as dipyramidole, potentiated responses to purines and nerve stimulation (for reviews, see Burnstock, 1972; Burnstock et al., 1979; Burnstock, 1981). However, it now seems likely that the enteric nervous system also functions with a number of peptides as neurotransmitters. Some of these peptides, especially VIP, mimic the actions of ATP, and in fact ATP may coreside in the same nerve terminals as the peptides. Thus, there is still controversy surrounding the idea that ATP functions in the usual sense as a neurotransmitter in the gut (Campbell and Gibbons, 1979; Hills et al., 1983; Su, 1983).

1.3. Defining Receptors for Purines

Most of the physiological actions of purines are receptor-mediated. Burnstock (1978) initially described two distinct receptors. Receptors at which *adenosine* was more potent than *ATP* were labeled P_1, while at P_2 receptors the agonist potencies were reversed, and ATP was more potent. The P_1 receptor, but not the P_2 receptor is antagonized by the methylxanthines such as theophylline and caffeine. Subsequent studies have revealed at least two distinct subtypes of the P_1 adenosine receptor based upon effects of adenosine on adenylate cyclase activity. Londos and Wolff (1977) described an extracellular R regulatory receptor site requiring an unsubstituted ribose. It was found that some R receptors activated adenylate cyclase while other R receptors were inhibitory to adenylate cyclase. These were called R_a and R_i respectively by Londos and Wolff, and A_2 and A_1 respectively by Van Calker et al. (1979). To avoid any further confusion in the nomenclature, we will use the designation P_2 as the receptor most sensitive to ATP, and A_1 and A_2 for adenosine receptors as defined above and in Table 1.

Using autoradiographic techniques it has been possible to localize adenosine receptors to specific portions of the rat CNS (Goodman et al., 1983;

Table 1. Purine Receptors[a]

Receptor	Agonist Potency	Antagonists	Metabolic Effect	Physiological Effect
P_2	ATP > ADP > AMP > Ad	Arylazido-aminopropionyl ATP	Stimulation of prostaglandin synthesis	Relaxation and hyperpolarization of guinea pig taenia coli, increase in g_K
$P_1 = A_1 + A_2$	Ad > AMP > ADP > ATP			
A_1	CHA > L-PIA > 2-Cl-Ads > Ads-CPC > D-PIA	8-phenyl theophylline, caffeine	Inhibition of cyclic AMP in brain membranes	Inhibition of field EPSP in hippocampus, inhibition of $g_{Ca^{2+}}$ (?)
A_2	Ads-CPC > NECA 2-Cl-Ads > L-PIA > D-PIA	8-phenyl theophylline, caffeine	Stimulation of cyclic AMP in brain membranes and coronary tissue	Relaxation and dilation of blood vessels, inhibition of calcium spikes in vascular smooth muscle and cardiac muscle

[a]Abbreviations: Ad, adenosine; CHA, cyclohexyladenosine; PIA, phenylisopropyl adenosine; 2-Cl-Ads, 2-chloroadenosine; Ads-CPC, adenosine 5'-cyclopropyl carboxyimide; NECA, N-6-ethylcarboxymide-adenosine. (See Burnstock, 1978; Daly, et al., 1983.)

Geiger et al., 1984). The ligand employed was [³H]cyclohexyladenosine. Adenosine receptors were associated with granule cell terminals in the cerebellum, retinal ganglion cell terminals in the superior colliculus, and neurons in the dorsal horn of the spinal cord. Some of these experiments suggest a presynaptic locus for the receptors and are consistent with a role for adenosine in the regulation of neurotransmitter release as discussed later in this chapter.

1.4. Metabolism of Purines

Nucleotides are ubiquitous in all tissues of the body. Within various regions of the brain it is possible to measure only minimal differences in the regional distributions of adenosine and ATP (Phillis and Wu, 1983). This result should not be surprising since these substances are also central to energy metabolism and gene expression. Thus, Fig. 2 details the principal

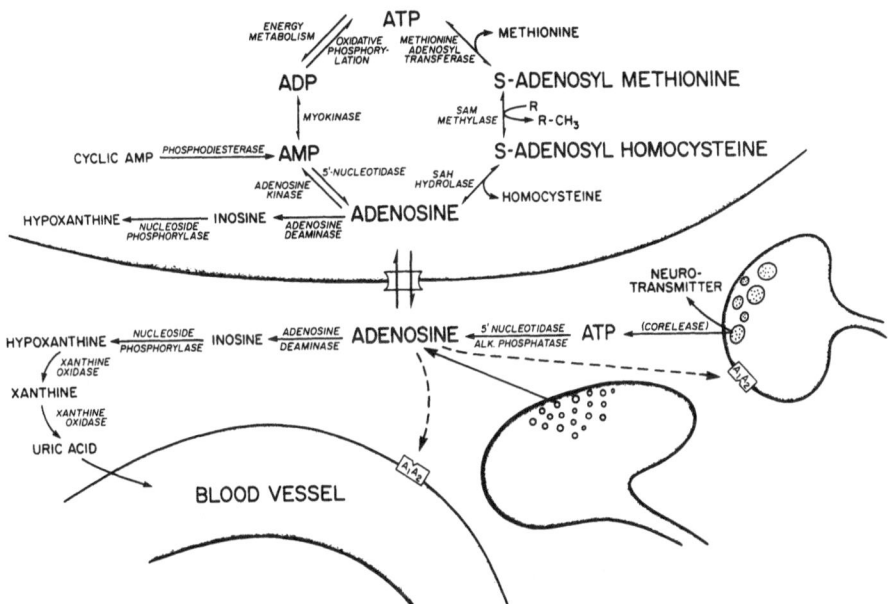

Figure 2. Summary of purine actions and metabolism. Adenosine released from neural or non-neural sources may act at surface adenosine receptors of the A_1 or A_2 type to regulate adenylate cyclase and/or mediate a physiological response such as inhibition of transmitter release from nerve terminals or a change in the contractility of blood vessels. Extracellular adenosine may be taken up into cells where it is converted by adenosine deaminase and nucleoside phosphorylase to inosine and hypoxanthine, or phosphorylated by adenosine kinase and myokinase to ATP. Extracellular adenosine can also be degraded by deamination and subsequent conversion to urate. S-adenosyl homocysteine, which may be formed via a series of reactions involving the methylation of ATP, is an important source of adenosine released under physiological conditions. When tissue levels of adenosine and homocysteine are high, this reaction, mediated by SAH hydrolase, is reversed to form S-adenosyl homocysteine.

metabolic pathways by which adenosine and ATP are synthesized and degraded. Of significance is the potential for a substantial contribution that methylation makes to adenosine production in the cell. Secondly, it is clear that a system of enzymes on the outside surface of neurons and glia (ectoenzymes) function to rapidly degrade released ATP and adenosine. Since no uptake mechanism exists for ATP, its degradation to adenosine is essential for recovery of the purine moiety, an energy-saving measure. Otherwise, the released purines are metabolized to uric acid and excreted by the kidneys.

2. PHYSIOLOGICAL ACTIONS OF ADENOSINE

Most of the observations that follow are based on the effects of *exogenous* adenosine in various experimental systems. This approach carries the risk that any results represent simple pharmacologic actions that may be unrelated to an intact functioning system releasing *endogenous* adenosine. With these reservations in mind, the following discussion suggests a role for endogenous adenosine under presumably more physiological circumstances yet to be fully characterized.

2.1. Neuronal Electrophysiology

2.1.1. Sympathetic Ganglion

The superior cervical ganglion is a useful model system for studies of receptor-mediated modulation of synaptic transmission at neuronal synapses (McAfee, 1982). This preparation can be maintained *in vitro* for hours, offering a convenient means to experimentally manipulate the composition of the bathing media. Unlike brain, it is simple in gross structure, having well-defined input and output nerves and a cholinergic synapse whose pharmacology has been well characterized. Using intracellular recording techniques, Henon and McAfee (1983a) found that adenosine inhibited calcium-dependent potentials in postganglionic neurons (Figs. 3A and 3B). Adenosine and its analogs inhibited, in a dose-dependent fashion, the calcium-component of the action potential and the hyperpolarizing afterpotential (HAP). The HAP is generated primarily by a Ca^{2+}-dependent K^+ conductance triggered by Ca^{2+} influx during the action potential. It appears that adenosine inhibits Ca^{2+} conductances in sympathetic neurons, thus antagonizing those processes dependent upon Ca^{2+} influx. In other tissues, adenosine appears to function by activating the hyperpolarizing outward K^+ currents. However, this does not appear to be an important mechanism in sympathetic ganglia since adenosine only weakly and inconsistently hyperpolarized postganglionic neurons.

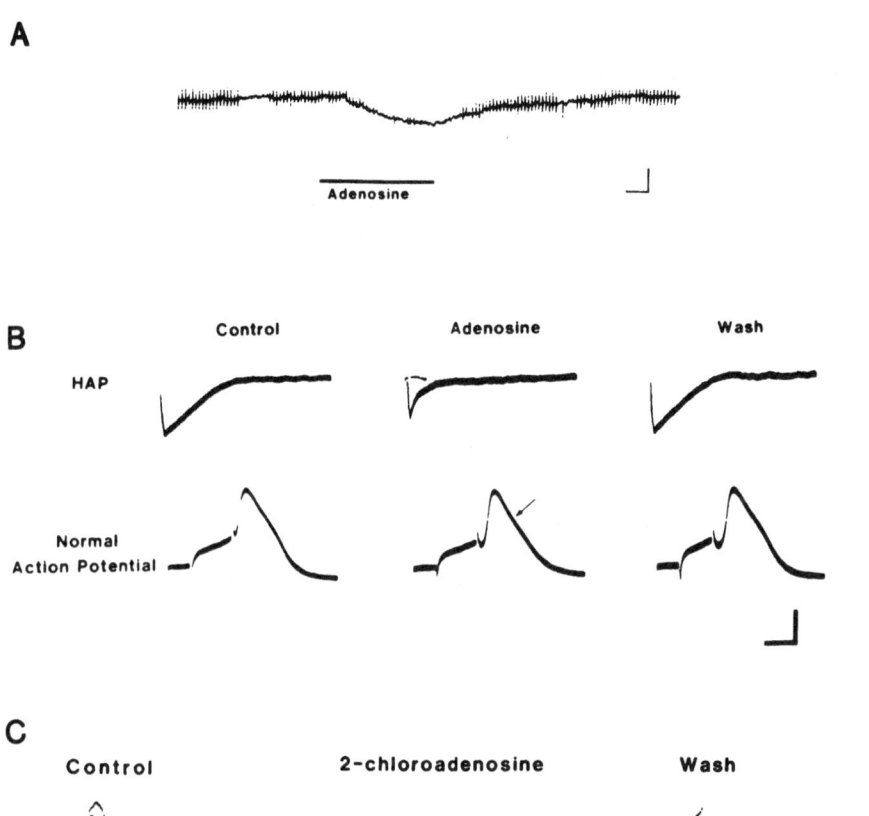

Figure 3. Electrophysiological effects of adenosine in the superior cervical ganglion. (A) Hyperpolarization of a postganglionic neuron in response to bath applied 10 μM adenosine for 5 min (bar). Vertical lines on the record are evoked action potentials attenuated by the low-frequency response of the chart recorder. Calibrations are 5 mV, 1 min. Resting potential was -59 mV and the input impedance (60MΩ) did not change in the presence of adenosine (not shown). (B) Adenosine (250 μM) reversibly reduced the hyperpolarizing afterpotential (HAP) that follows the spike (top trace) and a Ca^{2+}-dependent shoulder in the falling phase of the action potential in postganglionic neurons (lower trace). Calibrations: top, 5 mV, 100 msec; bottom, 20 mV, 2 msec. Resting potential, -52 mV. (C) Each panel shows five superimposed intracellularly recorded responses to single stimulus pulses delivered at 20-sec intervals to the preganglionic nerve. Left, in normal Locke's solution; center, in the presence of 5 μM 2-chloroadenosine; right, recovery of the EPSP amplitude following a 20-min wash in normal Locke's solution. A presynaptic action is indicated by the reversible reduction in amplitude of the nicotinic fast EPSP by 5 μM 2-chloroadenosine. Calibrations: 4 mV, 20 msec. Resting potential -59 mV. (From Henon and McAfee, 1983b, with permission.)

The response to adenosine occurs as a result of activation of specific adenosine receptors, since the effects of adenosine were antagonized by theophylline, a competitive receptor antagonist. Dipyridamole, a blocker of adenosine uptake, potentiated the effects of adenosine on sympathetic neurons as predicted if adenosine is, in part, inactivated by an uptake mechanism. Adenosine effects were mimicked by cyclic AMP, but this response was inhibited by the enzyme adenosine deaminase, which is specific for adenosine and does not act on cyclic AMP. It is clear then, that the effects of cyclic AMP must result from degradation of cyclic AMP to adenosine and subsequent activation of adenosine receptors. Furthermore, it is clear that other mechanisms such as enzymatic degradation function to inactivate released adenosine.

It is not known whether adenosine receptors act directly to inhibit the Ca^{2+} current or whether they act indirectly via a second messenger to affect Ca^{2+} or cyclic nucleotide metabolism. Adenosine does not stimulate cyclic AMP production in sympathetic ganglia (Roch and Kalix, 1975), but it has not yet been determined whether adenosine might *inhibit* adenylate cyclase. In either case, the concentrations of adenosine analogs required for inhibition of Ca^{2+} currents are at least an order of magnitude higher than that required to inhibit adenylate cyclases at A_1 receptors. Phillis and Wu (1981) have suggested that the receptor subtype mediating inhibition of Ca^{2+} fluxes may be cyclase independent and may represent an additional adenosine receptor subtype. Further studies will be required to determine the relationship, if any, of cyclic AMP to the physiologic responses of adenosine (Stone, 1981).

Adenosine was also shown to have presynaptic effects in the superior cervical ganglion (Henon and McAfee, 1983b). The nicotinic fast EPSP was reversibly reduced by the adenosine analogs (Fig. 3C). These agents are presumed to act presynaptically since they do not affect postsynaptic responses to exogenous cholinergic agonists. If adenosine also inhibits the voltage-dependent Ca^{2+} currents on the presynaptic nerve terminals, as it was found to do postsynaptically, it would of course limit Ca^{2+} influx required for the release of acetylcholine.

The presence of adenosine receptors at both pre- and postsynaptic sites has profound implications for regulation of synaptic efficacy. Recently, adenosine was shown to facilitate ganglionic transmission during repetitive stimulation of the preganglionic nerve (Henon and McAfee, 1983b; Henon and McAfee, 1983c). These effects of adenosine were also Ca^{2+} dependent. Perhaps adenosine functions as a "high-pass filter", inhibiting single or weak synaptic inputs but facilitating transmission of higher frequency events. This is an action particularly appropriate for a stress-related response.

2.1.2. Cerebral Cortex

Following the initial observations by Phillis et al. (1974) that adenosine inhibited spontaneous firing of cortical neurons (Fig. 4A), the physiological effects of adenosine on cortical neurons were investigated by intracellular

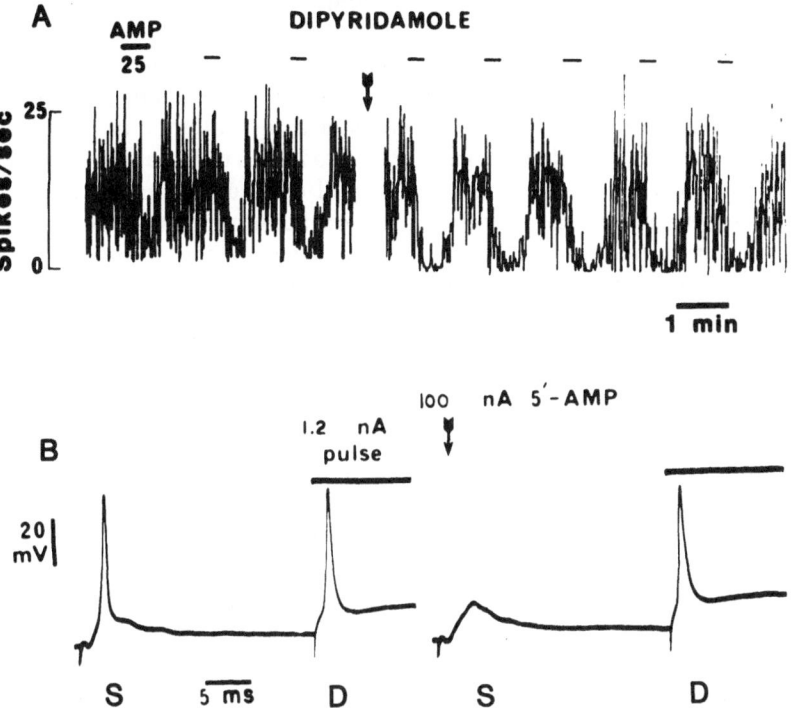

Figure 4. (A) A rate-meter recording from a spontaneously firing cerebral cortical neuron that is inhibited during the iontophoretic application of 5′AMP (bars). The magnitude and duration of the inhibition was potentiated by the intravenous administration of dipyridamole (0.1 mg/kg) to block adenosine uptake (arrow). (B) Intracellular action potentials recorded from a cerebral cortical neuron. Left pair: Action potentials were synaptically evoked (S) by stimulation of the adjacent cortex and then by a depolarizing current pulse (1.2 nA) passed directly (D) through the cell membrane from the microelectrode. Right pair: During the application of 5′AMP (100 nA), the EPSP evoked by cortical stimulation is too small to elicit an action potential, but the threshold for action potential generation by a direct current pulse is unaltered. Voltage calibration, 20 mV; time calibration, 5 msec. (From Phillis et al., 1979a, with permission.)

recording techniques (Edstrom and Phillis, 1976; Phillis et al., 1979a). In these experiments, the nucleotide adenosine 5′-monophosphate was applied by iontophoresis from double-barrel pipettes glued to the intracellular recording electrode. The purinergic agonist was shown to hyperpolarize single cortical neurons without significantly affecting membrane resistance or action potential threshold. This effect was unlike the response to GABA, which produced a hyperpolarization with a marked decrease in membrane resistance. The hyperpolarization produced by 5′-AMP was accompanied by a reduction in the amount of synaptic activity. In fact, synaptic responses were inhibited by 5′-AMP, but not responses to direct depolarization through the microelectrode (Fig. 4B). These results suggest that in the cortex, purinergic agents act primarily at presynaptic sites to reduce the release of the excitatory neurotransmitter.

Phillis et al. (1979b) were also able to present evidence for the release and action of endogenous purines in the brain. Adenosine deaminase inhibitors, such as deoxycoformycin (see Table 2), and adenosine uptake blockers, such as dipyridamole (see Table 2), were found to have inhibitory effects of their own on the spontaneous activity of cortical neurons. Furthermore, methylxanthines had excitatory effects on spontaneous firing, suggesting tonic inhibition by endogenous adenosine. These observations may provide a rationale for the well-known action of caffeine as a CNS stimulant.

Since responses to adenine nucleotides were potentiated by agents that prevent the deamination and uptake of adenosine, it is considered likely that their actions result from nucleotide hydrolysis to adenosine and then activation of adenosine receptors. This idea is supported by the observation that the alpha, methylene isosteres 5'ADP and 5'ATP, which are resistant to hydrolysis and cannot form adenosine, do not affect the excitability of cortical neurons.

Adenosine derivatives were also shown to reduce synaptic potentials evoked by stimulation of the lateral olfactory tract (LOT) in slices from the olfactory cortex. Adenosine inhibited EPSPs but did not affect propagation of action potentials in the presynaptic axon or the membrane properties of the postsynaptic neurons (Kuroda and Kobayashi, 1980). These observations are also consistent with the idea that adenosine inhibits release of neurotransmitters. An interesting property of the adenosine effect in olfactory cortex occurs following its washout where EPSP amplitudes are potentiated above control levels. This action of adenosine was mimicked by dibutryl cyclic AMP and 8-bromocylic AMP, which increased EPSP amplitude by 20–30%. Perhaps adenosine acts at one type of receptor (A_1) to inhibit Ca^{2+} influx required for transmitter release and at another receptor (A_2) to stim-

Table 2. Adenosine Pharmacology

Receptor agonists
  Adenosine, N^6-cyclohexyladenosine,[a] N^6-L-isopropyladenosine,[a]
  D-phenylisopropyladenosine, 2-chloroadenosine,
  adenosine 5'-carboxamide,[b]
  adenosine 5'-cyclopropylcarboxamide[b]

Receptor antagonists
  Theophylline, caffeine, 8-phenyltheophylline, 8-phenyl-1,3-dialkylxanthine

Uptake blockers
  Dipyridamole, hexobendine, nitrobenzylthioinosine

Adenosine deaminase inhibitors
  Deoxycoformycin, erythro-9(2-hydroxyl-3-nonyl) adenine hydrochloride (EHNA)

---

[a]Highest potency at A_1 adenosine receptors
[b]Highest potency at A_2 adenosine receptors

ulate cyclic AMP production, which persists upon washout of adenosine to facilitate transmitter release.

To address the question of how adenosine might regulate the release of a neurotransmitter, several laboratories (Riberio et al., 1979; Kuroda and Kobayashi, 1980; Wu et al., 1982) have examined the effects of adenosine on ^{45}Ca uptake into synaptosomal preparations of cerebral cortex. In these studies, adenosine inhibited the ^{45}Ca uptake induced by potassium depolarization by 20–60%. Conversely, dibutryl cyclic AMP stimulated ^{45}Ca uptake to 190% of control (Kuroda and Kobayashi, 1980). These results are consistent with the idea that adenosine can regulate the release of neurotransmitter, a calcium-dependent process, over a broad range.

2.1.3. Hippocampus

The hippocampal slice preparation has been an extremely useful one in which to address the question of whether or not adenosine is truly a neuronal signal molecule in the CNS. Hippocampal neurons are especially sensitive to the iontophoretic application of adenosine. However, it is important to know, not only that adenosine can produce pharmacological responses, but that these effects can be elicited at physiologically relevant concentrations, and, moreover, that they mimic endogenously released transmitter. The slice preparation has the advantage over in vivo iontophoretic techniques since it is possible to bathe the tissue with a known concentration of agonist, which permits quantitative receptor characterization. The hippocampus has a well-defined synaptic input, and a number of in vitro studies have demonstrated adenosine inhibition of evoked synaptic responses. Furthermore, adenosine and its derivatives meet several of the criteria established for classifying a substance as a neurotransmitter in this preparation. Adenosine is taken up and synthesized by nerve terminals, and released during neuronal stimulation (Schubert and Kreutzburg, 1974). In elegant histochemical studies, Schubert et al (1979) have shown that the distribution of 5′nucleotidase in the hippocampus is correlated with the sites of adenosine or adenine nucleotide release. 5′Nucleotidase is the key enzyme for production of adenosine from 5′-AMP and is associated primarily with glial cell membranes. Thus, not only are purines released from hippocampal neurons but there is a system of ectoenzymes for their degradation to adenosine and a mechanism for adenosine uptake.

In extracellular records from the hippocampal slice, Schubert and Mitzdorf (1979) showed that adenosine inhibited both a population spike response and a field EPSP elicited by stimulation of striatum radiatum afferents (Fig. 5). They concluded from current source density analysis that adenosine actions were primarily on presynaptic elements. Intracellular recordings (Siggins and Schubert, 1981) from the CA_1 neurons revealed a postsynaptic action of adenosine, but only at relatively high concentrations. While low concentrations (5 μM) of adenosine had no effect on postsynaptic membrane properties, higher concentrations (10–20 μM) significantly hyperpolarized

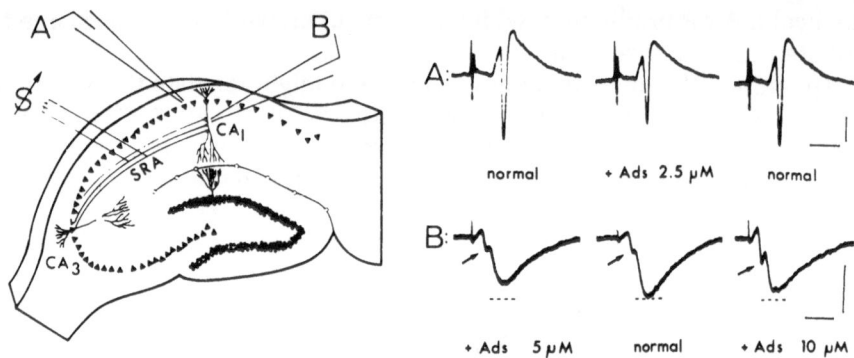

Figure 5. Hippocampal slice preparation showing electrode positions for the stimulation and extracellular recording of (A) population spikes from the somal layer and (B) the field EPSP from the dendritic layer. In (B) the arrows indicate the magnitude of the fiber volley input in response to stimulation of the stratum radiatum. Note that when the stimulus strength was maintained constant, 5 μM adenosine substantially inhibited the field EPSP (left). However, the stimulus strength had to be greatly increased in 10 μM adenosine (right) to generate a response similar in magnitude to the normal (center). Calibration: 5 msec, 1 mV. (From Schubert and Mitzdorf, 1979, with permission.)

the neurons. In about half the cells there was a small but detectable decrease in membrane resistance. The hyperpolarizing action of adenosine on CA_1 neurons was further characterized by Segal (1982), who determined that the hyperpolarization had a reversal potential of -90 mV. This suggests that an increase in potassium conductance is the underlying ionic mechanism. The hyperpolarization persisted when synaptic input was blocked by Co^{2+} and Mn^{2+} or by low Ca^{2+} and high Mg^{2+}, confirming that this is a postsynaptic effect.

In addition to activating K^+ conductances, adenosine inhibits Ca^{2+} spikes in hippocampal neurons (Proctor and Dunwiddie, 1983). It was clearly shown that adenosine increased the threshold for the generation of the Ca^{2+} spike. Proctor and Dunwiddie argue that a K^+ conductance increase occurring on remote dendrites could raise the threshold for Ca^{2+} spikes initiated in the dendrites without showing a detectable conductance increase at the somal level. An alternative hypothesis is that adenosine directly affects the Ca^{2+}-conductance mechanism.

Reddington et al. (1982) characterized and compared the pharmacology of the electrophysiological response (depression of evoked EPSPs), with the pharmacological properties of radioligand binding to adenosine receptors. Until very recently, radioligand binding to adenosine receptors was not feasible because ligands were displaced by endogenous adenosine and were subject to degradation by endogenous adenosine deaminase. The development of ligands such as 2-chloroadenosine and cyclohexyladenosine (CHA), which are resistant to uptake and degradation by adenosine deaminase, was a major breakthrough for the characterization of adenosine receptors. The order of agonist potency for inhibition of the evoked EPSP was found to be similar to that for the displacement of [³H]-CHA binding in rat brain membranes. The authors conclude that the pharmacology of this adenosine receptor is characteristic of an A_1 subtype based on rank ordering of agonist potencies (Table 1).

Adenosine receptors mediate inhibition of adenylate cyclase, but there is no evidence to relate this effect in a causative way to depression of the EPSP. In fact, Reddington and Schubert (1979) tested the idea that stimulation of adenylate cyclase and inhibition of the population spike were mediated by the same receptors. While adenosine and 2-chloroadenosine were equipotent in stimulating cyclic AMP production, 2-chloroadenosine was much more potent than adenosine in inhibiting the population spike. It was concluded that different receptors mediated the two responses.

In summary, adenine nucleotides meet several of the requirements for a neurotransmitter. In the hippocampus, there is evidence for release, enzyme systems for degradation at the site of release, and a mechanism for reuptake. A specific receptor-mediated physiological effect has been demonstrated, and there is also evidence for tonic regulation of excitability by endogenous adenosine. Since neither ATP nor adenosine mimics the effects of nerve stimulation, it is possible that their role is to modulate the effects of the primary transmitter. The modulatory effects are expressed as a presynaptic regulation of transmitter release and a postsynaptic influence on neuronal excitability.

2.2. Cardiovascular Effects

Adenosine appears to be important in the regulation of local blood flow, especially in the heart and brain. The cellular mechanisms by which it acts in these tissues seem similar to those in nervous tissue. Adenosine is released from the myocardium under conditions of stress or vigorous exercise that place an increased oxygen demand on the heart (Watkinson et al., 1979) or during pathological ischemia (Schrader et al., 1977; Winn et al., 1981). Adenosine has several actions on the heart. It produces coronary vasodilation with a consequent increase in coronary blood flow. It reduces sinus rhythm and A-V conduction velocity, which would decrease the metabolic demand of the heart. These are appropriate and protective responses to stress. However, during myocardial infarction, the amount of adenosine release may be so great as to be maladaptive, producing A-V conduction block and ventricular standstill (Belardinelli et al., 1983).

Studies of cardiac myocytes cocultured with sympathetic neurons have produced results that are consistent with the idea that endogenous adenosine plays a physiologic role in regulation of cardiovascular excitability (Potter et al., 1982). Repetitive stimulation of the sympathetic neurons could inhibit myocytes in a nonadrenergic, noncholinergic fashion. This effect was antagonized by 8-phenyltheophylline and adenosine deaminase. These studies clearly indicate that a purinergic transmitter can be released from single sympathetic neurons and induce a hypolarization in heart cells, but the exact identity of the transmitter is unknown.

The blood–brain barrier effectively shields CNS tissue from circulating adenosine. This is aided by the vascular endothelium, which is especially effective in removing adenosine from the blood by uptake and metabolism. However, it is clear that hypoxia and ischemia cause production and release of adenosine from brain cells into the extracellular fluid, and this produces profound effects on both neuronal discharge and local blood flow. It seems likely that under these conditions, adenosine, as it does in the heart, can protect the brain from damage by increasing blood flow and thus oxygen delivery, and by reducing neuronal discharge and thus oxygen demand (Berne et al., 1983; Phillis and Wu, 1983).

The cellular mechanism of these effects of adenosine are at least in part due to inhibition of Ca^{2+} influx. Adenosine inhibits Ca^{2+}-dependent action potentials in vascular smooth muscle and myocardium and uptake of Ca^{2+} by these tissues from the bathing media (Schrader et al., 1975; Rubio et al., 1983).

Adenosine has also been shown to mediate an increase in resting K^+ conductance in the frog sinus venosus (Hartzell, 1979). This results in hyperpolarization and reduced sinus rhythm. Adenosine actions in this preparation are probably receptor-mediated since they were antagonized by methylxanthines, and were potentiated by adenosine uptake blockers.

In addition to its effects on ionic permeability, adenosine appears to act as a modulator of the action of other autonomic neurotransmitters in autonomic neurons (Burnstock, 1981; Henon and McAfee, 1983b). Through an unknown mechanism, adenosine clearly antagonizes the cardiovascular effects of β-adrenergic receptor activation, including contractile responses, cyclic AMP production, and protein phosphorylation (Fig. 6; Schrader et al., 1977; Dobson and Fenton, 1983).

3. PHYSIOLOGICAL ACTIONS OF ATP

The role of ATP as a neurotransmitter or modulator is less well established than that for adenosine. One reason for this is the lack of an armamentarium of specific pharmacologic agents acting at ATP receptors such as those for adenosine A_1 and A_2 receptors. Another reason lies in the multitude of electrogenic or inotropic responses to ATP. Exogenous ATP depolarizes some cells and hyperpolarizes others. ATP specifically augments K^+ conductances in some systems and specifically inhibits K^+ conductances in others.

Study of the action of ATP in a given tissue ideally begins by demonstrating that it interacts with a specific receptor. Since ATP can be rapidly

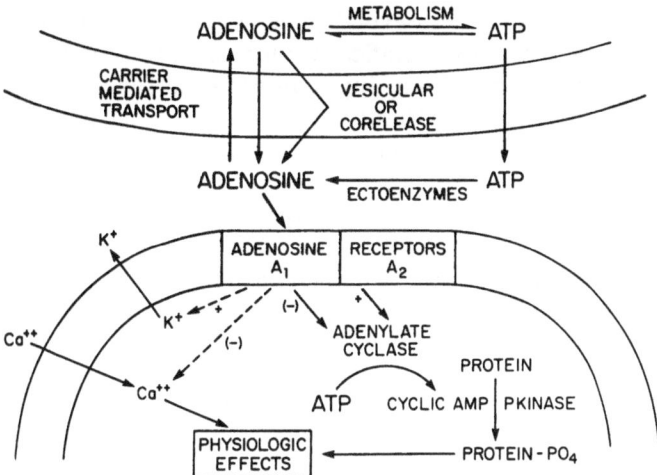

Figure 6. A diagram summarizing the purine modulation of physiologic activity. Extracellular adenosine may be released directly from neurons or derived from released ATP. Adenosine acts at A_1 receptors that inhibit adenylate cyclase and/or at A_2 receptors that stimulate adenylate cyclase to increase the production of cyclic AMP, and this leads to protein phosphorylation via protein kinase. Receptor activation may also change the membrane permeability of the target cell to K^+ or Ca^{2+} or may affect intracellular Ca^{2+} metabolism. All of these actions can influence the physiological properties of the target cell. Reuptake of adenosine is accomplished by carrier-mediated transport in a system of facilitated diffusion. Diffusion normally is inward because intracellular adenosine levels are kept low by rapid metabolism to ATP.

broken down to adenosine, it is important to prove that the receptor is selective for ATP rather than adenosine. Moreover, the effects of ATP should not be blocked by methylxanthines, which are specific antagonists for adenosine receptors. Some investigators in this field argue that responses specific to ATP should not be affected by adenosine uptake blockers and exogenous adenosine deaminase inhibitors. However, it seems likely that ATP, once released, is normally metabolized to adenosine and taken up or metabolized further, and then cleared by the circulation (see Fig. 2). Thus, this pathway for terminating the action of ATP might indeed be sensitive to agents that affect the metabolism of adenosine.

While ATP has potent actions on central neurons, these effects can often be related to the metabolism of ATP to adenosine and subsequent activation of A_1 and A_2 adenosine receptors. However, ATP itself also has potent effects on peripheral neurons and muscle, especially in the autonomic and gastrointestinal system.

3.1. Neuronal Electrophysiology

Studies in bullfrog sympathetic ganglia (Akasu et al., 1983) clearly show that ATP, and not adenosine, depolarizes postganglionic neurons in a concentration-dependent manner. Several lines of evidence lead to the conclusion that ATP depolarizes by specifically depressing K^+ conductances. ATP causes an increase in membrane input impedance (decreased membrane conductance). Moreover, the current-voltage curves constructed in the presence and absence of ATP intersect at -92 mV, near the K^+ equilibrium potential. Further studies indicate that ATP affects two distinct potassium conductances, the delayed rectifier and the M current (see Chapter 6). As evidence in favor of an action on the delayed rectifier, it was found that ATP reduced the peak amplitude of the spike afterpotential and the rate of decay of the action potential (i.e., there was broadening of the spike). In voltage-clamp experiments, ATP, as expected, reduced the outward current evoked by depolarizing voltage commands. However, when the delayed rectifier was for the most part blocked by tetraethylammonium (TEA), there was still an effect of ATP on the delayed outward current (Fig. 7). Further voltage-clamp

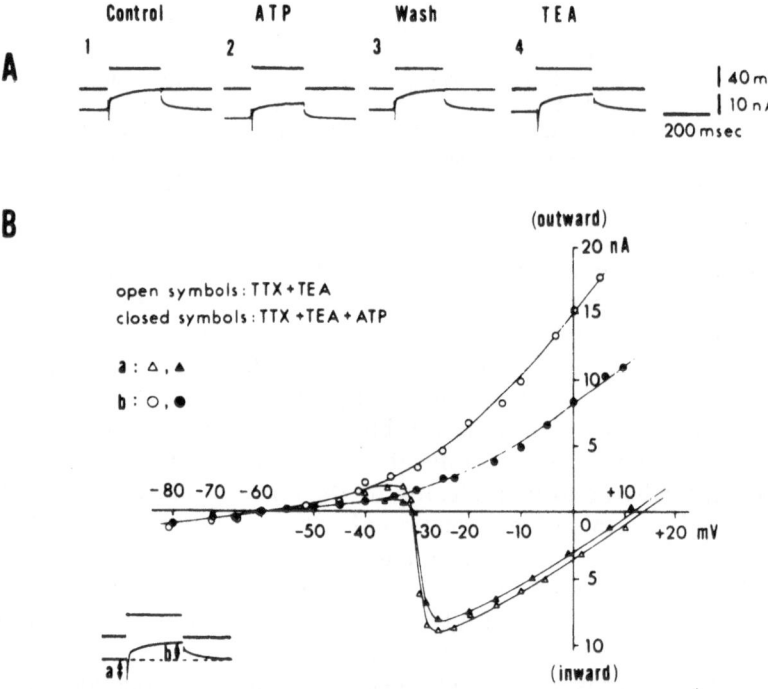

Figure 7. (A) Voltage-clamp records from neurons of the bullfrog sympathetic ganglion in the presence of tetrodotoxin to block the fast sodium current. The slow outward current was markedly reduced by 100 μM ATP and recovered following washout. Upper trace in each panel shows membrane potential, lower trace is the membrane current. (B) The I-V relationships of the slow inward Ca^{2+} current and the slow outward current in bullfrog postganglionic neurons bathed in tetraethylammonium (TEA; 20 μM). ATP markedly suppressed the outward current amplitudes (circles) but did not reduce the inward current (triangles). (From Akasu et al., 1983, with permission.)

recordings demonstrated that this was due to inhibition of the M current. Thus, ATP seems to affect both a TEA-sensitive potassium conductance involved in spike repolarization, and the TEA-insensitive M current that has been implicated in the control of excitability. However, due to the lack of specificity of TEA, more detailed voltage-clamp studies are required to better identify the specific membrane currents underlying the response to ATP and to exclude the involvement of calcium-dependent potassium conductances.

ATP also seems to function as a modulator of transmission at nicotinic synapses. Of importance in this regard is the observation of Silinsky (1975) that stimulation of motor nerves results in corelease of ATP in proportion to the synaptic (ACh) response at the neuromuscular junction. In the bullfrog sympathetic ganglion, ATP reduces release of ACh but increases the sensitivity of the nicotinic receptor (Akasu et al., 1981). These actions of ATP should theoretically result in facilitation of repetitive synaptic activity in a manner analogous to the effects on adenosine and norepinephrine in sympathetic ganglia (Henon and McAfee, 1983b). Reduced afterpotentials allow shorter interspike intervals and higher frequency discharge rates. Since cholinergic terminals in the ganglion and the neuromuscular junction release a surfeit of ACh, inhibiting release reduces the excessive postsynaptic conductance increases that would otherwise short-circuit the membrane and inactivate Na^+ conductances necessary for neuronal discharge. Unfortunately, such studies have not been specifically applied to ATP, and the role of this substance in neuron–neuron synaptic physiology remains speculative.

3.2. Smooth Muscle

The purinergic nerve hypothesis arose from the finding that ATP mimicked the inhibitory actions on the guinea pig *taenia coli* produced by stimulation of nonadrenergic, noncholinergic nerves (Bennett et al., 1963; Small and Weston, 1979). When cholinergic and adrenergic transmission were blocked by guanethidine and atropine, large transitory hyperpolarizations ("inhibitory junction potentials") were produced in response to single stimulus pulses. This led to cessation of spontaneous spike discharges and relaxation (Fig. 8). Since these inhibitory junction potentials (IJPs) were abolished by low concentrations of TTX, they were of neuronal origin and not the result of direct stimulation of the muscle. Stimulation of nònadrenergic, noncholinergic nerves produces similar inhibitory potentials in smooth muscle throughout the gastrointestinal tract including the jejunum, the colon, the guinea pig stomach, and the avian gizzard.

ATP is more potent than ADP and much more potent than AMP or adenosine in mimicking the IJP and the relaxation of intestinal smooth muscle (Jager and Schevers, 1980). Like other P_2 receptor-mediated responses, ATP effects are antagonized by quinidine, 2-substituted imidazolines,

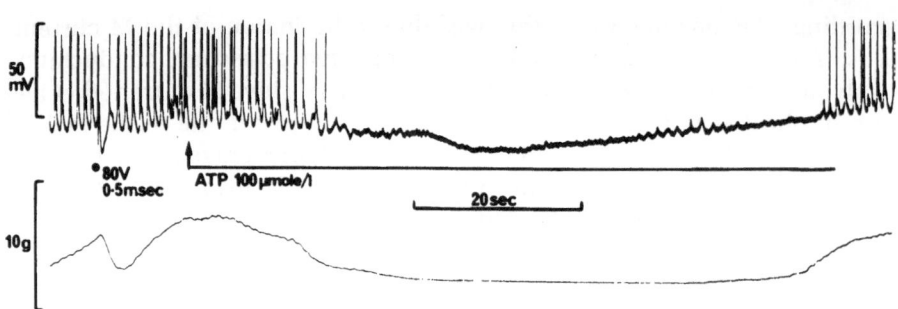

Figure 8. Simultaneous intracellular recording of membrane potential (upper trace) and mechanical activity (lower trace) in guinea pig taenia caeci. Hyoscine (0.3 μM) was present throughout. Field stimulation (●) evoked an inhibitory junction potential characterized by hyperpolarization and abolition of spontaneous spike activity (upper trace) and relaxation (lower trace). ATP (100 μM; arrow) mimicked stimulation. (From Small and Weston, 1979, with permission.)

2', 2 pyridilisatogen, and apamin, but none of these are competitive antagonists at the receptor. Arylazido aminopropionyl-ATP is a noncompetitive light-activated ATP analog that appears to be specific for ATP receptors. Surprisingly, this substance antagonizes responses to exogenous ATP on *taenia coli* but does not antagonize responses to inhibitory nerve stimulation (Westfall et al., 1982). This result suggests that ATP is not the substance that mediates nerve-induced inhibition. However, before the purinergic hypothesis can be discarded here, the investigator must establish that their ATP analog actually penetrates the synaptic cleft.

The pattern of smooth muscle innervation and the electrical coupling between muscle cells has complicated investigations of the mechanisms underlying the IJPs. The amplitudes of the inhibitory potentials, normally about 10–20 mV, were shown to depend on the extracellular K^+ concentration (Bennett et al., 1963), suggesting that the response was mediated by an increase in K^+ conductance. However, proof of a conductance increase by intracellular recording techniques proved infeasible since measurements of input resistance on the postsynaptic membrane were largely obscured by the large amount of membrane coupled in the smooth muscle syncytium. Using the sucrose gap technique, Tomita (1972) found a linear relationship between the amplitude of the IJP and membrane potential changes produced by polarizing currents applied to the whole tissue. This demonstrated that the IJP was the result of a conductance increase. The conductance was little affected by changes in external Cl^- but was increased by removal of K^+, a finding that is consistent with a conductance increase to K^+. The inhibitory potential was eliminated by hyperpolarizing the membrane to potentials approximating the potassium equilibrium potential. In addition, Den Hertog and Jager (1975) measured ion fluxes during the IJP, confirming a selective increase in membrane K^+ permeability.

ATP is not always inhibitory and may even be released from other than purely purinergic nerves (Burnstock, 1981; Hills et al., 1983). For example,

ATP is stored with catecholamines in granules. Stimulation of certain autonomic tissues causes release of both catecholamines and ATP. Finally, many target cells contain receptors for both ATP and norepinephrine. Westfall and his associates argue convincingly from this kind of evidence that ATP is a cotransmitter that acts synergistically with norepinephrine to excite the vas deferens (Fedan et al., 1981). The contractile response of the vas deferens to motor nerve (sympathetic-adrenergic) stimulation is biphasic. Sneddon and Westfall (1984), in an elegant series of physiological and pharmacological experiments, demonstrated that the initial contractile phase is induced by an ATP-generated excitatory junction potential. The later, more tonic phase, is mediated by noradrenergic activation of α-adrenergic receptors. Thus, there is considerable evidence that ATP is a neurotransmitter in the autonomic nervous system.

4. SUMMARY

We have presented a general overview of the basis for the idea that purines function as neurotransmitters. However, these substances may not always function in a classical fashion. For example, while adenosine may be released from nerves, it is also released from other metabolically active tissues (see Fig. 2). This nonneuronal adenosine is likely to act on local nervous tissue to modulate neuronal activity. In some cases, adenosine regulation may be implemented by release of ATP rather than adenosine. This substance is then metabolized in the extracellular space to adenosine, However, it is clear that specific receptors for ATP exist on nerve and muscle tissue, and this substance need not be metabolized further to have an effect on function. While better defined roles for these substances await further experimentation, it seems likely that purines are important to regulation of excitable tissue.

REFERENCES

Akasu, T., Hirai, K., and Koketsu, K., 1981, Increase of acetylcholine-receptor sensitivity by adenosine triphosphate: a novel action of ATP on ACh-sensitivity, Br. J. Pharmacol. **74**:505–507.

Akasu, T., Hirai, K., and Koketsu, K., 1983, Modulatory actions of ATP on membrane potentials of bullfrog sympathetic ganglion cells, Brain Res. **258**:313–317.

Belardinelli, L., West, A., Crampton, R., and Berne, R. M., 1983, Chronotropic and dromotropic effects of adenosine in: Regulatory Function of Adenosine (R. M. Berne, T. W. Rall, and R. Rubio, eds.), Nijhoff, Boston, pp. 377–398.

Bennett, M. R., Burnstock, K. G., and Holman, M. E., 1963, The effect of potassium and chloride ions on the inhibitory potential recorded in the guinea pig taenia coli, *J. Physiol. (Lond.)* **169**:33–34.

Berne, R. M., Winn, R. H., Knabb, T. M., Ely, S. W., and Rubio, R., 1983, Blood flow regulation by adenosine in heart, brain and skeletal muscles, in: *Regulatory Function of Adenosine* (R. M. Berne, T. W. Rall, and R. Rubio, eds.), Nijhoff, Boston, pp. 293–318.

Burnstock, G. 1972, Purinergic nerves, *Pharmacol. Rev.* **24**:509–572.

Burnstock, G. 1978, A basis for distinguishing two types of purinergic receptors, in: *Cell Membrane Receptors for Drugs and Hormones* (R. W. Straub and L. Bolis, eds.), Raven Press, New York, pp. 107–118.

Burnstock, G., 1981, Neurotransmitters and trophic factors in the autonomic nervous system, *J. Physiol. (Lond.)* **313**:1–35.

Burnstock, G., Campbell, G., Satchell, D., and Smythe, A., 1970, Evidence that adenosine triphosphate or a related nucleotide is the transmitter substance released by non-adrenergic inhibitory nerves in the gut, *Br. J. Pharmacol.* **40**:668–688.

Burnstock, G., Hökfelt, T., Gershon, M. D., Iversen, L. L., Kosterlitz, H. W., and Szurszewski, J. H., 1979, Non-adrenergic, non-cholinergic autonomic neurotransmission mechanisms, *Neurosci. Res. Program Bull.* **17**:3.

Campbell, G., and Gibbons, J. L., 1979, Noradrenergic noncholinergic transmission in the autonomic nervous system: purinergic nerves, in: *Trends in Autonomic Pharmacology*, Vol. 1 (S. Kalsner, ed.), Urban and Schwarzenberg, Baltimore, pp. 103–144.

Daly, J. W., Butts-Lamb, P., and Padgett, W., 1983, Subclasses of adenosine receptors in the central nervous system: Interaction with caffeine and related methylxanthines, *Cell Mol. Neurobiol.* **3**:69–80.

Den Hertog, A., and Jager, L. P., 1975, Ion fluxes during the inhibitory junction potential in the guinea pig taenia coli, *J. Physiol. (Lond.)* **250**:681–691.

Dobson, J. G., and Fenton, R. A., 1983, Antiadrenergic effects of adenosine in the heart, in: *Regulatory Function of Adenosine* (R. M. Berne, T. W. Rall, and R. Rubio, eds.) Nijhoff, Boston, pp. 363–376.

Drury, A. N., and Szent-Gyorgyi, A., 1929, The physiological activity of adenosine compounds with especial reference to their action upon the mammalian heart, *J. Physiol. (Lond.)* **68**:213–237.

Edstrom, J. P., and Phillis, J. W., 1976, The effects of AMP on the potential of rat cerebral cortical neurones, *Can. J. Physiol. Pharmacol.* **54**:787–790.

Fedan, J. S., Hogaboom, G. K., O'Donnell, J. P., Colby, J., and Westfall, D. P., 1981, Contribution by purines to the neurogeneic response of the vas deferens of the guinea pig, *Eur. J. Pharmacol.* **69**:41–53.

Geiger, J. D., LaBella, F. S., and Nagy, J. I., 1984, Characterization and localization of adenosine receptors in rat spinal cord, *J. Neurosci.* **4**:2303–2310.

Goodman, R. R., Kuhar, M. J., Hester, L., and Snyder, S. H., 1983, Adenosine receptors: Autoradiographic evidence for their location on axon terminals of excitatory neurons, *Science* **222**:967–969.

Hartzell, H. C., 1979, Adenosine receptors in frog sinus venosus: Slow inhibitory potentials produced by adenine compounds and acetylcholine, *J. Physiol. (Lond.)* **293**:23–49.

Henon, B. K., and McAfee, D. A., 1983a, The ionic basis of adenosine receptor actions on postganglionic neurones in the rat, *J. Physiol. (Lond.)* **336**:607–620.

Henon, B. K., and McAfee, D. A., 1983b, Modulation of calcium currents by adenosine receptors on mammalian sympathetic neurons, in: *Regulatory Function of Adenosine* (R. M. Berne, T. W. Rall, and R. Rubio, eds.), Nijhoff, Boston, pp. 455–466.

Henon, B. K., and McAfee, D. A., 1983c, Facilitation of repetitive synaptic activity in postganglionic neurons by adenosine and noradrenalin, *Soc. Neurosci. Abst.* 1143.

Hills, J. M., Collis, C. S., and Burnstock, G., 1983, The effects of vasoactive intestinal polypeptide on the electrical activity of guinea-pig intestinal smooth muscle, *Eur. J. Pharmacol.* **88**:371–376.

Holton, F. A., and Holton, P., 1954, The capillary dilator substances in dry powders of spinal roots; a possible role of adenosine triphosphate in chemical transmission from nerve endings. *J. Physiol. (Lond.)* **126**:124–140.

Jager, L. P., and Schevers, J. A. M., 1980, A comparison of effects evoked in guinea-pig taenia caecum by purine nucleotides and by 'purinergic' nerve stimulation, *J. Physiol. (Lond.)*, **299:**75–83.

Kuroda, Y., and Kobayashi, K., 1980, Post-tetanic potentiation can be mediated by adenosine-induced increase of cyclic AMP in the presynaptic terminal, *Proc. Intn. Union Physiol. Soc.* **14:**534.

Londos, C., and Wolff, J., 1977, Two distinct adenosine-sensitive sites on adenylate cyclase, *Proc. Natl. Acad. Sci. USA* **74:**5482–5486.

McAfee, D. A., 1982, Superior cervical ganglion: Physiological consideration, in: *Cholinergic Biology: Model Cholinergic Synapses* (I. Hanin and M. Goldberg, eds.) Raven Press, New York pp. 191–211.

Phillis, J. W., and Wu, P. H., 1981, The role of adenosine and its nucleotides in central synaptic transmission, *Prog. Neurobiol.* **16:**187–239.

Phillis, J. W., and Wu, P. H., 1983, The role of adenosine in central neuromodulation, in: *Regulatory Function of Adenosine* (R. M. Berne, T. W. Rall, and R. Rubio, eds.), Nijhoff, Boston, pp. 419–439.

Phillis, J. W., Kostopoulos, G. K. and Limacher, J. J., 1974, Depression of corticospinal cells by various purines and pyrimidines, *Can. J. Physiol. Pharmacol.* **52:**1226–1229.

Phillis, J. W., Edstrom, J. P., Kostopoulos, G. K., and Kirkpatrick, J. R., 1979a, Effects of adenosine and adenine nucleotides on synaptic transmission in the cerebral cortex, *Can. J. Physiol. Pharmacol.* **57:**1289–1312.

Phillis, J. W., Kostopoulos, G. K., Edstrom, J. P., and Ellis, S. W., 1979b, Role of adenosine and adenine nucleotides in central nervous function, in: *Physiological and Regulatory Functions of Adenosine and Adenine Nucleotides* (H. P. Baer, and G. I. Drummond, eds.) Raven Press, New York, pp. 343–349.

Potter, D. D., Furshpan, E. J., and Landis, S. C., 1983, Transmitter status in cultured rat sympathetic neurons: Plasticity and multiple function, *Fed. Proc.* **42:**1626–1632.

Proctor, W. R., and Dunwiddie, T., 1983, Adenosine inhibits calcium spikes in hippocampal pyramidal neurons *in vitro*, *Neurosci. Lett.* **35:**197–201.

Reddington, M., and Schubert, P., 1979, Parallel investigations of the effects of adenosine on evoked potentials and cyclic AMP accumulation in hippocampus slices of the rat, *Neurosci. Lett.* **14:**37–42.

Reddington, M., Lee, K. S., and Schubert, P., 1982, An A_1-adenosine receptor of evoked potentials in a rat hippocampal slice preparation, *Neurosci. Lett.* **28:**275–279.

Riberio, J. A., Sa-Almeida, A. M., and Namorado, J. M., 1979, Adenosine and adenosine triphosphate decrease Ca^{++} uptake by synaptosomes stimulated by potassium, *Biochem. Pharmacol.* **28:**1297–1300.

Roch, P., and Kalix, P., 1975, Adenosine 3′, 5′-monophosphate in bovine superior cervical ganglion: Effect of high extracellular potassium, *Biochem. Pharmacol.* **24:**1293–1296.

Rubio, R., Knabb, M. T., Tsukada, T., and Berne, R. M., 1983, Mechanisms of action of adenosine on vascular smooth muscle and cardiac cells, in: *Regulatory Function of Adenosine* (R. M. Berne, T. W. Rall, and R. Rubio, eds.), Nijhoff, Boston, pp. 319–332.

Schrader, J., Rubio, R., and Berne, R. M., 1975, Inhibition of slow action potentials of guinea pig atrial muscle by adenosine: A possible effect on Ca^{2+} influx, *J. Mol. Cell Cardiol.* **7:**427–433.

Schrader, J., Haddy, F. J., and Gerlach, E., 1977, Release of adenosine, inosine, and hypoxanthine from the isolated guinea pig heart during hypoxia, flow-autoregulation and reactive hyperemia, *Pflügers Arch.* **369:**1–6.

Schubert, P., and Kreutzburg, G. W., 1974, Axonal transport of adenosine and uridine derivatives and transfer to postsynaptic neurons, *Brain Res.* **76:**526–530.

Schubert, P., and Mitzdorf, U., 1979, Analysis and quantitative evaluation of the depressive effect of adenosine on evoked potentials in hippocampal slices, *Brain Res.* **172:**186–190.

Schubert, P., Komp, W., and Kreutzberg, G. W., 1979, Correlation of 5′-nucleotidase activity and selective transneuronal transfer of adenosine in the hippocampus, *Brain Res.* **168:**419–424.

Segal, M., 1982, Intracellular analysis of a postsynaptic action of adenosine in the rat hippocampus, *Eur. J. Pharmacol.* **79:**193–199.

Siggins, G. R., and Schubert, P., 1981, Adenosine depression in hippocampal neurons *in vitro*:

An intracellular study of dose-dependent actions on synaptic and membrane potentials, *Neurosci. Lett.* **23**:55–60.

Silinsky, E. M., 1975, On the association between transmitter secretion and the release of adenine nucleotides from mammalian motor nerve terminals, *J. Physiol. (Lond.)* **247**:145–162.

Small R. C., and Weston, A. H., 1979, Intramural inhibition in rabbit and guinea pig intestine, in: *Physiological and Regulatory Functions of Adenosine* (H. P. Baer, and G. I. Drummond, eds.) Raven Press, New York, pp. 45–60.

Sneddon, P., and Westfall, D. P., 1984, Pharmacological evidence that adenosine triphosphate and noradrenaline are co-transmitters in the guinea-pig vas deferens, *J. Physiol. (Lond.)* **347**:561–580.

Stone, T. W., 1981, Physiological roles for adenosine and adenosine 5'-triphosphate in the nervous system, *Neuroscience* **6(4)**:523–555.

Su, C., (1983), Purinergic neurotransmission and neuromodulation, *Am. Rev. Pharmacol. Toxicol.* **23**:397–411.

Tomita, T., 1972, Conductance changes during the inhibitory potential in the guinea pig taenia coli, *J. Physiol. (Lond.)* **225**:693–703.

Van Calker, D., Muller, M., and Hamprecht, B., 1979, Adenosine regulates via two different types of receptors, the accumulation of cyclic AMP in cultured brain cells, *J. Neurochem.* **33**:999–1005.

Watkinson, W. P., Foley, D. H., Rubio, R., and Berne, R. M., 1979, Myocardial adenosine formation with increased cardiac performance in the dog, *Am. J. Physiol.* **236**:H13–H21.

Westfall, D. P., Hogaboom, G. K., Colby, J., O'Donnell, J. P., and Fedan, J. S., 1982, Direct evidence against a role of ATP as the nonadrenergic, noncholinergic inhibitory neurotransmitter in guinea pig taenia coli, *Proc. Natl. Acad. Sci, USA* **79**:7041–7045.

Winn, H., Rubio, G. R., and Berne, R. M., 1981, The role of adenosine in the regulation of cerebral blood flow, *J. Cereb. Blood Flow Metab.* **1**:239–244.

Wu, P. H., Phillis, J. W., and Thierry, D. L., 1982, Adenosine receptor agonist inhibit K^+-evoked Ca^{2+} uptake by rat cortical synaptosomes, *J. Neurochem.* **39**:700–708.

Index